Vertical Alveolar Ridge Augmentation in Implant Dentistry
A Surgical Manual

This book is dedicated to my wife, Marina, for her sacrifices and unlimited love, and our children, Deana and Antony, who provided the light and drive to make this book possible.

Vertical Alveolar Ridge Augmentation in Implant Dentistry

A Surgical Manual

Edited by

Len Tolstunov, DDS, DMD

Private Practice, Oral and Maxillofacial Surgery, San Francisco, California, USA
Assistant Clinical Professor, Department of Oral and Maxillofacial Surgery, UCSF and UOP Schools of Dentistry, San Francisco, California, USA

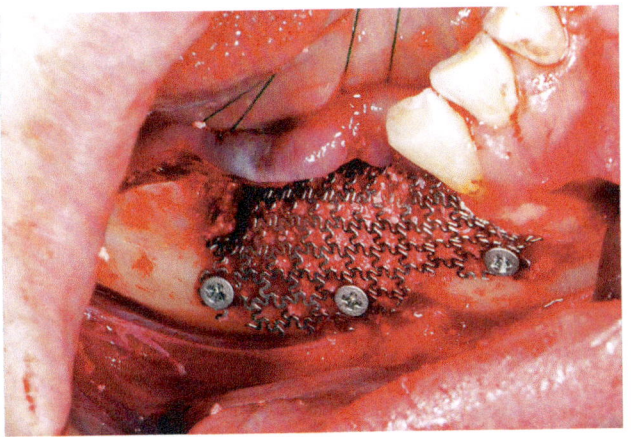

WILEY Blackwell

Copyright © 2016 by John Wiley & Sons, Inc. All rights reserved

Published by John Wiley & Sons, Inc., Hoboken, New Jersey
Published simultaneously in Canada

No part of this publication may be reproduced, stored in a retrieval system, or transmitted in any form or by any means, electronic, mechanical, photocopying, recording, scanning, or otherwise, except as permitted under Section 107 or 108 of the 1976 United States Copyright Act, without either the prior written permission of the Publisher, or authorization through payment of the appropriate per-copy fee to the Copyright Clearance Center, Inc., 222 Rosewood Drive, Danvers, MA 01923, (978) 750-8400, fax (978) 750-4470, or on the web at www.copyright.com. Requests to the Publisher for permission should be addressed to the Permissions Department, John Wiley & Sons, Inc., 111 River Street, Hoboken, NJ 07030, (201) 748-6011, fax (201) 748-6008, or online at http://www.wiley.com/go/permission.

The contents of this work are intended to further general scientific research, understanding, and discussion only and are not intended and should not be relied upon as recommending or promoting a specific method, diagnosis, or treatment by health science practitioners for any particular patient. The publisher and the author make no representations or warranties with respect to the accuracy or completeness of the contents of this work and specifically disclaim all warranties, including without limitation any implied warranties of fitness for a particular purpose. In view of ongoing research, equipment modifications, changes in governmental regulations, and the constant flow of information relating to the use of medicines, equipment, and devices, the reader is urged to review and evaluate the information provided in the package insert or instructions for each medicine, equipment, or device for, among other things, any changes in the instructions or indication of usage and for added warnings and precautions. Readers should consult with a specialist where appropriate. The fact that an organization or web site is referred to in this work as a citation and/or a potential source of further information does not mean that the author or the publisher endorses the information the organization or web site may provide or recommendations it may make. Further, readers should be aware that Internet web sites listed in this work may have changed or disappeared between when this work was written and when it is read. No warranty may be created or extended by any promotional statements for this work. Neither the publisher nor the author shall be liable for any damages arising therefrom.

For general information on our other products and services or for technical support, please contact our Customer Care Department within the United States at (800) 762-2974, outside the United States at (317) 572-3993 or fax (317) 572-4002.

Wiley also publishes its books in a variety of electronic formats. Some content that appears in print may not be available in electronic formats. For more information about Wiley products, visit our web site at www.wiley.com.

Library of Congress Cataloging-in-Publication Data

Names: Tolstunov, Len, editor.
Title: Vertical alveolar ridge augmentation in implant dentistry : a surgical
  manual / edited by Len Tolstunov.
Description: Ames, Iowa : John Wiley & Sons Inc., 2016. | Includes index.
Identifiers: LCCN 2015036875 | ISBN 9781119082590 (cloth)
Subjects: | MESH: Alveolar Ridge Augmentation—methods. | Bone
  Transplantation. | Dental Implantation—methods.
Classification: LCC RK667.I45 | NLM WU 600 | DDC 617.6/93—dc23 LC record available at http://lccn.loc.gov/2015036875

Background cover image: GettyImages-92816396/AbleStock.com

10 9 8 7 6 5 4 3 2 1

Contents

Contributors vii
Preface ix
Acknowledgments xi
Introduction xiii

Section I: Introduction

1. Introduction and Bone Augmentation Classification 3
   Len Tolstunov

2. Applied Surgical Anatomy of the Jaws 7
   Rabie M. Shanti and Vincent B. Ziccardi

3. Prosthetic Comprehensive Oral Evaluation in Implant Dentistry: Team Approach 14
   Steven J. LoCascio

4. Orthodontic Therapy in Implant Dentistry: Orthodontic Implant Site Development 30
   Ali Borzabadi-Farahani and Homayoun H. Zadeh

5. Radiographic Evaluation of the Alveolar Ridge in Implant Dentistry. Cone Beam Computed Tomography 38
   Sanjay M. Mallya

6. Classification of Alveolar Ridge Defects in Implant Dentistry 52
   Patrick Palacci

7. Alveolar Ridge Augmentation: An Algorithmic Approach 61
   Alan S. Herford, Katina Nguyen, and Ayleen Rojhani

8. The Fourth Dimension of 3D Surgical Alveolar Ridge Reconstruction: Bone and Soft Tissue Grafting to Compensate for Dynamic Craniofacial Changes Associated with Aging 71
   Oded Bahat, Richard Sullivan, Fereidoun Daftary, Ramin Mahallati, and Peter S. Wöhrle

Section II: Guided Bone Regeneration (GBR) with Particulate Graft for Vertical Alveolar Ridge Defects

9. Dental Implant Site Development with Particulate Bone Grafts and Guided Bone Regeneration 81
   Flavia Q. Pirih and Paulo M. Camargo

10. Vertical Augmentation of the Alveolar Ridge with Titanium-Reinforced Devices (Protected Bone Regeneration) 93
    Tetsu Takahashi and Kensuke Yamauchi

11. Pedicled Sandwich Plasty (Osteotomy) with Particulate Inlay Graft for Vertical Alveolar Ridge Defects 110
    Rolf Ewers

12. Piezoelectric Surgery for Atrophic Mandible: Vertical Ridge Augmentation with Sandwich Osteotomy Technique and Interpositional Allograft 121
    Dong-Seok Sohn

Section III: Subantral Grafting (Sinus Lift) for Vertical Ridge Augmentation in the Posterior Maxilla

13. Implant Diagnosis and Treatment Planning for the Posterior Edentulous Maxilla 135
    Douglas E. Kendrick

14. Crestal Sinus Floor Elevation: Osteotome Technique 144
    Michael Beckley and Len Tolstunov

15. Flapless Crestal Sinus Augmentation: Hydraulic Technique 152
    Byung-Ho Choi

16. Piezoelectric Surgery for Atrophic Maxilla: Minimally Invasive Sinus Lift and Ridge Augmentation, Role of Growth Factors 161
    Dong-Seok Sohn

17. Sinus Floor Elevation and Grafting: The Lateral Approach 178
    Michael Beckley and Len Tolstunov

18. Posterior Maxillary Sandwich Osteotomy Combined with Sinus Floor Grafting for Severe Alveolar Atrophy 186
    Ole T. Jensen

19. Management of Complications of Sinus Lift Procedures 194
    Douglas E. Kendrick

Section IV: Alveolar Distraction Osteogenesis for Vertical Alveolar Ridge Augmentation

20. Distraction Osteogenesis for Implant Site Development: Diagnosis and Treatment Planning 201
    Stephanie J. Drew

21. Alveolar Distraction Osteogenesis for Vertical Ridge Augmentation: Surgical Principles and Technique 222
    Shravan Renapurkar and Maria J. Troulis

22. Management of Maxillary and Mandibular Post-Traumatic Alveolar Bone Defects with Distraction Osteogenesis Technique 229
    Adi Rachmiel and Dekel Shilo

23. Management of Complications of Alveolar Distraction Osteogenesis Procedure 238
    Stephanie J. Drew

Section V: Autogenous Block Bone Grafting for Vertical Alveolar Ridge Augmentation

24. Vertical Alveolar Ridge Augmentation with Autogenous Block Grafts in Implant Dentistry 274
    Vishtasb Broumand, Arash Khojasteh, and J. Marshall Green III

Section VI: Free Bone Flaps and Osseointegrated Implants for Mandibular and Maxillary Alveolar Bone Reconstruction

25 Mandibular and Maxillary Alveolar Bone Reconstruction with Free Bone Flaps and Osseointegrated Implants 275
Edward I. Chang and Matthew M. Hanasono

Section VII: Soft Tissue Grafting for Implant Site Development

26 Soft Tissue Grafting for Implant Site Development: Diagnosis and Treatment Planning 285
Georgios A. Kotsakis, Suheil Boutros, and Andreas L. Ioannou

27 Soft Tissue Grafting Techniques in Implant Dentistry 291
Suheil Boutros and Georgios A. Kotsakis

28 Management of Complications Associated with Soft Tissue Grafting in Implant Dentistry 308
Fawad Javed, Suheil Boutros, and Georgios A. Kotsakis

Section VIII: Tissue Engineering of the Alveolar Complex

29 Alveolar Bone Augmentation via In situ Tissue Engineering 315
Robert E. Marx

30 Bone Marrow Aspirate: Rationale and Aspiration Technique 323
Dennis Smiler

31 Alveolar Complex Regeneration 335
Nelson Monteiro and Pamela C. Yelick

Index 343

Contributors

Oded Bahat, BDS, MSD
Diplomate
American Board of Periodontology
Beverly Hills, CA, USA

Michael L. Beckley, DDS
Assistant Clinical Professor
Department of Oral and Maxillofacial Surgery
University of the Pacific, Arthur A. Dugoni School of Dentistry Private Practice, Oral and Maxillofacial Surgery, Livermore, CA, USA

Ali Borzabadi-Farahani, DDS, MSCD MORTH RCS(ED)
Fellowship Craniofacial Orthodontics (CHLA/USC)
Associate Clinical Teacher, Orthodontics
Warwick Dentistry
Warwick Medical School
University of Warwick
Coventry, UK

Locum Consultant Orthodontist
NHS England, UK

Visiting Professor
Department of Orthodontics
School of Dentistry
Shahid Beheshti University of Medical Sciences
Tehran, Iran

Suheil Boutros, DDS, MS
Private Practice
Limited to Periodontics and Implants Surgery
Grand Blanc, MI, USA

Vishtasb Broumand, DMD, MD
Private Practice, Oral and Maxillofacial Surgery
Phoenix, AZ, USA

Adjunct Assistant Clinical Professor
Department of Oral and Maxillofacial Surgery
University of Florida College of Dentistry
Gainesville, FL, USA

Clinical Assistant Professor of Oral Maxillofacial Surgery
A.T. Still University
MD Anderson Cancer Center
Arizona School of Dentistry and Oral Health
Mesa, AZ, USA

Paulo M. Camargo, DDS, MS, MBA
Professor
Tarrson Family Endowed Chair in Periodontics
Associate Dean of Clinical Dental Sciences
UCLA School of Dentistry
Los Angeles, CA, USA

Edward I. Chang, MD
Assistant Professor
Department of Plastic Surgery
The University of Texas MD Anderson Cancer Center
Houston, TX, USA

Byung-Ho Choi, DDS, PHD
Professor
Department of Oral and Maxillofacial Surgery
Yonsei University Wonju College of Medicine
Wonju, South Korea

Fereidoun Daftary, DDS, MSD
Clinical Practice, Center for Implant and Esthetic Dentistry Beverly Hills, California, USA

Stephanie J. Drew, DMD
Private Practice
The New York Center for Orthognathic and Maxillofacial Surgery
West Islip
New York, USA

Assistant Clinical Professor
Stony Brook University
Hospital and Hofstra Medical School
New York, USA

Rolf Ewers, MD, DMD, PHD
Chairman
University Hospital for Cranio Maxillofacial and Oral Surgery
Medical University of Vienna
Vienna, Austria

J Marshall Green III, DDS
Lieutenant US Navy
Fellow
Maxillofacial Oncology and Reconstructive Surgery
Division of Oral and Maxillofacial Surgery
University of Miami, Miller School of Medicine
Miami, FL, USA

Matthew M. Hanasono, MD
Professor
Department of Plastic Surgery
The University of Texas MD Anderson Cancer Center
Houston, TX, USA

Alan S Herford, DDS, MD, OMFS
Chair and Professor
Oral and Maxillofacial Surgery Department
Loma Linda University
Loma Linda, CA, USA

Andreas L. Ioannou, DDS
Dental Fellow
Department of Developmental and Surgical Sciences
Division of Periodontology
University of Minnesota
Minneapolis, MN, USA

Fawad Javed, BDS, PHD
Division of General Dentistry
Eastman Institute for Oral Health
University of Rochester
New York, NY, USA

Ole T. Jensen, DDS, MS
Adjunct Professor
School of Dentistry
University of Utah
Salt Lake City, UT, USA

Douglas E. Kendrick, DDS
Department of Oral and Maxillofacial Surgery
The University of Iowa Hospitals and Clinics
Iowa City, IA, USA

Arash Khojasteh, DMD, MS
Associate Professor
Department of Oral and Maxillofacial Surgery
Director
Dental Research Center, Dental School
Shahid Beheshti University of Medical Sciences
Tehran, Iran

George A. Kotsakis, DDS, MS
Assistant Professor
Department of Periodontics
University of Washington
Seattle, WA, USA

Steven J. LoCascio, DDS
Clinical Associate Professor
Department of Oral and Maxillofacial Surgery
University of Tennessee Graduate School of Medicine
Knoxville, TN, USA

Clinical Assistant Professor
Department of Prosthodontics
Louisiana State University Health Sciences Center
School of Dentistry
New Orleans, LA, USA

Full Time Private Practice, Limited to Prosthodontics and Maxillofacial Prosthetics
Knoxville, TN, USA

Ramin Mahallati, DDS
Clinical Practice, Center for Implant and Esthetic Dentistry
Beverly Hills, CA, USA

Sanjay M. Mallya, BDS, MDS, PHD
Associate Professor and Program Director
Section of Oral and Maxillofacial Radiology
UCLA School of Dentistry
Los Angeles, CA, USA

Robert E. Marx, DDS
Professor of Surgery and Chief
Division or Oral and Maxillofacial Surgery
University of Miami Miller School of Medicine
Miami, FL, USA

Nelson Monteiro, PHD
Postdoctoral Fellow
Department of Orthodontics
Division of Craniofacial and Molecular Genetics
Tufts University School of Dental Medicine
Boston, MA, USA

Katina Nguyen, DDS, OMFS
Research Fellow
Oral and Maxillofacial Surgery Department
Loma Linda University
Loma Linda, CA, USA

Patrick Palacci, DDS
Brånemark Osseointegration Center Marseille, France
Visiting Professor
Boston University
Boston, MA, USA
Visiting Professor
Andrés Bello University Santiago de Chile
Chile
Visiting Professor
Maimónides University
Buenos Aires, Argentina

Flavia Q. Pirih, DDS, PHD, MS
Assistant Professor
Section of Periodontics
UCLA School of Dentistry
Los Angeles, CA, USA

Adi Rachmiel, DMD, PHD
Professor
Department of Oral and Maxillofacial Surgery
Rambam Health Care Campus
Haifa, Israel
Bruce Rappaport Faculty of Medicine Technion–Israel
Institute of Technology
Haifa, Israel

Shravan Renapurkar, BDS, DMD
Assistant Professor
Department of Oral and Maxillofacial Surgery
Virginia Commonwealth University
Richmond, VA, USA

Ayleen Rojhani, DDS: OMFS
Senior Resident
Oral and Maxillofacial Surgery Department
Loma Linda University
Loma Linda, CA, USA

Rabie M. Shanti, DMD, MD
Fellow in Head and Neck Oncologic Surgery/
Microvascular Reconstructive Surgery
Department of Oral and Maxillofacial/Head and Neck Surgery
Louisiana State University Health Sciences Center
Shreveport, LA, USA

Dekel Shilo, DMD, PHD
Department of Oral and Maxillofacial Surgery
Rambam Health Care Campus
Haifa, Israel

Dennis Smiler, DDS, MSCD
Oral and Maxillofacial Surgeon
Encino, CA, USA

Dong-Seok Sohn, DDS, PHD
Professor and Chair
Department of Oral and Maxillofacial Surgery
Daegu Catholic University
School of Medicine
Daegu, Korea

Richard Sullivan, DDS
Vice-President
Clinical Technologies
Nobel Biocare North America
Yorba Linda, CA, USA

Tetsu Takahashi, DDS, PHD
Professor and Chairman
Department of Oral and Maxillofacial Surgery
Tohoku University Graduate School of Dentistry
Sendai, Miyagi, Japan

Len Tolstunov, DDS, DMD
Private Practice, Oral and Maxillofacial Surgery
San Francisco, CA, USA
Assistant Clinical Professor
Department of Oral and Maxillofacial Surgery
UCSF and UOP Schools of Dentistry
San Francisco, CA, USA

Maria J. Troulis, DDS, MS
Chief of Service
Department of Oral and Maxillofacial Surgery
Massachusetts General Hospital, Walter C. Guralnick
Professor and Chair of Oral and Maxillofacial Surgery
Harvard School of Dental Medicine
Boston, MA, USA

Peter S. Wöhrle, DMD, MMEDSC
Clinical Practice, Newport Beach, CA, USA

Kensuke Yamauchi, DDS, PHD
Lecturer
Department of Oral and Maxillofacial Surgery
Tohoku University Graduate School of Dentistry
Sendai, Miyagi, Japan
Vice Director
Dental Implant Center, Tohoku University Hospital
Sendai, Japan

Pamela C. Yelick, PHD
Professor
Department of Orthodontics
Director
Division of Craniofacial and Molecular Genetics
Tufts University School of Dental Medicine
Boston, MA, USA

Homayoun H. Zadeh, DDS, PHD
Associate Professor and Director
Division of Periodontology
Laboratory for Immunoregulation and Tissue Engineering
Diagnostic Sciences Dental Hygiene
University of Southern California
Los Angeles, CA, USA

Vincent B. Ziccardi, DDS, MD, FACS
Professor and Chair/Program Director, Assistant Dean of Hospital Affairs
Department of Oral and Maxillofacial Surgery
Rutgers School of Dental Medicine
Newark, NJ, USA

Preface

"Education is not a learning of facts, but training of the mind to think,"
Albert Einstein.

"Anatomy is destiny,"
Sigmund Freud.

Implant Dentistry (Oral Implantology) is a constantly evolving dental and surgical clinical practice and science. There are a variety of books that come out every year on different aspects of this surgical–restorative discipline. Large hardcover textbooks with a name containing at least two words *implant* and *dentistry* heavily dominate shelves of medical/dental bookstores of many publishing companies and subsequently homes of many dentists who are happy to dedicate themselves to a lifelong learning. For different reasons, these expensive and authoritative books are often not top sellers. These books often become "shelve-bound", collecting dust but more importantly providing little practical use in spite of their original intent.

During my professional dental graduate and oral and maxillofacial surgery postgraduate studies in three universities, I have always enjoyed more practical books - clinical manuals. These usually smaller medical, surgical, and dental books in a hard or soft cover were my mobile knowledge friends that I could take with me anywhere and study "on the go" in any setting. Arguably, these friendly manuals are preferred by most medical and dental students, residents, and doctors alike.

A good example of this type of clinically relevant practical book for me has always been *Rapid Interpretation of EKG's* by Dale Dubin, MD. This is by far one of the most widely read and studied medical books by any medical or dental practitioner who had to learn about electrocardiography (EKG). This outstanding book is now in its successful 6th Edition and has always been a No.1 Best Seller. Why? I believe this is not only because it is a brilliantly written book accompanied by easy to follow photos, graphs, and tables, as well as quizzes and interactive courses, but also because of the book's immense practicality and relevance for any health science student or practitioner or often a lay reader/learner.

The book that you are holding in your hands is an attempt to write this sort of book, a very clinically relevant surgical manual, a practical guide on the WHY and HOW of the alveolar bone augmentation in implant dentistry, a "take to the operative room" book full of clinically oriented chapters that can be easily understood and followed.

In the middle of writing this book, due to an enormous amount of accumulated techniques for the alveolar ridge augmentation, Dr. Ole Jensen (whom I consider my mentor and who wrote an Introduction for this book) suggested that it would be an impossible and confusing task to demonstrate to doctors, residents, and students all these amazing surgical techniques in a single book volume. The size of this book would be enormous and practicality of having something very relevant with you and being able to "carry it around" would be a daunting task. That is how slowly the concept of two volumes (two books, really) evolved where horizontal and vertical ridge augmentation techniques in a style of a surgical manual-atlas full of case reports and illustrative photos are described in separate books.

The first book (Book I) contains multiple surgical techniques intended for mainly width-deficient alveolar ridges and thus the book is, in general, about the horizontal ridge augmentation; the second book, *Vertical Alveolar Ridge Augmentation in Implant Dentistry: A Surgical Manual* (Book II) contains a variety of surgical procedures designed for height (and volume) deficient alveolar ridges and therefore is about vertical and three-dimensional ridge augmentation. Both books do not claim to be a complete all-inclusive dissertation of all alveolar bone augmentation techniques. That would be impossible and impractical. Many surgical techniques are being proposed almost daily on the pages of peer-review oral surgical, periodontal, implant, and general dental journals and other publications. They are also often modified from the original versions with the discovery of new instrumentation and advances in computer technology. Two books approach was a logical (we thought) attempt to "split" the presented material into horizontal and vertical surgical techniques for the sake of learning.

Our goal with these two intrinsically linked books was to present a variety of commonly used and sometimes less known surgical techniques from a different point of view in a clear and concise manner with photographs and illustrations, and supplemented by case reports. Each book starts with the applied surgical anatomy and embryology of the jaws, move through diagnosis and treatment planning, which includes a team approach with restorative practitioner (prosthetic chapter) and often an orthodontic colleague (orthodontic implant side development chapter), and then move to a variety of hard (and even soft) tissue augmentation techniques. Each book ends with a glance into the future (quickly becoming a present-day reality), like tissue engineering, stem-cell technology, and organ regeneration. All these chapters were written by top-notch surgical specialists (surgeons–researchers–lecturers) from around the globe in the area of their particular expertise.

A reader of any skill or knowledge- a surgical resident or a new dental practitioner, an experienced periodontist or an oral and maxillofacial surgeon- pay a special attention to the following three surgical concepts presented in these books:

1. Soft tissue versus hard tissue augmentation, or a combined hard–soft tissue augmentation approach that is often needed in the esthetic zone.
2. Static versus dynamic bone augmentation of the alveolar ridge (block graft versus distraction osteogenesis, or ridge-split versus orthodontic forced eruption, or guided bone regeneration (GBR) versus periosteal expansion osteogenesis).
3. Two-dimensional versus three-dimensional versus four-dimensional (predicting future bone changes associated with aging) bone augmentation.

As the editor and one of many contributors of these two surgical manuals, I hoped to accomplish the intended goal of these two books - to present a clinically relevant surgical material that would be read and re-read many times during your career and, therefore, would undoubtedly benefit your patients. If this will happen, I will consider myself a happy man.

Len Tolstunov

Acknowledgments

I would like to express my sincere gratitude to all 70 individuals from around the globe (from 10 countries) who became contributors to these two books (65 chapters in total) for their unselfish sharing of their knowledge, expertise, talent, and time. This was a volunteer army of top-notch professionals who sacrificed their own personal time to contribute to these books and thus to dental and medical education. In the process of book writing and production, many of them have become my friends and genuine collaborators whom I admire and look up to.

I especially would like to acknowledge my wife, Marina, who had to occupy her life with new hobbies and interests to fill the gap that her husband created for two full years by not being around all the time and spending numerous hours in the office occupied with this project. Marina is the love of my life and I would be remiss forgetting her sacrifices, which are numerous. My kids, Deana and Antony, were a daily part of my comfort zone that I needed so much in order to express myself clearly, genuinely, and completely on the pages of this book.

I also would like to thank the representatives of John Wiley & Sons for their skillful and patient daily guidance through the uncharted (for me) territory of writing my first professional book. They are Rick Blanchette, Commissioning Editor, Teri Jensen, Editorial Assistant, and Jenny Seward and Catriona Cooper, Senior Project Editors. Patricia Bateson, an academic copyeditor, was instrumental in carrying out a thorough screening of each chapter to make sure it was written in correct English and the content made understandable sense. Shikha Pahuja at the final stage of book production was essential in working with each contributor and the editor to make sure that each and every chapter is ready for the publication. I am very grateful to these Wiley professionals for their exemplary work and meticulous attention to details. Brittany King, our book artist-illustrator, deserves special accolades for her artistry in medical illustrations and patience in dealing with those who need them.

I am also very grateful to my dear staff at our Van Ness Oral and Maxillofacial Surgery Center in San Francisco, who helped me to run my full-time surgical practice simultaneously with full-time book writing without major distress. They are Vilma Mejia, Liliya Kaganovsky, Marina Tolstunov, and Ann Siebert.

Many professional teachers and colleagues have unknowingly contributed to this book through the education they have provided to me. They include teachers and oral surgeons at the Moscow Medical Stomatological Institute in Moscow, Russia, the University of the Pacific in San Francisco, and the University of California San Francisco.

Introduction

In modern implant-driven oral rehabilitation, alveolar bone deficiency is defined by what is necessary for successful dental implant osseointegration. This need for adequate quantity and quality of bone has led to the development of several innovative methods for alveolar ridge augmentation. At the same time, improved implant technology, like computer-guided implant placement methods, have lessened the need for complex augmentation procedures. The practitioner may ask what is needed for a specified treatment without regard to full regeneration of hard tissue. Where once large-scale reconstruction was considered, now minimally invasive surgical procedures are employed. The clinician then may ask what kind of minimally invasive procedures can and should be performed to support a restoratively driven implant treatment plan. This book will attempt to answer this question.

In addition to osseointegration, there are other factors to consider, including regaining alveolar form and associated esthetic gingival contour – effects termed *orthoalveolar form*. Orthoalveolar form, however, implies that the alveolar process and associated soft tissues are restored to ideal form and function with alveolar arches in functional occlusal relationship, including alveolar width and height and gingival drape essential for osseointegration and subsequent long-term function of dental implants. This means that the alveolus is not only restored to its original form but also often increased in bone mass and quality of soft tissue to accommodate dental implants. It is important to be familiar with a variety of surgical procedures in order to achieve an orthoalveolar form. This book will attempt to demonstrate these techniques.

Practitioners sometimes lose sight of what they need to accomplish. Completion of a surgical grafting procedure may not be needed for the prescribed implant procedure. Final restoratively driven surgical outcome according to a precise implant treatment plan helps to keep the whole dental team on track of what is needed to accomplish in each particular case. The surgeon must visualize where implant elements need to be placed, decide if the bone mass is needed there to support implants, and graft accordingly. This requires preprosthetic planning, which may include the use of surgical guide or navigation. The plan may prescribe staged or simultaneous grafting, even secondary grafting after implant placement. Whatever the plan, surgical efforts should attempt to gain added bone stock within the envelope of function, choosing a surgical method that has a biological basis for success. This book will attempt to illustrate these methods.

The surgical method of grafting is judged by early and late healing events but include the concepts of consolidation, functional remodeling, resistance to resorption, and bioactive capability for osseointegration. An ideal bone graft should therefore be well consolidated, undergo remodeling without significant resorption, and be well vascularized. Bone graft substitutes, like alloplasts, xenografts, and possibly allografts, may not fully integrate with native bone. Various forms of autografts, recombinant biomimetics, and autologous cell-based therapies may have an improved biological basis but require advanced surgical skills and technical support. This book will attempt to describe these therapies.

The quest for ideal bone graft is continuing. New techniques are constantly being introduced to simplify, improve, or expand indications for alveolar reconstruction. Currently, surgical techniques for implant-driven alveolar ridge augmentation can be classified into four broad categories. These would include: (1) guided tissue and bone regeneration (with or without titanium-reinforced devices), (2) block grafting (extraoral and intraoral), (3) ridge-split with formation of osteoperiosteal (pedicled) flaps, and (4) distraction osteogenesis. Alveolar ridge deficiency can also be classified according to defect morphology such as vertical defects, horizontal defects, combination defects, and complete absence of bone. Science and practice of alveolar ridge reconstruction is still a descriptive surgical discipline with numerous variables to consider, not the least of which is the "patient factor" that includes the patient's general medical condition, patient's wishes and desires (wants and needs), and patient's cooperation. This book will attempt to address these factors of importance.

Another factor to consider in any surgery is the healing capacity of the host's recipient site being grafted. In many cases, it can be more important than the type of material used for grafting. If the site is well vascularized and the grafting procedure is done well, complete incorporation of the bone graft may occur. Interestingly, in 1668, the very first bone graft (harvested from a dog) worked so well that it could not be removed when the patient asked for it to be removed for religious reasons at a later date. Failure of a bone graft, often attributed to the material used, probably happens more often due to host site healing deficiency or flawed surgical technique rather than the intrinsic property of the graft material per se.

One factor that has become extremely important is simplification of treatment, that is, economy of surgery, management, and expenditure. This means that the social contract between patient and physician has narrowed to favor minimally invasive procedures, shortened treatment times, simplified surgical management, and affordability. This is why an immediate function implant treatment has become so prevalent, even in the face of simultaneous bone grafting. The difficulty with simplification is proper diagnosis, comprehensive treatment planning, and adequate training. In addition, consensus on bone grafting and decision-making process are often limited to experience-based case report knowledge and lacking level I and II evidence-based controlled studies that are frequently difficult to find.

The purpose of this clinically oriented book in two volumes is to demonstrate the various techniques of implant-driven horizontal (Book I) and three-dimensional/vertical (Book II) alveolar bone augmentation treatment in use today in an easy to follow, step-by-step format. An international and multidisciplinary group of surgical specialists, well known in their own fields, will present various surgical methods that will be illustrated graphically and supplemented by multiple intraoperative photographs. Benefits, risks, alternatives and complications of each technique will be demonstrated and scientific references will be provided, giving a reader a true insight into each surgical technique. This, hopefully, will help a reader to improve the knowledge of a selected technique as well as broaden the scope of surgical modalities that can be successfully employed in his or her practice. If you are a true learner, this book is for you.

Ole T. Jensen

SECTION I

Introduction

CHAPTER 1
Introduction and Bone Augmentation Classification

Len Tolstunov

Private Practice, Oral and Maxillofacial Surgery, San Francisco, California, USA
Department of Oral and Maxillofacial Surgery, UCSF and UOP Schools of Dentistry, San Francisco, California, USA

Brånemark's discovery of osseointegration arguably became one of the most significant events in dentistry in the twentieth century [1, 2]. It could be stated that this discovery divided dentistry into two periods: pre-implant era or era of symptomatic (symptom-driven) dentistry and an implant era or era of physiologic dentistry. In the first period, restorative dentistry had only two meaningful treatment options for failed teeth or edentulous jaws: removable dentures and fixed bridges. Both removable dentures and fixed bridges relied on support of adjacent teeth and underlying alveolar mucosa with little consideration for bone preservation.

For the last 50 years of the second and modern period of dentistry, restorative (reconstructive) dentistry has been utilizing physiologic treatment by replacing missing or failing teeth with bone-anchored (osseointegrated) endosseous implants that have an ability to maintain the alveolar bone in a similar manner to a natural dentition. A new principle of bone preservation was based on the concept of endosseous bone loading (EBL). Dental implants also removed an unnecessary load from adjacent teeth, thus decreasing and eliminating deteriorating effects of removable and fixed tooth-borne prostheses on natural dentition, strengthening masticatory function, and improving esthetics and patient's comfort.

Initially surgically driven, implant dentistry was concerned mainly with an implant integration of dental implants. It was soon to become clear that in order to properly *restore* endosseously placed implants, they have to be inserted into the bone in a restoratively driven position, identical or close to where the natural teeth used to be, even if bone was no longer available in the area. Implant dentistry has emerged as a prosthetically driven surgical–restorative discipline.

In the last few decades, it became clear that success of implant dentistry and longevity of dental implants depend on three factors ("implant triangle"). These factors are: (1) a proper restoratively driven placement of implants, (2) the presence of a sufficient amount of bone stock, a foundation for the osseointegration, and (3) the presence of healthy peri-implant soft tissue for proper implant hygiene and maintenance. Missing any one component of the implant triangle tends to eventually result in compromise of implant health or longevity, and can often lead to implant failure.

The presence of bone atrophy or resorption due to tooth loss and trauma (among many other factors) has led to the development of a variety of implant-driven bone augmentation procedures in a single or staged fashion. This two-volume book is about bone augmentation techniques applicable to implant dentistry. A variety of bone augmentation procedures for the deficient (atrophied) alveolar bone has been proposed in the literature [3–5] and are described in these two books. Each method has its indications and contraindications, its proponents and opponents. The following four alveolar ridge reconstruction techniques are frequently used in oral implantology and are described in this book:

1 Guided bone regeneration (GBR) with particulate bone graft [6, 7].
2 Onlay (veneer) extraoral (hip, rib, calvarium) [8] and intraoral (chin, ramus, posterior mandible, zygomatic buttress, maxillary tuberosity) [9–11] block bone graft.
3 Ridge-split/bone graft and sandwich osteotomy [12–14].
4 Alveolar distraction osteogenesis [15, 16].

To simplify learning of the surgical techniques, the editor (Tolstunov) of this book divided them roughly into two categories: horizontal augmentation and vertical (volumetric) augmentation. Book I inspects horizontal bone augmentation of alveolar ridges with bone *width* deficiency and Book II scrutinizes vertical bone augmentation of alveolar ridges with bone *height* loss. Both books do not claim to be a complete all-inclusive dissertation of all alveolar bone augmentation techniques. That would be impossible and impractical. Many surgical techniques are being proposed almost daily on the pages of peer-review oral surgical, periodontal, implant, and general dental journals and other publications. They are also often modified from the original versions with the discovery of new instrumentation and computer technology.

Classifications tend to simplify learning of a certain subject. They often give a reader a "bird's-eye view" of the complex topic. There is a variety of different classifications of alveolar bone augmentation in implant dentistry. Table 1.1 demonstrates the editor's classification. Based on years of teaching, practicing and in the process of writing this book, we offer the classification that can, hopefully, be well understood by students, surgical residents, and doctors, and be *conceptually* robust from the biologic point of view. Examine Table 1.1 after finishing this chapter.

The editor's recommendation for readers of this two-volume book is to open the book on any chapter that seems clinically relevant at that particular moment and read/learn/study the technique thoroughly. Targeted (selective) reading is common and productive in medical literature. After finishing one chapter, you might want to come back later to the same chapter to re-think its content. Then, move on to another chapter on a different type of

Vertical Alveolar Ridge Augmentation in Implant Dentistry: A Surgical Manual, First Edition. Edited by Len Tolstunov.
© 2016 John Wiley & Sons, Inc. Published 2016 by John Wiley & Sons, Inc.

Table 1.1 Classification of alveolar ridge augmentation procedures through bone grafting in implant dentistry (both vertical and horizontal).

Types	Graft donor site	Type of augmentation	Graft type, flap type, and graft revascularization	Graft consolidation	Augmenting tissues
I. Inlay (interpositional) bone graft: **A. Particulate** 1. GBR (three–four-wall tooth socket or bone defect)	None or autogenous (if used)	Static	**Free graft** Limited mucoperiosteal flap; endosteal (mainly) revascularization	Woven-to-lamellar; starts with bone formation	Hard tissue
2. Ridge-split or pedicled sandwich osteotomy (two-wall horizontal or vertical bone defect)			Osteomucoperiosteal vascular flap [17–19]; two-to-three surfaces of vascularization: endosteal – from both split bone surfaces plus periosteal (lingual- for vertical, buccal- for horizontal) [20]		
3. Sinus lift (subantral augmentation)			No flap (crestal approach) or mucoperiosteal flap (lateral approach); endosteal and periosteal neovascularization (sinus membrane plays a role of periosteum)		
4. Tent-pole technique with autogenous cortical block bone			Mucoperiosteal flap; tenting block graft does not get vascularity and tends to resorb		
B. Block	Local (intraoral) or distant (extraoral)		No flap; endosteal (mainly) revascularization	Woven-to-lamellar; starts with bone resorption	
II. Onlay (juxtaposed) bone graft: **A. Particulate** 1. GBR (one–two-wall socket or bone defect) or subperiosteal tunnel	None or autogenous (local or distant)	Static	**Free graft**; mucoperiosteal flap; endosteal (mainly) revascularization initially, additional vitality from reattached periosteum comes in 3-4 weeks.	Woven-to-lamellar; starts with bone formation	Hard tissue
2. Tent-pole technique with Ti-mesh, screws or implants [21–23]			Endosteal (mainly) revascularization of the particulate graft		
B. Block	Local (intraoral) or distant (extraoral)		Endosteal (mainly) revascularization of the block graft	Woven-to-lamellar; starts with bone resorption	
III. Alveolar distraction osteogenesis	None	Dynamic	**No graft, mucoperiosteal flap** Endosteal (mainly) and periosteal revascularization (lingual or palatal)	Callus formation, similar to fracture healing, *intramembranous* (mostly) ossification followed by bone remodeling	Hard and soft tissue (simultaneously distracted/ expanded)
IV. Free bone flap transfer (with microvascular anastomosis)	Distant	Static	**Free bone–soft tissue flap** Microanastomosis between local (recipient) and distant (donor) vascular networks plus endosteal (recipient) revascularization	Callus formation, similar to fracture healing, *endochondral* ossification followed by bone remodeling	Hard and soft tissue (simultaneously transferred)

(horizontal or vertical) augmentation for comparison, as well as read current literature on this subject. This might help you to eventually select the technique that suits *you* (feels best in *your* hands). Always remember the biologic rationale of each procedure when selecting the one to help your particular patient.

For a novice dental surgeon or an experienced dental practitioner while studying surgical methods and techniques, I would suggest paying special attention to the following:

1 Soft tissue versus hard tissue augmentation: what is needed and what is the priority, especially in the esthetic zone.
2 Static versus dynamic bone augmentation techniques: block graft versus distraction osteogenesis, ridge-split versus orthodontic forced eruption, etc.
3 Two-dimensional (2D), three-dimensional (3D), and, finally, "four-dimensional" (4D) tissue augmentation: horizontal or vertical (2D) versus volumetric (3D) versus time-dependent bone and soft tissue grafting (considering the fourth dimension), with emphasis on aging changes that can be predicted and prevented by thoughtful augmentation techniques (especially, in the anterior maxilla).

Use this book as a surgical reference guide or manual at any locations – at the university, home, or in the operative room – and let us know what you liked or did not like, and what you would change, add, or delete in future editions of this book. We want each new edition to be better that the one before. Good luck on your learning journey for the benefit of your patients.

I. Particulate bone grafting

1. For INLAY grafts consider xenograft, possibly with autogenous bone (including bone morphogenetic protein (BMP)). Ideally, implant neck and apex are to be positioned in the native bone while the implant body is to be surrounded by the grafted bone. Primary implant stability in the native bone is important.
2. For ONLAY grafts consider mixed xeno-allograft, possibly with autogenous bone (including BMP). Implant neck is to be surrounded by the grafted bone, while the implant body is to be placed into the native bonewith good primary stability (30 + NCm) at the time of insertion.

Tenting procedures for the particulate graft

1. **Cortical autogenous tenting.** Detached free cortical bone block in width or height-deficient ridges is used for a 2D augmentation with a particulate graft positioned in between the cortical block and basal (native) bone as an INLAY graft. Separated cortical "tenting" free bone has no blood supply initially and 4-5 weeks later-some re-established periosteal source of revascularization only, which limits its survival and increases its impending resorption. Both endosteal and periosteal revascularization are provided for the particulate graft that has a good survival potential.
2. **Ti-mesh tenting.** Titanium mesh is used for 3D (volumetric) reconstruction of the collapsed ridge and functions as a scaffold protective device for the particulate graft underneath. The particulate graft is placed in ONLAY fashion on top of native bone. Endosteal revascularization is provided for the particulate graft that has a good survival potential.
3. **Periosteal tenting**
   (a) **Screw tenting:** a soft tissue matrix is tented by metal screws for space creation for the particulate graft placed in ONLAY fashion on top of native bone. Both 2D and 3D ridge augmentations are possible (horizontally and vertically positioned screws). Endosteal and periosteal revascularizations are provided for the particulate graft that has a good survival potential.
   (b) **Implant tenting:** a soft tissue envelope is tented by dental implants for space creation for the particulate graft placed in ONLAY fashion on top of native bone. A 2D ridge augmentation in height-deficient ridges is possible. Endosteal and periosteal revascularization are provided for the particulate graft that has a good survival potential.

II. Block bone grafting

Onlay or inlay, horizontal, vertical or combination (J-graft), fixation screws and plates. Secondary bone resorption often occurs.

III. Alveolar distraction osteogenesis

Horizontal or vertical, specific distractor devices.

IV. Free distant *bone flap* transfer with microvascular anastomosis

Vertical and horizontal, plates and screws.

Graft Revascularization implies bone healing (from angiogenesis to mineralization and ossification) from the particular vascular source:
1. **Endosteal** (central or centrifugal). Bone-to-bone healing (ossification) through angiogenesis. This applies to any onlay or inlay grafts and also for a gap osteotomy created by osteoperiosteal flaps (as in the ridge-split procedure). This is a dominant source of blood supply needed for free bone graft survival.
   (a) **Particulate graft:** internal "coagulum" is converted into the woven bone; fast revascularization through bone formation.
   (b) **Block graft:** plasmatic imbibition to block graft; slow revascularization through resorption.
2. **Periosteal** (peripheral or centripetal). Periosteal proximal angiogenesis to the grafted bone that is exposed to the juxtaposed periosteum (as in an onlay block graft). This is a supplementary source of blood supply needed for free bone graft survival.
3. **Microvascular anastomosis.** The best source of blood supply. Vascular free graft with hard and soft tissue transfer. The endosteal and periosteal sources are also established and are supplementary.

References

1. Brånemark P-I, Zarb G, Albrektsson T: *Tissue-Integrated Prostheses*. Quintessence Publishing Company, Chicago, IL, 1985.
2. Brånemark P-I, Hansson B, Adell R, et al: *Osseointegrated Implants in the Treatment of the Edentulous Jaw. Experience for a 10-Year Period*. Almqvist & Wiksell International, Stockholm, Sweden, 1977.
3. Aghaloo TL, Moy PK: Which hard tissue augmentation techniques are the most successful in furnishing bony support for implant placement? *Int J Oral Maxillofac Implants* 2007;**22**(Suppl):49–70.
4. McAllister BS, Haghighat K: Bone augmentation techniques. *J Periodontol* 2007;**78**(3):377–396.
5. Chiapasco M, Zaniboni M, Boisco M: Augmentation procedures for the rehabilitation of deficient edentulous ridges with oral implants. *Clin Oral Implants Res* 2006;**17**(Suppl 2):136–159.
6. Buser D, Brägger U, Lang NP, et al: Regeneration and enlargement of jaw bone using guided tissue regeneration. *Clin Oral Implants Res* 1990;**1**(1):22–32.
7. Annibali S, Bignozzi I, Sammartino G, et al: Horizontal and vertical ridge augmentation in localized alveolar deficient sites: a retrospective case series. *Implant Dent* 2012;**21**(3):175–185.
8. Keller EE, Triplett WW: Iliac bone grafting: a review of 160 consecutive cases. *J Oral Maxillofac Surg* 1987;**45**(1):11–14.
9. Bedrossian E, Tawfilis A, Alijanian A: Veneer grafting: a technique for augmentation of the resorbed alveolus prior to implant placement. A clinical report. *Int J Oral Maxillofac Implants* 2000;**15**(6):853–858.
10. Pikos MA: Mandibular block autografts for alveolar ridge augmentation. *Atlas Oral Maxillofac Clin North Am* 2005;**13**(2):91–107.
11. Tolstunov L: Maxillary tuberosity block bone graft: innovative technique and case report. *J Oral Maxillofac Surg* 2009;**67**(8):1723–1729.
12. Simion M, Baldoni M, Zaffe D: Jawbone enlargement using immediate implant placement associated with a split-crest technique and guided tissue regeneration. *Int J Periodontics Restorative Dent* 1992;**12**:462–473.
13. Scipioni A, Bruschi GB, Calesini G: The edentulous ridge expansion technique: a five-year study. *Int J Periodontics Restorative Dent* 1994;**14**:451–459.
14. Jensen OT, Cullum DR, Baer D: Marginal bone stability using 3 different flap approaches for alveolar split expansion for dental implants: a 1-year clinical study. *J Oral Maxillofac Surg* 2009;**67**(9):1921–1930.
15. McCarthy JG: The role of distraction osteogenesis in the reconstruction of the mandible in unilateral craniofacial microsomia. *Clin Plast Surg* 1994;**21**(4):625–631.
16. Chin M, Toth BA: Distraction osteogenesis in maxillofacial surgery using internal devises: review of five cases. *J Oral Maxillofac Surg* 1996;**54**(1):45–53.

17 Jensen OT, Ellis E: The book flap: a technical note. *J Oral Maxillofac Surg* 2008;**65** (5):1010–1014.
18 Jensen OT, Mogyoros R, Owen Z, et al: Island osteoperiosteal flap for alveolar bone reconstruction. *J Oral Maxillofac Surg* 2010;**68**(3):539–546.
19 Casap N, Brand M, Mogyros R, et al: Island osteoperiosteal flaps with interpositional bone grafting in rabbit tibia: preliminary study for development of new bone augmentation. *J Oral Maxillofac Surg* 2011;**69**(12):3045–3051.
20 Ewers R, Fock N, Millesi-Schobel G, Enislidis G: Pedicled sandwich plasty: a variation on alveolar distraction for vertical augmentation of the atrophic mandible. *Br J Oral Maxillofac Surg* 2004;**42**:445–447.
21 Le B, Rohrer MD, Prasad HS: Screw "tent-pole" grafting technique for reconstruction of large vertical alveolar ridge defects using human mineralized allograft for implant site preparation. *J Oral Maxillofac Surg* 2010 Feb;**68**(2):428–435.
22 Kuoppala R, Kainulainen VT, Korpi JT, et al: Outcome of treatment of implant-retained overdenture in patients with extreme mandibular bone resorption treated with bone grafts using a modified tent pole technique. *J Oral Maxillofac Surg* 2013 Nov;**71**(11):1843–1851.
23 Korpi JT, Kainulainen VT, Sandor GK, et al: Long-term follow-up of severely resorbed mandibles reconstructed using tent pole technique without platelet-rich plasma. *J Oral Maxillofac Surg* 2012 Nov;**70**(11):2543–2548.

CHAPTER 2
Applied Surgical Anatomy of the Jaws

Rabie M. Shanti[1] and Vincent B. Ziccardi[2]

[1]Department of Oral and Maxillofacial/Head and Neck Surgery, Louisiana State University Health Sciences Center, Shreveport, Louisiana, USA
[2]Department of Oral and Maxillofacial Surgery, Rutgers School of Dental Medicine, Newark, New Jersey, USA

In order to perform vertical augmentation of the maxillary and/or mandibular alveolus safely in preparation for placement of endosseous implants, one must consider adjacent anatomic structures, as well as the variability of the location of these structures and their relationship with adjacent structures secondary to skeletal development, inherent anatomic variations, and changes of the bony anatomy related to bone atrophy from aging and/or tooth loss. An appreciation of the anatomy of the jaws will allow the clinician to perform the procedures and techniques safely that are presented in this textbook.

Dental implant surgery and augmentation of the alveolar ridge when necessary is performed by a variety of dental practitioners and specialists with various levels of surgical training and clinical experiences; however, irrespective of clinical training all healthcare provision should have a mastery of anatomic structures within the relevant anatomic subsite. This knowledge is critical to avoid unnecessary morbidity to the patient and medical litigation. Figure 2.1a and b highlight cases in which there was gross error in the placement of endosseous implants within the maxilla and mandible as a result of inadequate appreciation of the local anatomy.

The maxilla and mandible are located within the oral cavity. The oral cavity by definition extends from the cutaneous–vermillion junction of the upper and lower lip with the hard–soft palate junction serving as the superior–posterior border, the anterior tonsillar pillars serving lateral–posterior borders, and the circumvallate papillae serving as the posterior–inferior border. All anatomic structures posterior to these anatomic borders (e.g., the base of the tongue, palatine tonsils, soft palate) are part of the oropharynx. The oral cavity provides a multitude of physiologic functions including: mastication, provision of salivary lubricants and buffers, mediation of the oral preparatory and oral transit phases of swallowing, special taste sensations, immunologic defenses mediated via innate immunity, speech, protection of adjacent deep anatomic structures, and contributing to human behavioral communication and interaction. Due to these varied and complex physiologic and social functions, the oral cavity is composed of a myriad of hard and soft tissue structures within a locally compact space in order to allow the execution of these highly organized functions. Furthermore, due to the complex interplay of these structures even a minor disturbance in an anatomic structure of the oral cavity will result in morbidity to the patient. Therefore, in this chapter we will review in detail the anatomic structures serving as the bony bases of the oral cavity, the maxilla and mandible, and also significant adjacent anatomic structures, which must be considered when performing surgical procedures on or within the maxillomandibular complex.

Anatomy of the mandible

Foramina and canals

The mandible is the only freely mobile bone as well as the densest bone within the craniofacial skeleton. The mandible articulates with the skull base via the temporomandibular joints. The mandible is an aesthetically prominent bone due to a mental protuberance, which is a bony prominence in the chin region located inferior to the mandibular incisors. The mandible is a "U-shaped" bone when viewed from above or below.

The mandible contains three named foramina: *mandibular foramen*, *mental foramen*, and *lingual foramen*. Clinically, the mental foramen becomes significant when performing procedures in the premolar region, such as placement of endosseous implants or alveolar ridge augmentation. However, the mandibular foramen is not of concern with procedures related to endosseous implants for restoration of dentition, due to the foramen being situated at a significant distance from the mandibular dentition. However, the mandibular foramen does become significant when performing operations on the ascending ramus of the mandible, such as sagittal split ramus osteotomy or vertical ramus osteotomy. The lingual foramen is a small foramen located along the medial surface of the mid-line of the mandible. Unlike the other two named foramina of the mandible, the lingual foramen is an arterial foramen, meaning that its contents are vascular rather than neurovascular, as is the case of the mandibular foramen and mental foramen. The lingual foramen in the dentate mandible is located towards the inferior border. Small perforating vessels enter the lingual foramen, which arises from anastomotic branches of the right and left sublingual arterial branches of the lingual artery.

The mandibular foramen allows entry of the inferior alveolar neurovascular bundle into the mandible, which is located along the medial surface of the mandibular ramus 15–20 mm inferior to the

Vertical Alveolar Ridge Augmentation in Implant Dentistry: A Surgical Manual, First Edition. Edited by Len Tolstunov.
© 2016 John Wiley & Sons, Inc. Published 2016 by John Wiley & Sons, Inc.

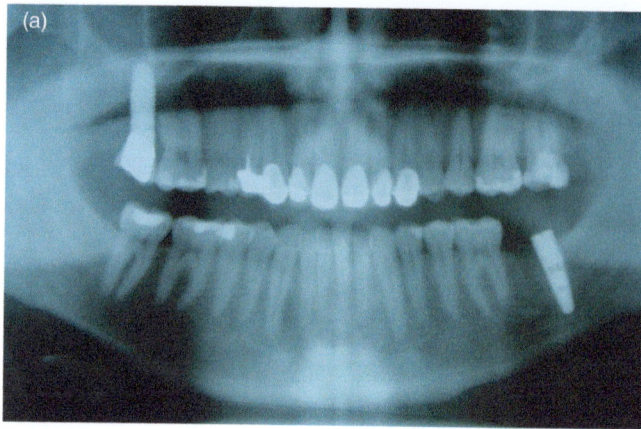
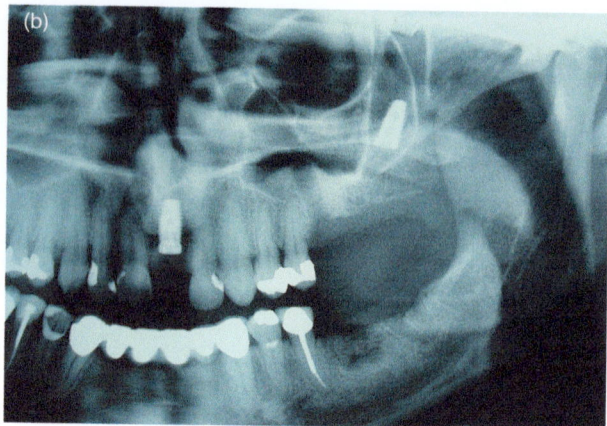

Figure 2.1 (a) Orthopantomogram of implant in the mandibular left second molar position that violates the mandibular canal. (b) Orthopantomogram of implant displaced into left maxillary sinus, status – post-internal (crestal) sinus lift with an attempt to implant placement in the position of the maxillary left first molar.

sigmoid notch. The mandibular foramen is the beginning of the mandibular canal, which is a canal that runs obliquely downward and forward within the ramus of the mandible. The mandibular canal begins at the level of the mandibular foramen and for its first 8–10 mm, the canal typically runs close to the lingual cortex [1]. As the mandibular canal descends within the ramus it takes on a more central position. As the canal moves forward it will typically be positioned closer to the inferior border of the mandible until it passes the second molar and first molar teeth. The most inferior position of the canal is also its most lingual position, which is in between the second molar and first molar region (Figure 2.2) [1]. Once, the canal reaches its most inferior position it will then ascend towards the mental foramen, traveling toward the buccal cortex. Eventually, the mandibular canal will fork into the mental canal and incisive canal, which house the mental nerve and incisive nerve, respectively. Multiple, rare, variations of the mandibular canal have been reported, with the bifid mandibular canal being the most commonly observed anatomic variation of the mandibular canal with a reported incidence of 15.6% [2]. Four variations of the mandibular canal (Figure 2.3), with the retromolar canal variation being the most common occurring in 52.5% cone beam computed tomography (CBCT) scans [3, 4]. Trifid canals have also been reported. The true prevalence of these anatomic variations has only become recently known due to the advent and prevalence of CBCT [4].

The mental canal deviates superiorly towards the mental foramen. The mental foramen is spatially located within the same vertical plane as the infraorbital foramen. The vertical location of the mental foramen within the dentate mandible is consistent, with the foramen being located almost halfway between the tip of the alveolar process and the inferior (lower) border of the mandible; however, this could change with atrophy of the mandible. The transverse position of the mental foramen is varied with slightly conflicting distribution patterns depending on whether the studies utilize radiographic imaging or cadaveric dissection specimens [5, 6]. Von Arx and colleagues reported that the majority (56%) of mental foramina are located between the apices of the first and second premolar teeth and the remaining 35.7% of mental foramina are positioned below the second premolar tooth [5]. Furthermore, each mental foramen is on average 25 mm from the mid-line of the mandible. An accessory mental foramen has been reported to exist in 1.4–10% of patients [7].

The incisive canal will extend anterior to the mental canal and foramen, and houses the mandibular incisive nerve. The incisive canal is not always readily apparent radiographically. Pires and colleagues identified that the mandibular incisive canal was visualized in 83% of cone beam computed tomography scans, while on panoramic radiographs it was only identified in 11% of radiographs [8].

Neurovascular structures

In order to understand conceptually the innervation patterns of the maxilla and mandible, one must consider the embryologic origin of the jaws. Both the maxilla and mandible are first branchial arch derivatives; similarly, the *trigeminal nerve* is a first branchial arch structure. Therefore, the sensory innervation of the maxilla and mandible is provided by the trigeminal nerve as a result of a shared embryologic derivation. The trigeminal nerve is the largest of the twelve cranial nerves, and while the trigeminal nerve captures the entirety of the sensory information from the maxilla and mandible, there are additional neural structures that provide sensory and/or motor innervation to soft tissue structures within the oral cavity, such as *chorda tympani* (branch of seventh cranial nerve), *vagus nerve* (tenth cranial nerve), and *hypoglossal nerve* (twelfth cranial nerve). However, these are typically distant enough from the mandible to not be at risk from injury while performing vertical ridge augmentation within the alveolus of the mandible. Below we will discuss clinically significant nerves, which either receive sensory input from the mandible and associated structures (i.e., teeth) or lie in close proximity to the mandible (Figure 2.4).

Each of the two trigeminal nerves leaves the brain at the level of the pons. The trigeminal nerve then descends laterally to join the ipsilateral trigeminal (Gasserian or semilunar) ganglion located

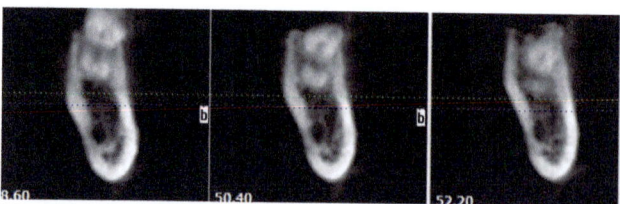

Figure 2.2 Coronal cross-section of cone beam computed tomography depicting most inferior and lingual position of mandibular canal as it traverses the mandible.

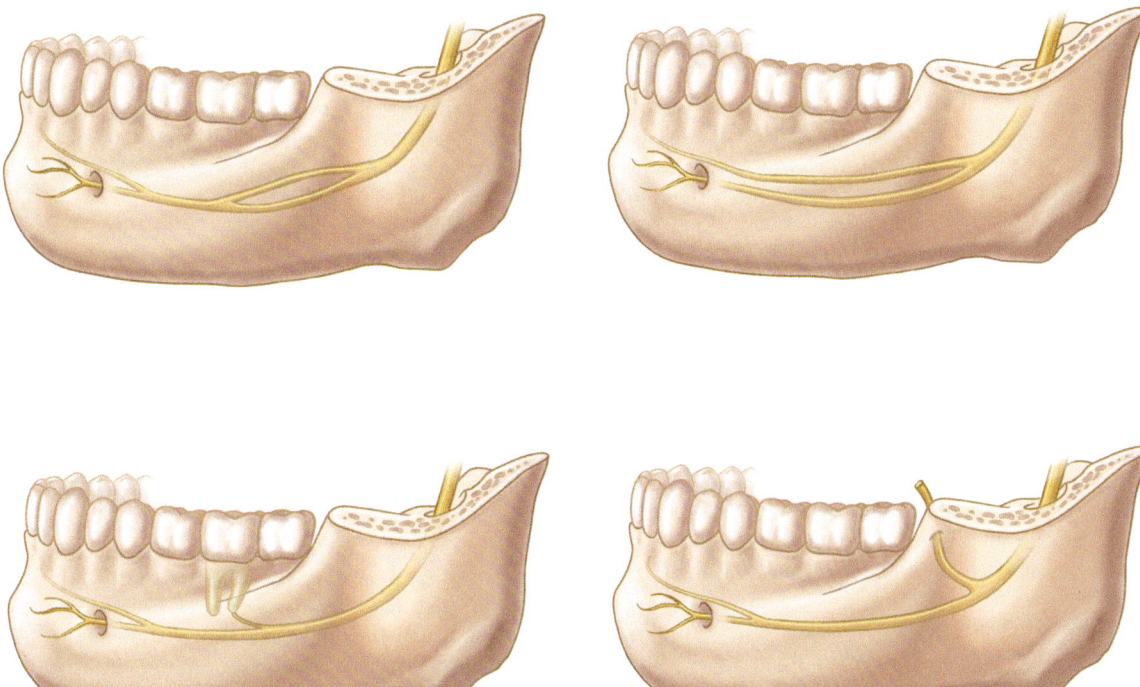

Figure 2.3 Anatomic variation of mandibular canal. Adapted from Naitoh M, et al., *International Journal of Oral and Maxillofacial Implants*, 2009 [3].

within the trigeminal (Meckle) cave, which is a cerebrospinal fluid containing an arachnoidal pouch near the apex of the petrous portion of the temporal bone. It is at the level of the trigeminal (Gasserian or semilunar) ganglion that the trigeminal nerve branches into three large nerve trunks: (1) ophthalmic division (V1), (2) maxillary division (V2), and (3) mandibular division (V3). The ophthalmic division (V1) is the smallest of the three and only receives sensory information from facial structures outside the oral cavity. However, the maxillary (V2) and mandibular (V3) divisions receive all of the sensory input from the jaws.

The *inferior alveolar nerve* (IAN) is a mixed (sensory and motor) nerve, which is the largest terminal branch of the mandibular division (V3). The IAN is primarily a sensory nerve; however, it gives off a motor branch, the nerve to the mylohyoid (mylohyoid nerve), which innervates the anterior belly of the digastric muscle and mylohyoid muscle. The IAN branches from the mandibular division (V3) at a level just below the lower head of the lateral pterygoid muscle, and then descends within the pterygomandibular space (lateral to the medial pterygoid muscle and sphenomandibular ligament) and also in a parallel route that is posterior and lateral to the lingual nerve. The IAN will enter the mandible via the mandibular foramen located on the medial surface of the ascending ramus of the mandible. Encasing the IAN just before it enters the mandibular foramen is the sphenomandibular ligament.

Through its course within the mandible, the IAN is accompanied by the inferior alveolar artery, vein, and lymphatic vessels. Anatomic studies have indicated there are often multiple inferior alveolar veins, which lie superior to the nerve. The inferior alveolar artery appears to be solitary and is generally located medial to the nerve [9]. Throughout its intrabony course, the IAN it will give off many small branches, which will receive sensory input from molar and premolar teeth, as well as their associated periodontal ligaments and alveolar bone. The IAN will eventually divide into the incisive and mental nerves in the vicinity of the premolar teeth.

The "anterior loop" of the IAN has been the subject of much debate [10]. When present, the anterior loop begins after the incisive branches from the IAN, with the remaining portion of the IAN running below and past the mental foramen, and then looping back towards the mental foramen to become the mental nerve. The anterior loop has been identified in 48% of study subjects, with a mean length and length range of 0.89 mm and 0–5.7 mm, respectively [11]. When performing surgery within the posterior mandible (i.e., placement of dental endosseous implants, ridge augmentation, etc.), one must always consider the relationship of the proposed operative procedures to the IAN. As the nerve cannot be visualized by standard radiographic techniques (i.e., plain

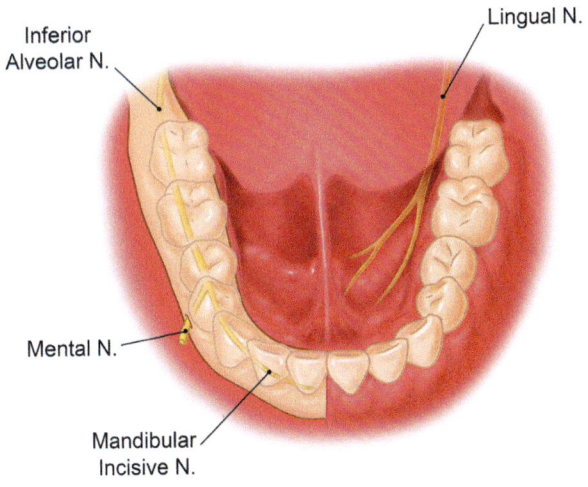

Figure 2.4 Major sensory nerves located within the oral cavity, which lie in close proximity to the mandible.

film radiography, cone beam computed tomography), a general recommendation of maintaining 2 mm from the superior lamina dura of the mandibular canal will avoid injury to the nerve unless there exists an anatomic variation, which was not readily detected on radiographic imaging. The following radiograph highlights a case where the mandibular canal was violated during such procedures when the patient presents with anesthesia of the inferior alveolar nerve distribution (Figure 2.1a). Of note, being that the mental and incisive nerves are terminal branches of the IAN, injury to the IAN within the body of the mandible will result in neurosensory deficits of all structures innervated by the IAN portion distal to the site of injury, as well as the mental and incisive branches.

The *mental nerve* is a strictly sensory nerve and, as previously discussed, is a terminal branch of the inferior alveolar nerve. The nerve begins within the mandible and then courses superiorly along an oblique angle to exit the mandible via the mental foramen. Subsequently, as the nerve exits the mental foramen it is surrounded by a tough sheath, and immediately divides into three branches deep to the depressor anguli oris muscle (Figure 2.5a and b). These branches receive sensory input from the skin of the chin, vestibular gingiva, mandibular facial gingiva, and skin and mucosa of the lower lip. The presence of these small distal nerve branches complicates augmentation of the alveolar ridge in the premolar region, and therefore consideration of the incision design and augmentation technique should take the mental nerve and its branches into account.

One must always consider the position of the mental foramen and branches of the mental nerve, for the incidence of permanent neurosensory disturbance within the mental nerve distribution subsequent to placement of dental implants has been reported in between 7 and 10% of cases [12]. Furthermore, in the atrophic mandible the position of the mental foramen will be variable dependent on the degree of bone atrophy. In cases of severe atrophy of the mandible the foramen could be located along the ridge of the mandible, which must be considered when making a crestal incision and/or performing dissection in the vicinity of the foramen. Even a minor disturbance within the mental nerve distribution could result in varying degrees of morbidity, including lower lip biting, drooling, and/or impaired speech.

As previously discussed, anterior to the mental foramen the mandibular canal is referred to as the incisive canal. The incisive canal houses the mandibular *incisive nerve*, which receives sensory input from the ipsilateral first premolar tooth, canine tooth, lateral incisor, and central incisor teeth. The nerve and its canal have been found to end below the ipsilateral lateral incisor tooth in the majority of patients. Difficulty in detecting the nerve and the canal past this region has been attributed to the nerve dispersing into microscopic tributaries [13]. Injury to the incisive nerve is generally not clinically relevant to patients and is sometimes sacrificed with trigeminal nerve reconstructive surgery. This allows ridge augmentation within the mental interforaminal region to be performed with little risk of post-operative neurosensory disturbances.

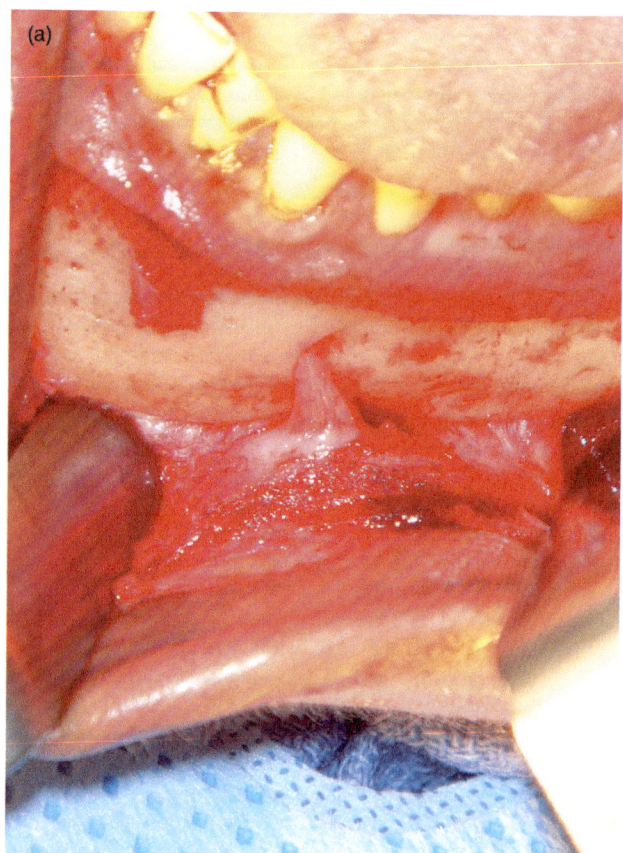 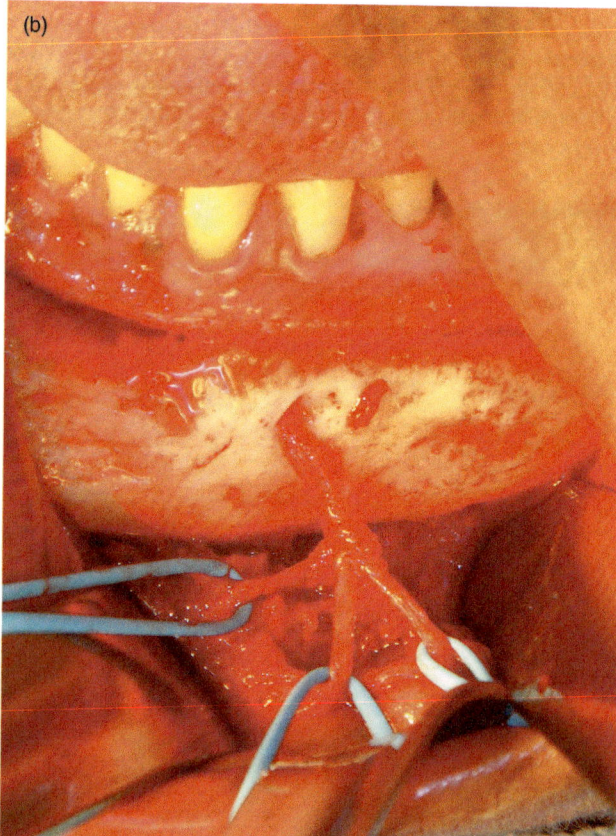

Figure 2.5 (a) Clinical photograph of the mental nerve with the overlying depressor anguli oris muscle. (b) Clinical photograph of the skeletonized mental nerve and its three branches.

Lastly, the *lingual nerve* must be considered when performing procedures within the posterior mandible. As a peripheral branch of the mandibular division (V3) of the trigeminal nerve, the lingual nerve receives sensory input from the anterior two-thirds of the tongue. While the *glossopharyngeal nerve* (ninth cranial nerve) receives the sensory input from the posterior one-third of the tongue, there is a zone of overlap between these two nerves within the posterior aspect of the anterior two-thirds of the tongue. Within the lingual nerve travels the chorda tympani, which is a nerve that arises from the *facial nerve* (seventh cranial nerve) and is responsible for the sensation of taste from the anterior two-thirds of the tongue and also provides secretory motor innervation to the ipsilateral submandibular and sublingual gland via presynaptic parasympathetic fibers terminating within the submandibular ganglion. The lingual nerve is given off the mandibular division just caudal to the foramen ovale; subsequently, it descends medial to the medial surface of the ramus of the mandible towards the anterior two-thirds of the tongue. During its course to the tongue it will cross with the submandibular duct in the area of the mandibular first and second molar teeth. However, in the region of the third molar the lingual nerve could be intimately associated with the lingual cortex of the mandible and the lingual alveolar crest. Miloro and colleagues reported that on magnetic resonance imaging (MRI) the in the third molar region the lingual nerve was in direct contact with the lingual cortical plate in 25% of patients, and above the lingual alveolar crest in 10% of patients [14]. Furthermore, Pogrel and colleagues identified that the mean distance between the lingual nerve and the lingual crest in the transverse plane is 3.45 mm ± 1.48 mm and the mean vertical distance between the lingual nerve and the lingual alveolar crest is 8.32 mm ± 4.05 mm (Figure 2.6) [15]. The variation of the relationship of the lingual nerve with the lingual cortex and lingual alveolar crest was not statistically consistent between the right nerve and the left nerve [15].

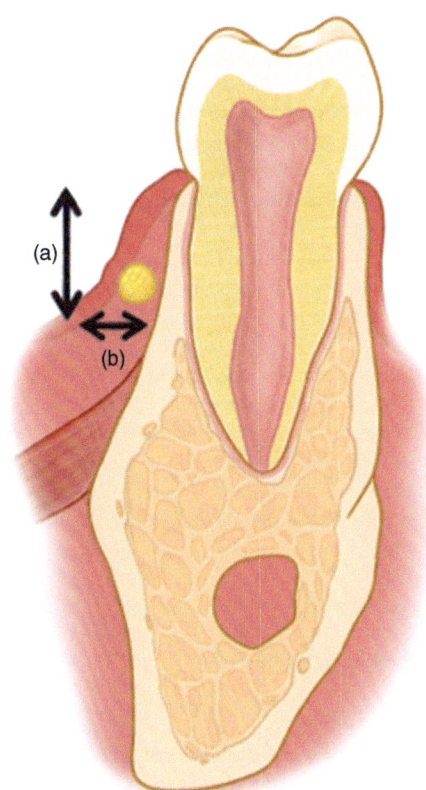

Figure 2.6 Relationship of lingual nerve and lingual crest of mandible: (a) 8.32 mm ± 4.05 mm and (b) 3.45 mm ± 1.48 mm. Adapted from Pogrel MA, et al., *Journal of Oral and Maxillofacial Surgery*, 1995 [15], reproducedwith permission from Elsevier.

Critical vascular structures

When performing reconstructive procedures at the level of the mandibular alveolus in general local neural structures (i.e., inferior alveolar nerve, mental nerve, mandibular incisive nerve, and lingual nerve) are of greatest concern. While injury to these peripheral nerve branches could pose significant morbidity to the patient, injury to local vascular structures could result in a life-threatening hemorrhagic situation secondary to airway embarassment [16]. When it comes to critical vascular structures when performing alveolar ridge augmentation and/or placement of endosseous implant no region of the mandible is as critical as the lingual cortex of the anterior mandible. There have been more than a dozen cases reported in the English literature of a life-threatening hemorrhage secondary to placement of endosseous implants into the mandible [16, 17]. The sublingual artery and the submental artery are the two arterial branches at risk of injury if the lingual cortex of the anterior mandible is perforated. In this section, we will discuss the anatomy of these two arterial branches and also the inferior alveolar artery, which must be considered when operating within the posterior region of the mandible.

The sublingual artery is one of the four branches of the lingual artery. The lingual artery is the third branch of the external carotid artery system. The lingual artery is given off at the level of C3 and ascends toward the greater cornu of the hyoid bone. The lingual artery has a total of four branches, which are the dominant arterial supplies to the tongue and floor of the mouth. The four branches are the suprahyoid branch of the lingual artery, deep lingual artery (ranine artery), sublingual artery, and the dorsal lingual branch of the lingual artery. The sublingual artery runs within the floor of mouth in between the ipsilateral mylohyoid muscle and the genioglossus muscle. At the level of the anterior lingual alveolar mucosa the sublingual artery will anastomose with its contralateral counterpart [16].

When operating within the anterior mandible, "perforating" the lingual cortex not only poses the risk of injury to the sublingual artery but also the submental artery. The submental artery is the largest branch of the facial artery. The facial artery is a branch of the external carotid artery. During its ascent the facial artery travels through the submandibular gland, and once it emerges through the gland the facial artery will give off the submental artery. This artery will travel anteriorly on the mylohyoid muscle, eventually anastomosing with the sublingual artery and with the mylohyoid artery [16]. In hopes of further elucidating the vascular anatomy along the lingual surface of the anterior mandible, Hofschneider and colleagues dissected 34 human cadavers [18]. In this study, the authors concluded that within this anatomic territory the sublingual artery was identified in 71% of cadaver specimens, and a large branch of the submental artery was identified in 41% of cadaver specimens. Of note, the branch of the submental artery had perforated the mylohyoid muscle in order to reach the anterior floor of the mouth. Therefore, when operating in the anterior mandible one must take precautions to not "perforate" through the lingual cortical plate, as within this region lies arterial branches of the lingual artery and submental artery, which have enough flow to result in the development of an expanding sublingual hematoma that could result in immediate airway embarrassment.

As previously discussed in the *neurovascular structures* section, the mandibular canal houses the *inferior alveolar nerve, inferior alveolar artery, inferior alveolar vein*, and *lymphatics*. While life-threatening hemorrhage from the inferior alveolar artery is extremely rare, it is still a known phenomenon [19]. The inferior alveolar artery is a branch of the internal maxillary artery and enters the mandible via the mandibular foramen. As the artery travels within the mandibular canal it gives off numerous branches to the teeth. Although this is an artery with a highly consistent anatomy, Jergenson and colleagues reported a case of an inferior alveolar artery arising from the external carotid artery [20]. In this cadaver specimen, the contralateral inferior alveolar artery originated from the internal maxillary artery. As previously discussed, the anatomic studies by Pogrel and colleagues described a condition within the mandibular canal where there are often multiple inferior alveolar veins that lie superior to the inferior alveolar nerve, while the inferior alveolar artery appears to be solitary and is located medial to the nerve [9].

Anatomy of the maxilla

Foramina and canals

Just as is the case with the mandible, the maxilla contains important foramina that transmit nerves and blood vessels in the vicinity of the dentoalveolar complex. These foramina include the *incisive foramen, greater palatine foramen, lesser palatine foramen*, and *infraorbital foramen*. The incisive foramen, also known as the nasopalatine foramen or anterior palatine foramen, is located in the mid-line of the anterior hard palate, immediately posterior to the maxillary central incisor teeth, and transmits the right and left greater palatine arteries from the oral cavity to branches of the sphenopalatine artery within the nasal cavity, as well as the right and left nasopalatine nerves from the nasal cavity to the oral cavity. The incisive foramen is the terminus of the incisive canal (also known as the nasopalatine canal). The right and left incisive canals end at the incisive foramen, and there is only one incisive foramen. The incisive canal in essence connects the floor of the anterior nasal cavity with the oral cavity. The greater palatine foramen is located along the posterior aspect of each of the palatine bones, always palatal to the maxillary molar dentition.

The greater palatine foramen transmits the ipsilateral greater palatine nerve and the greater palatine artery and vein. Most anatomic studies have determined that the most common location of the greater palatine foramina is medial opposite to the maxillary second or third molar. Westermoreland and colleagues observed that in 57% of dry human skulls the foramen was opposite to the third molar [21]. Furthermore, Sujatha and colleagues observed that in 85.9% of dry human skulls this foramen was opposite to the third molar [22]. The greater palatine canal transmits the descending palatine artery, which becomes the greater palatine artery as it emerges from the foramen. Likewise, the descending palatine nerve emerges from the greater palatine foramen as the greater palatine nerve.

The lesser palatine foramen is always situated posterior to the greater palatine foramen. The lesser palatine foramen transmits the lesser palatine nerve and blood vessels. Lastly, the infraorbital foramen is located along the anterior maxillary wall. It transmits the infraorbital nerve, artery, and vein. As previously mentioned, the infraorbital foramen lies along the same vertical plane as the mental foramen. The infraorbital nerve emerges approximately 10 mm below the infraorbital rim and may be encountered with surgical procedures of this region.

Maxillary sinus

The maxillary sinus is the largest of the four paired paranasal sinuses. Its anatomic dimensions are 33 mm high, 23 mm wide, and 34 mm in anteroposterior length. It is described as a pyramidal-shaped structure, being the lateral nasal wall. The sinus is lined by Schneiderian, which consists of pseudostratified ciliated columnar epithelium. The thickness of the Schneiderian membrane ranges from 0.13 to 0.5 mm. The drainage system of the maxillary sinus is via the medial meatus. Normal anatomic variants found within the maxillary sinus are bony septations. Velasquez-Plata and colleagues reported that these bony septations within the maxillary occur with an incidence of 24% [23]. The neurovascular architecture of the maxillary sinus consists of the anterior superior alveolar, posterior superior alveolar, and infraorbital arteries and nerves providing the blood supply and innervation to the maxillary sinus. A complex arcade exists between the arteries making up the arterial architecture of the maxillary sinus. Kqiku and colleagues described the presence of an intarosseous anastomosis in 100% and an extraosseous anastomosis in 90% of cases [24].

Growth of the alveolar process

Within the maxilla and mandible the alveolar processes function to support teeth and their associated structures. This interplay begins at the time of tooth and jaw development. The alveolar bone will typically mature with elongation and function of teeth. This unique interplay between the alveolar bone and teeth is highlighted in cases where there is congenital tooth agenesis and the alveolar bone does not develop at all [25]. Likewise, in situations of tooth loss, the alveolar bone will undergo resorption, which if not addressed could result in complete loss of the alveolar bone in the edentulous sites. Within the posterior maxilla this could result in pneumatization of the maxillary sinus.

Conclusion

The alveolar ridge of the maxilla and mandible is surrounded by many vascular structures, which, in the case of iatrogenic injury, could result in significant bleeding and in certain situations in life-threatening hemorrhage. Additionally, multiple nerves surround the alveolar ridge of the jaws and their injury could result in lasting and painful neurosensory deficits. Therefore, in-depth knowledge of the local anatomy allows clinicians to appropriately treatment plan their case and be mindful of critical neurovascular structures in order to execute the reconstructive surgical treatment plan effectively and safely.

References

1 Pogrel MA, Kahnberg KE, Andersson L: *Essential of Oral and Maxillofacial Surgery*. Wiley-Blackwell, New Jersey, 2014.

2 Kuribayashi A, Watanabe H, Imaizumi A, et al: Bifid mandibular canals: cone beam computed tomography evaluation. *Dentomaxillofac Radiol* 2010;**39**:235–239.

3 Naitoh M, Hiraiwa Y, Aimiya H, et al: Observation of bifid mandibular canal using cone-beam computerized tomography. *Int J Oral Maxillofac Implants* 2009;**24**:155–159.

4 Kang JH, Lee, KS, Oh MG, et al: The incidence and configuration of the bifid mandibular canal in Koreans by using cone-beam computed tomography. *Imaging Science in Dentistry* 2014;**44**:53–60.

5. von Arx T, Friedli M, Sendi P, et al: Location and dimensions of the mental foramen: a radiographic analysis by using cone-beam computed tomography. *J Endod* 2013;**39**:1522–1528.
6. Udhaya K, Saraladevi KV, Sridhar J: The morphometric analysis of the mental foramen in adult dry human mandibles: a study on the South Indian population. *J Clin Diagn Res* 2013;**7**:1547–1551.
7. Balcioglu HA, Kocaelli H: Accessory mental foramen. *N Am J Med Sci* 2009;**1**:314–315.
8. Pires CA, Bissada NF, Becker JJ, et al: Mandibular incisive canal: cone beam computed tomography. *Clin Implant Dent Relat Res* 2012;**14**:67–73.
9. Pogrel MA, Dorfman D, Fallah H: The anatomic structure of the inferior alveolar neurovascular bundle in the third molar region. *J Oral Maxillofac Surg* 2009;**67**:2452–2454.
10. Greenstein G, Tarnow D: The mental foramen and nerve: clinical and anatomical factors related to dental implant placement: a literature review. *J Periodontol* 2006;**77**:1933–1943.
11. Apostolakis D, Brown JE: The anterior loop of the inferior alveolar nerve: prevalence, measurement of its length and a recommendation for interforaminal implant installation based on cone beam CT imaging. *Clin Oral Implants Res* 2012;**23**:1022–1030.
12. Wismeijer D, van Waas MA, Vermeeren JI, et al: Patients' perception of sensory disturbances of the mental nerve before and after implant surgery: a prospective study of 110 patients. *Br J Oral Maxillofac Surg* 1997;**35**:254–259.
13. Vu DD, Brockhoff HC, Yates DM, et al: Course of the mandibular incisive canal and its impact on harvesting Symphysis bone grafts. *J Oral Maxillofac Surg* 2015;**73**:e1–258.
14. Miloro M, Halkias LE, Slone HW, et al: Assessment of the lingual nerve in the third molar region using magnetic resonance imaging. *J Oral Maxillofac Surg* 1997;**55**:134–137.
15. Pogrel MA, Renaut A, Schmidt B, et al: The relationship of the lingual nerve to the mandibular third molar region: an anatomic study. *J Oral Maxillofac Surg* 1995;**53**:1178–1181.
16. Woo BM, Al-Bustani S, Ueeck BA: Floor of mouth hemorrhage and life-threatening airway obstruction during immediate implant placement in the anterior mandible. *Int J Oral Maxillofac Surg* 2006;**35**:961–964.
17. Givol N, Chaushu G, Helamish-Shani T, et al: Emergency tracheostomy following life-threatening hemorrhage in the floor of mouth during immediate implant placement in the mandibular canine region. *J Periodontol* 2000;**71**:1893–1895.
18. Hofschneider U, Tepper G, Gahleitner A, et al: Assessment of the blood supply to the mental region for reduction of bleeding complications during implant surgery in the intraforaminal region. *Int J Oral Maxillofac Implants* 1999;**14**:379–383.
19. Pham N, Sivapatham T, Hussain MS, et al: Particle embolization of the bilateral superior and inferior alveolar artery for life threatening dental socket hemorrhage. *J Neurointerv Surg* 2012;**4**:e20.
20. Jergenson MA, Norton NS, Pack JM, et al: Unique origin of the inferior alveolar artery. *Clin Anat* 2005;**18**:597–601.
21. Westmoreland EE, Blanton PL: An analysis of the variation in position of the greater palatine foramen in the adult human skull. *Anat Rec* 1982;**204**:383–388.
22. Sujatha N, Manjunath KY, Balasubramanyam V: Variations of the location of the greater palatine foramina in dry human skulls. *Indian J Dent Res* 2005;**16**:99–102.
23. Velasquez-Plata D, Hovey LR, Peach CC, et al: Maxillary sinus septa: a 3-dimensional computerized tomographic scan analysis. *Int J Oral Maxillofac Implants* 2002;**17**:854–860.
24. Kqiku L, Biblekaj R, Weiglein AH, et al: Arterial blood architecture of the maxillary sinus in dentate specimens. *Croat Med J* 2013;**54**:180–184.
25. Dixon AD, Hoyte DA, Ronning O: *Fundamentals of Craniofacial Growth*. CRC Press, LLC, Florida, 1997.

CHAPTER 3

Prosthetic Comprehensive Oral Evaluation in Implant Dentistry: Team Approach

Steven J. LoCascio

Department of Oral and Maxillofacial Surgery, University of Tennessee Graduate School of Medicine, Knoxville, Tennessee, USA
Department of Prosthodontics, Louisiana State University Health Sciences Center, School of Dentistry, New Orleans, Louisiana, USA
Full Time Private Practice, Limited to Prosthodontics and Maxillofacial Prosthetics, Knoxville, Tennessee, USA

History and the team approach

Partial and complete edentulism are clinical conditions that have created functional and esthetic challenges for men and women alike over many centuries. The simple loss of teeth can result in disabilities and handicaps for many patients due to their inability to speak and chew properly. Over the past hundred years, the dental profession has continually searched for products, procedures, and techniques to help liberate these patients from the suffering associated with the loss of their dentition.

Since its accidental discovery in 1952 by Dr. P.I. Brånemark, and subsequent introduction to dentistry in the late 1970s and early 1980s, osseointegration has revolutionized how dentists treat patients. Early work among different investigators consisted of treatment with blade, transosteal, and subperiosteal implants. It was the design of these implants that allowed their placement in atrophic jaws without vertical or horizontal augmentation procedures. Their use nonetheless demonstrated various levels of success, complications, and failures [1–9]. It was, however, the simple concept of intimate bone formation around root form endosteal titanium fixtures, without ingrowth of soft tissue, that has predictably helped thousands of patients get back to living near-normal lives. Without argument, it can be safely stated that the endosseous dental implant is the single greatest advance that dentistry has seen in the last century. Utilization of a few endosseous implants can significantly improve a patient's quality of life by replacing missing teeth, restoring a smile and facilitating the ability to chew and function without experiencing pain and embarrassment [10, 11].

When patients were first treated with dental implants more than three decades ago, the focus of treatment was surgical. Suffice it to say, implants were surgically placed with little consideration as to the prosthetic end result. Implants were positioned in the jaws of patients where the best quantity and quality of bone was located. Treatments were considered successful if the implant(s) integrated and prosthetic teeth were secured to the fixtures. It was not long before the realization surfaced that the mere biologic integration of an endosseous implant was only the beginning of what was truly needed for optimal patient care and ideal treatment outcomes. In addition to a macromechanical and micromechanical interlocking of osseous tissue around titanium, implants need to be functionally and esthetically integrated. This means that the role implants play is merely to retain and/or support a removable (partial or complete) or fixed (single or multiple unit) dental prosthesis. It is the design and fabrication of removable prostheses that assist in achieving functional and esthetic integrated results for the removable patient. In addition, it is the design and fabrication of a fixed prosthesis as well as the surrounding hard and soft tissues that assist in achieving functional and esthetic integrated results for the fixed patient. For these reasons, since the time implants were introduced to dentistry, there has been a gradual paradigm shift in treatment approaches from a primarily surgical focus to a prosthetically driven discipline.

Bone grafting has a very lengthy history in regards to the selection of materials and techniques. As discussed by Horowitz et al., dental surgeons are faced with many choices at the time of extraction, ridge augmentation, or sinus grafting, including the type of material used (particulate, putty, or block), the site or mode of entry (flap or flapless), the source of bone replacement materials (autogenous, allogeneic, alloplast, or xenografts), the use of growth enhancers, the specific characteristic of the graft material, and the barrier type [12]. The material and techniques selected should allow for the best predictability in maintaining, repairing, or regenerating an appropriate volume and characteristic of bone for each clinical case. It should be noted, however, that prior to embarking upon the surgical grafting decision tree, the treatment plan should begin by determining the specific number and the desirable location of the implants needed. It is the final prosthesis (design and prosthetic goal) that should drive every surgeon's decision making. The best implant outcomes are achieved with a *team* approach involving the patient, dental surgeon, restorative doctor, and laboratory technician. It is the patient that communicates what he or she wants, and it is the remaining three team members who are charged with the task of developing a joint plan that provides the patient with not necessarily just what is wanted but more importantly what is needed. It is imperative to understand that patients are great at knowing what they want; however, it is rare that they completely understand what they need. Every clinical team must develop a befitting treatment approach that will result in the most predictable outcome for each individual patient. In the event that patient expectations are unrealistic, it is the responsibility of the dental surgeon and

---

Vertical Alveolar Ridge Augmentation in Implant Dentistry: A Surgical Manual, First Edition. Edited by Len Tolstunov.
© 2016 John Wiley & Sons, Inc. Published 2016 by John Wiley & Sons, Inc.

restorative doctor to educate the patient as to the potential shortcomings and limitations of therapy. All team members, including the patient, must understand which goals are attainable and which goals are not.

Vertical and horizontal osseous tissue preservation or rebuilding should be directed by the specific prosthetic needs. The question that needs to be asked is who gets what? In other words, who will be treated with a crown and bridge type of fixed prosthesis? Who will be treated with a fixed–detachable hybrid prosthesis? Who will require a removable prosthesis? Does the patient need a flange for esthetics? Does the patient have a high or low smile line? What is the current bone volume? It is the answer to these simple questions that will dictate the additive or subtractive osseous surgical needs. When it is determined that the bone volume is insufficient, surgical plans and patient treatments should include predictable bone building procedures. If the surgical needs are not predictable, it may be necessary to choose an alternative prosthetic design. Conversely, some cases may have an excess of bone volume. These are the cases that may require bone trimming and removal. Finally, when considering prosthetic designs for patients, it should be understood that what can be predictably accomplished in the mandible cannot always be extrapolated to the maxillary arch.

Vertical space requirements

This prosthetic chapter belongs to the book volume that deals with vertical ridge augmentation. Surgical-restorative requirements of the presence of vertical bone stock for implant insertion and sufficient vertical prosthetic space for successful restorative element in implant dentistry are very important to understand.

The concept of restorative dimension requirements has been discussed in the literature [13, 14]. Different prostheses have different vertical space requirements. As a general rule, the needed restorative space is consistent for both the maxilla and the mandible since it is the prosthesis that dictates the space requirements. The three different prosthetic designs for consideration here are: (1) crown and bridge fixed prostheses, (2) fixed hybrid dentures, and (3) removable overdenture prostheses with a primary bar and a secondary superstructure. For the latter, the greatest amount of vertical space is needed due to the appropriate "stacking" of a variety of materials required in its construction. It is recommended that approximately 15 to 17 mm of vertical space be available for this primary bar overdenture. The space is measured from the residual soft tissue to the opposing occlusion and should allow for enough space between the primary bar and the soft tissue (approximately 2 mm), the bar itself (3 mm minimum), the nylon attachments and their associated metal housings (approximately 2 mm), the denture base resin superior and inferior to any secondary reinforcement casting (2–4 mm total), the secondary casting itself (1 mm), the prosthetic teeth (approximately 2–4 mm), and the cold cure resin used to connect the attachment housings to the denture base resin (1 mm) (Figure 3.1). Some primary bar overdenture cases may require less vertical restorative space (approximately 11 mm total) if secondary reinforcement castings are not utilized [15].

When determining the ideal vertical level of osseous tissue for overdenture prostheses, one must remember that an average of 2–3 mm of soft tissue covers the bone. Thus, when a patient requires a primary bar overdenture prosthesis, vertical grafting may be needed only in those cases that exhibit severe atrophy. In these extremely atrophic cases, 10–12 mm of resulting vertical height may be needed to place implants of a minimal length. For cases with mild

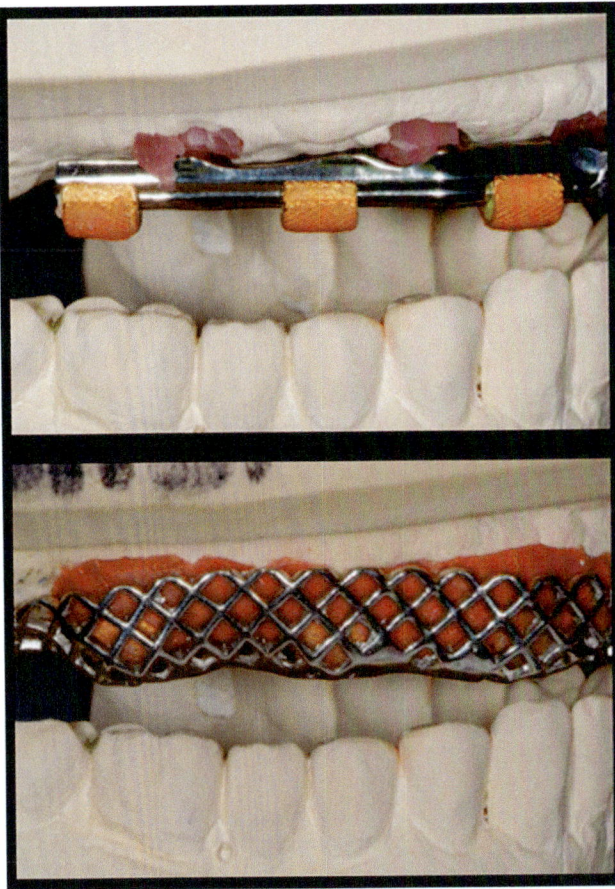

Figure 3.1 Implant-supported primary bar overdentures require the greatest amount of vertical restorative space for the appropriate "stacking" of materials.

to moderate atrophy, subtractive surgical procedures may be needed to allow for the appropriate vertical "stack." This involves removal of enough vertical hard tissue to provide for the 17–20 mm of space needed from the osseous crest to the opposing occlusion. Some rare edentulous maxillary cases may require both subtractive and additive surgical procedures. A great example of this scenario may be seen with patients that have excessive vertical down positioning of the posterior tuberosity with adequate bony height. These clinical cases may require vertical reduction of the posterior bone on the oral side along with sinus augmentation to build vertical height on the sinus side (Figure 3.2a to e).

Fixed crown and bridge prostheses need the least amount of vertical space since we are creating a restoration that closely mimics the height and width proportions of natural teeth. These restorations need approximately 7 to 13 mm of vertical height from the residual soft tissue to the opposing occlusion posteriorly and from the residual soft tissue to the incisal edge anteriorly (Figure 3.3a and b). The average interarch clearance for fixed prostheses has been reported as 10 mm [15]. Finally, hybrid denture prostheses need an intermediate volume of space. It has been recommended that 13 to 15 mm is the ideal vertical height for these prostheses [16]. This vertical volume allows for the appropriate veneering of prosthetic teeth and pink prosthetic material over and/or around traditional CAD/CAM titanium metal frames while maintaining accessibility for hygiene (Figure 3.4).

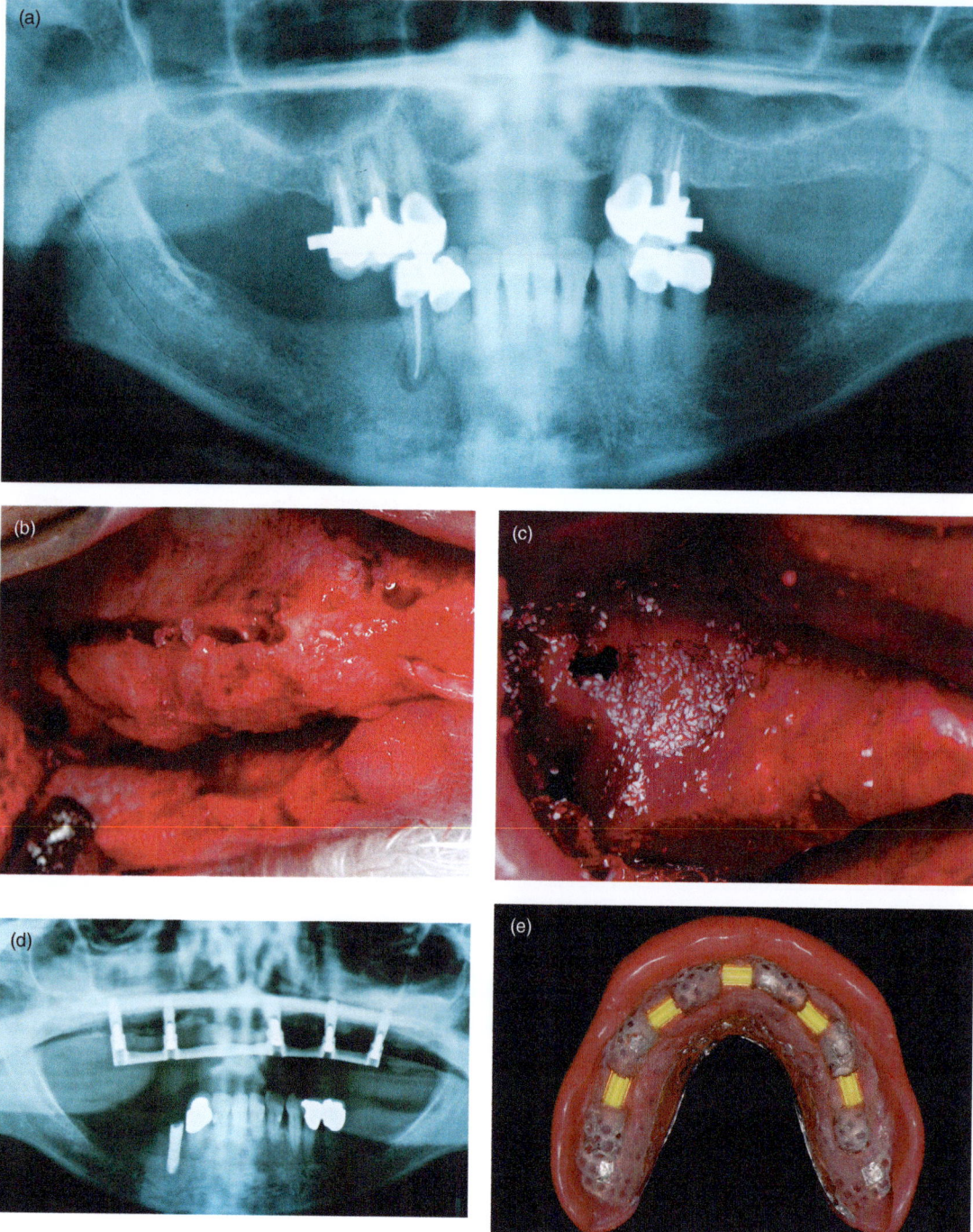

Figure 3.2 (a) The hopeless maxillary dentition will be removed followed by treatment with an implant-supported overdenture. (b) Posterior maxillary hard tissue excess is reduced on the oral side of the sinus to facilitate the vertical space needed for the planned implant-supported primary bar overdenture. (c) Augmentation is performed on the sinus side with an open window technique to build the needed volume for placement of the endosseous implants. (d) Post-treatment radiograph. (e) Intaglio of the definitive maxillary prosthesis. Grafting and implant surgery by Dr. Charles Shanks, Maryville, TN. Reproduced with permission from Dr. Charles Shanks.

The edentulous patient

When an edentulous patient presents for treatment, the first decision to be made is what type of prosthesis is best for that specific patient. At times, clinicians can be too quick in rendering treatment recommendations without adequately examining and diagnosing each individual edentulous case. It is easy to hypothesize that fixed restorations are always better when compared to removable restorations since they seem to represent an end result that closely mimics a natural dentition. In addition, when comparing prostheses to natural dentitions, common sense may dictate that patients should have greater satisfaction with prostheses that have partial palatal coverage. However, is this really true? In other words, do fixed restorations and/or prostheses with an open palate always provide the most satisfactory prosthetic results for the edentulous

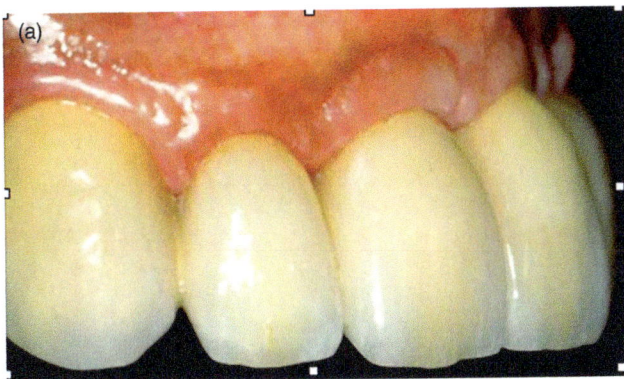
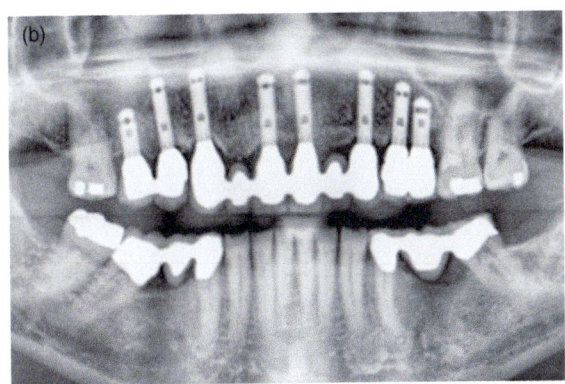

Figure 3.3 (a) Definitive implant-supported ceramometal prosthesis in a minimally atrophic edentulous maxilla. Note the natural emergence of the prosthetic teeth through the soft tissue. Approximately 7–13 mm of vertical restorative space is recommended for these crown and bride designs. (b) Ten-year follow-up radiograph. Implant surgery by Dr. Mike Block, New Orleans, LA.

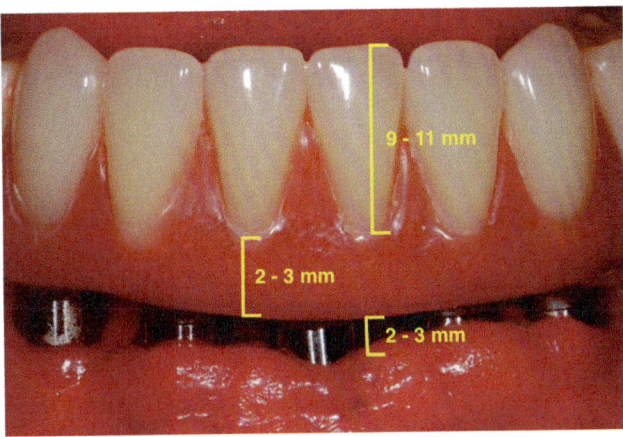

Figure 3.4 Hybrid denture prostheses need approximately 13–15 mm of vertical restorative space. Implant Surgery by Dr. Joshua Campbell, Oak Ride, TN.

patient? Moreover, are implants always needed to provide patient-based satisfactory treatment results?

In 2003, Heydecke et al. reported on patient satisfaction of maxillary fixed and removable prostheses [17]. This was a within-subject comparison study that included the patient's ultimate choice of prostheses. Patients that were previously treated with mandibular implants were accepted into this study. Four to six implants were placed in the maxillary arch. Half of the patients received a fixed prosthesis first and half of the patients received a removable prosthesis first. Following two months of functioning, the prostheses were exchanged. The second prostheses were also worn for two months. In this study, patient ratings of general satisfaction (compared to natural teeth) were measured with visual analog scales (VAS) and information about the patient's physical and psychosocial function and overall health was measured with category scales (CAT). The psychometric measurements consisted of general satisfaction, comfort, ability to speak, stability, esthetics, ease of cleaning, occlusion, and chewing ability. Removable overdentures received higher ratings than fixed prostheses in this study. In fact, more than two times the number of patients chose to keep the removable overdenture. The authors concluded that maxillary overdentures on multiple implants might provide patients with better function and overall satisfaction than fixed prostheses.

Another patient-based outcome investigation by de Albuquerque et al. was reported in 2000 [18]. This was a crossover trial to measure differences in patient satisfaction of maxillary overdentures with and without palatal coverage. Totally edentulous French-speaking patients who had worn complete maxillary and mandibular dentures for at least five years were accepted into this study. Four implants were placed in the maxilla and four implants were placed in the mandible. The four data-gathering periods for this study were as follows: (1) new maxillary and mandibular complete dentures, (2) maxillary complete denture opposing a mandibular fixed restoration, (3) maxillary overdenture prosthesis with full palatal coverage opposing a mandibular fixed restoration, and (4) maxillary overdenture prosthesis with partial palatal coverage opposing a mandibular fixed restoration. Patient comparisons of treatments were evaluated with VAS and CAT scales. The authors of this study reported no significant differences between treatments in the four periods of the trial, suggesting that patients may be equally satisfied with maxillary overdenture prostheses regardless of whether they are fabricated with or without palatal coverage. It must be noted that the ratings given to the maxillary implant prostheses were not significantly higher than for new conventional maxillary prostheses. This suggests that maxillary implant prostheses may not be the ideal treatment of choice for patients with good bony support. In other words, patients that have excellent bony support may be treated satisfactorily with conventional maxillary complete dentures.

The two investigations mentioned above clearly illustrate the point that each edentulous patient must undergo detailed diagnostic procedures including clinical interviews with chief complaint and history gathering, digital imaging (two-dimensional and/or three-dimensional) examinations, and diagnostic wax-ups [15,16,19]. The treating restorative clinician is responsible for correlating the objective clinical findings and condition of the current prosthesis (es) with the patient's chief complaint. If the patient is wearing a poorly designed and/or ill-fitting denture prosthesis, it may be indicated to fabricate a new provisional denture prosthesis to complete the diagnosis. The importance of fabricating new complete provisional denture prostheses, as part of the diagnostic phase of treatment, cannot be understated or overemphasized. In 1971, Dr. Earl Pound introduced the "branching" concept of denture fabrication [20, 21]. The provisional or trial denture described in this technique can be utilized to evaluate smile and profile esthetics,

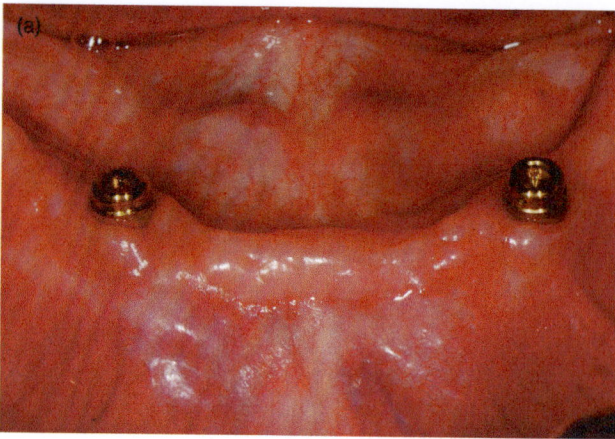
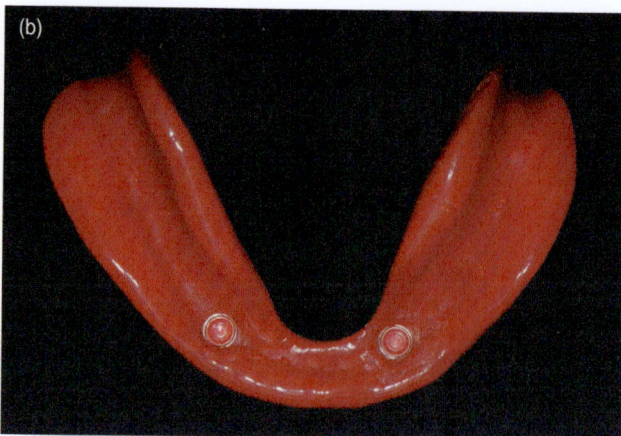

Figure 3.5 (a) The non-splinted stud attachments on two anterior implants assist in denture retention. (b) Intaglio of the definitive implant-retained overdenture prosthesis. Implant surgery by Dr. Robert Cain, Oak Ridge, TN. Reproduced with permission from Dr. Robert Cain.

phonetics, vertical dimension of occlusion, vertical dimension of speech, tolerance of material thickness, support, stability, retention, comfort, and overall patient satisfaction. This initial phase of treatment begins by selecting the correct size and shape of anterior teeth followed by positioning them within the frame of the lips based on esthetics and speech. The location of these teeth are critical because it is the incisal edge position of teeth 8 and 9 that determines the proper restorative occlusal plane for both maxillary and mandibular arches. Initial treatment results with conventional provisional dentures will greatly assist in determining the type and design of the prosthesis(es) required, the number and position of implants, and finally the need for surgical additive tissue procedures (grafting) versus subtractive tissue procedures (bone removal).

Treatment options for the edentulous mandible

The general treatment options for the edentulous mandible include: (1) conventional denture, (2) implant-retained overdenture, (3) implant-supported overdenture, and (4) fixed hybrid denture with or without immediate occlusal loading. If the edentulous patient does not achieve total satisfaction with conventional provisional denture prosthesis, then treatment with dental implants may be indicated.

An implant-retained mandibular overdenture typically utilizes two implants positioned in the anterior mandible for the purpose of assisting with the retention of the denture prosthesis (Figure 3.5a and b). The functional loads of chewing are supported by the tissue posteriorly, which means the implants are utilized only to help retain the prosthesis.

An implant-supported mandibular overdenture usually requires at least four implants positioned between both mental foramen. A primary bar is fabricated with distal extensions for the purpose of supporting the functional loads of chewing posteriorly (Figure 3.6a and b). This prosthetic design is indicated for those patients who suffer from constant pain from denture pressure. Implants for these patients should be positioned with a large anterior/posterior (AP) spread between the mental foramen when posterior atrophy

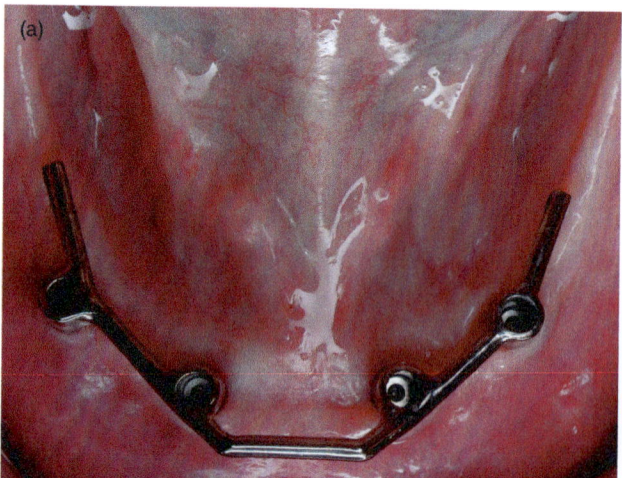
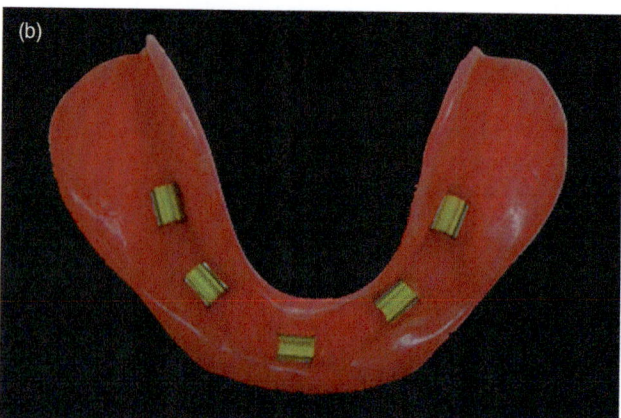

Figure 3.6 (a) A primary bar is secured to four interforaminally positioned implants for an implant-supported mandibular overdenture prosthesis. (b) The intaglio of the definitive mandibular implant-supported overdenture prosthesis. Implant surgery by Dr. Jack Gotcher, Knoxville, TN.

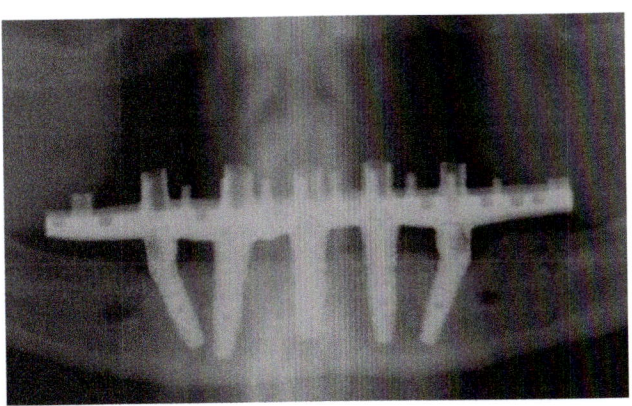

Figure 3.7 Implants can be positioned at angles, up to approximately 30 degrees, to develop a greater AP spread. Implant Surgery by Dr. Joshua Campbell, Oak Ride, TN.

precludes placement of implants posterior to the foramen. Patients that require this form of treatment typically suffer from moderate to severe atrophy.

A hybrid mandibular denture prosthesis requires placement of four or more implants with a maximum AP spread. In atrophic cases, the dental implants are generally placed in the anterior mandible due to the lack of vertical height of bone over the inferior alveolar nerve posteriorly. A fixed, one-piece full-arch prosthesis can be secured to these implants with retaining screws and is indicated for those patients who cannot tolerate the base resin flange material associated with overdenture prostheses or for those patients who have a desire to have a restoration that is not removable. This can be accomplished with a delayed protocol or immediately following extraction of the remaining mandibular teeth. Cases that involve extraction and immediate placement will usually require removal of vertical bone height to satisfy the vertical restorative space requirements previously discussed. Patients with moderate mandibular atrophy will need minimal alveolar reduction only to reduce the "knife edge" occlusal osseous tissue to a level that allows an appropriate ridge width for placement of implants. For this prosthesis, the distal implants can be placed vertically or at angles with angle correction, up to approximately 30 degrees, to increase the AP spread of the implants (Figure 3.7). The anterior mandible must have enough vertical height to place implants with sufficient lengths to support the entire mandibular prosthesis. For patients who have suffered severe mandibular atrophy, vertical bone building may be necessary in order to place implants of minimal lengths. It has been suggested that four or more implants with a minimum length of 10 mm be utilized in the anterior mandible for implant-supported overdentures and implant-supported fixed prostheses [22–24]. Advanced mandibular atrophy can be a significant surgical challenge. When the vertical height of the mandible is insufficient, vertical grafting is needed. A variety of surgical techniques have been utilized including staged reconstruction with autogenous onlay grafts, inferior border grafts, and interpositional grafts [25–30]. In 2002, Marx described a vertical augmentation tenting technique [31]. This procedure involves an extra oral transcutaneous submental approach with placement of four to six dental implants positioned between the mental foramina with a large AP spread. The periosteum and soft tissue is reflected to provide for adequate soft tissue expansion. The dental implants are placed and secured to the inferior border of the mandible extending approximately 9 to 11 mm above the original level of bone. Corticocancellous bone harvested from the iliac crest is positioned around the implants that function as "tent poles" to support the overlying periosteum and soft tissue. Sagging and/or contraction of the soft tissue over unsupported grafts can lead to resorption of the grafted bone. This technique utilizes the dental implants to support the overlaying soft tissue during the healing and consolidation of the graft. Following graft consolidation and implant integration, the implants can be traditionally uncovered and subsequently restored with an implant-supported overdenture or hybrid denture prosthesis. This tenting technique has been described as a safe and effective method to reconstruct the severely resorbed mandible [32] (Figure 3.8a to d).

When implants are positioned in the anterior mandible due to advanced posterior resorption, it is possible to design and fabricate implant-supported prostheses (hybrid dentures and primary bar overdentures) with cantilever extensions for the purpose of establishing posterior occlusion. This cantilever can extend posteriorly approximately 1½ times the AP spread of the implants [33]. This spread is measured from the mid-portion of the mid-line implant(s) and a line drawn through the distal aspect of both distal-most implants. If, for example, the AP spread measures 10 mm, the cantilever can be extended 15 mm ($1.5 \times 10\,mm = 15\,mm$) (Figure 3.9). Shackelton et al. engaged in study that was prompted by several instances of component fracture and other prosthodontic problems with an implant-supported prosthesis [34]. The purpose of this investigation was to determine whether a relationship existed between the survival time of the prostheses and the lengths of their posterior cantilever segments, regardless of the AP spread of the implants. The authors reported that prostheses with cantilever lengths of 15 mm or less survived significantly better than prostheses with cantilever lengths greater than 15 mm. Finally, in 2000, Sadowsky and Caputo reported on load transfer characteristics of different mandibular overdenture designs, with and without edentulous ridge contact [35]. In this study the loaded cantilever bar generated the greatest stress to the distal ipsilateral implant, without intimate contact of the extension base. This study concluded that simulated tissue contact with the extension base of the mandibular overdenture prostheses demonstrated low stress transfer to the ipsilateral terminal abutment when loaded. These studies illustrate that hybrid dentures and implant-supported primary bar overdenture prostheses with appropriate cantilever lengths and distal base extension tissue support for the overdentures are predictable designs when implants are positioned in the anterior mandible. Therefore, when needed, vertical grafting for these two prosthetic designs should be focused in the anterior and not the posterior mandible.

Treatment options for the edentulous maxilla

Treatment of the edentulous maxilla poses unique challenges that include smile esthetics, profile esthetics, phonetics, and hygiene access [36, 37]. It can be easily stated that treatment of the edentulous maxilla may be the greatest challenge in dentistry. Top-down planning is crucial for any dental restoration, but no more critical than when treatment planning the edentulous maxilla. The surgical and restorative team should plan the case from the incisal edge or the occlusal plane instead of from the osseous tissue. Through a diagnostic work-up, the ideal position of the prosthetic teeth is established and the resulting interocclusal restorative

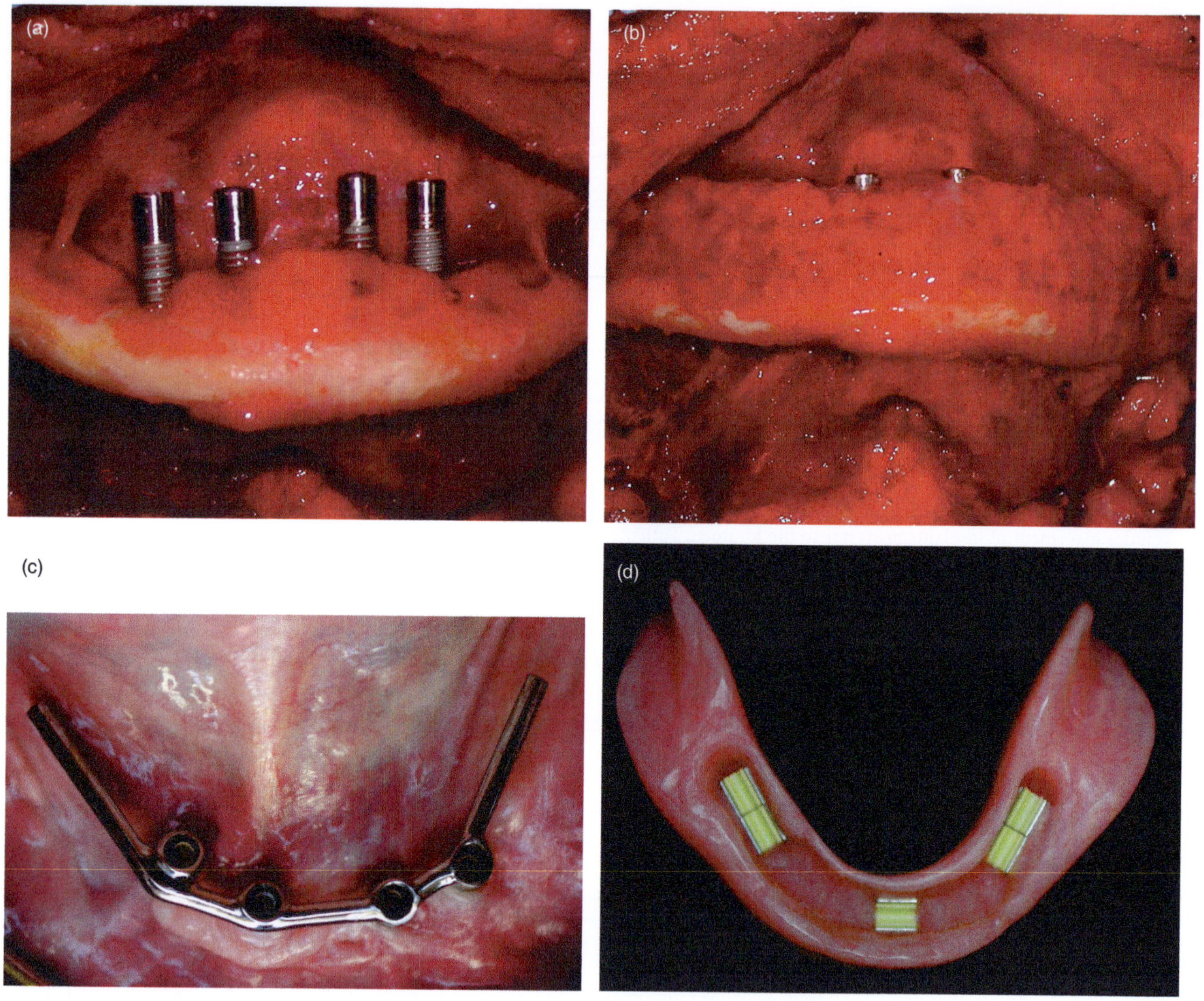

Figure 3.8 (a) Four endosseous implants are positioned interforaminally extending above the existing bone level to support the overlying soft tissue. (b) Autogenous bone is positioned around all implants. (c) Definitive implant-supported primary bar. (d) Intaglio of the definitive implant-supported mandibular overdenture prosthesis. Grafting and implant surgery by Dr. Eric Carlson, Knoxville, TN.

dimension available for that maxillary arch can be determined [19]. Next, the appropriate prosthetic design for the maxilla can be selected. The final maxillary prosthesis will dictate surgical decisions regarding the number and positions of implants and whether the patient needs osseous tissue grafting versus bone removal.

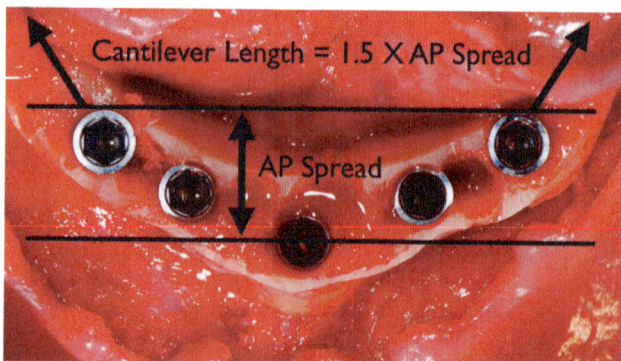

Figure 3.9 Cantilever length formula for implant-supported prostheses.

The general treatment options for the edentulous maxilla are similar to those of the edentulous mandible with a few exceptions. The maxillary options include: (1) a conventional denture, (2) an implant-retained overdenture, (3) an implant-supported overdenture, (4) a fixed hybrid denture with or without immediate occlusal loading, and (5) a fixed crown and bridge splint with or without immediate occlusal loading. As is the case with treatment of the edentulous mandible, if a patient does not achieve reasonable satisfaction with a new provisional maxillary denture prosthesis, implants may be needed to achieve optimal results. It must be understood, however, that some form of denture prosthesis (conventional, implant-retained, or implant-supported [38]) is indicated when the patient requires a flange for lip support and its resulting facial/profile esthetics.

An implant-retained maxillary overdenture utilizes approximately four endosseous implants placed anteriorly, from the mid-line area to the piriform rims bilaterally. These implants assist in the retention of the denture prosthesis [39]. The literature does not contain much evidence regarding the success rates of non-splinted implants in the edentulous maxilla with implant-retained

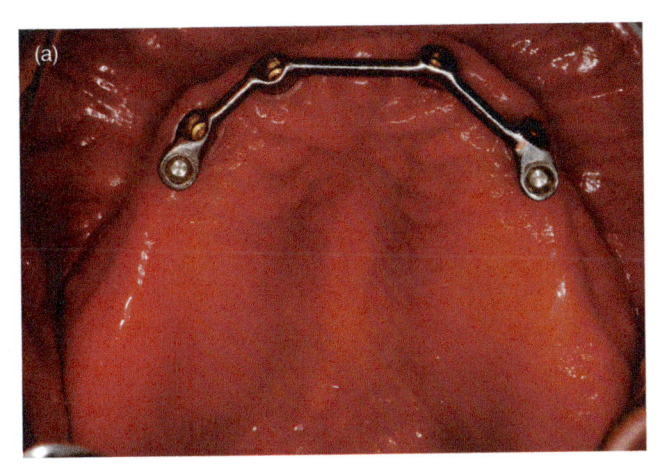

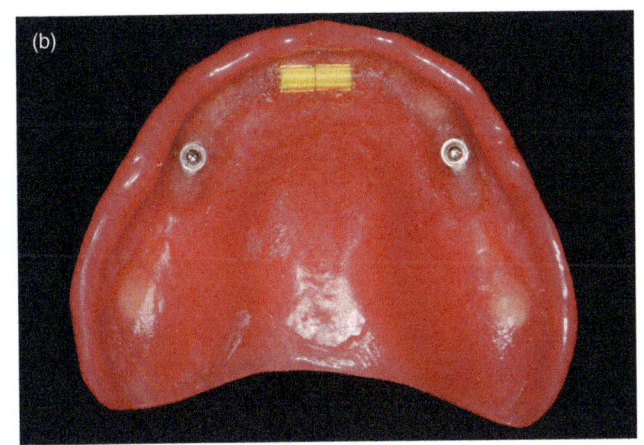

Figure 3.10 (a) A primary bar is secured to four anterior implants for an implant-retained maxillary overdenture prosthesis. (b) The intaglio of the definitive maxillary implant-retained overdenture prosthesis. Implant surgery by Dr. Jack Gotcher, Knoxville, TN.

overdenture prostheses. It can be hypothesized that if the edentulous maxilla has an extremely favorable bone type with excellent volume, and the implants can be positioned with relative parallelism, then an overdenture supported by non-splinted implants may be a viable option [40]. However, there may be very few maxillary arches requiring implants that fit in this classification, suggesting that most implant-retained maxillary prostheses are fabricated with splinted primary bars on four implants [39] (Figure 3.10a and b). With these cases, the majority of the retention is supplied by the proper design and construction of the prosthesis. Specifically, the proper height and thickness of the flanges, the accuracy of the intaglio, the design and finish of the polished surfaces, and the occlusion all play critical roles in retention of implant-retained maxillary overdentures. To that point, full palatal coverage is mandatory for ideal retention of maxillary implant-retained overdentures. When a primary bar is utilized with this type of prosthesis, the 15–17 mm of vertical restorative space is required where the bar is positioned as previously discussed.

If a patient cannot tolerate the palatal base material, a horseshoe design is desired, or the need for total implant support exists for functional loading (mastication and/or parafunction), then an implant-supported overdenture prosthesis may be indicated. If the patient has no objections to this type of removable appliance, then approximately six implants should be positioned in the edentulous maxilla. There are two design concepts to consider here: (1) one continuous primary bar or (2) two separate posterior bars. As with any primary bar overdenture, the vertical restorative space required is 15–17 mm whether the implants are located anteriorly and/or posteriorly.

In 2008, a retrospective study by Krennmair et al. was published in the literature [41]. The purpose of this investigation was to evaluate implant-supported maxillary overdentures using either an anterior or a posterior maxillary implant placement. No statistical differences in implant survival rates were seen between either the anterior (98.4%) and posterior (97.4%) group or the non-grafted (98.0%) and grafted (97.5%) implants. The authors concluded that high survival rates can be achieved for implants placed in the anterior or posterior (grafted or non-grafted) maxilla to support overdenture prostheses. Although the overall post-treatment maintenance of the integrated retentive prosthetic elements was relatively low for both groups, the need for clip activation or renewal was two times more common in the posterior group than in the anterior group. Since retention has been shown to be one of two ideal predictors of satisfaction for patients with overdenture prostheses [42], it may be optimal to place maxillary implants with a large AP spread with a continuous cross-arch primary bar to help maintain attachment retentive values over an extended period of time (Figure 3.11a and b). This means that adequate vertical bone volumes may be needed for implant placement in both the anterior and posterior areas of the maxilla to produce optimal long-term prosthetic results for maxillary overdentures supported by implants.

Fixed restorative options for the edentulous maxilla include hybrid denture prostheses and crown and bridge designs. These restorative designs must satisfy both smile and profile esthetics, support optimal phonetics, and allow for hygiene access. Accomplishing these three requirements may be most difficult with maxillary hybrid dentures [36, 37]. If a fixed restoration requires pink prosthetic material for smile or profile esthetics, it is imperative that the transition of the prosthetic pink material to the natural gingival soft tissue is either indistinguishable to the human eye or hidden beneath the lip with the highest smile. Improved and more suitable products are constantly being introduced to dentistry, but, due to the difficulties and challenges with color and shading of pink prosthetic material, hiding the "pink to pink" margin under the lip may provide for the most predictable esthetic results. If a patient has a high smile line and/or needs material extended facial and superior to the residual maxillary edentulous ridge for any reason, the intaglio surface of the prosthesis will have a concave design. This concavity will prevent the required access for appropriate hygiene. The result will be plaque buildup and debris accumulation (Figure 3.12a, b, and c). If a hybrid denture cannot be fabricated with a convex or flat intaglio surface, then the treating clinicians should consider an alternative prosthetic design such as a crown and bridge fixed prosthesis or an implant-supported overdenture (Figure 3.12d, e, and f). If a patient has minimal atrophy with excellent bone volume, the ideal fixed option may be a crown and bridge design since the optimal vertical space required for this restoration is minimal (approximately 7 to 13 mm). It should be noted that if immediate occlusal loading is planned for the edentulous maxilla, the decision for vertical bone reduction should be based on the planned definitive prosthesis and not the immediate load provisional prosthesis. In other words, a definitive crown and bridge prosthesis will require no

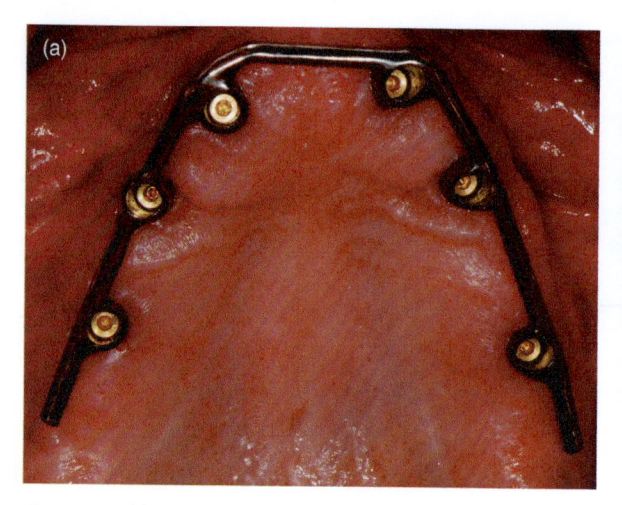

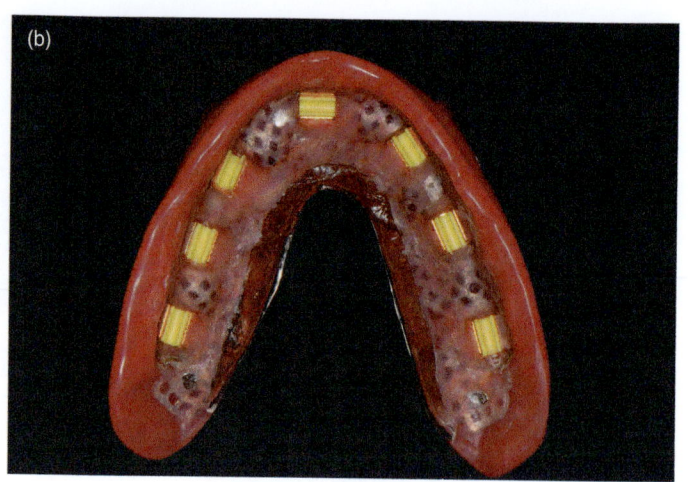

Figure 3.11 (a) A primary bar is secured to six implants with a large AP spread for an implant-supported maxillary overdenture prosthesis. (b) The intaglio of the definitive maxillary implant-supported overdenture prosthesis. Note the horseshoe design. Implant Surgery by Dr. Danny Adkins, Knoxville, TN.

vertical reduction while a hybrid denture will require enough vertical reduction to allow for the 13–15 mm of restorative space previously discussed (Figure 3.13a to e).

The partially edentulous patient

Treatment of the partially edentulous patient follows the same esthetic, phonetic, and hygiene access principles and vertical space requirements as was previously described for the completely edentulous patient. The general treatment options for the partially edentulous maxilla and mandible include: (1) a fixed crown and bridge prosthesis, (2) a partial hybrid denture prosthesis, and (3) an implant and tooth-supported "overpartial." When the patient has both a high smile line and severe vertical ridge deficiency, an overpartial denture design may be the optimal choice of prosthesis for esthetic and hygiene reasons (Figure 3.14a to d). Partial hybrid denture prostheses may be considered as treatment options for those partially edentulous clinical situations with average to severe atrophy, when the patient has limited smile lines, where full flanges are not needed, and the prosthetic pink to natural pink interface can be hidden under the patient's lip with the most animated smile. One additional factor to consider when treating partially edentulous maxillary patients with partial hybrids is the need to esthetically manage the transition of the prosthetic teeth to the natural teeth (prosthetic white to natural white) and possibly the prosthetic pink to the natural teeth (prosthetic pink to natural white) (Figure 3.15a to e). If the transition of any prosthetic material (white or pink) to natural tissue (gingiva or teeth) cannot be successfully managed esthetically or effectively hidden under the lip in a high smile line situation, then the treating clinician should avoid choosing a partial hybrid denture design. To that point, partial hybrid dentures may be a better choice for treatment in the posterior maxilla when compared to the anterior maxilla. Some partially edentulous residual ridges exhibit moderate to severe atrophy, but still have enough vertical and horizontal bone volume to place implants of adequate lengths for overpartial or hybrid designs. These ridges do not need to be grafted. However, when vertical bone volume is insufficient to support implants of minimal lengths for an overpartial or partial hybrid denture, vertical augmentation should be performed only to build enough bone to support the implants in question. All soft tissue esthetics will be provided by the proper design of the pink colored prosthetic material used in these two prosthetic options. If a partially edentulous patient has minimal atrophy with excellent bone volume, a traditional crown and bridge prosthetic design can be considered, as discussed for the completely edentulous patient. The vertical space required for this restorative option is the same 7 to 13 mm previously described.

Biologic width and soft tissue esthetics

Prior to considering grafting for partially edentulous crown and bridge cases, it is important to be mindful of the basic principles that propel anterior esthetics. Earlier in this chapter it was stated that dental implants need to be both functionally and esthetically integrated. To understand what drives esthetics around dental implants, it is necessary to understand what drives esthetics around natural teeth. Esthetics is driven by both the teeth and surrounding gingival tissue. A pleasing and esthetic smile with a natural or restored dentition displays teeth that have acceptable proportions, color and shade, surface texture, contours, morphology, and, most importantly, symmetry across the mid-line [43]. In addition, the gingival soft tissues must appear healthy, provide for appropriate tooth length, and display reasonable symmetry [43]. When a patient has short clinical crowns, poor length to width ratios, uneven gingival levels, or suffers from altered passive eruption, elective esthetic crown lengthening surgery may be indicated to lengthen the clinical crowns of the teeth to enhance smile esthetics. This may be done with or without restorative treatments. It has been established in the literature that a certain biologic width exists around natural teeth [44, 45]. Thus, when crown lengthening is indicated the crestal position of bone may need to be altered to achieve optimal soft tissue results. Biologic width is reestablished following surgical crown lengthening surgery where the supracrestal connective tissue regenerates above the crestal osseous tissue and the connective tissue covers itself with junctional epithelium [46].

The principles that drive esthetics around dental implants are very similar to those of natural teeth. It is the ideal proportions, color and shade, surface texture, contours and morphology of the restoration(s), as well as symmetry across the mid-line along with the symmetry and healthy appearance of the gingival tissues, that

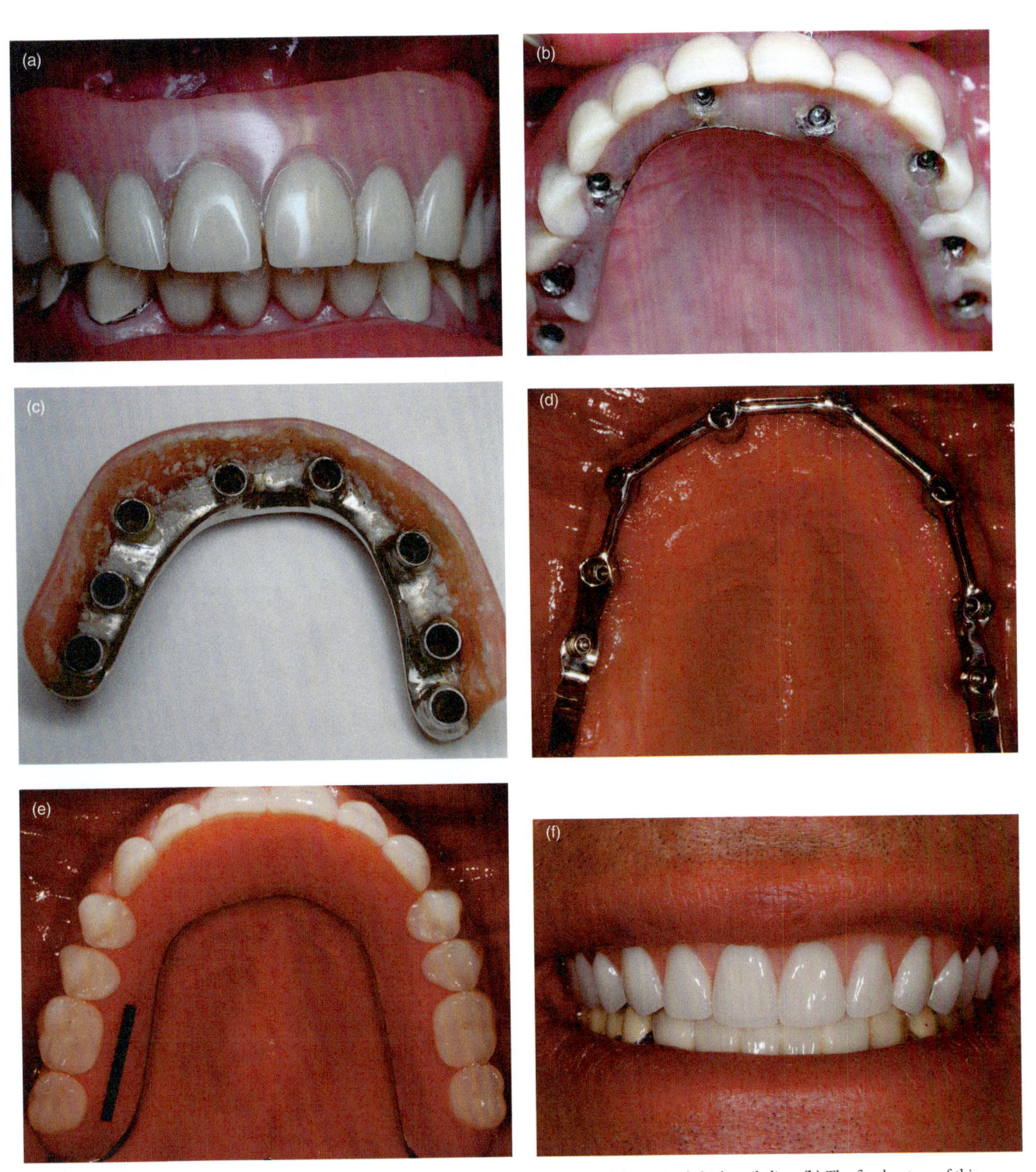

Figure 3.12 (a) A flange was used with this maxillary hybrid denture prosthesis because of the patient's high smile line. (b) The fixed nature of this specific prosthesis makes hygiene access impossible. (c) Note the plaque and debris buildup on the intaglio of the prosthesis. (d) Corrective prosthetics included fabrication of a primary bar to support an overdenture superstructure. (e) Occlusal view of the new maxillary implant-supported locking bar prosthesis. (f) Post-treatment smile. Implant surgery by Dr. Carroll Shanks, Maryville, TN.

provide for optimal esthetic results with dental implants. There are reports that demonstrate the establishment of biologic width around implants [47–51]. When an inflammatory cell infiltrate is established around an implant the connective tissue migrates apically to shield the bone, the bone resorbs, and the connective tissue is covered with junctional epithelium. Data exist suggesting that biologic width not only exists around implants but that it is a physiologically formed and stable dimension as is found around natural teeth [50, 51]. Suffice it to say, biologic width is the driver for crestal bone remodeling and the support scaffolding for the overlying gingival soft tissue. Where biologic width is supra crestal around natural teeth, biologic width is subcrestal around dental

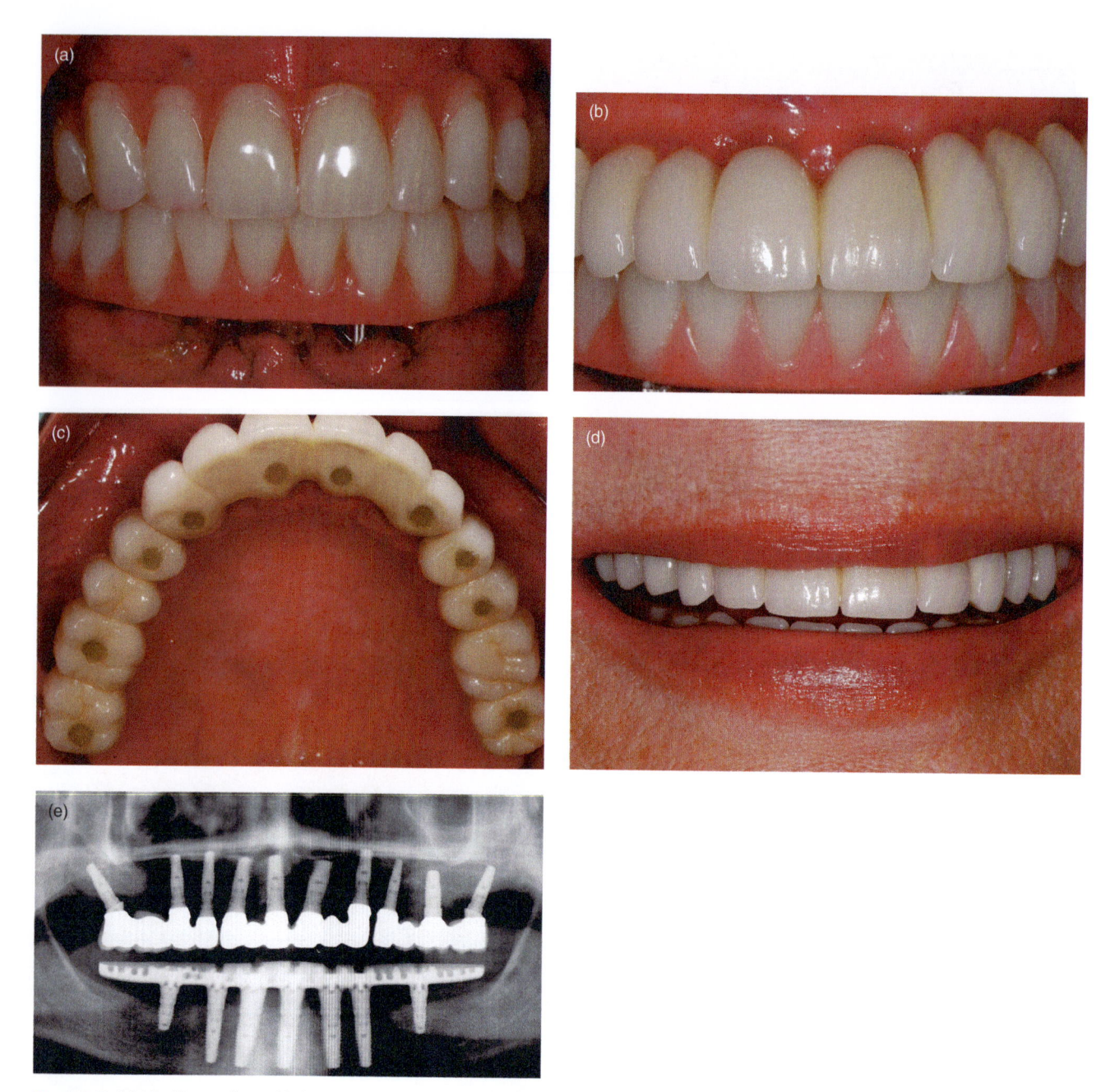

Figure 3.13 (a) Maxillary and mandibular immediate load prostheses. (b) Definitive maxillary ceramometal screw-retained fixed prosthesis and definitive mandibular resin to titanium CAD/CAM hybrid denture prosthesis. (c) Occlusal view of the maxillary screw retained implant-supported ceramometal splints. (d) Post-treatment smile. (e) Post-treatment radiograph. Grafting and implant surgery by Dr. Joshua Campbell, Oak Ridge, TN.

implants. This explains the observation of circumferential bone loss around dental implants to the first one or two threads following the introduction of a microgap to the oral environment. Finally, it is the surrounding bone and the contours of the existing restoration that drive the level and contour of the gingival tissue around dental implants [52]. To that point, when a crown and bride restoration is planned for a partially edentulous situation, the treating surgeon must take care to preserve as much bone as possible. Some clinical situations may require vertical and horizontal augmentation procedures to provide for the appropriate bone volume to support the implant(s) as well as the required gingival tissue.

The single implant supported crown

The restoration of either a single natural tooth or a single implant in the anterior maxilla poses unique esthetic challenges. To achieve a satisfactory result the single restoration must be indistinguishable from the natural teeth in a patient's smile. In addition, the soft tissues around the restored tooth or implant must appear healthy and closely match the soft tissue around the contralateral tooth. The symmetrical appearance of the soft tissue becomes more critical as the edentulous site gets closer to the mid-line.

What drives the vertical height of soft tissue around dental implants? As was stated previously, it has been recognized that

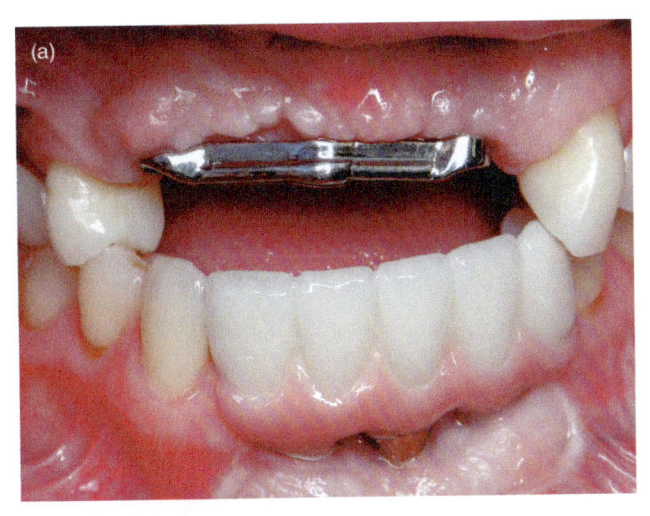

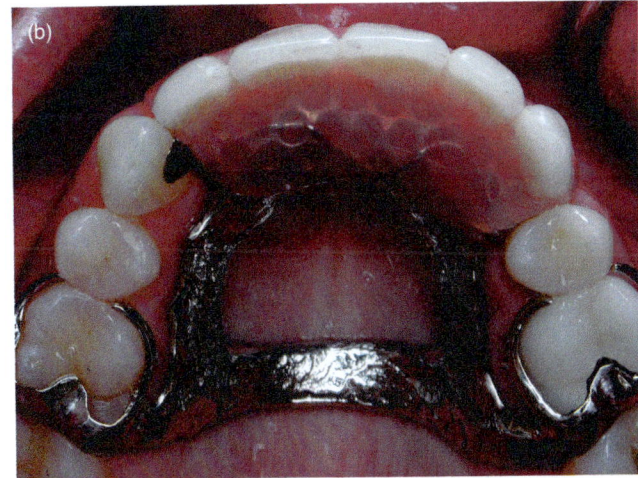

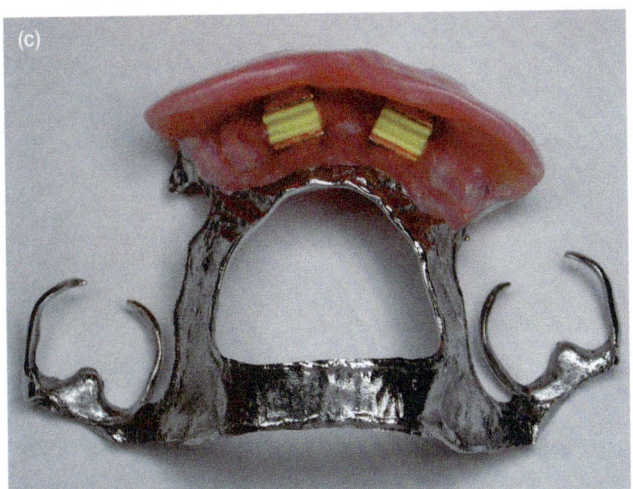

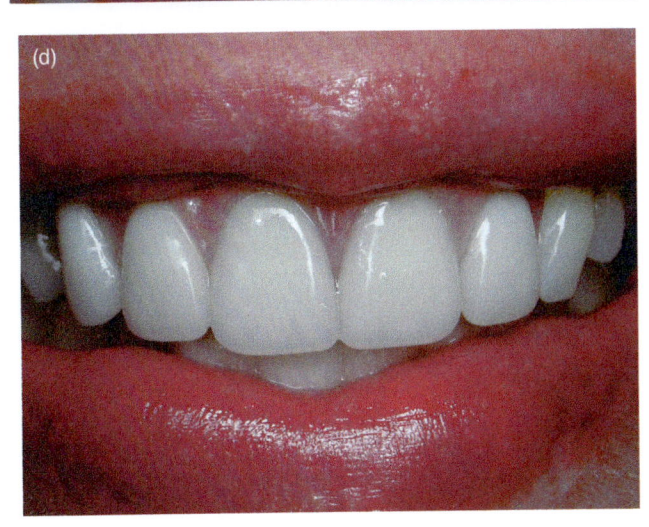

Figure 3.14 (a) As a result of trauma, this patient suffered loss of teeth and the supporting osseous tissue. Note the anterior primary bar to support an overpartial denture prosthesis. (b) Occlusal view of the definitive maxillary overpartial denture prosthesis. (c) The intaglio of the maxillary overpartial denture prosthesis. (d) Post-treatment smile. Implant surgery by Dr. Kevin Gross, Maryville, TN.

biologic width is established around a dental implant when a microgap is introduced to the oral environment [47–49]. The result is loss of bone circumferentially around the implant, 1.5 to 2 mm apical to the implant abutment junction [53]. If the implant is positioned at least 1.5 mm away from the adjacent natural tooth, the bone loss around the implant does not affect the interproximal bone on the natural tooth. Maintenance of the bone around the natural tooth is critical since it is this bone that supports the soft tissue between the implant and the natural tooth. Studies measuring the vertical height of the interdental papilla in patients have been reported in the literature. In a natural tooth investigation, Tarnow et al. reported that if the distance from the inferior portion of the contact point between two teeth to the crestal bone is 5 mm or less, a papilla could be expected to fill in 98% of the time or greater [54]. If that distance increases by just 1 mm to a distance of 6 mm, a papilla would be expected to fill in only 56% of the time or greater [54]. Choquet described the tissue height between implant restorations and natural teeth [55]. In this study it was stated that, if the distance from the inferior portion of the contact point between an implant restoration and an adjacent natural tooth was 5 mm or less, a papilla would fill in 88% of the time or greater. If that distance increases by just 1 mm to a distance of 6 mm, a papilla would fill in only 50% of the time or greater. Thus, when planning implant restorations with or without grafting, it is important to understand that it is the vertical height of bone on the adjacent teeth that drives the vertical height of interproximal soft tissue. In addition, a restorative crown design with long contacts may be needed to enhance esthetic results when there is a vertical deficiency of interproximal bone. When the facial or interproximal crestal bone height on a natural tooth is deficient, elective orthodontic extrusion can be considered to bring the bone height more coronal to enhance the resulting soft tissue height [56].

The osseous tissue around an endosseous implant also supports the vertical height of soft tissue located on the facial surface of the implant. Grunder et al. have recommended that at least 2 mm of bone be present on the facial of a dental implant to support and stabilize the gingival tissue buccal to that implant [57]. This suggests that most edentulous sites may need horizontal osseous grafts to maximize and maintain the vertical volume of facial gingival tissue. If there is less than 2 mm of bone on the facial surface of an implant, bone loss from biologic width establishment may result in loss of vertical height of facial soft tissue. These situations may have poor esthetic results and need surgical and restorative corrective procedures. The clinical case depicted in Figure 3.16a to d demonstrates

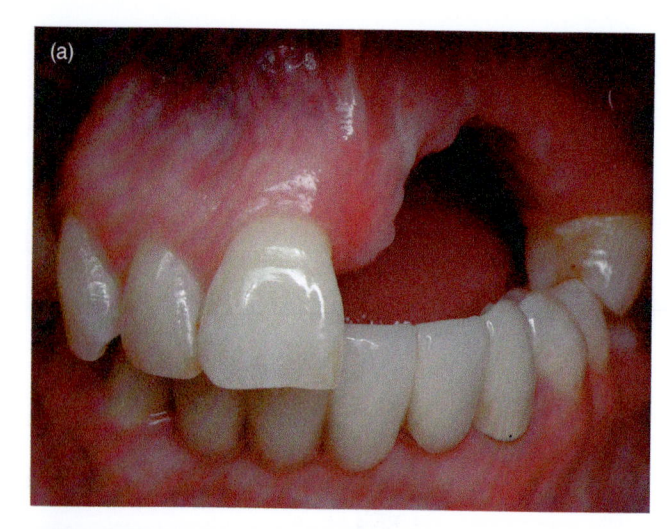

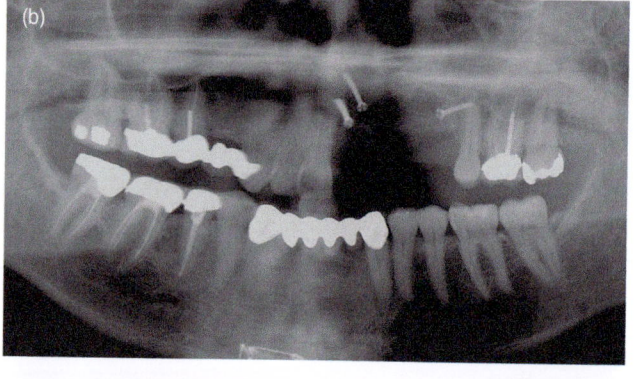

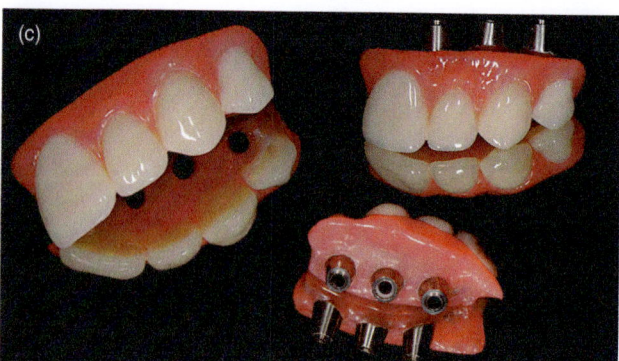

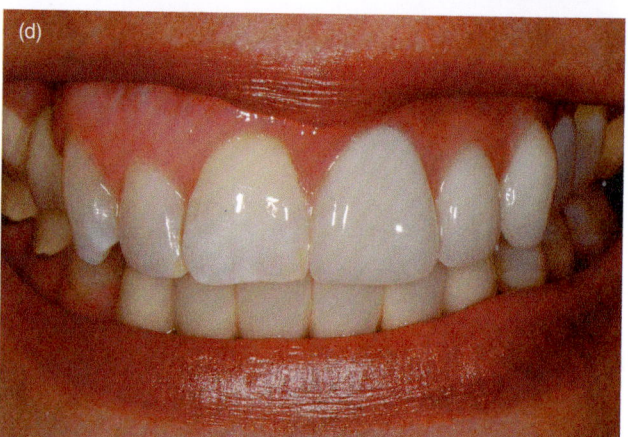

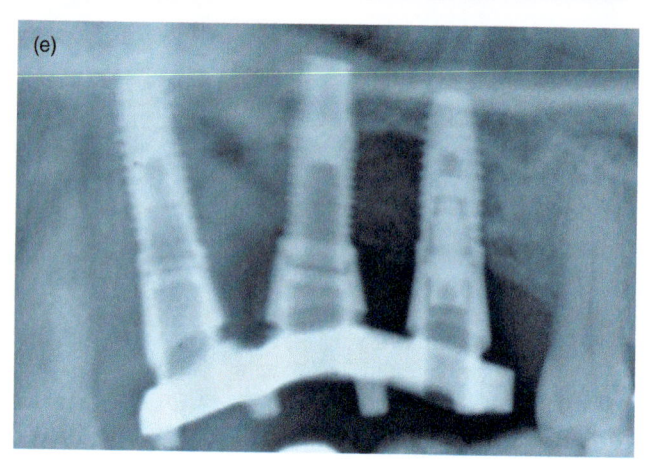

Figure 3.15 (a) As a result of trauma this patient suffered loss of teeth and the supporting osseous tissue. (b) A block graft was performed to build the vertical volume of bone needed to support endosseous implants of acceptable lengths. (c) Three views of the definitive "wrap around" CAD/CAM hybrid denture prosthesis design. (d) Post-treatment smile. The "pink to pink," "white to white," and "pink to white" interfaces were effectively managed in this case. (e) Post-treatment radiograph. Grafting and implant surgery by Dr. David Johnson, Oak Ridge, TN.

an unacceptable esthetic result that is directly related to the vertical soft tissue deficiency on the facial surface of the implant. In this case, the facially positioned implant created a three-walled bony defect (mesial, distal, and lingual) and surgical correction of the vertical height of facial tissue is easily managed with horizontal grafting. The vertical height of facial tissue regenerated and illustrated in the final result can be considered a "vertical illusion," resulting from the horizontal rebuilding procedure and proper positioning of a new implant. It is important to understand that the limiting factor for predicting the resulting vertical height of the soft tissue is the bone on the adjacent natural teeth. Finally, subsequent soft tissue grafting may be needed in cases to improve the quality of keratinized tissue at the site.

Multiple implant supported crowns

The vertical volume of bone between two adjacent implants is vital in maintaining the soft tissue height between the implants. When biologic width is established around two adjacent implants, an interimplant distance of 3 mm or greater results in lateral bone loss that does not overlap [58]. The result is minimal crestal bone loss between the two implants. Even when implants are positioned

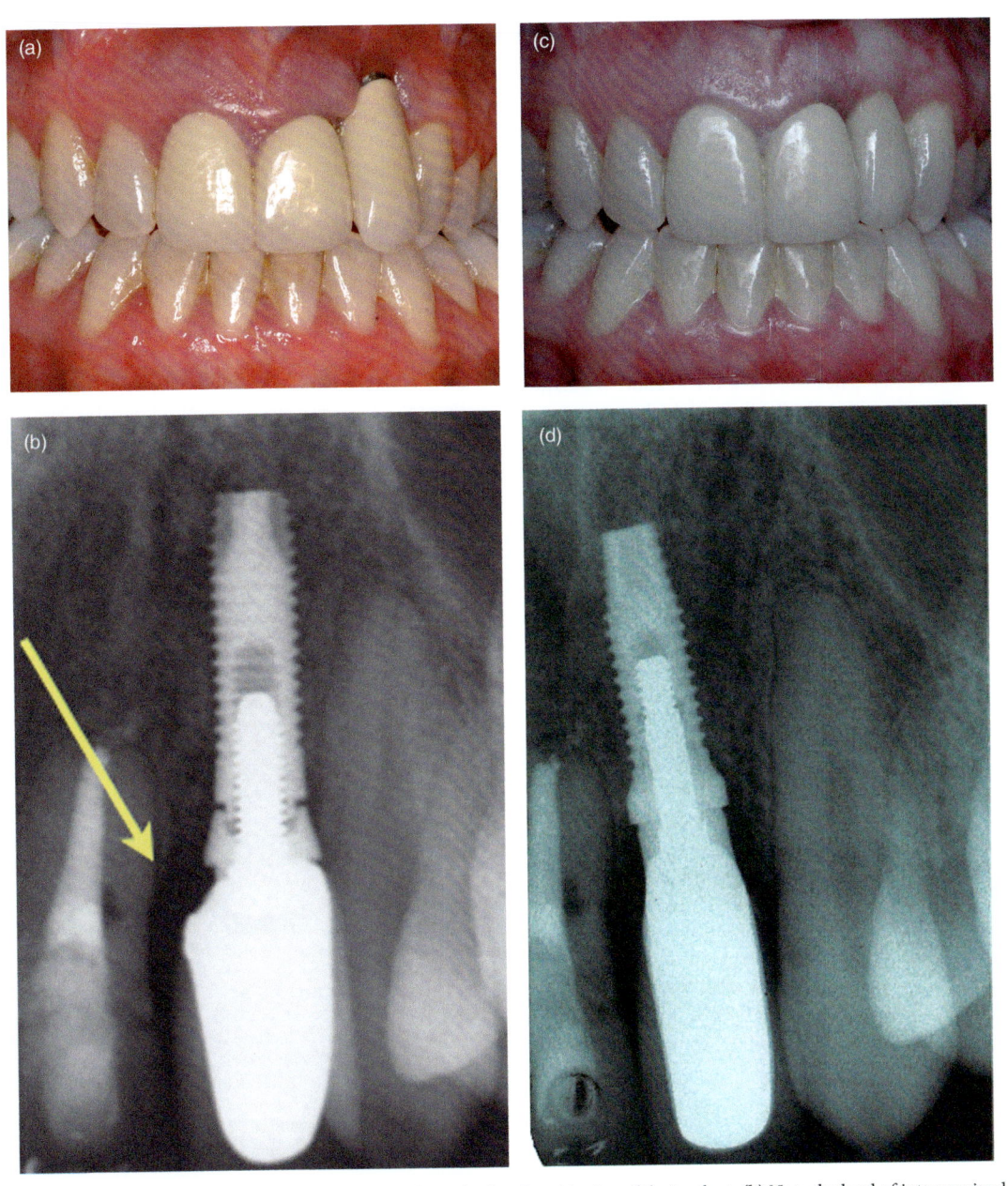

Figure 3.16 (a) Poor esthetics resulting from vertical tissue loss from the facial positioning of the implant. (b) Note the level of interproximal bone on the adjacent central incisor. (c) Post-corrective surgical and restorative treatment result. (d) Post-treatment radiograph. Corrective surgery by Dr. James Madigan, Knoxville, TN.

side by side with the required distance of 3 mm or greater between them, we can expect only 2 mm, 3 mm, or 4 mm, with an average of 3.4 mm, of soft tissue covering this crestal bone [59]. This means that there may be a 1 to 3 mm discrepancy in soft tissue height when comparing the soft tissue between an implant and a natural tooth and the tissue between two perfectly positioned adjacent implants. The greater the discrepancy of soft tissue heights across the midline, the less pleasing the smile will be. In these situations, decisions need to be made as to whether grafting is needed or indicated, or whether other interdisciplinary treatment options need to be explored.

When planning implant restorations for multiple missing teeth, consideration must be given to the vertical volume of hard and resulting soft tissue. Clinical cases that have both high smile lines and partially edentulous sites of moderate to severe atrophy may be difficult to manage esthetically with surgical grafting. Vertical grafting techniques for the partially edentulous patient include onlay block grafts [60–63], particulate grafts [64–67], screw tent pole particulate grafts [68], distraction osteogenesis [69], grafting with titanium mesh trays [70, 71], or a combination of techniques [71–73]. The question to be asked is not only how much bone is needed for the successful long-term integration of the implants but will the resulting volume of tissue satisfy the vertical height needed for an esthetic result? During the diagnostic phase of treatment, the restorative doctor must first determine the appropriate volume of tissue that is needed to provide acceptable tooth proportions (length/width ratios). Next, the clinical team must ascertain the short- and long-term predictability of any vertical grafting procedure. If the volume of tissue building is deemed impossible or unpredictable, then a restorative design with pink prosthetic material may be the optimal choice for the patient. It must be noted that a pre-treatment diagnostic work-up with a detailed wax-up will greatly assist in determining the ideal restorative design. As previously discussed, hiding the pink prosthetic margin is critical in achieving acceptable esthetic results. When artificial gingival material is needed, vertical reduction of anterior bone may be indicated to hide the "pink to pink" interface.

Conclusion

The ordinary loss of a single tooth or multiple teeth can have negative effects on a patient's ability to chew and smile. Endosseous dental implants have played an instrumental role in helping replace missing teeth, thus restoring masticatory function as well as a patient's smile. An adequate volume of bone is needed to place implants of specific widths and lengths. Some clinical cases will require staged treatment approaches that include *vertical and/or horizontal osseous augmentation* procedures in order to build the needed volume of bone prior to any implant surgery. Conversely, some cases may require *vertical reduction* of osseous tissue prior to the placement of dental implants. All implant cases need to be surgically planned with the end result in mind. Simply put, all implant cases must be restoratively driven. It is the attentive and detailed pre-treatment restorative planning that will assist in determining what prosthetic option and design is ideal for each individual case. The prosthetic plan will dictate the number of implants required, the position of the implants, and the need for hard tissue building or reduction. Favorable treatment results can only be achieved utilizing a team approach that embraces a collaborative surgical and restorative effort. Communication amongst all team members is crucial in helping patients achieve healthy and attractive smiles.

Acknowledgments

Dr. Steven LoCascio wishes to acknowledge his wife, Christl, and two sons, Steven, Jr. and Brandon, for their unrelenting support. The author is also grateful for the collaborative efforts of all the surgeons who participated in the care of patients presented in this chapter.

References

1 Linkow LI: The blade vent – a new dimension in endosseous implantology. *Dent Concepts* 1968 Spring; 11(2):3–12.
2 Linkow LI, Donath K, Lemons JE: Retrieval analyses of a blade implant after 231 months of clinical function. *Implant Dent* 1992 Spring;1(1):37–43.
3 Linkow LI, Wagner JR: Management of implant-related problems and infections. *J Oral Implantol* 1993;19(4):321–335.
4 Dal Carlo L, Pasqualini ME, Carinci F, Corradini M, Vannini F, Nardone M, Linkow LI: A brief history and guidelines of blade implant technique: a retrospective study on 522 implants. *Annals of Oral and Maxillofacial Surgery* 2013 Feb; 1(1):3.
5 Bodine RL, Yanase RT, Bodine A: Forty years of experience with subperiosteal implant dentures in 41 edentulous patients. *J Prosthet Dent* 1996 Jan;75(1):33–44.
6 Schou S, Pallesen L, Hjørting-Hansen E, Pedersen CS, Fibaek B: A 41-year history of a mandibular subperiosteal implant. *Clin Oral Implants Res* 2000 Apr;11(2):171–178.
7 Bosker H, van Dijk L: The transmandibular implant: a 12-year follow-up study. *J Oral Maxillofac Surg* 1989 May;47(5):442–450.
8 Verhoeven JW, Cune MS, Van Kampen FM, Koole R: The use of the transmandibular implant system in extreme atrophy of the mandible; a retrospective study of the results in two different hospital situations. *J Oral Rehabil* 2001 Jun;28(6):497–506.
9 Bosker H, Jordan RD, Sindet-Pedersen S, Koole R: The transmandibular implant: a 13-year survey of its use. *J Oral Maxillofac Surg* 1991 May;49(5):482–492.
10 Awad MA, Locker D, Korner-Bitensky N, Feine J: Measuring the effect of intra-oral implant rehabilitation on health-related quality of life in a randomized controlled clinical trial. *J Dent Res* 2000;79:1659–1663.
11 Jofre J, Castiglioni X, Lobos CA: Influence of minimally invasive implant-retained overdenture on patients' quality of life: a randomized clinical trial. *Clin Oral Implants Res* 2013;24:1173–1177.
12 Horowitz RA, Leventis MD, Rohrer MD, Prasad HS: Bone grafting: history, rationale, and selection of materials and techniques. *Compendium of Continuing Education in Dentistry* 2014 Nov–Dec;35(Special Issue 4):1–13.
13 Phillips K, Wong KM: Vertical space requirements for the fixed detatchable implant supported prosthesis. *Compendium of Continuing Education in Dentistry* 2002;23(8):750–756.
14 Lee CK, Agar JR: Surgical and prosthetic planning for a two-implant-retained mandibular overdenture: a clinical report. *J Prosthet Dent* 2006;95(2):102–105.
15 Carpentieri, J, Drago C: *Treatment of the edentulous and partially edentulous maxilla: clinical guidelines. JIRD* 2011;3(1):7–17.
16 LoCascio S, Salinas T: Rehabilitation of an edentulous mandible with an implant-supported prosthesis. *Pract Periodont Aesthet Dent* 1997;9(3):357–370.
17 Heydecke G, Boudrias P, Awad M, de Albuquerque RF, Lund JP, Feine JS: Within- subject comparisons of maxillary fixed and removable implant prostheses: patient satisfaction and choice of prostheses. *Clin Oral Impl Res* 2003;14:125–130.
18 de Albuquerque RF, Lund JP, Larivee J, de Grandmont P, Gauthier G, Feine JS: Within-subject comparison of maxillary long-bar implant-retained prostheses with and without palatal coverage: patient-based outcomes. *Clin Oral Impl Res* 2000;11:555–565.
19 Bedrossian E, Sullivan RM, Malo P: Fixed-prosthetic implant restoration of the edentulous maxilla: a systematic pretreatment evaluation method. *J Oral Maxillofac Surg* 2008;66:112–122.
20 Pound E, Murrell GA: An introduction to denture simplification. *J Prosthet Dent* 1971;26(6):570–580.
21 Pound E, Murrell GA: An introduction to denture simplification: Phase vII. *J Prosthet Dent* 1973;29(6):598–607.
22 Brånemark PI, Svensson B, van Steenberghe D: Ten-year survival rates of fixed prostheses on four or six implants ad modum Brånemark in full edentulism. *Clin Oral Implants Res* 1995;6(4):227–231.
23 Gallucci GO, Doughtie CB, Hwang JW, et al: Five year results of fixed implant-supported rehabilitations with distal cantilevers for the edentulous mandible. *Clin Oral Implants Res* 2009;20(6):601–607.
24 Eliasson A: On the role of number of fixtures, surgical technique and timing of loading. *Swed Dent J Suppl* 2008; (197):3–95.
25 Baker RD, Terry BC, Davis WH, et al: Long-term results of alveolar ridge augmentation. *J Oral Surg* 1979;37:486.
26 Davis WH, Martinoff JT, Kaminshi RM: Long-term follow up of transoral rib grafts for mandibular atrophy. *J Oral Maxillofac Surg* 1984;42:606.
27 Verhoeven JW, Cune MS, Terlou M, et al: The combined use of endosteal implants and iliac crest onlay grafts in the severely atrophic mandible: a longitudinal study. *Int J Oral Maxillofac Surg* 1997;26:5.
28 Finn RA, Bell WH, Brammer JA: Interpositional "grafting" with autogenous bone and coralline hydroxyapatite. *J Maxillofac Surg* 1980;8:217.
29 Härle F: Visor osteotomy to increase the absolute height of the atrophied mandible. A preliminary report. *J Maxillofac Surg* 1975;3:257.
30 Stoelinga PJ, Tideman H, Berger JS, et al: Interpositional bone graft augmentation of the atrophic mandible: A preliminary report. *J Oral Surg* 1978;36:30.
31 Marx RE, Shellenberger T, Wimsatt J, Correa P: Severely resorbed mandible: predictable reconstruction with soft tissue matrix expansion (tent pole) grafts. *J Oral Maxillofac Surg* 2002;60:8.
32 Korpi JT, Kainulainen VT, Sándor GK, Oikarinen KS: Long-term follow-up of severely resorbed mandibles reconstructed using tent pole technique without platelet-rich plasma. *J Oral Maxillofac Surg* 2012;70:2543–2548.
33 English CE: The critical A-P spread. *The Implant Society* March–April 1990;1(1): 2–3.

34. Shackleton JL, Carr L, Slabbert JC, Becker PJ: Survival of fixed implant-supported prostheses related to cantilever lengths. *J Prosthet Dent* 1994;71:23–26.
35. Sadowsky SJ, Caputo AA: Effect of anchorage systems and extension base contact on load transfer with mandibular implant-retained overdentures. *J Prosthet Dent* 2000;84:327–334.
36. Jemt T: Failures and complications in 391 consecutively inserted fixed prostheses supported by Brånemark implants in edentulous jaws: a study of treatment from the time of prosthesis placement to the first annual checkup. *Int J Oral Maxillofac Implants* 1991;6:270.
37. Schnitman P: The profile prosthesis: an aesthetic fixed implant-supported restoration for the resorbed maxilla. *Pract Periodont Aesthet Dent* 1999;11:143.
38. Fortin Y, Sullivan RM, Rangert B: The Marius implant bridge: surgical and prosthetic rehabilitation for the completely edentulous upper jaw with moderate to severe resorption: a 5-year retrospective clinical study. *Clin Implant Dent Relat Res* 2002;4:69.
39. Williams BH, Ochiai KT, Hojo S, Nishimura R, Caputo AA: Retention of maxillary implant overdenture bars of different designs. *J Prosthet Dent* 2001;86:603–607.
40. Cavallaro JS, Tarnow DP: Unsplinted implants retaining maxillary overdentures with partial palatal coverage: Report of 5 consecutive cases. *Int J Oral Maxillofac Implants* 2007;22:808–814.
41. Krennmair G, Krainhofner M, Piehslinger E: Implant-supported maxillary overdentures retained with milled bars: maxillary anterior versus maxillary posterior concept – A retrospective study. *Int J Oral Maxillofac Implants* 2008;23:343–352.
42. Ettinger R, Jakobsen J: A comparison of patient satisfaction and dentist evaluation of overdenture therapy. *Community Dent Oral Epidemiol* 1997;25:223–227.
43. Chiche G, Pinault A: *Esthetics of Anterior Fixed Prosthodontics*. Quintessence Publishing Co., 1994.
44. Gargulio AW, Wentz FM, Orban B: Dimensions and relations of the dentogingival junction in humans. *J Perio* 1961;32:261–267.
45. Vacek JS, Gher ME, Assad DA, Richardson AC, Giambarresi L: The dimension of the human dentogingival junction. *I J Perio Rest Dent* 1994;14(2):155–165.
46. Oakley E, Rhyu I, Karatzas S, Gandini-Santiago L, Nevins, M, Caton J: Formation of biologic width following crown lengthening in nonhuman primates. *I J Perio Rest Dent* 1999;19(6):529–541.
47. Berglundh T, Lindhe J: Dimension of the periimplant mucosa. *J Clin Periodontol* 1996;23:971–973.
48. Ericsson I, Nilner K, Klinge B, Glantz P: Radiological and histological characteristics of submerged and nonsubmerged implants. *Clin Oral Impl Res* 1996;7:20–26.
49. Abrahamsson I, Berglundh T, Lindhe J: The mucosal barrier following abutment dis/reconnection. *J Clin Periodontol* 1997;24:568–572.
50. Cochran DL, Hermann JS, Schenk RK, Higginbottom FL, Buser D: Biologic width around titanium implants. A histometric analysis of the implant–gingival junction around unloaded and loaded nonsubmerged implants in the canine mandible. *J Periodontol* 1997;68:186–198.
51. Hermann JS, Buser D, Schenk RK, Higginbottom FL, Cochran DL: Biologic width around titanium implants. A physiologically formed and stable dimension over time. *Clin Oral Impl Res* 2000;11:1–11.
52. Priest G: Predictability of soft tissue form around single-tooth implant restorations. *Int J Perio Rest Dent* 2003;23:19–27.
53. Lazarra RJ, Porter SS: Platform switching: a new concept in implant dentistry for controlling postrestorative crestal bone levels. *I J Perio Rest Dent* 2006;26:9–17.
54. Tarnow DP, Magner AW, Fletcher P: The effect of the distance from the contact point to the crest of bone on the presence or absence of the interproximal papilla. *J Periodontol* 1992;63:995–996.
55. Choquet V, Hermans M, Adriaenssens P, Daelemans P, Tarnow DP, Malevez C: Clinical and radiographic evaluation of the papilla level adjacent to single-tooth dental implants. A retrospective study in the maxillary anterior region. *J Periodontol* 2001;72:1364–1371.
56. Chambrone L, Chambrone LA: Forced orthodontic eruption of fractured teeth before implant placement: case report. *J Can Dent Assoc* April 2005;71(4):257–261.
57. Grunder, U, Gracis S, Capelii M: Influence of the 3-D bone-to-implant relationship on aesthetics. *I J Perio Rest Dent* 2005;25:113–119.
58. Tarnow DP, Cho SC, Wallace SS: The effect of inter-implant distance on the height of inter-implantbone crest. *J Periodontal* 2000;71:546–549.
59. Tarnow D, Elian N, Fletcher P, Froum S, Magner A, Cho S, Salama M, Salama H, Garber D: Vertical distance from the crest of bone to the height of the interproximal papilla between adjacent implants. *J Periodontol* 2003;74:1785–1788.
60. Misch CM: Comparison of intraoral donor sites for onlay grafting prior to implant placement. *Int J Oral Maxillofac Implants* 1997;12:767.
61. Rasmusson L, Meredith N, Kahnberg KE, et al: Effects of barrier membranes on bone resorption and implant stability in onlay bone grafts. An experimental study. *Clin Oral Implants Res* 1999;10:267.
62. Proussaefs P, Lozada J, Rohrer MD: A clinical and histologic evaluation of a block onlay graft in conjunction with autogenous particulate and inorganic bovine mineral (Bio-Oss): a case report. *Int J Periodontont Restor Dent* 2002;22:567.
63. Keller EE, Tolman DE, Eckert S: Surgical-prosthodontic reconstruction of advanced maxillary bone compromise with autogenous onlay block bone grafts and osseointegrated endosseous implants: a 12 year study of 32 consecutive patients. *Int J Oral Maxillofac Implants* 1999;14:197.
64. Buser D, Dula K, Belser UC, et al: Localized ridge augmentation using guided bone regeneration. II. Surgical procedure in the mandible. *Int J Periodontics Restorative Dent* 1995;15:10.
65. Buser D, Dula K, Hirt HP, et al: Lateral ridge augmentation using autografts and barrier membranes: a clinical study with 40 partially edentulous patients. *J Oral Maxillofac Surg* 1996;54:420.
66. Buser D, Dula K, Hess D, et al: Localized ridge augmentation with autografts and barrier membranes. *Periodontol 2000* 1999;19:151.
67. Misch CM, Misch CE: The repair of localized severe ridge defects for implant placement using mandibular bone grafts. *Implant Dent* 1995;4:261.
68. Le B, Rohrer R, Prassad H: Screw "tent-pole" grafting technique for reconstruction of large vertical alveolar ridge defects using mineralized allograft for implant site preparation. *J Oral Maxillofac Surg* 2010;68:428–435.
69. Jensen OT, Cockrell R, Kuhike L, et al: Anterior maxillary alveolar distraction osteogenesis: a prospective 5-year clinical study. *Int J Oral Maxillofac Implants* 2002;17:52.
70. Louis PJ, Gutta R, Said-Al-Naief N, et al: Reconstruction of the maxilla and mandible with particulate bone graft and titanium mesh for implant placement. *J Oral Maxillofac Surg* 2008;66:235.
71. Thor A: Reconstruction of the anterior maxilla with platelet gel, autogenous bone and titanium mesh: a case report. *Clin Implant Dent Relat Res* 2002;4:150.
72. Simion M, Jovanovic SA, Tinti C, et al: Long-term evaluation of osseointegrated implants inserted at the same time or after vertical ridge augmentation: a retrospective study on 123 implants with 1–5 year follow-up. *Clin Oral Implants Res* 2001;12:35.
73. Fugazzotto PA: Report of 302 consecutive ridge augmentation procedures: technical considerations and clinical results. *Int J Oral Maxillofac Implants* 1998;13: 358

CHAPTER 4

Orthodontic Therapy in Implant Dentistry: Orthodontic Implant Site Development

Ali Borzabadi-Farahani[1] and Homayoun H. Zadeh[2]

[1]Orthodontics, Warwick Dentistry, Warwick Medical School, University of Warwick, Coventry, UK
NHS England, UK
Department of Orthodontics, School of Dentistry, Shahid Beheshti University of Medical Sciences, Tehran, Iran
Formerly, Craniofacial Orthodontics, Children's Hospital Los Angeles and Center for Craniofacial Molecular Biology, University of Southern California, Los Angeles, California, USA
[2]Division of Periodontology, Laboratory for Immunoregulation and Tissue Engineering, Diagnostic Sciences and Dental Hygiene, University of Southern California, Los Angeles, California, USA

Introduction

The optimal aesthetic and function of implants requires placement of implants in a proper relationship to the planned restoration with adequate bone volume and mucosa [1–4]. Where the bone and soft tissues are defective due to pathologic diseases, varieties of reconstructive surgeries have been utilized. These procedures have generally been successful in augmenting bone and soft tissues, but the most challenging conditions are vertical augmentation of alveolar bone and soft tissue. Potential morbidity of surgical augmentation procedures presents an additional drawback of these procedures. Orthodontic therapy can often serve an adjunctive role in optimizing implant sites. The objective of this chapter is to review some of the orthodontic strategies that can be employed in preparation for implant therapy.

Orthodontic implant site development

Where implants are required, overeruption of opposing teeth or drift of adjacent teeth into the edentulous space (future implant site) is common. Space analysis will be required during the diagnosis phase in an effort to determine the optimal proportions and position of the teeth. The next step is to decide on the particular restorative scheme, that is, screw- versus cement-retained restoration, in an effort to determine the planned position and axial orientation of the implant. For a 4 mm diameter implant, approximately 8 mm of mesiodistal space is required for optimum implant placement [3, 4]. This corresponds to 2 mm bone thickness around the implant for optimal results in terms of soft tissue aesthetics and long-term survival [3–6]. Similarly, approximately 8 mm of vertical space is required from the crest of the alveolar bone to the occlusal surface of the opposing teeth to fabricate and design a prosthetic crown [5]. The fixed orthodontic appliances may be used for uprighting and space opening. If implant placement is a part of the definitive treatment plan, appropriate root positioning should be monitored by periodic radiographic assessments during orthodontic site development. Aiming for the ideal crown position, that is, crown torque and crown tip, can be misleading and would not often lead to sufficient interradicular space and root parallelism suitable for implant placement. Therefore, orthodontic tooth movement should be guided by a three-dimensional need of the implant site dictated by the radiographical facts.

Mini-implants [7], skeletal anchors, or temporary anchorage devices (TADs), which are typically placed in the interradicular alveolar locations or in the palate, have been introduced during the last two decades to reinforce the anchorage. They can be used along with the fixed braces to intrude the overerupted teeth, adjust spaces mesiodistally, such as in mandibular molar protraction or maxillary posterior distalization, and upright tilted teeth adjacent to the edentulous space (Figure 4.1a) [8, 9]. TADs are pure titanium or titanium alloy [10] bone screws with a polished endosseous surface body as osseointegration is not intended, complicating removal of the TADs, as well as increasing the risk of fracture at removal [11–13]. The body dimensions of a TAD are 1.5–2 mm in diameter and 6–10 mm in length [14], and in general they are used for tooth movements over a period of 6–8 months. Compared to endosseous implants, TADs rely more on mechanical retention within the cortical layers of alveolar and palatal bones rather than osseointegration [14]. As a tooth is extruded, a clockwise moment at the centre of resistance of the tooth, which is closer to the apex in a periodontally compromised tooth, will move the apex in a facial direction. The utilization of a counter-torqueing moment, that is, rectangular wires or brackets with negative torque, has been suggested [40] to minimize the risk of fenestration/dehiscence formation on the facial bone plate. This strategy is expected to yield coronal movement of tissues, improvement/formation of the interproximal papilla [34], and formation of peri-implant keratinized tissue, which initially resembles an inflamed tissue as sulcular epithelium undergoes keratinization [19, 35, 45, 46].

Insertion often requires a small amount of local anesthetic injection, using a self-drilling screwdriver [14]. Subsequently, TADs can

---

Vertical Alveolar Ridge Augmentation in Implant Dentistry: A Surgical Manual, First Edition. Edited by Len Tolstunov.
© 2016 John Wiley & Sons, Inc. Published 2016 by John Wiley & Sons, Inc.

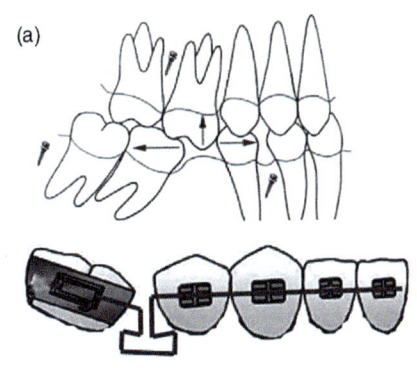

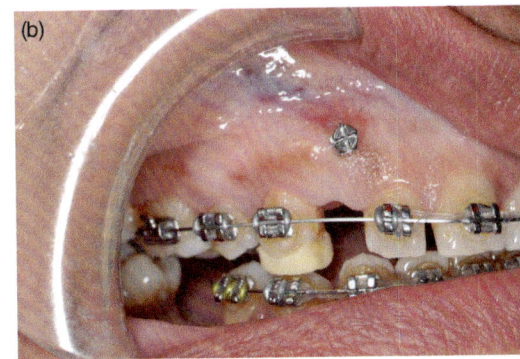

Figure 4.1 Temporary anchorage devices (TADs) and orthodontic mechanics can be used for implant site development (a). A TAD has been placed distal to the maxillary right lateral incisor (b) to facilitate space closure in the maxillary right canine area. This was due to the presence of an ectopic and palatally placed canine in an adult patient, which was surgically removed. An orthodontic space opening in the maxillary right first bicuspid area, which could be used for a single unit implant placement, as well as first bicuspid substitution were suggested. Source: J. Kishabay, K. Daroee and D. Casione. Reproduced with permission from J. Kishabay, K. Daroee and D. Casione.

be immediately loaded for anchorage reinforcement. Many adult patients require delicate space planning and orthodontic tooth movements prior to implant placement (Figure 4.1b). Within that context, a recent clinical trial [15] claims that TADs provide a safe and versatile, minimally invasive, anchorage technique, which is not reliant on patient cooperation and is more reliable for maximum anchorage reinforcement than conventional anchorage supplementation.

Orthodontic extrusion

Elimination of infrabony defects resulting from periodontal disease [16] or treating teeth considered non-restorable due to crown fracture (subgingival) or subgingival dental caries [17, 18] have been cited as the earliest indications of orthodontic extrusion. The available evidence on implant site development by orthodontic extrusion has been reviewed previously [19–37] (Table 4.1). Orthodontic extrusion of non-restorable or periodontally compromised teeth has been used in patients (age ranges of 19–62 years) to increase the hard and soft tissue (i.e., increase the keratinized attached gingiva) volumes in the implant site [20–37], reduce or eliminate vertical or buccolingual bone volume deficiencies, and obviate/reduce the need for hard and soft tissue augmentation procedures [19]. The so-called "orthodontic extrusive remodelling" or "orthodontic forced extraction" has been described by Salama and Salama [23], where hopeless teeth were extruded to the point of extraction, aiming at forming hard and soft tissues along the vector of tooth movement.

Alveolar ridge augmentation techniques are more predictable in restoring the width of an alveolar ridge than its height [38]. Techniques such as guided bone regeneration (GBR), distraction osteogenesis, and onlay bone grafting have been used for vertical bone augmentation [38], though these methods are technically demanding, with varying degrees of success. The GBR and distraction osteogenesis have been shown to be successful in achieving 2–8 mm and 5–15 mm of vertical bone gain, respectively [39]. The most commonly reported complication for GBR has been barrier membrane exposure with the reported incidence of 0–45.5%. For distraction osteogenesis, a high percentage of complications (10–75.7%) has been reported, including the fracture of the distractor, infection of the distraction chamber, fractures of transported or basal bone, slight resorption of the transported fragment, soft tissue dehiscence, and premature or delayed consolidation as well as fibrous non-union, to name a few [39]. Moreover, it is difficult to control the vector of movement of the transported bone, resulting in vertically expanded bone, which is sometimes in an undesirable position.

Orthodontic extrusion is one of the most reliable and relatively non-invasive means of gaining vertical bone augmentation, as well as papilla regeneration (reformation) [40]. This is particularly true in the maxillary anterior region where vertical bone augmentation is challenging. A review of the literature reveals various orthodontic extrusion treatment protocols [19]. However, good plaque control, elimination of periodontitis, the existence of at least one-third to one-fourth of the apical attachment, use of rectangular archwires to create controlled vertical and facial extrusive tooth movement, and a sufficient stabilization period have been cited as necessary requirements for a successful forced eruption [23, 26, 40, 41]. Light and constant extrusive forces of 15 and 50 g for anterior and posterior teeth have been recommended, respectively [19]. Orthodontic extrusion is done at a rate of 1–2 mm per month, and a stabilization period of 1 month for each millimeter extruded (typically 4–6 months) has been recommended [19, 40, 42, 43]. When a periodontally compromised tooth is extruded, torquing [19, 26] and tipping of the tooth toward the angular bone defect are often necessary and increase the alveolar bone volume in that region [35, 40]. An animal study reported that 80% of the vertical tooth movement, in the direction of tooth extrusion, occurred in the attached gingiva [44]. As a tooth is extruded, a clockwise moment at

Table 4.1 Clinical situations in which orthodontic extrusion can be used for implant site development.

Periodontally hopeless tooth with vertical bone loss presenting with Class II or III tooth mobility
Extensive coronal or recurrent subgingival caries
Traumatic vertical root fracture presenting with extensive vertical and horizontal bone loss
Severe gingival recession presenting with loss of interdental papilla and alveolar bone loss
History of failure of surgical periodontal treatment or unsuccessful endodontic treatment presenting with endodontic–periodontal lesions
Poor crown-to-root ratio
Severe external root resorption

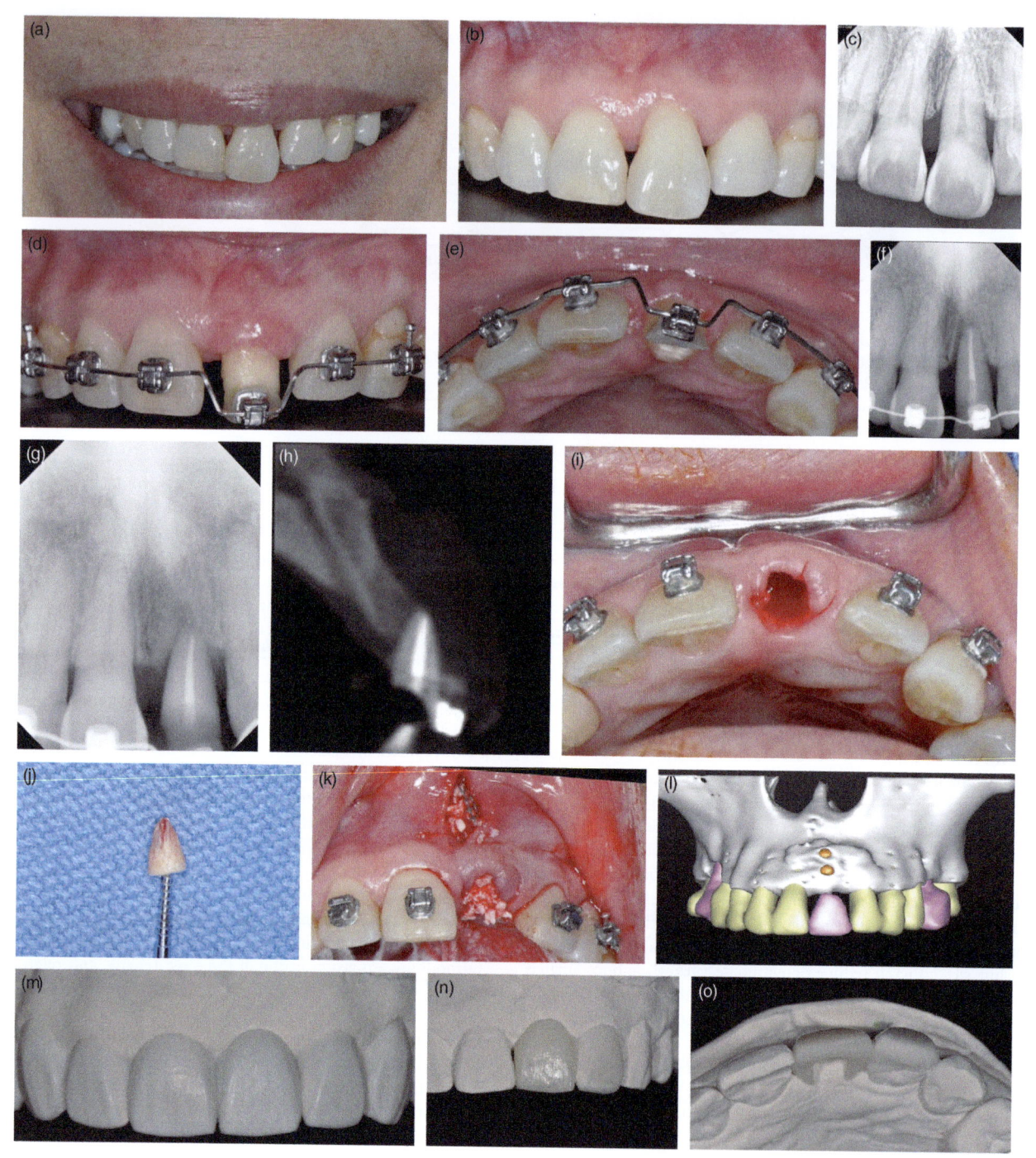

Figure 4.2 Pre-operative clinical (**a** and **b**) and radiographic (**c**) images of a patient in need of orthodontic extrusion. Note the palatal crown position of the maxillary left central incisor, using a rectangular wire, leading to forced vertical and facial (root) eruption at the conclusion of orthodontic therapy (**d** and **e**) aimed at bone augmentation in the labial part of the socket that is frequently very thin [83]. Periapical radiographs during and after orthodontic therapy (**f** and **g**). The cross-sectional reconstruction of CBCT at the end of orthodontic therapy showing vertical and facial forced eruption (**h**). Extraction socket (**i**) and extracted maxillary left central incisor (**j**). The VISTA technique [47] (**k**). CBCT following bone augmentation (**l**). Diagnostic wax-up (**m**) that was used for fabrication of the surgical guide (**n** and **o**). Immediate post-operative radiograph (**p**) and clinical image (**q**) of the implant placed in the central incisor position. Virtually designed CAD/CAM abutment (**r** and **s**). A ceramometal restoration (**t** and **u**). Source: J. Kishabay, K. Daroee and D. Casione. Reproduced with permission from J. Kishabay, K. Daroee and D. Casione.

the centre of resistance of the tooth, which is closer to the apex in a periodontally compromised tooth, will move the apex in a facial direction. The utilization of a counter-torqueing moment, that is, rectangular wires or brackets with negative torque, has been suggested [40] to minimize the risk of fenestration/dehiscence formation on the facial bone plate. This strategy is expected to yield coronal movement of tissues, improvement/formation of the interproximal papilla [34], and formation of peri-implant keratinized tissue, which initially resembles an inflamed tissue as sulcular epithelium undergoes keratinization [19, 35, 45, 46].

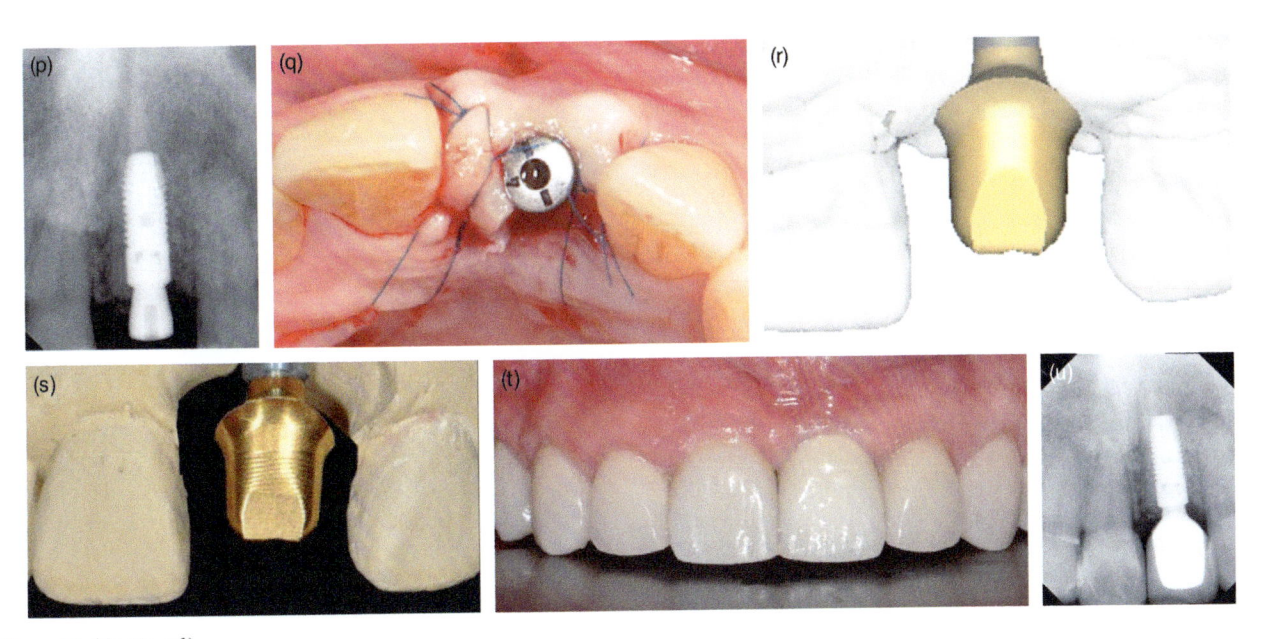

Figure 4.2 (Continued)

Using orthodontic extrusion for implant site development often requires prior root canal treatment to manage the sensitivity or pulpal exposure during occlusal tooth reduction [45]. Vertical crown height reduction of the tooth that is to be extruded is also necessary to eliminate occlusal interferences and contact to the opposing arch [40, 47]. Following the extraction of an extruded compromised tooth, immediate implant placement or additional horizontal bone augmentation should be followed to eliminate the risk of further bone resorption and soft tissue loss [40].

Figure 4.2 shows a clinical case where orthodontic extrusion was utilized to optimize the alveolar ridge in preparation for implant therapy. Pre-operative clinical (Figure 4.2a and b) and radiographic (Figure 4.2c) examination revealed severe periodontitis, associated vertical alveolar bone loss, Miller class 3 recession defect, and supraeruption of the maxillary left central incisor. Orthodontic extrusion of the maxillary left central incisor was performed, moving the tooth in a coronal (Figure 4.2d) and palatal (Figure 4.2e) directions. The tooth was extruded at a rate of 1 mm per month, followed by 6 months of maintenance to stabilize the newly formed alveolar bone. Periapical radiographs in Figure 4.2f and g provide evidence for correction of the angular defects of interproximal bone of the maxillary left central incisor. Cross-sectional reconstruction of the cone beam computerized tomography (CBCT) image taken following 6 months of active orthodontic movement and 6 months of maintenance revealed significant vertical down-growth of alveolar bone (Figure 4.2h). However, since the width of the alveolar bone was only 5.5 mm, it was decided to perform horizontal augmentation of the alveolar bone to optimize the implant site. To that end, the tooth was extracted (Figure 4.2i and j) and GBR was performed (Figure 4.2k). Access to the facial alveolar bone was accomplished by vestibular incision subperiosteal tunnel access (VISTA) technique [48]. This entailed making a 1 cm vertical incision in the vestibule over the mid-line frenum. Subperiosteal tunnel access was made to expose the facial plate. Two 1.5 mm × 8 mm tenting screws (Salvin Dental Specialties, Charlotte, NC) were partially inserted into the facial plate in such a manner that half of the screw was anchored into the bone and the remaining half was left above the bone (not shown). Deproteinated bovine bone mineral (Bio-Oss, Geistlich Pharma North America, Princeton, NJ) was placed over the facial plate of the maxillary left central incisor, as well as neighboring teeth. Six months later, a CBCT view was taken to evaluate the adequacy of augmented bone (Figure 4.2l). The alveolar ridge volume was determined to be optimal at this point. Though horizontal bone augmentation was required, orthodontic extrusion aided in optimizing the alveolar ridge topography. Prior to placement of the implant, a diagnostic wax-up was performed to design the proportion of the future restorations in the esthetic zone (Figure 4.2m). A surgical guide was fabricated based on the wax-up (Figure 4.2n and o) to facilitate positioning the implant based on available guidelines of 3 mm apical and 2 mm palatal of the cervical contour of the planned restoration [49, 50]. Utilizing the guide, an implant (Astra Tech Osseospeed, 4.0 mm × 11 mm) was placed (Figure 4.2p). Figure 4.2q shows that in order to optimize the peri-implant soft tissue, the crestal incision was placed palatal of the crest. Before approximation of the flap, a palacci incision [51] was made on the facial and rotated mesially.

A computer-aided design/computer-aided machining (CAD/CAM) abutment (ATLANTIS abutment, DENTSPLY Implants, Mölndal, Sweden) with full anatomic contour was designed virtually (Figure 4.2r) and milled (Figure 4.2s). A ceramometal restoration was fabricated and delivered (Figure 4.2t and u). The restoration of this patient with compromised periodontal and dental conditions involved an interdisciplinary team of periodontist, orthodontist, restorative dentist, laboratory technician, and CAD/CAM service. This approach required careful planning, coordination, and execution to ensure the outcome desired by the patient. At each step, a decision tree was formulated and a variety of available options was considered among relevant team members. Although orthodontic extrusion was employed to improve osseous topography prior to implant placement, this was not the only reason for orthodontic therapy. Orthodontic therapy was utilized in this case as part of the comprehensive care to optimize the spacing and position of remaining teeth, in preparation for the restoration.

Orthodontic extrusion, as with any technique, has pros and cons. On the positive side, orthodontic extrusion can vertically translate the bone at the alveolar crest and provide native bone for implant placement. However, the drawbacks of this technique include the added length of time required for orthodontic tooth extrusion, the cost of additional prior endodontic therapy, as well as the fact that the vertically translated bone may not have sufficient buccolingual volume. This latter point was illustrated in the previous case. Therefore, the clinician is advised to consider these pros and cons in selecting an appropriate technique, which will be suited to the requirement of a given clinical situation.

Tooth preservation and delayed orthodontic space opening

When placement of implants in the near future is not feasible for patients with missing teeth, it is advisable to maintain the retained primary teeth or compromised teeth. This is because some reduction in the buccolingual and vertical dimensions of the alveolar ridge occurs in the edentulous sites with congenitally absent teeth [43] or following tooth extractions [52–56]. Previous research has shown that after extraction of primary mandibular second molars, the ridge narrows by 25% during the first 4 years and after 7 years the buccolingual ridge width atrophy reaches 30% [52]. As can be seen in a patient with multiple missing teeth (Figure 4.3), there is an obvious difference in the alveolar bone height between the lower right side (arrow), where the patient lost a primary molar(s), and the left side. However, maintaining the primary tooth on the lower left side led to some arrested vertical bone development (Figure 4.3). Early identification of the arrested vertical alveolar development, which can be severe, is also important and early removal of retained primary teeth and space closure may be advisable (Figure 4.4) to obviate the need for future implant placement and prevent overeruption of opposing teeth.

Human and animal studies confirm that extraction ridge defect is primarily in the buccal aspects [52, 57, 58], and the reduction in the width of an alveolar ridge is greater than the loss of height [56]. A 6 month randomized clinical trial reported a reduction in ridge width and height of 2.6 mm and 0.9 mm, respectively, after non-molar tooth extractions [58]. This bone defect, which can be avoided by maintaining the retained primary teeth, often requires bone augmentation or demands more lingual or palatal placement of implants. As can be seen in Figure 4.5a through g, preserving, extruding, and restoring a permanent tooth with a crown fracture or a severely damaged crown (due to decay or tooth wear) is another

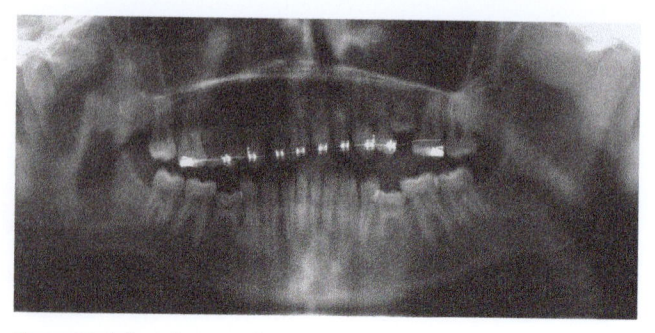

Figure 4.4 Infraocclusion and arrested vertical bone development in the maxillary and mandibular second bicuspid areas are evident.

strategy during adolescence to maintain the alveolar bone volume prior to implant placement. Figure 4.5 illustrates preserving, extruding, and restoring the maxillary right central incisor with a crown fracture (Figure 4.5a and b) in a 14-year-old boy. Although the prognosis of the tooth was poor, implant therapy was not advised at an early age [59]. Therefore, the crown was restored (Figure 4.5c) and after root canal treatment, orthodontic extrusion was performed (Figure 4.5d and e). The tooth was restored following orthodontic extrusion (Figure 4.5f and g) and was maintained for almost 10 years.

Edentulous sites often have some degree of atrophy that requires augmentation prior to implant placement. To optimize restorative positions, an orthodontic space opening may be required to create the desired space for implants. However, the newly created edentulous ridge may undergo atrophy during the prolonged period [60–62], although 2 years after tooth movement, opening changes are minimal [61]. This bone defect can be seen in areas such as missing maxillary lateral incisors or mandibular premolars, common sites for congenitally absent teeth [63]. Literature suggests that to avoid the surgical ridge atrophy and future requirement for augmentation at the site of congenitally absent maxillary lateral incisors, the distalization of canines should be postponed until after the age of 13 years [64] or near the end of skeletal growth [65]. However, this approach has been disputed [61]. Therefore, so far as possible, the time gap between the orthodontic space opening and implant placement should be reduced to avoid further ridge resorption.

The orthodontic implant site switching

Extraction of teeth, in particular in the absence of a ridge preservation procedure, can lead to significant atrophy of the alveolar ridge [66]. Various surgical techniques have been developed for augmentation of the alveolar bone. Orthodontic therapy has been proposed as an alternative to surgical intervention in enhancing atrophic edentulous sites adjacent to natural teeth. The orthodontic movement of teeth toward an adjacent atrophic edentulous alveolar ridge is accompanied by movement of the alveolar bone associated with the tooth [65, 67–72]. This leads to expansion of the alveolar bone, potentially obviating the need for surgical ridge augmentation. The application of orthodontic therapy for the enhancement of adjacent atrophic alveolar bone has been termed orthodontic implant site switching (OISS) [5, 73]. In carefully selected cases, this can eliminate or minimize the need for surgical augmentation (Figure 4.6). This procedure has been associated with minimal changes in the periodontal support of the transposed tooth [74] and,

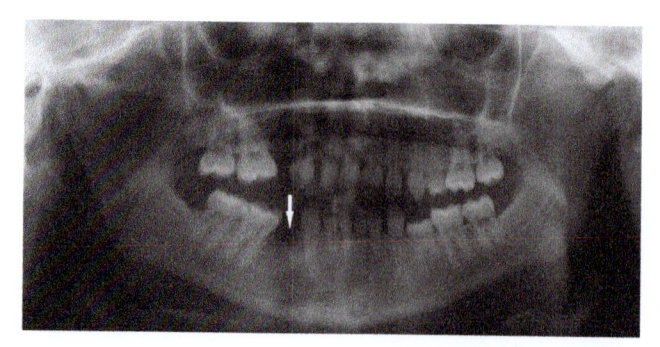

Figure 4.3 A patient with multiple missing teeth, including the maxillary and mandibular bicuspids, showing vertical bone deficiency in the right mandibular bicuspid area (arrow).

Orthodontic Therapy in Implant Dentistry **35**

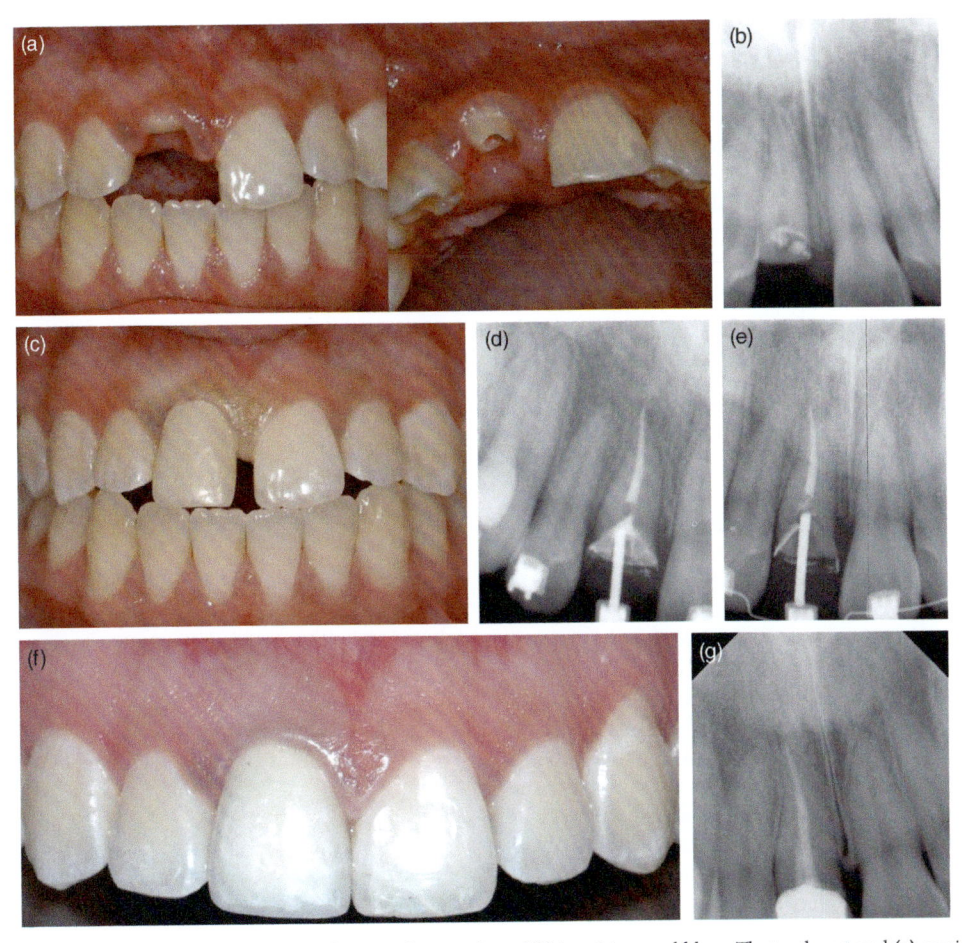

Figure 4.5 Preserving a maxillary right central incisor with crown fracture (**a and b**) in a 14-year-old boy. The tooth restored (**c**) received root canal treatment, orthodontic extrusion (**d and e**), restored following orthodontic extrusion (**f and g**), maintained for almost 5 years after finishing orthodontic treatment.

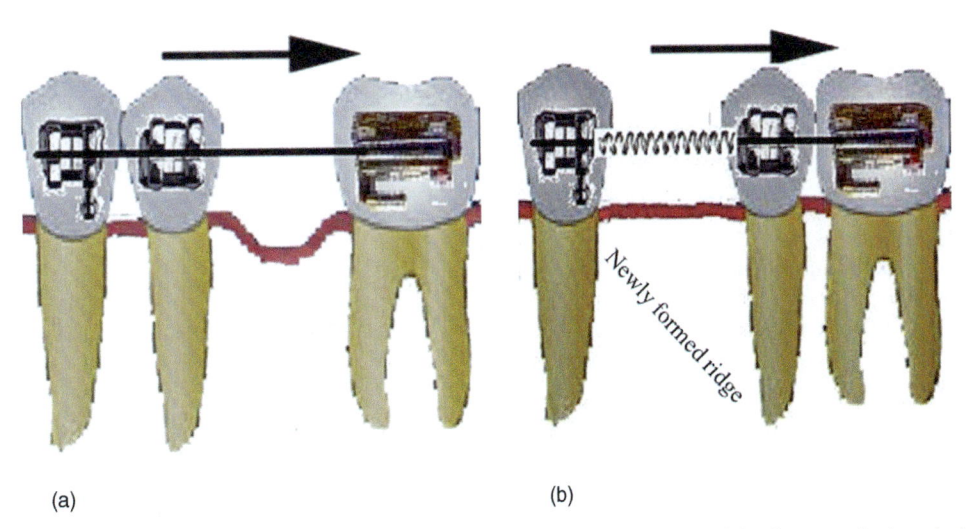

Figure 4.6 The orthodontic implant site switching [5, 73] uses tooth movement to generate a new bone. (**a**) A first premolar is pushed distally into the second premolar position, where bone volume deficiency exists. (**b**) New bone is generated in the first premolar position and can be used for implant placement, obviating the need for bone grafting.

by using adjacent teeth as a stimulus for alveolar-site development, the need for a bone graft may be eliminated [70]. The OISS can be used in common sites for congenital tooth agenesis [63] to generate sufficient bone volume in the maxillary and mandibular lateral incisor or premolar regions. For instance, mesialization of the second premolar into the narrowed and deficient site of a missing first premolar (or vice versa) leaves behind an alveolar ridge with adequate bone volume, eliminating bone grafting before implant placement [65, 70, 72]. Orthodontic tooth movement in edentulous ridge areas has been described in a case series [72] reporting mean increases of 1.6 and 0.8 mm in the thickness of the buccolingual alveolar ridge width, at the retention stage, at the 2 and 5 mm crestal level, respectively. These increases were associated with minimal changes at 1 year follow-up [72].

Orthodontic retention

Provision of retention after orthodontic space opening or orthodontic implant site switching (OISS) is vital for maintaining the implant site. In children, several years can elapse between completion of orthodontic treatment and initiation of implant therapy. Consequently, a rigid bonded retainer or a fixed resin-bonded bridge restoration should be provided after the successful orthodontic implant site development because positional changes of teeth adjacent to implant sites are common [75]. The overeruption of the unopposed teeth into the edentulous space can also compromise the future prosthetic treatment [76]. With regard to the implant site, positional changes such as the root reapproximation of the adjacent teeth [77, 78], tilting of adjacent crowns into the implant site [77, 78], and overeruption of unopposed molars [76] should be prevented.

The study of the post-retention root position of maxillary central incisors and canines has revealed that 11% of patients experience relapses, significant enough to prevent implant placement in that area [78]. This relapse can potentially compromise or prevent future implant placement, requiring further orthodontic treatment to facilitate implant placement. Previous research has demonstrated that removable retainers are not efficient at maintaining the dimensions of edentulous space [78] and, therefore, placement of a rigid bonded wire or a fixed–fixed resin-bonded bridge is recommended. This prevents root approximation during the retention stage or overeruption of unopposed molars following tooth loss [70, 78].

Summary

Complications and morbidity of surgical alveolar ridge augmentation have been observed in association with both donor sites (i.e., hematoma, altered sensation of teeth, mucosa and skin, postoperative pain) and recipient sites (i.e., graft or membrane exposure, graft loss, graft displacement, infection) [79–82]. Moreover, surgical ridge augmentation has biologic limitations, particularly with regard to vertical ridge augmentation [40]. The potential of orthodontic treatment as an alternative/adjunct to overcome some of these limitations may be beneficial to clinicians. Currently, no comparison has been made between the effectiveness of the surgical bone augmentation techniques and orthodontic alternatives, and each of these methods of implant site development has advantages and disadvantages [83]. Future multicenter randomized clinical trials are required to address this question. In the meantime, clinicians are advised to weigh the pros and cons of each of the methods available for implant site development in an effort to select an appropriate treatment strategy for each case.

Acknowledgments

The authors acknowledge the contribution of the interdisciplinary team to the clinical care of patients, whose cases are illustrated in Figures 4.1 and 4.2, namely Dr. John Kishabay (orthodontist), Dr. Kathy Daroee (restorative dentist), and Mr. Domenico Casione (dental technician). The authors are grateful to Allen Press for granting permission to reprint excerpts from previously published material (*Journal of Oral Implantology* 2012;**38**:779–791 and 2015;**41**:501–508).

References

1 Le B, Nielsen B: Esthetic implant site development. *Oral Maxillofac Surg Clin North Am* 2015;27:2835.
2 Tarnow DP, Cho SC, Wallace SS: The effect of inter-implant distance on the height of inter-implant bone crest. *J Periodontol* 2000;71:546–549.
3 Spray JR, Black CG, Morris HF, Ochi S: The influence of bone thickness on facial marginal bone response: stage 1 placement through stage 2 uncovering. *Ann Periodontol* 2000;5:119–128.
4 Le BT, Borzabadi-Farahani A: Labial bone thickness in area of anterior maxillary implants associated with crestal labial soft tissue thickness. *Implant Dent* 2012;21:406–410.
5 Borazabadi-Farahani A: Orthodontic considerations in restorative management of hypodontia patients with endosseous implants. *J Oral Implantol* 2012;38:779–791.
6 Le BT, Borzabadi-Farahani A, Pluemsakunthai W: Is buccolingual angulation of maxillary anterior implants associated with the crestal labial soft tissue thickness? *Int J Oral Maxillofac Surg* 2014;43:874–878.
7 Creekmore T, Eklund M: The possibility of skeletal anchorage. *J ClinOrthod* 1983;4:266–269.
8 Skeggs RM, Benson PE, Dyer F: Reinforcement of anchorage during orthodontic brace treatment with implants or other surgical methods. *Cochrane Database of Systematic Reviews* 2007, Issue 3, Art. No.: CD005098.
9 Reynders R, Ronchi L, Bipat S: Mini-implants in orthodontics: a systematic review of the literature. *Am J Orthod Dentofac Orthop* 2009;13:564.e1–19.
10 Carano A, Leonardo P, Velo S, Incorvani C: Mechanical properties of three different commercially available miniscrews for skeletal anchorage. *Prog Orthod* 2005;6:82–97.
11 Chen YJ, Chen YH, Lin LD, Yao CC: Removal torque of miniscrews used for orthodontic anchorage – a preliminary report. *Int J Oral Maxillofac Implants* 2006;21:283–289.
12 Jolley TH, Chung CH: Peak torque values at fracture of orthodontic miniscrews. *J Clin Orthod* 2007;41:326–328.
13 Kravitz ND, Kusnoto B: Risks and complications of orthodontic miniscrews. *Am J Orthod Dentofacial Orthop* 2007;131(Suppl 4):S43–S51.
14 Cousley RR, Sandler PJ: Advances in orthodontic anchorage with the use of mini-implant techniques. *Br Dent J* 2015;218(3):E4.
15 Sandler J, Murray A, Thiruvenkatachari B, Gutierrez R, Speight P, O'Brien K: Effectiveness of 3 methods of anchorage reinforcement for maximum anchorage in adolescents: a 3-arm multicenter randomized clinical trial. *Am J Orthod Dentofac Orthop* 2014;146:10–20.
16 Brown IS: The effect orthodontic therapy has on certain types of periodontal defects. I. Clinical findings. *J Periodontol* 1973;4:742–756.
17 Ingber JS: Forced eruption. I. A method of treating isolated one and two wall infrabony osseous defects – rationale and case report. *J Periodontol* 1974;45:199–206.
18 Ingber JS: Forced eruption: part II. A method of treating nonrestorable teeth – periodontal and restorative considerations. *J Periodontol* 1976;47:203–216.
19 Korayem M, Flores-Mir C, Nassar U, Olfert K: Implant site development by orthodontic extrusion: a systematic review. *Angle Orthod* 2008;78:752–760.
20 Mantzikos T, Shamus I: Forced eruption and implant site development: soft tissue response. *Am J Orthod Dentofacial Orthop* 1997;112:596–606.
21 Mantzikos T, Shamus I: Case report: forced eruption and implant site development. *Angle Orthod* 1998;68:179–186.
22 Buskin R, Castellon P, Hochstedler JL: Orthodontic extrusion and orthodontic extraction in preprosthetic treatment using implant therapy. *Pract Periodontics Aesthet Dent* 2000;12:213–219.
23 Salama H, Salama M: The role of orthodontic extrusive remodelling in the enhancement of soft and hard tissue profiles prior to implant placement: a systematic approach to the management of extraction site defects. *Int J Periodontics Restorative Dent* 1993;13:312–333.

24 Mantzikos T, Shamus I: Forced eruption and implant site development: an osteophysiologic response. *Am J Orthod Dentofacial Orthop* 1999;**115**:583–591.
25 Ostojic S, Sieber R, Borer K, Lambrecht JT: Controlled orthodontic extrusion with subsequent implantation [in French, German]. *Schweiz Monatsschr Zahnmed* 2005;**115**:222–231.
26 Zuccati G, Bocchieri A: Implant site development by orthodontic extrusion of teeth with poor prognosis. *J Clin Orthod* 2003;**37**:307–311.
27 Nozawa T, Sugiyama T, Yamaguchi S, et al: Buccal and coronal bone augmentation using forced eruption and buccal root torque: a case report. *Int J Periodontics Restorative Dent* 2003;**23**:585–591.
28 Danesh-Meyer MJ, Brice DM: Implant site development using orthodontic extrusion: a case report. *NZ Dent J* 2000;**96**:18–22.
29 González López S, Olmedo Gaya MV, Vallecillo Capilla M: Esthetic restoration with orthodontic traction and single tooth implant: case report. *Int J Periodontics Restorative Dent* 2005;**25**:239–245.
30 Biggs J, Beagle JR: Pre-implant orthodontics: achieving vertical bone height without osseous grafts. *J Indiana Dent Assoc* 2004;**83**:18–19.
31 Celenza F: The development of forced eruption as a modality for implant site enhancement. *Alpha Omegan* 1997;**90**:40–43.
32 Chambrone L, Chambrone LA: Forced orthodontic eruption of fractured teeth before implant placement: case report. *J Can Dent Assoc* 2005;**71**:257–261.
33 Chandler KB, Rongey WF: Forced eruption: review and case reports. *Gen Dent* 2005;**53**:274–277.
34 Lin CD, Chang SS, Liou CS, Dong DR, Fu E: Management of interdental papillae loss with forced eruption, immediate implantation, and root-form pontic. *J Periodontol* 2006;**77**:135–141.
35 Uribe F, Taylor T, Shafer D, Nanda R: A novel approach for implant site development through root tipping. *Am J Orthod Dentofacial Orthop* 2010;**138**:649–655.
36 Makhmalbaf A, Chee W: Soft- and hard-tissue augmentation by orthodontic treatment in the esthetic zone. *Compend Contin Educ Dent* 2012;**33**:302–306.
37 Amato F, Mirabella AD, Macca U, Tarnow DP: Implant site development by orthodontic forced extraction: a preliminary study. *Int J Oral Maxillofac Implants* 2012;**27**:411–420.
38 Esposito M, Grusovin MG, Coulthard P, Worthington HV: The efficacy of various bone augmentation procedures for dental implants: a Cochrane systematic review of randomized controlled clinical trials. *Int J Oral Maxillofac Implants* 2006;**21**:696–710.
39 Rocchietta I, Fontana F, Simion M: Clinical outcomes of vertical bone augmentation to enable dental implant placement: a systematic review. *J Clin Periodontol* 2008;**35**(Suppl 8):203–215.
40 Hochman MN, Chu SJ, Tarnow DP: Orthodontic extrusion for implant site development revisited: a new classification determined by anatomy and clinical outcomes. *Semin Orthod* 2014;**20**:208–227.
41 Kokich VG, Kokich VO: Interrelationship of orthodontics with periodontics and restorative dentistry. In: Nanda R (ed.), *Biomechanics and Esthetic Strategies in Clinical Orthodontics*. Elsevier, St. Louis, MO, 2005, pp. 348–372.
42 Rose TP, Jivraj S, Chee W: The role of orthodontics in implant dentistry. *Br Dent J* 2006;**201**:753–764.
43 Salama H, Salama M, Kelly J: The orthodontic–periodontal connection in implant site development. *Pract Periodontics Aesthet Dent* 1996;**8**:923–932.
44 Kajiyama K, Murakami T, Yokota S: Gingival reactions after experimentally induced extrusion of the upper incisors in monkeys. *Am J Orthod Dentofacial Orthop* 1993;**104**:36–47.
45 Kim SH, Tramontina VA, Papalexiou V, Luczyszyn SM: Orthodontic extrusion and implant site development using an interocclusal appliance for a severe mucogingival deformity: a clinical report. *J Prosthet Dent* 2011;**105**:72–77.
46 Celenza F: Implant interactions with orthodontics. *J Evid Based Dent Pract* 2012;**12**(Suppl 3):192–201.
47 Rasner SL: Orthodontic extrusion: an adjunct to implant treatment. *Dent Today* 2011;**30**:104,106,108–109.
48 Zadeh HH: Minimally invasive treatment of maxillary anterior gingival recession defects by vestibular incision subperiosteal tunnel access and platelet-derived growth factor BB. *Int J Periodontics Restorative Dent* 2011;**31**:653–660.
49 Cooper LF: Objective criteria: guiding and evaluating dental implant esthetics. *J Esthet Restor Dent* 2008;**20**:195–205.
50 Evans CD, Chen ST: Esthetic outcomes of immediate implant placements. *Clin Oral Implants Res* 2008;**19**:73–80.
51 Palacci P, Nowzari H: Soft tissue enhancement around dental implants. *Periodontol 2000* 2008;**47**:113–132.
52 Ostler M, Kokich V: Alveolar ridge changes in patients congenitally missing mandibular second molars. *J Prosthet Dent* 1994;**71**:144–149.
53 Pietrokovski J, Massler M: Alveolar ridge resorption following tooth extraction. *J Prosthet Dent* 1967;**17**:21–27.
54 Pietrokovski J, Sorin S, Hirschfeld Z: The residual ridge in partially edentulous patients. *J Prosthet Dent* 1976;**36**:150–158.
55 Schropp L, Wenzel A, Kostopoulos L, Karring T: Bone healing and soft tissue contour changes following single-tooth extraction: a clinical and radiographic 12-month prospective study. *Int J Periodontics Restorative Dent* 2003;**23**:313–323.
56 Van der Weijden F, Dell'Acqua F, Slot DE: Alveolar bone dimensional changes of post-extraction sockets in humans: a systematic review. *J Clin Periodontol* 2009;**36**:1048–1058.
57 Araujo MG, Lindhe J: Dimensional ridge alterations following tooth extraction. An experimental study in the dog. *J Clin Periodontol* 2005;**32**:212–218.
58 Iasella JM, Greenwell H, Miller RL, Hill M, et al: Ridge preservation with freeze-dried bone allograft and a collagen membrane compared to extraction alone for implant site development: a clinical and histologic study in humans. *J Periodontol* 2003;**74**:990–999.
59 Daftary F, Mahallati R, Bahat O, Sullivan RM: Lifelong craniofacial growth and the implications for osseointegrated implants. *Int J Oral Maxillofac Implants* 2013;**28**:163–169.
60 Uribe F, Chau V, Padala S, Neace WP, Cutrera A, Nanda R: Alveolar ridge width and height changes after orthodontic space opening in patients congenitally missing maxillary lateral incisors. *Eur J Orthod* 2013;**35**:87–92.
61 Nováčková S, Marek I, Kamínek M: Orthodontic tooth movement: bone formation and its stability over time. *Am J Orthod Dentofacial Orthop* 2011;**139**:37–43.
62 Spear FM, Mathews DM, Kokich VG: Interdisciplinary management of single-tooth implants. *Semin Orthod* 1997;**3**:45–72.
63 Vahid-Dastjerdi E, Borzabadi-Farahani A, Mahdian M, Amini N: Non-syndromic hypodontia in an Iranian orthodontic population. *J Oral Sci* 2010;**52**:455–461.
64 Beyer A, Tausche E, Boening K, Harzer W: Orthodontic space opening in patients with congenitally missing lateral incisors. *Angle Orthod* 2007;**77**:404–409.
65 Carmichael RP, Sándor GK: Dental implants in the management of nonsyndromal oligodontia. *Atlas Oral Maxillofac Surg Clin North Am* 2008;**16**:11–31.
66 Horváth A, Mardas N, Mezzomo LA, Needleman IG, Donos N: Alveolar ridge preservation. A systematic review. *Clin Oral Investig* 2013;**17**:341–363.
67 Zachrisson BU: Orthodontic tooth movement to regenerate new alveolar tissue of bone for improved single implant aesthetics. *Eur J Orthod* 2003;**25**:442.
68 Kokich VG: Maxillary lateral incisor implants: planning with the aid of orthodontics. *J Oral Maxillofac Surg* 2004;**62**(9 Suppl 2):48–56.
69 Gündüz E, Rodríguez-Torres C, Gahleitner A, Heissenberger G, Bantleon HP: Bone regeneration by bodily tooth movement: dental computed tomography examination of a patient. *Am J Orthod Dentofacial Orthop* 2004;**125**:100–106.
70 Kokich VG, Kokich VO: Congenitally missing mandibular second premolars: clinical options. *Am J Orthod Dentofacial Orthop* 2006;**130**:437–444.
71 Fudalej P, Kokich VG, Leroux B: Determining the cessation of vertical growth of the craniofacial structures to facilitate placement of single-tooth implants. *Am J Orthod Dentofacial Orthop* 2007;**131**(Suppl 4):S59–67.
72 Lindskog-Stokland B, Hansen K, Ekestubbe A, Wennström JL: Orthodontic tooth movement into edentulous ridge areas – a case series. *Eur J Orthod* 2013;**35**:277–285.
73 Borzabadi-Farahani A, Zadeh HH: Adjunctive orthodontic applications in dental implantology. *J Oral Implantol* 2015;**41**:501–508.
74 Diedrich PR, Fuhrmann RA, Wehrbein H, Erpenstein H: Distal movement of premolars to provide posterior abutments for missing molars. *Am J Orthod Dentofacial Orthop* 1996;**109**:355–360.
75 Petridis HP, Tsiggos N, Michail A, Kafantaris SN, Hatzikyriakos A, Kafantaris NM: Three-dimensional positional changes of teeth adjacent to posterior edentulous spaces in relation to age at time of tooth loss and elapsed time. *Eur J Prosthodont Restor Dent* 2010;**18**:78–83.
76 Lindskog-Stokland B, Hansen K, Tomasi C, Hakeberg M, Wennström JL: Changes in molar position associated with missing opposed and/or adjacent tooth: a 12-year study in women. *J Oral Rehabil* 2012;**39**:136–143.
77 Dickinson G: Space for missing maxillary lateral incisors – orthodontic perceptions. *Ann R Australian Coll Dent Surg* 2000;**15**:127–131.
78 Olsen TM, Kokich VG Sr: Post orthodontic root approximation after opening space for maxillary lateral incisor implants. *Am J Orthod Dentofacial Orthop* 2010;**137**:158.e1–158.e8.
79 Meraw SJ, Eckert SE, Yacyshyn CE, Wollan PC: Retrospective review of grafting techniques utilized in conjunction with endosseous implant placement. *Int J Oral Maxillofac Implants* 1999;**14**:744–747.
80 Serra FM, Cortez AL, Moreira RW, Mazzonetto R: Complications of intraoral donor site for bone grafting prior to implant placement. *Implant Dent* 2006;**15**:420–426.
81 Raghoebar GM, Timmenga NM, Reintsema H, Stegenga B, Vissink A: Maxillary bone grafting for insertion of endosseous implants: results after 12–124 months. *Clin Oral Implants Res* 2001;**12**:279–286.
82 Misch CM: Comparison of intraoral donor sites for onlay grafting prior to implant placement. *Int J Oral Maxillofac Implants* 1997;**12**:767–776.
83 Magkavali-Trikka P, Kirmanidou Y, Michalakis K, et al: Efficacy of two site-development procedures for implants in the maxillary esthetic region: a systematic review. *Int J Oral Maxillofac Implants* 2015;**30**:73–94.

CHAPTER 5

Radiographic Evaluation of the Alveolar Ridge in Implant Dentistry. Cone Beam Computed Tomography

Sanjay M. Mallya

Section of Oral and Maxillofacial Radiology, UCLA School of Dentistry, Los Angeles, California, USA

Introduction

Radiological evaluation of the jaws is a key component of the presurgical implant treatment planning process and contributes to the overall success of a dental implant-supported prosthesis. During the initial diagnostic phase, radiographic evaluation augments the clinical examination to provide a local assessment of the anatomical and architectural characteristics of the potential implant site and to provide an overall perspective of oral health as it pertains to the specific implant treatment plan. Imaging modalities that provide this radiological information include conventional periapical and panoramic radiographs and cone beam computed tomography (CBCT). Clinicians must be familiar with these imaging modalities, including their advantages and limitations, and the radiation dose considerations in their use. The appropriate use of these imaging modalities is important to develop an effective treatment plan and to minimize the risk of complications from implant placement.

Conventional radiography

Initial assessment of the dental implant patient is often accomplished with conventional two-dimensional imaging. For this purpose, periapical and panoramic radiographs are used. The overall diagnostic objectives of this initial examination are to provide a general assessment of the teeth and dentoalveolar structures. Panoramic radiography produces a single image that encompasses both the maxillary and mandibular dental arches. In this technique, the X-ray source and image receptor rotate around the patient creating a focal trough – a zone in which structures cast sharp images. In panoramic radiography, the images of structures outside this zone are blurred, and this enables selective imaging of structures within the curved dental arches without superimpositions from structures on the opposite side of the arch. Panoramic radiography provides broad anatomic coverage of the jaws, including the dentoalveolar arches, the maxillary sinuses, and the temporomandibular joints. It is a relatively easily accessible technology and a low-cost procedure, and thus is often used as the initial imaging examination of the dental implant patient. For this initial evaluation, panoramic radiography provides an overall assessment of the dental and periodontal health, including the marginal periodontal bone, the presence of periapical disease, and residual roots and pathology. A limitation of panoramic radiography is that it does not adequately depict fine anatomic details. For this reason, panoramic examination is often supplemented with bitewing and selected periapical radiographs to provide a more detailed evaluation of caries, marginal periodontal bone loss, and integrity of lamina dura and periodontal ligament space around carious or endodontically treated teeth, as well as a better evaluation of root tips and subtle apical periodontal pathology. Overall, this combined examination of panoramic and selected intraoral radiographs, as necessary, is adequate to provide diagnostic information for an initial assessment of the dental implant patient. This conventional radiological examination will provide a gross evaluation of the extent of residual ridge resorption, the proximity to adjacent vital structures such as the mandibular canal, the maxillary sinus, and the nasal cavity, angulation of the adjacent teeth, and approximate evaluation of the length of the edentulous span (Figure 5.1). All of these are important considerations in determining the feasibility and complexity of the implant treatment plan.

As with other forms of planar imaging, a major limitation of panoramic radiography is the two-dimensional nature of the information portrayed. It does not provide any information on the buccolingual dimensions of the edentulous ridge or the buccolingual relationships of anatomic structures. An important disadvantage of panoramic radiography, from the point of view of implant treatment planning, is the geometric distortion that is inherent in production of panoramic images. This geometric distortion limits the utility of measurements made on panoramic images. There are a number of factors that influence geometric distortion, including machine-specific factors, location of an object within the focal trough, the range of variation in the shape of dental arches, and angulation of the X-ray beam relative to the structures being imaged. However, many of these factors cannot be adequately controlled or adequately standardized. Importantly, the magnitude of horizontal and vertical magnification is unequal across the image. For this reason, mathematical correction of measurements to account for the various sources of geometric distortion is not feasible. Thus, measurements made on panoramic images, for example to determine the available height of the residual alveolar ridge, are inaccurate and unreliable. Given this limitation, panoramic radiography must not be used as the sole imaging examination for the comprehensive diagnostic and treatment planning tasks for dental implants.

Vertical Alveolar Ridge Augmentation in Implant Dentistry: A Surgical Manual, First Edition. Edited by Len Tolstunov.
© 2016 John Wiley & Sons, Inc. Published 2016 by John Wiley & Sons, Inc.

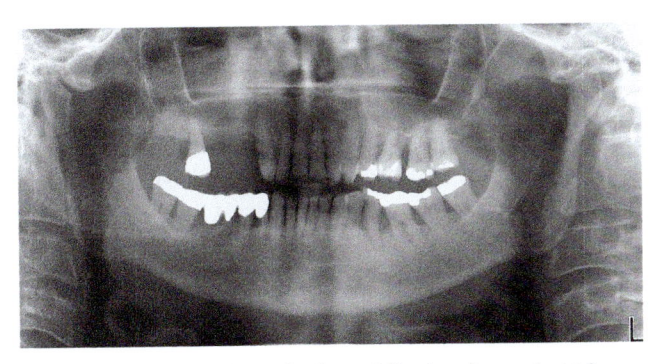

Figure 5.1 Panoramic radiograph of a partially edentulous patient taken as an initial examination for implant treatment planning. Note considerable resorption of the vertical height of the ridge in the right posterior maxilla and proximity to the maxillary sinus floor. Note the generalized moderate to severe marginal periodontal bone loss through both jaws. Adapted from Mallya and White, 2013. Reproduced with permission from Wiley.

Principles of cone beam computed tomography

Over the last 15 years, the advent of CBCT technology has revolutionized dentomaxillofacial diagnostic imaging. Technological advances now enable acquisition of high-resolution images with relatively low radiation doses. CBCT has diverse applications in dentomaxillofacial diagnosis, including assessment of potential implant sites, endodontic diagnosis and treatment planning, craniofacial assessment for orthognathic and orthodontic treatment planning, evaluation of the temporomandibular joints, paranasal sinus assessment, intraosseous pathology of the jaws, and evaluation of impacted teeth. To appropriately apply CBCT imaging for these diagnostic tasks, it is important that the clinician be familiar with the basic principles of CBCT image acquisition so that they can select patients who would benefit from this technology, and can optimize imaging protocols for specific diagnostic tasks.

Computed tomography (CT) is an imaging modality that generates cross-sectional images or "slices" of the body. The imaging equipment consists of an X-ray source and an array of detectors that are fixed within a gantry or on a C-arm. The radiation source-detector assembly rotates around the patient sequentially, acquiring planar projections at several different angles along the rotational arc. The total numbers of these two-dimensional basis projections vary from a few to several hundred. Each projection represents the pattern of X-ray attenuation by objects along the path of the X-ray beam. CT reconstruction algorithms use this attenuation data from all of the projections to reconstruct the spatial locations of the various objects within the imaged volume. This basic process of CT image generation is used by multidetector computed tomography (MDCT), used widely in medicine, and by dental CBCT units. In MDCT the radiation source is collimated to a narrow fan-shaped beam, and rotations of the gantry serially acquire contiguous and partially overlapping anatomic slices that are then assembled by the computer algorithms to generate an image volume. In CBCT, the radiation beam is collimated to a cone-shaped beam that encompasses a much broader region of the patient's anatomy. The rotation of the gantry acquires images of the entire volume, which is then reconstructed into individual slices. Although both MDCT and CBCT technologies use the same general principle to generate cross-sectional images, there are differences between these two technologies that have significance for dental applications. First, the spatial resolution of CBCT is typically higher than that of MDCT. The higher spatial resolution enables a more detailed evaluation of the dental and periodontal structures. Second, radiation doses from standard MDCT protocols are considerably higher than those from CBCT imaging procedures, and thus the detriment from radiation is significantly lower with CBCT.

CBCT offers considerable advantages over conventional periapical and panoramic imaging. A major limitation of periapical and panoramic radiography is the inherent two-dimensional nature of the images. In contrast, CBCT allows assessment of the anatomy in all three planes and can be reconstructed to provide information in virtually any plane. Second, conventional two-dimensional images are superimpositions of structures along the path of the X-ray beam, which is not the case with CBCT. Finally, there is an inherent geometric distortion of the image in both periapical and panoramic radiographs. In contrast, CBCT volumes are reconstructed without geometric distortion and thus permit accurate and reliable linear and angular measurements.

CBCT technical parameters

There are several dental CBCT units that differ in design, footprint, detector used, and the available fields of view (FOV). Importantly, there is considerable variation in the image quality and the patient radiation dose between these units, and also between individual imaging protocols of the same unit [1]. Clinicians must understand the influence of various technical components and technical parameters on image quality and radiation dose, and must optimize these parameters for specific diagnostic tasks on individual patients.

Image detector

The image detector captures X-ray photons that are transmitted through the patient to produce the two-dimensional basis projections that constitute the raw data for CT reconstruction. There are two types of digital detectors that are used in dental CBCT units. The earlier units used image intensifiers. This system uses a florescent screen to convert the X-ray photons to visible light photons, which are subsequently converted into electrons by a photocathode [2]. These electrons are accelerated by a series of electrodes and strike an output phosphor screen to produce a visible light image, which is then captured by a CCD camera. Given the multiple components, the entire image intensifier assembly is somewhat bulky. Additionally, due to designed restrictions, this system is subject to inherent and induced artifacts [2]. Notably, as the phosphor ages the intensity of the light produced upon X-ray photon capture decreases, and thus the image quality decreases during the lifetime of the image intensifier. Most currently available CBCT units use a flat-panel detector (FPD). This digital receptor uses a phosphor screen, typically made of cesium iodide or gadolinium oxysulfide, to convert X-ray photons to light photons, which are then read using a thin-film transistor array. FPDs have a greater sensitivity to X-rays and produce images with higher spatial and contrast resolution and with fewer artifacts, compared with image intensifiers [3].

Number of basis projections

As described above, a series of two-dimensional planar projections are acquired during rotation of the source and detector around the patient. The number of basis projections acquired varies between manufacturers, and also between imaging protocols of the same unit. The frame rate (projections acquired per unit time), the extent of the rotational arc, and the rotation time are interrelated factors that determine the number of projections acquired. In general, as the number of projections is increased, the spatial resolution and contrast resolution of the CT image is higher. However, increasing the number of projections also increases the radiation dose delivered to the patient. The balance between radiation dose and image quality is an important consideration for both the manufacturers and clinicians.

Some units offer the option of a "high-resolution" imaging protocol, where the number of projections acquired is increased. This requires a longer gantry rotation time and increases the chances of patient motion during imaging. Some CBCT units acquire projections using only a partial (typically 180°) rotational arc. Some high-end CBCT units offer the option of using either a complete 360° or a partial 180° arc for image capture. As described above, the impact of these imaging protocols on image quality should be considered. Some *in vitro* studies have demonstrated that the use of a partial 180° arc does not compromise diagnosis for vertical root fractures and simulated periapical lesions. However, the decreased number of basis projections decreases the contrast-to-noise ratio and increases image artifacts, such as those around metallic dental implants.

Field of view

The field of view (FOV) (Figure 5.2) is one of the most important protocol adjustments that must be determined by the clinician prescribing the CBCT scan. A smaller FOV exposes a smaller volume of patient tissue and decreases the radiation exposure compared with a larger FOV. Importantly, the spatial resolution of a smaller FOV scan is typically higher than that of a larger FOV scan. The FOV in a dental CBCT unit is typically categorized as limited or small (less than 5 cm), medium (5 to 15 cm), and large or full (greater than 15 cm). An important guiding principle is that the smallest FOV that provides adequate anatomic coverage for the diagnostic task must be used.

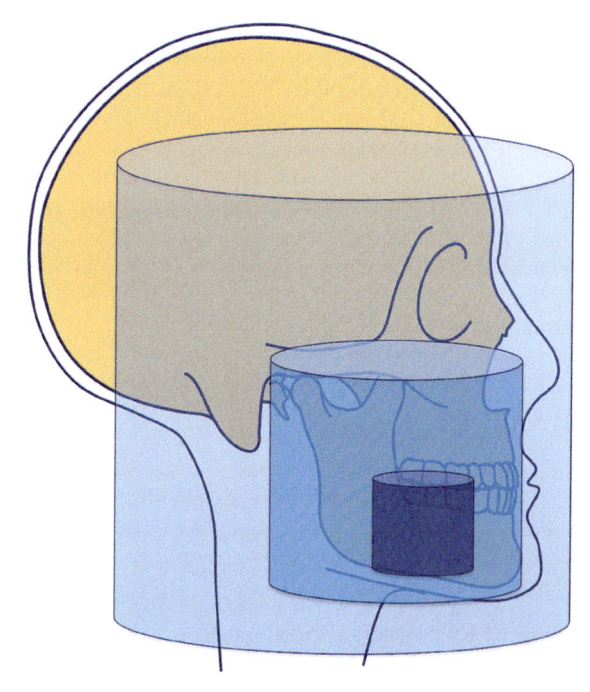

Figure 5.2 Fields of view. Schematic representation of the anatomical coverage for small (limited), medium (dentoalveolar), and large (craniofacial) fields of view. From Mallya SM, White SC: The Nature of Ionizing Radiation and the Risks from Maxillofacial Cone Beam Computed Tomography. Cone Beam Computed Tomography, John Wiley & Sons, Inc; 2013, pp. 25–41. Reproduced with permission from Wiley.

Voxel size

The voxel is the smallest three-dimensional data unit on a CBCT scan. In current CBCT systems the voxel size varies from 0.076 to 0.4 mm. In general, a smaller voxel size yields an image with higher spatial resolution. However, clinicians must recognize that voxel size is not the only determinant of image resolution. Many unit-specific parameters, such as the reconstruction algorithm used, reconstruction kernels, number of basis projections, etc., are more important determinants of the signal-to-noise ratio and spatial resolution. Thus, simply using a detector with a smaller voxel size does not necessarily yield an image with higher resolution.

X-ray exposure parameters

The X-ray tube voltage (kilovoltage, kV) and tube current (milli-amperes) must be adjusted for an individual, similar to the procedure for conventional radiography. In some CBCT units these parameters are fixed and cannot be controlled by the operator. Some CBCT units have a built-in automatic exposure control feature that customizes the tube current on a patient-specific basis. Such features are important for radiation dose reduction.

Diagnostic imaging objectives for implant treatment planning

Information from the patient history and clinical examination should be used to design an appropriate radiographic examination for an individual patient. Panoramic radiography is used for the initial radiographic evaluation of the dental implant patient and provides an overall assessment of the remaining dentition and the presence of residual roots or pathology at the edentulous sites. As needed, periapical radiographs may be used to supplement this information and provide a more critical analysis of the teeth and surrounding bone. Following this initial assessment, a more detailed evaluation of the edentulous site is needed to develop the pre-surgical implant treatment plan. This assessment requires some form of cross-sectional imaging to provide information in all three spatial planes. Approaches to cross-sectional imaging include conventional tomography, MDCT and CBCT. The American Academy of Oral and Maxillofacial Radiology (AAOMR) recommends, "any potential implant site should include cross-sectional imaging orthogonal to the site of interest" [4]. Considering radiation dose, cost, and spatial resolution, CBCT imaging is the modality of choice to provide this cross-sectional imaging. Clinicians must consider the various parameters described above to design a patient-specific CBCT imaging protocol. This must consider the anatomic coverage required to accomplish the diagnostic tasks at hand. In general, the smallest FOV that provides adequate anatomic coverage must be selected. Ideally, a radiographic stent should be used during CBCT imaging. This stent is made of acrylic and contains radiopaque markers that indicate the sites of proposed implant placement (Figure 5.3). The radiopaque markers may be simple gutta-percha cylinders or may be more elaborate markers that show the location and contours of the proposed restorations. This latter approach allows better collaboration between the restorative dentist, the radiologist, and the implant surgeon.

The specific diagnostic objectives of radiographic imaging are:

1 *To evaluate the morphology of the edentulous site and the amount of residual alveolar bone available for implant placement.* The amount of available bone volume is an important consideration in the implant treatment planning process. It guides decisions on the number of implants that can be placed at the edentulous span,

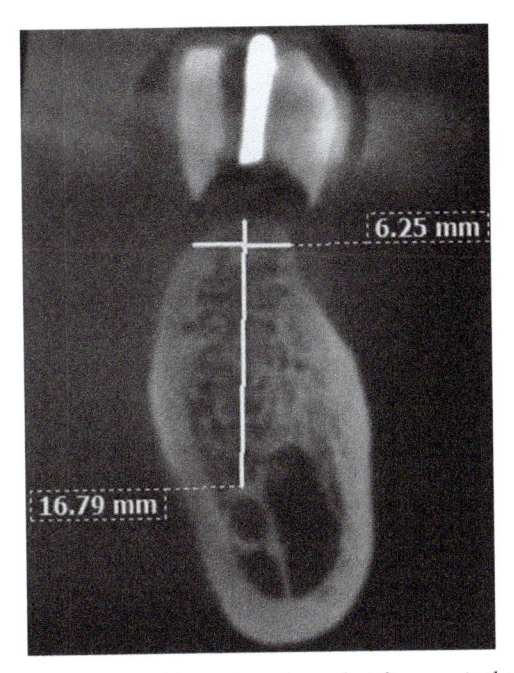

Figure 5.3 Cross-sectional image through an edentulous area in the mandible. The imaging stent incorporates a radiopaque marker and demonstrates the contours of the planned restoration. The measurements indicate the vertical height from the crest of the ridge to the superior cortication of the mandibular canal and the width of the ridge just below the crest.

consists of a thin shell of cortical bone that surrounds sparse and poorly mineralized trabecular bone. Types II and III have intermediate amounts of cortical bone with an adequate amount of well-mineralized trabecular bone. Currently, the quality of bone is assessed subjectively by visual radiographic evaluation. Based on the high success of dental implants, as reported in the literature, it is likely that this visual assessment of the implant site bone quality is adequate for clinical success of implant placement and osseointegration. This visual assessment must include an evaluation of cortical thickness, the trabecular radiodensity, and the presence of any sclerotic areas that may compromise implant placement (Figure 5.5).

The data in a CT scan is compartmentalized into discrete voxels, each represented by a numerical value or a CT number that describes the gray value of that voxel within the imaged volume. In MDCT units, the CT numbers are expressed as Hounsfield units (HUs), which express X-ray attenuation of a voxel relative to the attenuation of water. However, dental CBCT units do not use a standard scaling system. Importantly, the CT numbers in a CBCT unit are strongly influenced by several factors including exposure parameters, FOV, and the location of the object within the image volume [6–9]. Thus, measurement of CT numbers on a CBCT scan is not a reliable quantitative measure of the amount of X-ray attenuation and should not be used to infer the degree of mineralization of bone. Many software programs provide tools to measure the gray values either within a region of interest or at a specific point in the image, and clinicians must be wary of using these tools to make decisions on the bone quality.

as well as the positions and dimensions of the individual implants. CBCT imaging provides accurate measurements of the bucco-lingual width and vertical height of the residual alveolar ridge (Figure 5.3). These measurements allow the clinician to determine the available bone volume and, in particular, the maximum dimensions of the implant that can be placed at the site. Importantly, CBCT provides an assessment of the extent of buccolingual resorption, which is not evident on two-dimensional radiographs (Figure 5.4). Furthermore, measurement of the edentulous span provides guidance on the number of implants that can be placed. When deficiencies in bone volume are identified, the measurements provide an assessment of the degree of inadequacy that must be corrected and an indication of the type of surgical procedure needed to augment the alveolar ridge. For example, mild deficiencies may be amenable to augmentation with bone graft material or ridge expansion at the time of implant placement. Alternatively, severe deficiencies may require a more elaborate surgical augmentation, for example with block bone grafts or with sinus elevation.

2 *To evaluate the architecture and quality of the trabecular and cortical bone at potential implant sites.* In addition to bone volume, the local quality of bone is an important factor for implant success. Bone at the implant site should provide primary implant stability and a pre-implant environment that is conducive to osseointegration. Typically, the quality of bone is determined by a visual assessment that considers the amounts of trabecular and cortical bone at the implant site. The most widely used classification of bone quality is that proposed by Lekholm and Zarb [5], which categorizes bone into four types depending on the thickness of the cortical bone and the density of the trabecular bone. Type I bone is composed of almost entirely cortical bone, whereas type IV

3 *To identify anatomical structures and variations and pathological conditions that constrain implant placement.* An important aspect of evaluation of the edentulous site is to identify critical anatomical structures. These include the nasopalatine canal, incisive foramen, floor of the nasal cavity, maxillary sinus, mandibular canal, the mental foramen, and the lingual foramen. Critical evaluation of the location and course of the neurovascular canals is particularly important to prevent damaging these structures during implant placement. Typically, the cortical outlines of the structures are seen as radiopaque lines. However, in some patients, especially those with osteopenia or osteoporosis, the cortical boundaries may be thin or indistinct, and in these cases it is crucial to appropriately identify the lumen of the canal.

(a) *Nasopalatine canal and incisive foramen.* The nasopalatine canal is located in the mid-line, immediately palatal to the maxillary central incisors. It transmits the descending palatine artery and the nasopalatine nerve. The incisive foramen is the opening of this canal on the palate. The size and shape of the nasopalatine canal and the incisive foramen varies considerably. These structures are visualized on periapical and panoramic images. However, its course, and the relationship to the adjacent teeth, is best appreciated on sagittal and axial CBCT sections (Figure 5.6).

(b) *Nasal cavity.* The nasal cavity can be visualized as a radiolucent airspace above the palate. In the mid-line, the cavity is divided by the nasal septum. The floor of the nasal cavity is seen as crisp radiopaque lines. Thin bony projections called conchae arise from the lateral nasal wall. These bony projections are encased in a thick mucosal covering, called turbinates (Figure 5.7).

(c) *Maxillary sinus.* The maxillary sinus is one of the four paranasal sinuses – maxillary, ethmoid, sphenoid, and frontal sinuses. The orbital floor forms the roof of the maxillary sinus. The maxillary sinus floor is seen in the dentoalveolar bone, often

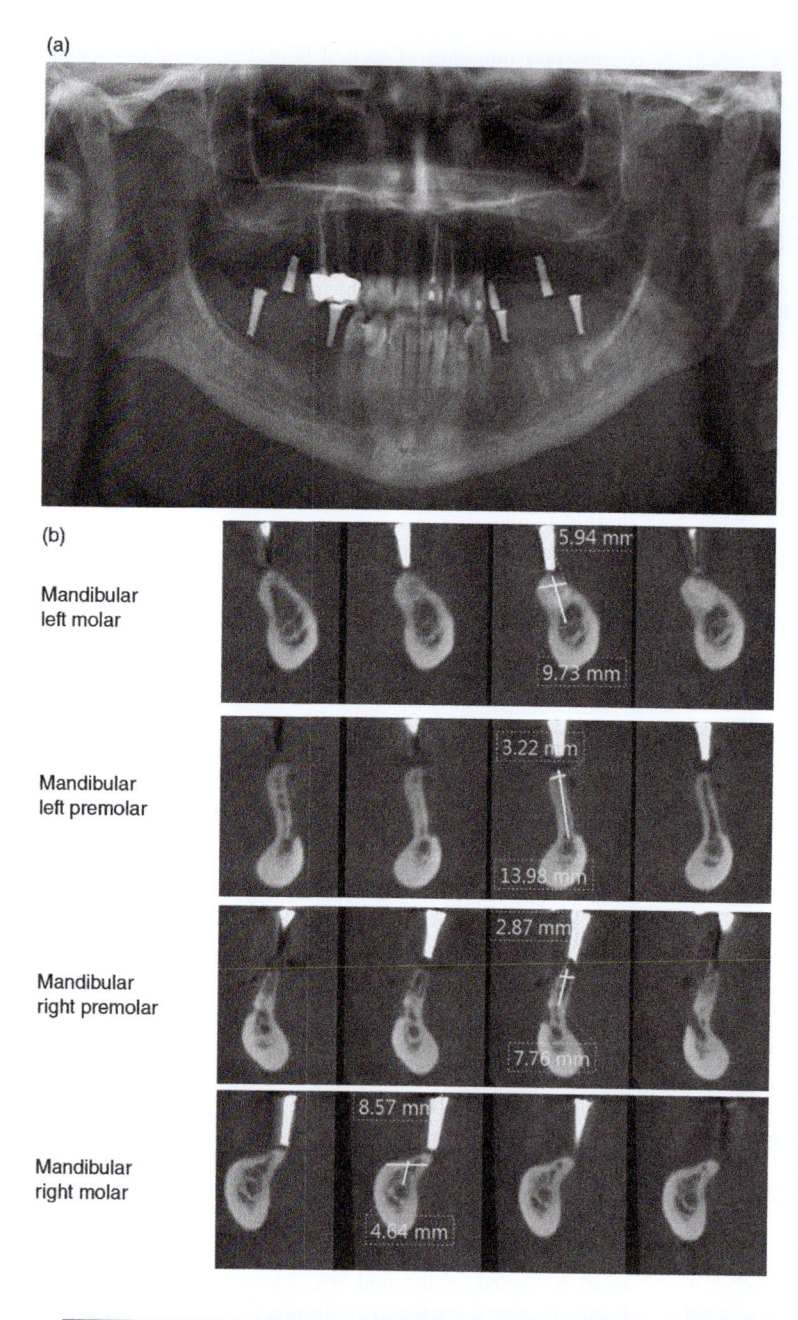

Figure 5.4 (a) Panoramic radiograph showing a partially edentulous maxilla and mandible. Radiopaque markers are used to indicate sites of implant placement. (b) CBCT cross-sections through the mandibular edentulous areas. Note marked resorption of the buccolingual dimensions of the residual ridge that is not evident on the panoramic radiograph.

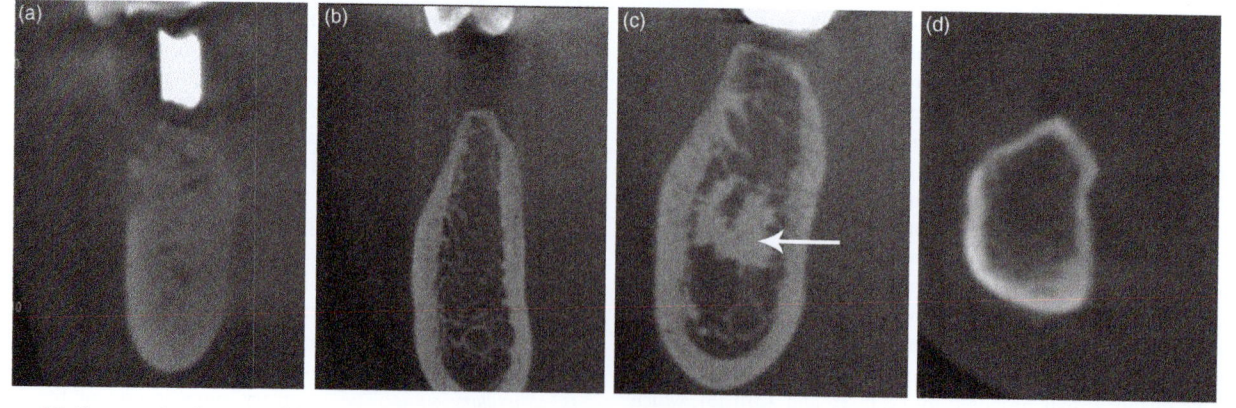

Figure 5.5 Cross-sectional images of the mandible of four different patients, demonstrating differences in bone quality. (a) Marked sclerosis involving the entire thickness of the mandible, extending from the crest to the inferior border. (b) Well-trabeculated bone with thick cortices. (c) Adequate thickness of cortical bone with adequate trabecular density at the crest. However, note an area of ostesclerosis (arrow). (d) Thin buccal and lingual cortices with sparse trabecular bone.

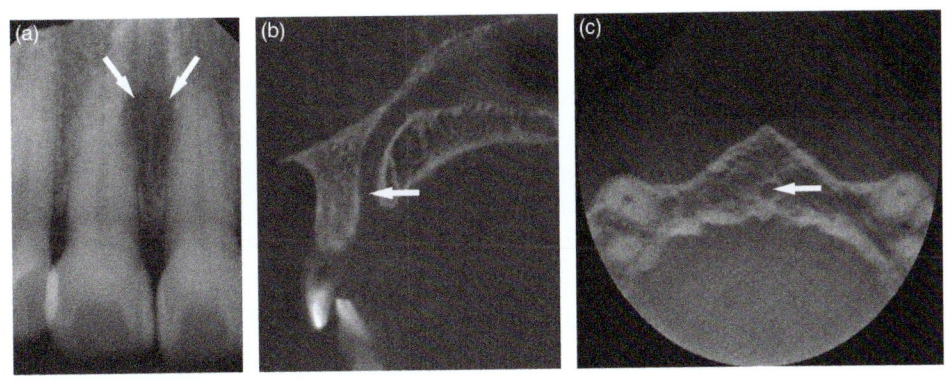

Figure 5.6 (a) Periapical radiograph showing the incisive foramen. (b) Midsagittal CBCT section showing the nasopalatine canal and incisive foramen. (c) Axial CBCT section showing the opening of the incisive foramen on the palate.

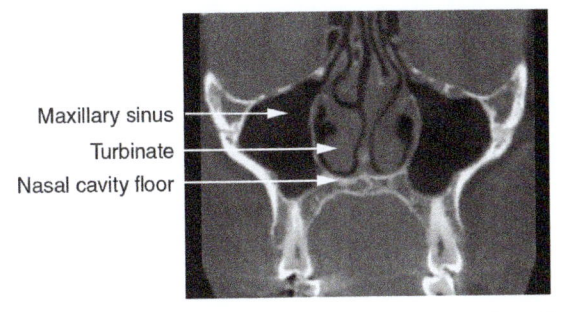

Figure 5.7 Coronal CBCT section showing the nasal cavity and maxillary sinuses.

contacting the lamia dura around the molar teeth and dipping into the interdental bone (Figure 5.8).

When maxillary sinus elevation is contemplated, the anatomy of the maxillary sinus must be evaluated with particular emphasis on the presence of the septa and neurovascular canals. Maxillary sinus septae arise from the floor or walls and extend into the sinus lumen (Figure 5.9). Depending on the length, they may partially divide the sinus into two or more cavities. The presence of the septae may increase the risk of perforation of the Schneiderian membrane, especially when using the lateral window approach for sinus augmentation. Additionally, depending on the location and height of the septa, the location of the lateral window may

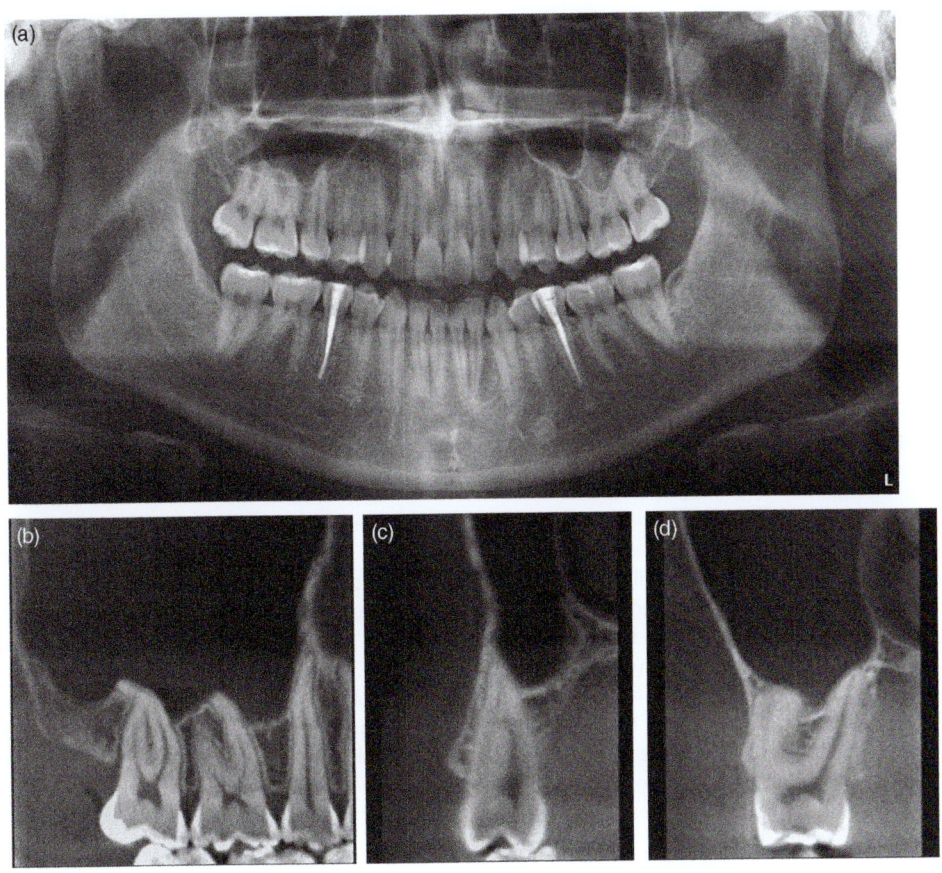

Figure 5.8 (a) Panoramic radiograph. The extent of the maxillary sinuses is clearly portrayed as radiolucent with a sharply demarcated radiopaque border. (b–d) Sagittal and coronal CBCT sections through the premolar and molar teeth showing the close relationship between the maxillary sinus floor and the tooth roots.

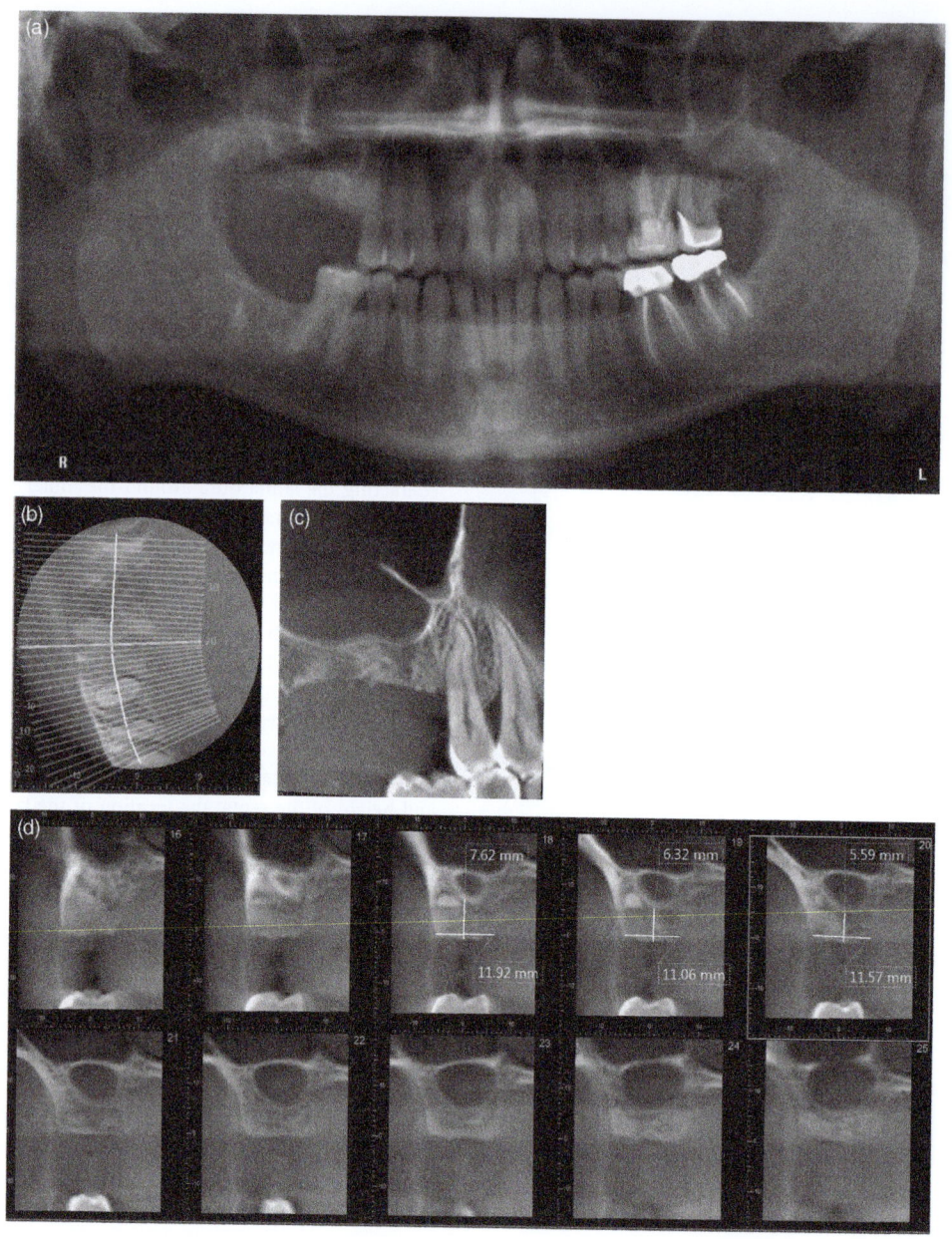

Figure 5.9 (a) Panoramic and (b–d) CBCT sections for implant planning in the maxillary right molar region. (b) Axial section showing locations of cross-sections depicted in panel D. (c) Sagittal section showing a septa arising from the floor in the anterior region of the maxillary sinus. (d) Panel of cross-sections that demonstrate the septa and the partial division of the maxillary sinus into locules. Also note the presence of a residual root.

need to be altered. Second, the location of the posterior superior alveolar artery within the lateral wall of the maxillary sinus must be identified (Figure 5.10). This is usually identified as an indentation or sometimes a discrete canal on the lateral wall of the maxillary sinus. Damage to this artery can cause excessive bleeding during surgery. It is important for the clinician to recognize that the vessel is recognized indirectly by the presence of an indentation on the lateral wall, and in the absence of this feature it is not possible to identify the vessel on CBCT scans. Thus, even in the absence of this radiographic feature, clinicians must contemplate potential complications from vessel damage.

(d) *Mandibular canal.* When planning implants in the posterior mandible, it is essential to identify the mandibular canal and trace its course through the mandibular ramus and body. On panoramic radiographs, the canal is seen as two distinct radiopaque lines extending from the ramus to the mental foramen, seen as an oval radiolucency, typically between the premolar roots (Figure 5.11). On cross-sectional CBCT images, the canal is seen as a round or oval lucency with well-corticated borders. Often, the cortication of the canal may be thin or indistinct. The relationship of the canal relative to the tooth roots and to the crest of the residual ridge must be assessed. Anatomic variations include bifid mandibular canals, an accessory mental foramen, and an anterior loop of the canal, where the canal extends anterior to the mental foramen, loops backward, and then exits through the mental foramen. Anatomic variations are often

Radiographic Evaluation of the Alveolar Ridge in Implant Dentistry 45

noted, for example bifurcation of the mandibular canal and the presence of additional foramina (Figure 5.12).

Sometimes, the mandibular incisive canal may be evident, seen as an anterior extension of the canal lumen beyond the mental foramen to the mandibular anterior region. Additionally, the opening of the lingual foramen, adjacent to the genial tubercles in the anterior mandible must be identified (Figure 5.13). The mandibular incisive neurovascular bundle supplies the anterior mandibular teeth. When the anterior mandible is edentulous, damage to the mandibular incisive nerve does not cause any neurological deficit. However, damage to the blood vessels may result in excessive bleeding, which may complicate implant placement.

(e) *Anatomic variants.* Other anatomic variations of importance in implant placement are undercuts on the alveolar ridge. These are typically noted on the lingual aspect of the posterior mandible (Figure 5.14) and on the buccal aspect of the anterior maxilla.

A less frequent, but clinically significant anatomic variation, is the canalis sinuosus, which houses the anterior superior alveolar neurovascular bundle. Sometimes this canal extends from the floor of the nasal cavity through the maxillary alveolar ridge to exit on to the palatal cortical plate (Figure 5.15). Depending on its size, damage to this vessel may result in excessive bleeding during implant placement at the site.

The edentulous site must also be evaluated critically for signs of pathology or altered bone architecture. For example, irregular lytic changes may suggest the presence of residual inflammation. Additionally, the presence of excessive sclerosis, for example

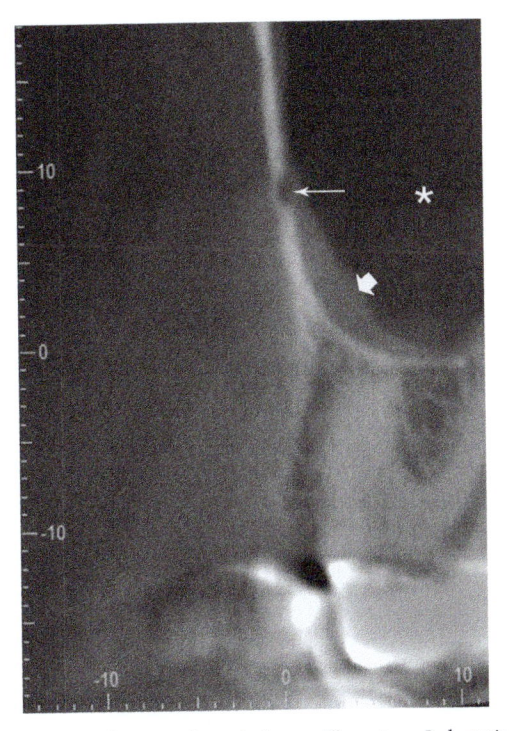

Figure 5.10 Coronal section through the maxillary sinus. Indentation of the posterior superior alveolar vessel into the wall of the maxillary sinus is noted (arrow). Also note trace mucosal thickening on the sinus floor (arrowhead). The lumen of the sinus is indicated by the asterisk.

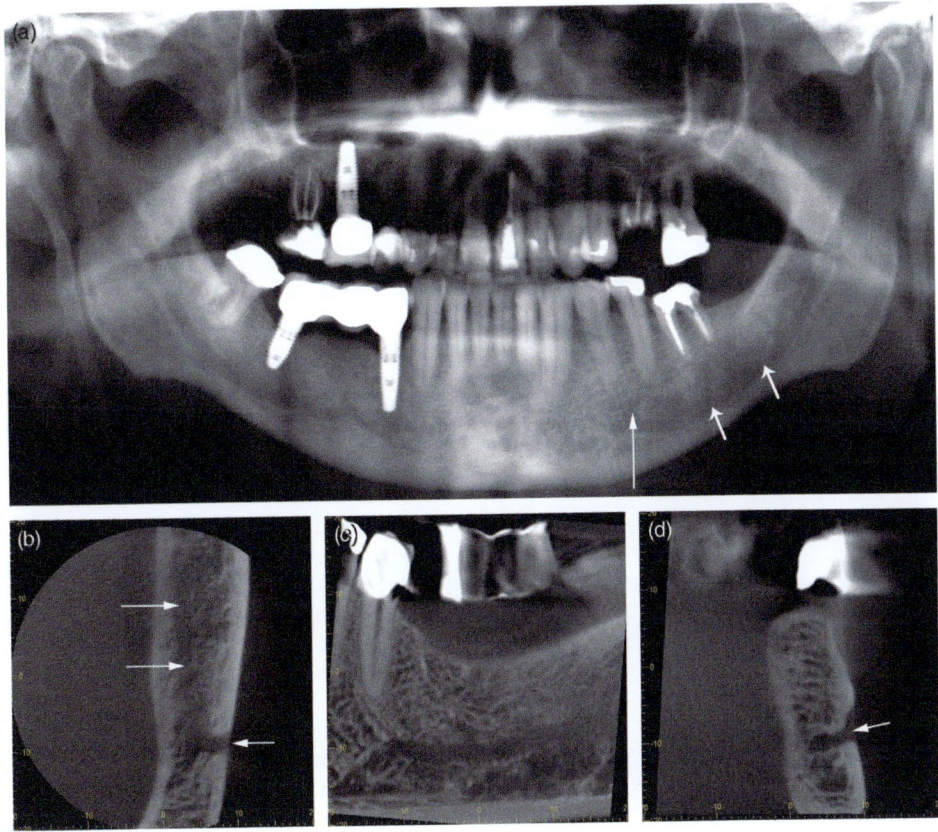

Figure 5.11 (a) Panoramic radiograph showing the course of the mandibular canal (short arrows) and the opening of the mental foramen (long arrow). (b–d) Axial, sagittal, and cross-sectional CBCT sections. Note how these sections provide a better assessment of the canal course and location of the mental foramen.

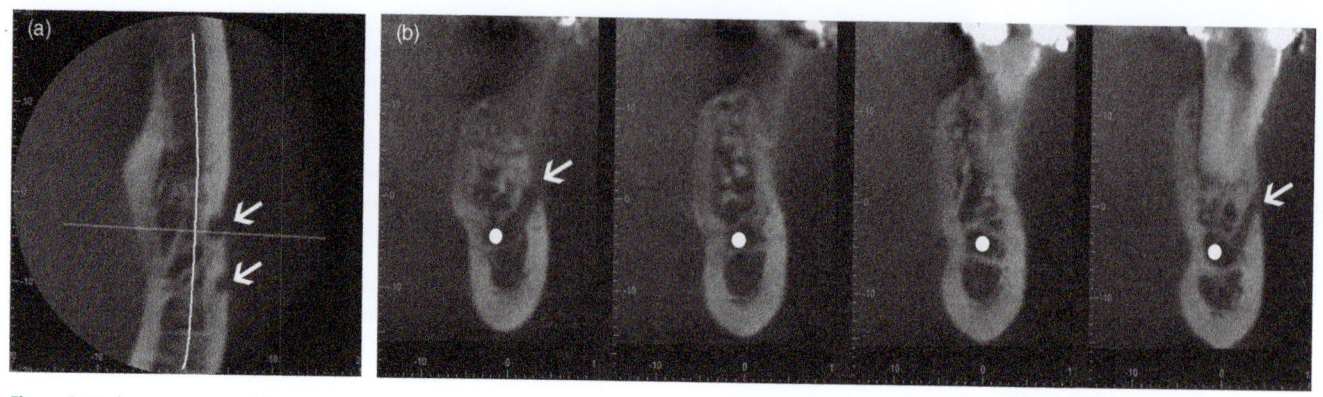

Figure 5.12 Accessory mental foramen. **(a)** Axial section of the mandibular left premolar region. **(b)** CBCT cross-sections showing the locations of the mandibular canal (white dot) and the exit of the mandibular canal to two discrete mental foramina (arrows).

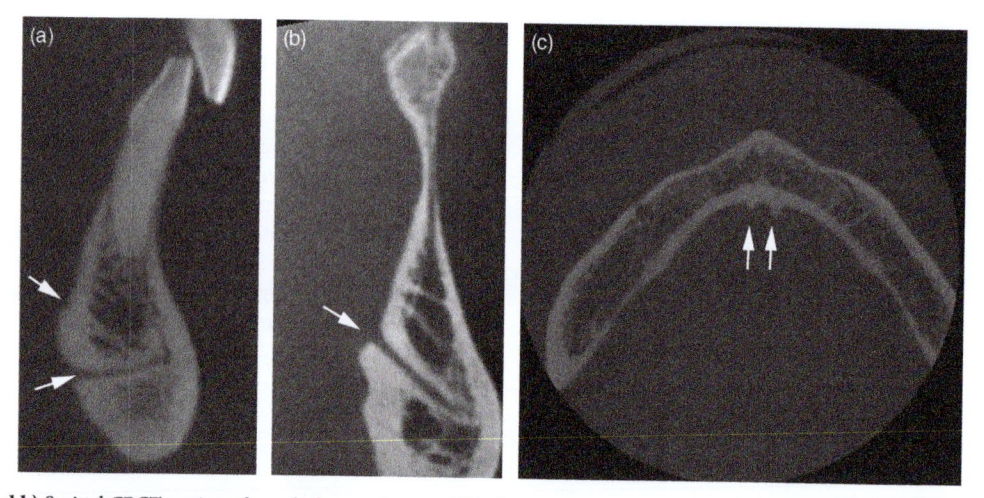

Figure 5.13 **(a and b)** Sagittal CBCT sections through the anterior mandible showing the locations and course of the lingual canals and lingual foramen. **(c)** The lingual foramen is typically located between the genial tubercles, seen as small protuberances from the lingual cortex of the anterior mandible in the mid-line.

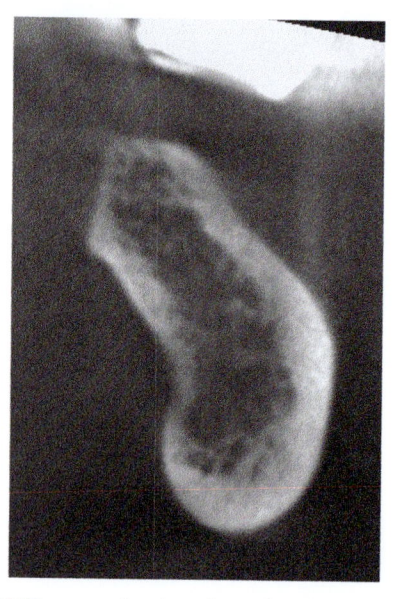

Figure 5.14 CBCT cross-section through an edentulous region in the mandibular molar region. Note the lingual inclination of the alveolar ridge and the marked undercut on the lingual aspect of the mandible.

from regions of osteosclerosis (Figure 5.16) or fibro-osseous lesions, may complicate implant placement.

4 *Pre-surgical and post-surgical evaluation of bone augmentation prior to implant placement.* When the initial clinical and CBCT assessment identifies a need for bone augmentation prior to implant placement, CBCT provides valuable information that guides selection and design of the augmentation procedure.

CBCT provides excellent visualization of pathological changes within the maxillary sinus, including thickening of the sinus mucosa, mucus retention phenomena, polyps and mucoceles (Figure 5.17). Depending on the FOV acquired, such sinus pathology may only be partially visualized on the CBCT scan. In these cases, it may be necessary to acquire an additional CBCT scan that encompasses all of the paranasal sinuses to assess the general sinus health as it pertains to the sinus graft procedure. When evaluating the sinus, the patency of the ostium must be assessed (Figure 5.18).

CBCT also allows evaluation of the location of the donor site for block grafts, such as the mandibular symphysis and ramus. For example, cortical bone grafts are often harvested from the posterior mandibular body. The buccolingual location and orientation of the mandibular canal must be assessed in order to

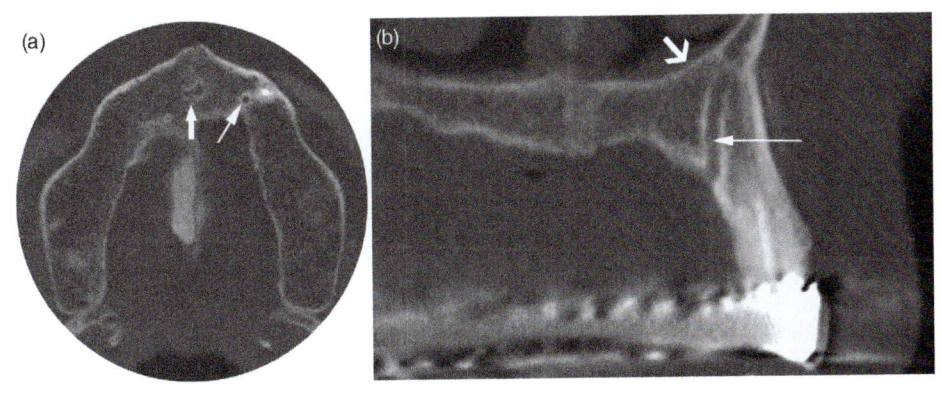

Figure 5.15 Canalis sinuosus. (a) Axial section through the maxillary alveolus showing the nasopalatine canals (solid arrow) and the canalis sinuosus (thin arrow), located palatal to the maxillary canine. (b) Cross-sectional slice showing the course of the canalis sinuosus (thin arrow) from the nasal floor (arrowhead) to the palatal cortex.

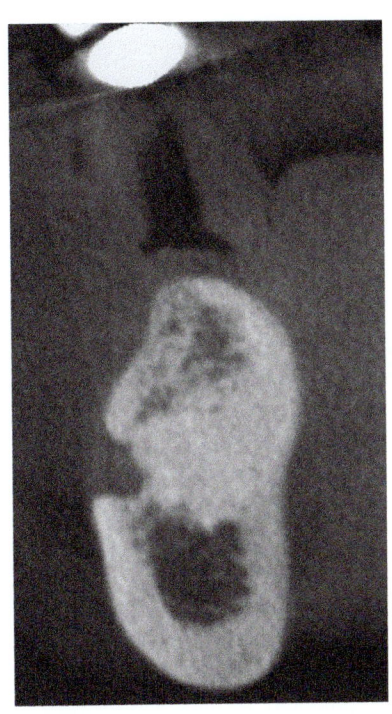

Figure 5.16 CBCT section showing the presence of a large area of osteosclerosis in the edentulous ridge. Due to reduced vascularity, this may complicate implant osseointegration.

determine the maximum thickness of the graft that can be harvested and to prevent damage to the inferior alveolar nerve.

CBCT should also be considered to evaluate the outcome of bone augmentation procedures (Figures 5.19 and 5.20). Evidence of successful augmentation includes an increase in the vertical and/or horizontal dimension of the alveolar ridge, successful integration of the allogenic or autologous graft into the underlying trabecular bone, and the absence of signs of any local inflammatory changes within and around the graft. Failure of sinus grafts may evoke inflammatory changes in the sinus mucosa, evidenced by mucosal thickening (Figure 5.21).

5 *To develop a prosthetically driven treatment plan that considers esthetics and function.* The overall success of implant-supported restorations depends not only on implant osseointegration but also on achieving hard and soft tissue contours that are esthetic and functional. This is particularly important when implants are placed within the esthetic zone. The use of well-fabricated radiographic stents that identify the locations and contours of the proposed restorations contributes to achieving this goal. More sophisticated approaches include the use of third-party software programs that use CBCT data to develop an implant treatment plan *in silico* (Figure 5.22) and to translate this plan into a computer-generated surgical guide. The use of such technology allows for more effective collaboration between clinicians involved in the diagnosis and treatment planning aspects of implant placement and restoration. The success of implants placed using computer-fabricated surgical guides is comparable to implants placed following conventional procedures. However, clinicians must be aware of the accuracy of such systems. A recent meta-analysis showed that the mean error in the planned versus placed position is 0.9 mm at the entry point and 1.3 mm at the implant apex, with a mean angular deviation of 3.5° [10]. Importantly, the range of these measurements was wide [10]. It is particularly important that clinicians consider the sources of error in the systems and appropriately plan for an adequate safety zone to avoid damage to critical structures such as neurovascular bundles.

6 *To evaluate post-surgical implant complications.* CBCT imaging is also of value in post-surgical evaluation of the implant, specifically to assess potential complications of implant placement. These include perforations of the cortical plates (Figure 5.23) or adjacent vital structures. An example of such a situation is a patient who develops pain, neurological deficit, or altered sensation following implant placement in the posterior mandible. In such situations, CBCT is the modality of choice to provide information on the potential damage to the mandibular canal. Likewise, patients who demonstrate implant mobility or signs of infection around the implant site should also be imaged using CBCT. In evaluating these scans, it is important that the clinician remember that beam-hardening artifacts around the metallic implant appear as radiolucent areas, and thus bone around the implant cannot be critically evaluated. Finally, all patients in whom implant retrieval is planned should be imaged with CBCT to assess the amount of bone around the implant and to evaluate the position of the implant in relation to adjacent critical structures such as neurovascular bundles, maxillary sinus, and the nasal cavity.

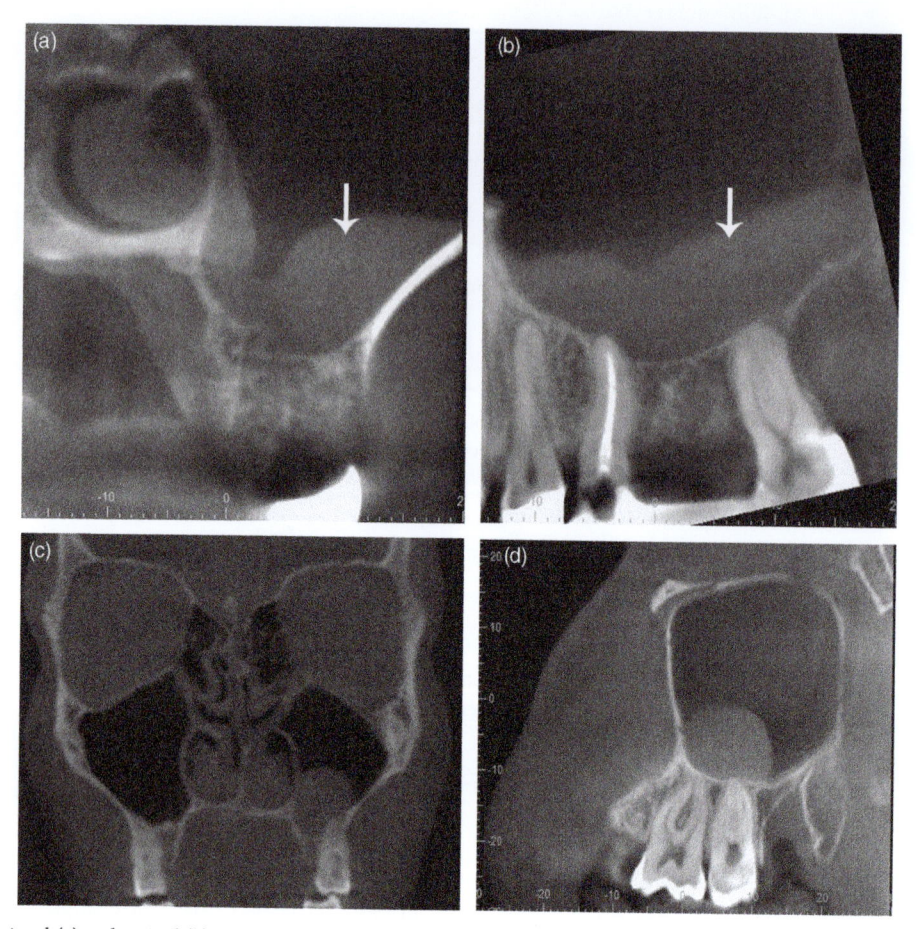

Figure 5.17 Cross-sectional (**a**) and sagittal (**b**) sections showing thickening of the maxillary sinus mucosa (arrow). The floor of the maxillary sinus is seen as an intact cortical line. (**c and d**) Dome-shaped radiopacities in the maxillary sinus with no evidence of bony displacement or destruction suggestive of mucous retention phenomenon.

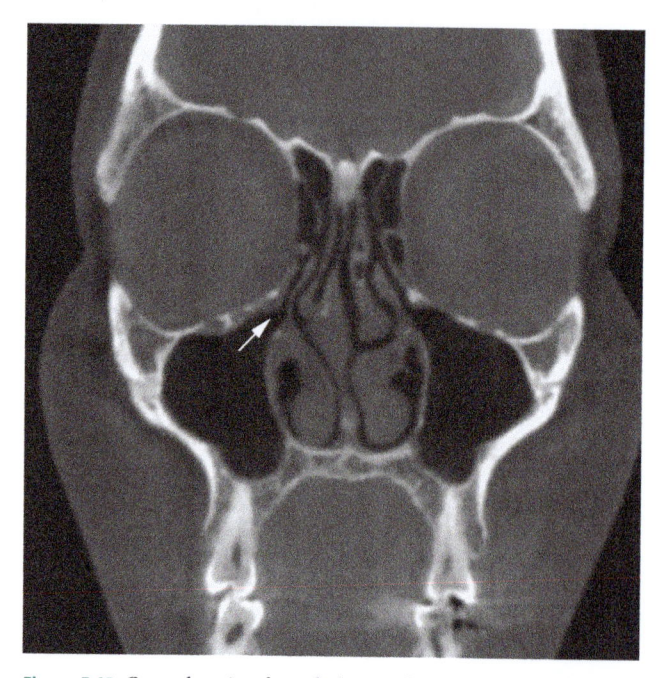

Figure 5.18 Coronal section through the maxillary sinuses. Note that both maxillary sinuses are clear without evidence of mucosal thickening or other soft tissue changes. The ostium on the right side is indicated with an arrow.

Radiation risks from CBCT examinations

The premise of all diagnostic radiological examinations is that the benefit from the procedure far outweighs the risks associated with radiation exposure. As described above, there is a strong rationale to use CBCT as an imaging modality for pre-surgical implant treatment planning and selected cases for evaluation of post-surgical complications from implant placement. There is vast literature on the radiation doses delivered by CBCT examinations. These dosimetric studies use tissue-equivalent anthropomorphic phantoms to measure the absorbed dose at specific organ sites, and this is then used to calculate the effective dose from a specific CBCT examination. It is important that the clinician understands the concept of effective dose – a unit used to convey the net detriment from a radiographic examination, which can be used to compare radiation risks between different modalities, imaging protocols, and radiographic procedures that expose different regions of the body. For example, the risk of a maxillofacial CBCT examination with an effective dose of 40 microSieverts is considered to be approximately 2 times higher than the risk from a panoramic radiograph with an effective dose of 20 microSieverts.

There is considerable variation in radiation doses from CBCT units from different manufacturers. Additionally, the magnitude of

Radiographic Evaluation of the Alveolar Ridge in Implant Dentistry | 49

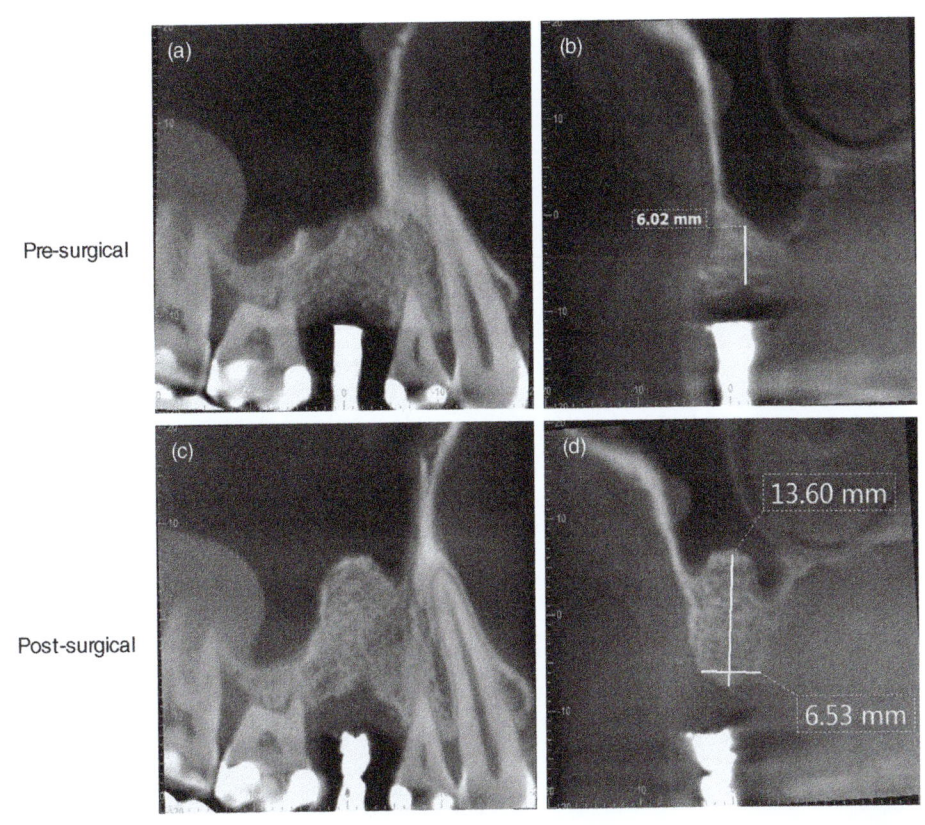

Figure 5.19 Sagittal (**a and c**) and cross-sectional (**b and d**) sections showing pre-surgical and post-surgical evaluation of the maxillary sinus. Note the heterogeneous graft material in c and d that blends into the adjacent trabecular bone. The augmentation procedure has yielded additional height and width for implant placement.

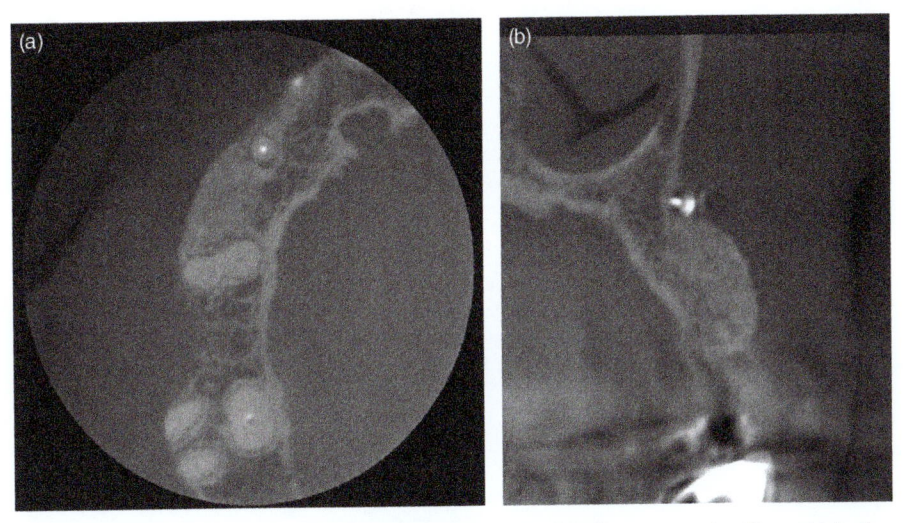

Figure 5.20 (**a**) Axial and (**b**) cross-sectional slices showing uptake of bone graft material used to augment the ridge width in the maxillary premolar region. Note how the graft material blends with the underlying trabecular bone.

radiation dose delivered is strongly dependent on the specific protocol used, particularly the FOV size. Table 5.1 summarizes the ranges of the effective doses for small, medium, and large FOV protocols. In conveying radiation doses to patients, it is useful to describe these doses relative to natural background radiation, and these are also included in Table 5.1.

Guidelines and position statements on CBCT use in diagnosis and treatment planning of the dental implant patient

Several professional organizations have developed guidelines for CBCT use in implant diagnosis and treatment planning. These include the AAOMR [4], Academy for Osseointegration [11],

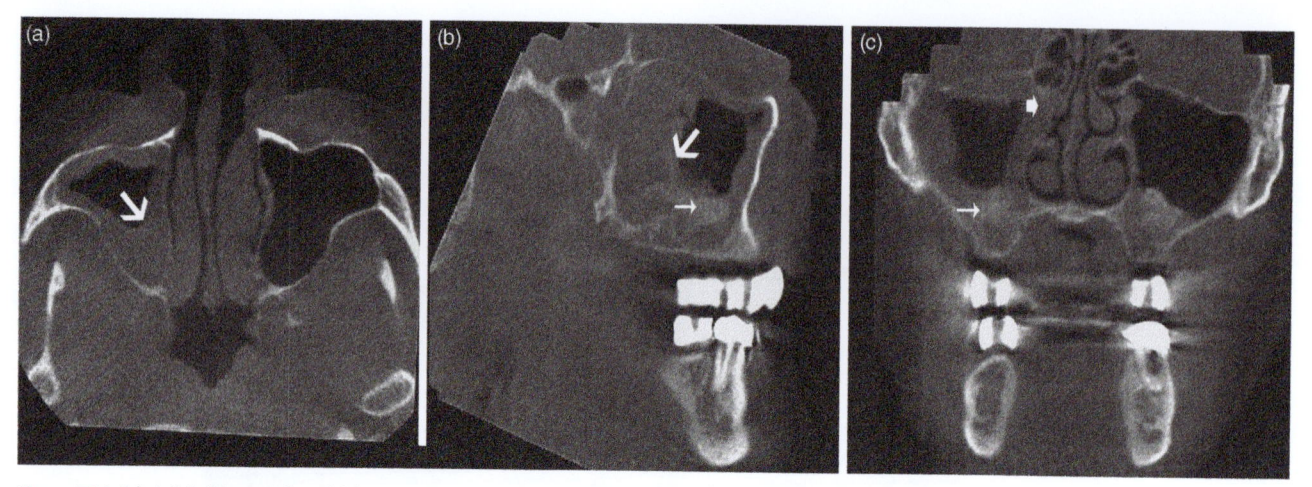

Figure 5.21 (a) Axial, (b) sagittal, and (c) coronal sections showing failure of uptake of the sinus graft material. Marked mucosal thickening (small arrows) is present, surrounding interspersed radiopaque graft material (large arrows). Note blockage of the right maxillary sinus ostium by the mucosal thickening (arrowhead).

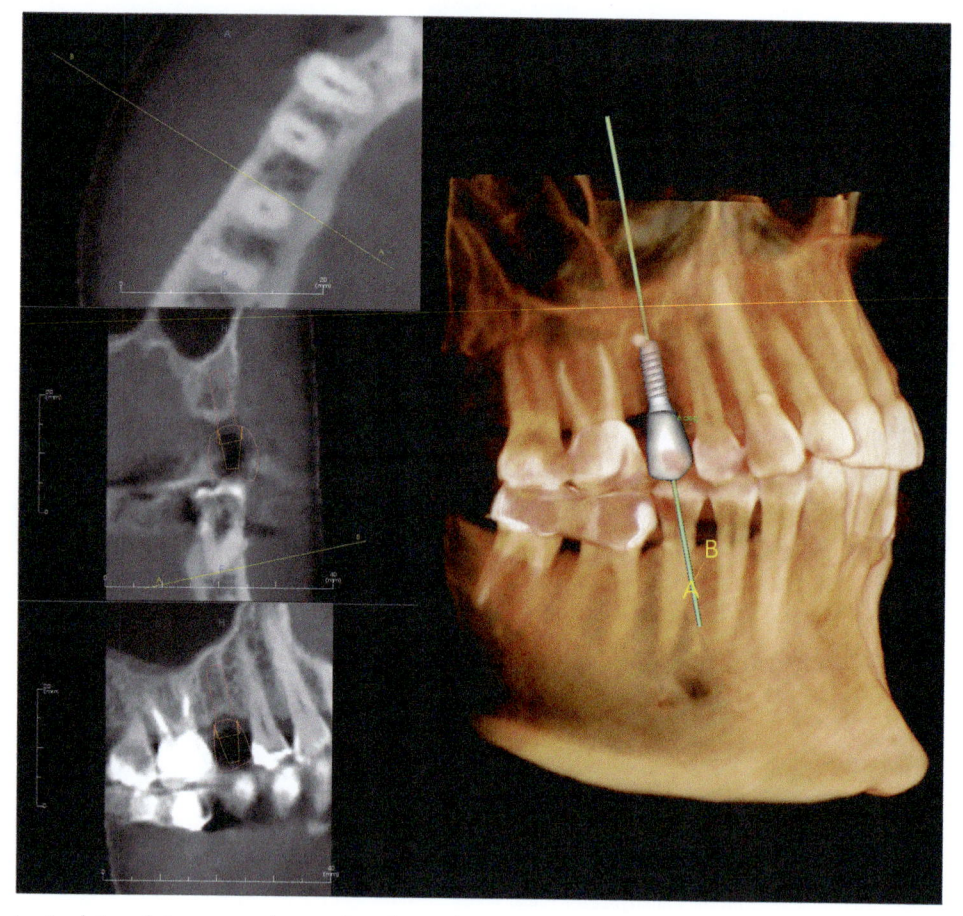

Figure 5.22 Computer simulation of placement and restoration of an implant using Anatomage *in vivo* software.

European Academy of Osseointegration [12], the International Congress of Oral Implantologists (ICOI) [13], and the International Team for Implantology (ITI) [14]. The AAOMR specifically recommends that CBCT be considered the imaging modality of choice for pre-surgical cross-sectional imaging of potential implant sites [4]. Likewise, the ICOI Consensus Panel concluded that "Because the 3-D information gained with CBCT scans cannot be obtained with other 2-D imaging modalities, it is virtually impossible to predict which treatment cases would not benefit from having this additional information before obtaining it" [13]. Given the strong recommendations from professional organizations regarding CBCT use, it would be prudent for

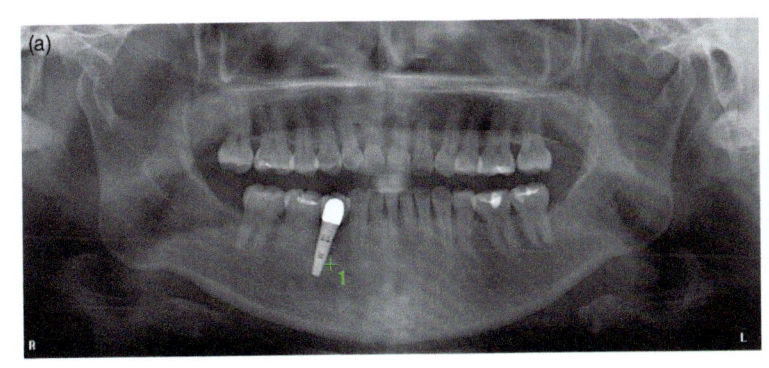

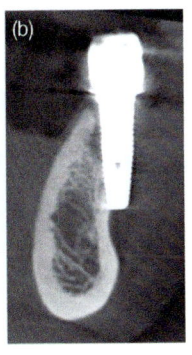

Figure 5.23 (a) Panoramic radiograph and (b) CBCT cross-sectional image taken to evaluate an implant placed in the mandibular right premolar region. Note perforation and a dehiscence defect along the lingual cortical plate. This is clearly evident on the CBCT scan but is not depicted in the panoramic radiograph.

Table 5.1 Effective doses from selected CBCT and dentomaxillofacial radiographic examinations.

Examination	Effective dose* (microSv)	Equivalent background radiation (days)†
CBCT small (limited) field of view	13–44	2–5
CBCT medium field of view		
Standard protocol	28–548	3–65
High resolution protocol	68–652	8–77
CBCT large field of view	30–1073	4–126
Intraoral radiographs		
Bitewings (PSP/F-speed, rectangular collimation)	5	0.6
(PSP/F-speed, rectangular collimation)	35	4
(PSP/F-speed, round collimation)	171	20
Panoramic (digital, CCD-based)	14–24	2–3
Lateral cephalometric (digital, PSP-based)	6	0.7

Adapted from Mallya SM, White SC: *The Nature of Ionizing Radiation and the Risks from Maxillofacial Cone Beam Computed Tomography. Cone Beam Computed Tomography*, John Wiley & Sons, Inc, 2013, pp. 25–41.
*Doses are rounded to the nearest whole number.
†Calculation of background equivalent days is based on an annual exposure of 3.1 milliSv. For doses above 10 microSv, the background equivalent days are rounded to the nearest whole number.

clinicians to prescribe CBCT imaging for pre-surgical evaluation of all dental implant patients. To that end, clinicians must also be aware of the clinical liabilities associated with acquiring CBCT images. In addition to the specific implant site, the entire CBCT scan must be evaluated for potential pathology. As needed, dentists who are not well versed with the full scope of CBCT imaging should seek the expertise of an appropriate specialist, such as an oral and maxillofacial radiologist, to provide a full interpretation of the imaged volume.

References

1. Pauwels R, Beinsberger J, Stamatakis H, Tsiklakis K, Walker A, Bosmans H, et al: Comparison of spatial and contrast resolution for cone-beam computed tomography scanners. *Oral Surg Oral Med Oral Pathol Oral Radiol* 2012;**114**(1):127–135.
2. Wang J, Blackburn TJ: The AAPM/RSNA physics tutorial for residents: X-ray image intensifiers for fluoroscopy. *Radiographics* 2000;**20**(5):1471–1477.
3. Seibert JA: Flat-panel detectors: how much better are they? *Pediatric Radiology* 2006;**36**(Suppl 14):173–181.
4. Tyndall DA, Price JB, Tetradis S, Ganz SD, Hildebolt C, Scarfe WC: Position statement of the American Academy of Oral and Maxillofacial Radiology on selection criteria for the use of radiology in dental implantology with emphasis on cone beam computed tomography. *Oral Surg Oral Med Oral Pathol Oral Radiol* 2012;**113**(6):817–826.
5. Lekholm U, Zarb GA: Patient selection and preparation. In: Branemark PI, Zarb GA, Albektsson T (eds.), *Tissue Integrated Prostheses Osseointegration in Clinical Dentistry*, 3rd edn. Quintessence Publishing Co., Chicago, IL, 1985, pp. 199–209.
6. Nomura Y, Watanabe H, Honda E, Kurabayashi T: Reliability of voxel values from cone-beam computed tomography for dental use in evaluating bone mineral density. *Clin Oral Implants Res* 2010;**21**(5):558–562.
7. Oliveira ML, Tosoni GM, Lindsey DH, Mendoza K, Tetradis S, Mallya SM: Influence of anatomical location on CT numbers in cone beam computed tomography. *Oral Surg Oral Med Oral Pathol Oral Radiol* 2013;**115**(4):558–564.
8. Oliveira ML, Tosoni GM, Lindsey DH, Mendoza K, Tetradis S, Mallya SM: Assessment of CT numbers in limited and medium field-of-view scans taken using Accuitomo 170 and Veraviewepocs 3De cone-beam computed tomography scanners. *Imaging Science in Dentistry* 2014;**44**(4):279–285.
9. Pauwels R, Nackaerts O, Bellaiche N, Stamatakis H, Tsiklakis K, Walker A, et al: Variability of dental cone beam CT grey values for density estimations. *Br J Radiol* 2013;**86**(1021):20120135
10. Bornstein MM, Al-Nawas B, Kuchler U, Tahmaseb A: Consensus statements and recommended clinical procedures regarding contemporary surgical and radiographic techniques in implant dentistry. *Int J Oral Maxillofac Implants* 2014;**29**(Suppl):78–82.
11. 2010 Guidelines of the Academy of Osseointegration for the provision of dental implants and associated patient care. *Int J Oral Maxillofac Implants* 2010;**25**(3):620–627.
12. Harris D, Horner K, Grondahl K, Jacobs R, Helmrot E, Benic GI, et al: E.A.O. guidelines for the use of diagnostic imaging in implant dentistry 2011. A consensus workshop organized by the European Association for Osseointegration at the Medical University of Warsaw. *Clin Oral Implants Res* 2012;**23**(11):1243–1253.
13. Benavides E, Rios HF, Ganz SD, An CH, Resnik R, Reardon GT, et al: Use of cone beam computed tomography in implant dentistry: the International Congress of Oral Implantologists consensus report. *Implant Dent* 2012;**21**(2):78–86.
14. Bornstein MM, Al Nawas B, Kuchler U, Tahmaseb A: Consensus statements and recommended clinical procedures regarding contemporary surgical and radiographic techniques in implant dentistry. *Int J Oral Maxillofac Implants* 2014;**29**(Suppl):78–82.

CHAPTER 6

Classification of Alveolar Ridge Defects in Implant Dentistry

Patrick Palacci

Brånemark Osseointegration Center, Marseille, France

Introduction

In 1985, Lekholm and Zarb [1] presented a classification of the jawbone based on shape and quality to be used to analyze implant anchorage. They described five groups of mandibular and maxillary cross-sectional shapes (Figure 6.1):

A. Most of the alveolar ridge is present.
B. Moderate residual ridge resorption has occurred.
C. Advanced residual ridge resorption has occurred (only basal bone remains).
D. Some resorption of the basal bone has started.
E. Extreme resorption of the basal bone has occurred.

The authors also described four groups of bone quality:

1. Almost the entire jawbone is composed of homogenous compact bone.
2. A thick layer of cortical bone surrounds dense trabecular bone.
3. A thin layer of cortical bone surrounds a core of dense trabecular bone.
4. A thin layer of cortical bone surrounds a core of low-density trabecular bone.

In addition to this classification, the thickness of the ridge mucosa also has to be considered. The classification of Lekholm and Zarb [1] helps to clarify the relationship between the surgical techniques to be used and jaw bone shape and quality. This classification determines the position and number of implants to be placed, as well as the need for additional surgeries in order to optimize implants positioning.

For example, in the presence of a Class A group an implant can be placed slightly forward while additive surgery is needed in order to be able to optimally place an implant in a Class D case.

Concerning bone quality, the surgeon has to focus on initial stability and needs to avoid any excess heat during drilling and implant insertion. This is why under or over preparation and the use of different implant diameters are considered.

According to Seibert [2, 3], ridge defects in edentulous regions can be divided into three classes (Figure 6.2):

1. Class I: loss of tissue in the buccolingual direction with normal height in the apical-coronal direction.
2. Class II: loss of the tissue in the apical-coronal direction, with normal width in the buccolingual direction.
3. Class III: a combination of Class I and Class II (loss of both height and width).

In the anterior maxilla, the position of the lip line (high or low), as well as the lip mobility, has to be considered. The architecture of the lip line, in combination with the mobility of the lip, determines the need for additional surgical procedures for an optimal aesthetic outcome [4].

Implant treatment becomes more challenging in the presence of a high lip line and significant lip mobility.

Implant position, shape, color, texture of the soft tissue (the presence or absence of interdental papillae), and quality of the final prosthetic restoration are of a great importance for the overall final result.

The interdental papilla is the part of the periodontal soft tissue between crowns of two teeth (Figure 6.3). The contact relationship between the teeth, the width of the proximal tooth surfaces, and the course of the CEJs define papilla's shape. Thus, in the anterior regions of the dentition, the interdental papilla assumes a pyramidal or conical shape.

Two major types of gingival architecture have been described in the literature (for example, Olsson and Lindhe, 1991 [5]; Olsson et al., 1993 [6]; and Seibert and Lindhe, 1997 [2]), namely the "scalloped-thin" and the "flat-thick" gingival architecture (Figure 6.4a and b, respectively). The gingival architecture is determined by many genetic and local factors, including the anatomy of the teeth and position and size of the contact surfaces of the teeth.

Palacci–Ericsson classification of the alveolar ridge

The use of a classification of the overall shape of the anterior maxilla (including the soft tissues) will help the practitioner to evaluate the anatomical conditions in implant treatment. This classification of the alveolar ridge is based on the amount of vertical and horizontal loss of soft tissue, hard tissue, or both, and can also be applied to other parts of the jaws. It is divided into four classes according to the vertical dimension and into four classes according to the horizontal dimension [7–9].

Based on *vertical* loss, Class I has intact or slightly reduced papillae (Figure 6.5). Class II has limited loss of the papillae

---

Vertical Alveolar Ridge Augmentation in Implant Dentistry: A Surgical Manual, First Edition. Edited by Len Tolstunov.
© 2016 John Wiley & Sons, Inc. Published 2016 by John Wiley & Sons, Inc.

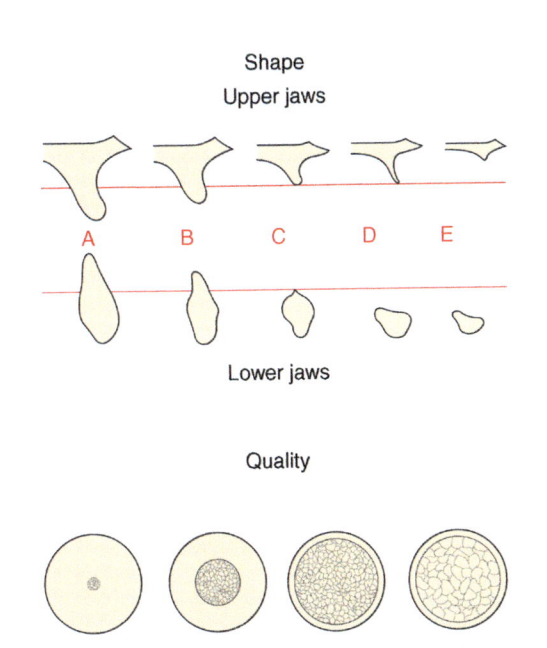

Figure 6.1 Bone shape and bone quality classification according to Lekholm and Zarb (1985) [1].

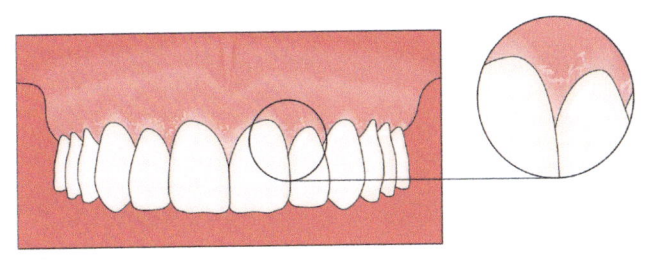

Figure 6.3 The interdental papilla.

- respect of the per-implant soft tissue,
- no additive surgeries are needed

Class IA cases are rare; most of the time hard and soft tissue resorption follows teeth extraction and after a few weeks we are more likely to be in presence of a Class IIB, where hard and soft tissues surgeries are needed.

However, in the presence of a simultaneous extraction and implant placement we can consider being in presence of a Class IA, where:

- atraumatic extraction of the teeth,
- ridge preservation technique,
- optimal positioning of the implants,
- additive soft tissue procedures (connective tissue grafts),
- optimal temporary restoration,
- optimal emergence profile respecting the blood supply,
- careful control of occlusal forces

are all needed for the success of the case.

(Figure 6.6). Class III has severe loss of the papillae (Figure 6.7), and Class IV represents absence of the papillae (Figure 6.8).

Based on *horizontal* loss, Class A shows intact or slightly reduced buccal tissue (Figure 6.9). Class B has limited loss of buccal tissue (Figure 6.10). Class C has severe loss of buccal tissue (Figure 6.11). Finally, Class D has extreme loss of buccal tissue, often in combination with a limited amount of attached mucosa (Figure 6.12). Of course, many combinations of the different classes occur, and each patient must be viewed as unique.

A good final outcome depends on the clinician's understanding of the complexity of the overall treatment. The anterior maxilla classification should be used to document the anatomical condition before treatment and will guide the clinician in choosing proper treatment options to reach the expected final result. Some treatments (for example, Class IA) normally require only proper implant placement and minimal soft tissue handling.

In a Class IA case, we are in the presence of intact and healthy papillae and an intact ridge. The keys to success in implant therapy are:

- optimal implant positioning,
- minimal invasive surgery,

Case 1: Figures 6.13 to 6.18

A fifty-seven years old female presents with an advanced periodontal disease with severe hard and soft tissue loss, more precisely in the anterior maxilla. There is a need for aesthetic and if possible an immediate temporary fixed restoration [10].

Four anterior incisors are carefully extracted using a periotome trying to avoid any ridge fracture or alteration. Three implants are inserted and the site of the upper left central incisor filled with biomaterial and connective tissue graft in order to preserve ridge volume [11, 12].

Voids between implants and alveolas are also filled with biomaterial in order to minimize the risk for bone resorption and maintain soft tissue volume as well as overall aesthetics of the case [13].

A reinforced temporary restoration is then placed (screw retained) with sufficient embrasures to maintain a soft tissue blood supply between the implants and papillae. Final restoration is in placed four months later, allowing optimal hygiene maintenance

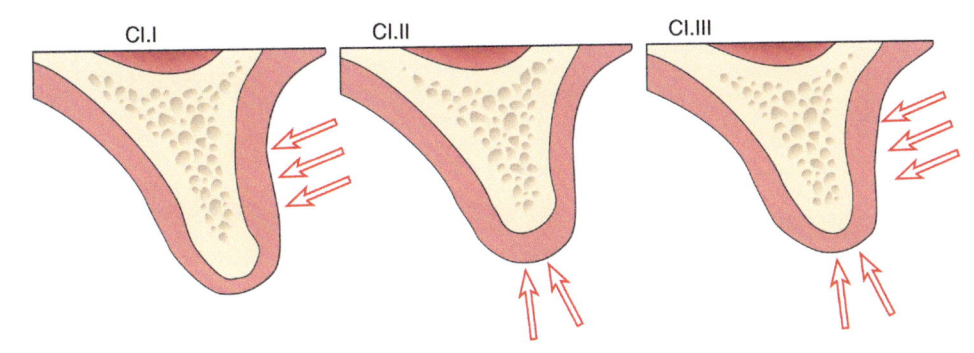

Figure 6.2 Ridge defect classification according to Seibert (1983) [3].

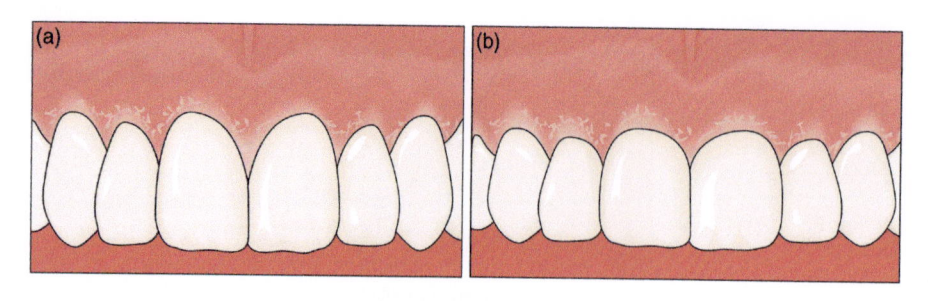

Figure 6.4 (a) "Scalloped-thin" gingival architecture. (b) "Flat-thick" gingival architecture.

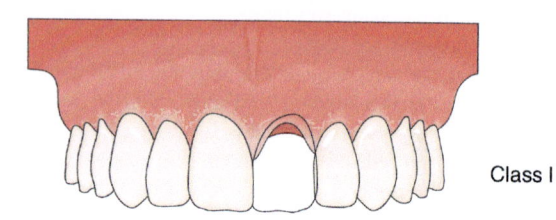

Class I

Figure 6.5 Class I.

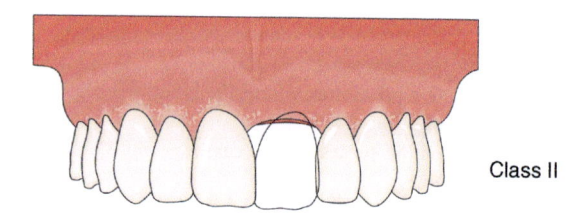

Class II

Figure 6.6 Class II.

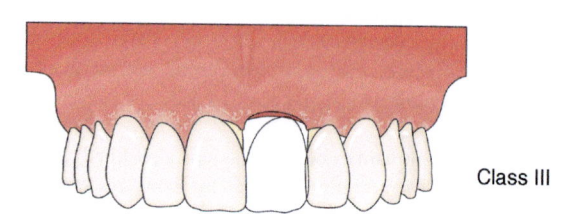

Class III

Figure 6.7 Class III.

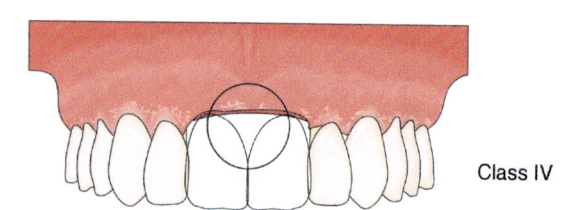

Class IV

Figure 6.8 Class IV.

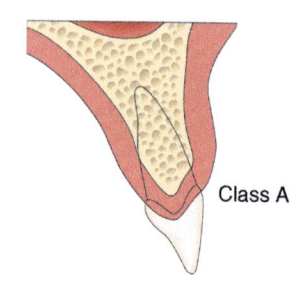

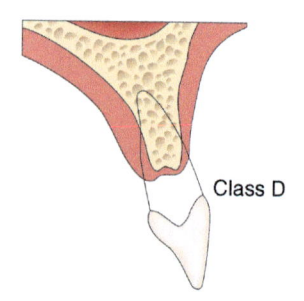

Class A

Figure 6.9 Class A.

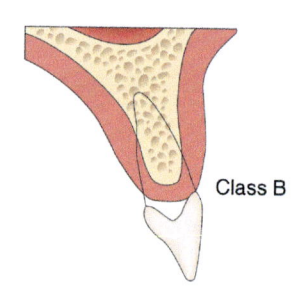

Class B

Figure 6.10 Class B.

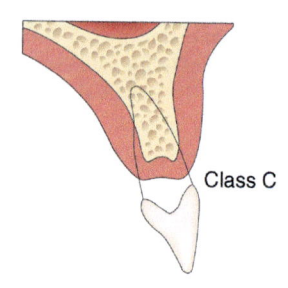

Class C

Figure 6.11 Class C.

Class D

Figure 6.12 Class D.

and aesthetics. Occlusion, extremely important, has to be carefully checked in order to maintain long-term osseointegration.

Acceptable results in Class IV, in contrast, may require additional hard and soft tissue surgical procedures prior to, at the time of, or after implant placement.

Classification of Alveolar Ridge Defects in Implant Dentistry

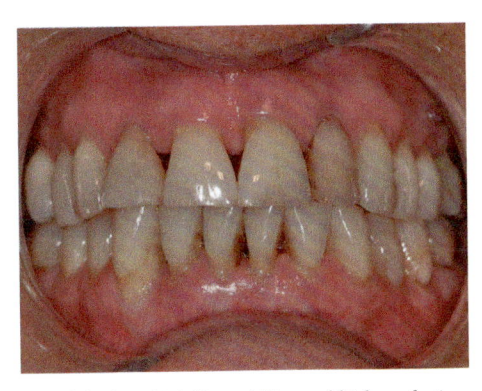

Figure 6.13 High lip line, high lip mobility, and high aesthetic expectations are the main characteristics of this case. Note the soft tissue loss following the periodontal disease.

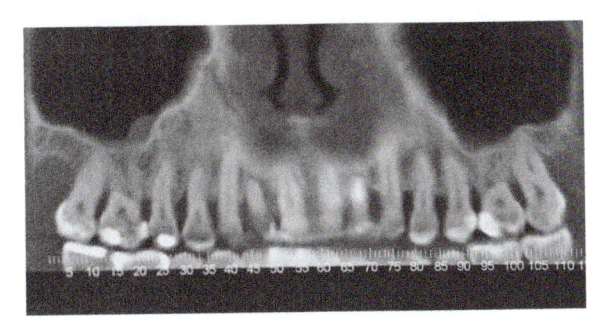

Figure 6.14 Radiographic examination. Note the significant hard tissue loss around the incisors.

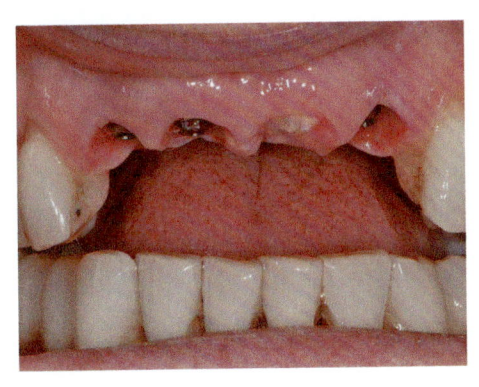

Figure 6.15 Flapless surgery performed in order to minimize tissue trauma. Site preservation technique combined with biomaterial filling and a connective tissue graft in the upper left central incisor region.

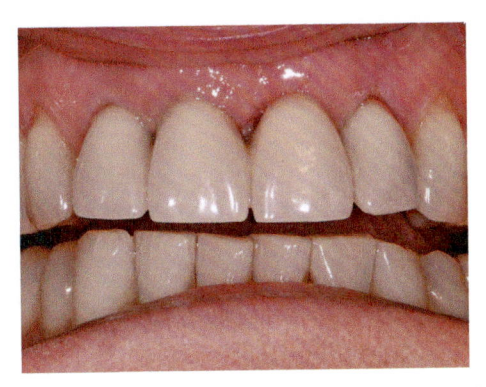

Figure 6.16 Temporary restoration in place. Note the presence of papillae two weeks post-op and the emergence profile emerging directly from the implants.

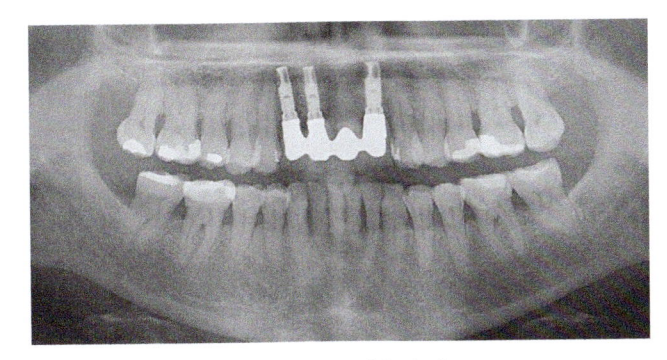

Figure 6.17 Radiographic examination of the final case.

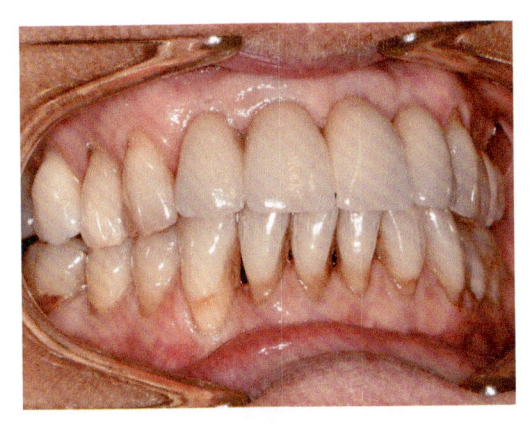

Figure 6.18 Clinical results after six years. Note the stability of the tissues.

Case 2: Figures 6.19 to 6.27

A forty-five years old man presents with a fractured upper right central incisor root resulting in an acute abscess and significant bone loss. The extraction of the root results in a ridge loss associated with the loss of the existing papillae [14, 15].

An autogenous bone graft (harvested from the chin) is performed as well as a connective tissue graft placed into the internal side of the flap at the time of implant installation in order to get enough soft tissue to be manipulated (papillae regeneration technique – Palacci) [6–10] at the time of abutment placement [16, 17]. A ceramic crown is then placed on a zirconia abutment in order to achieve a reliable aesthetic result.

This case, which could be presented as a Class IA before extraction, became a Class IIIC after extraction and bone resorption. It is almost impossible to jump from Class IIID to Class IA in one step. Bone ridge has to be augmented first in order to go from Class IIID to Class IIB; then with placement of an implant one can go from Class IIB to Class IA by soft tissue augmentation.

The benefits need to be noticed of, for example, a 2 mm gain by bone addition, and/or a 2 mm gain by soft tissue manipulation, and/or a 1–2 mm gain by crown lengthening of the adjacent teeth that makes a 5–6 mm gain of tissue that can make a significant difference.

This difference is extremely important in the aesthetic zone, being a key factor for the final aesthetic result.

No scientific evidence for the absolute need for attached mucosa from a functional or survival point of view has been presented (Wennström et al., 1994 [18]). However, from an esthetic and oral hygiene point of view, an adequate zone of attached peri-implant mucosa is preferable.

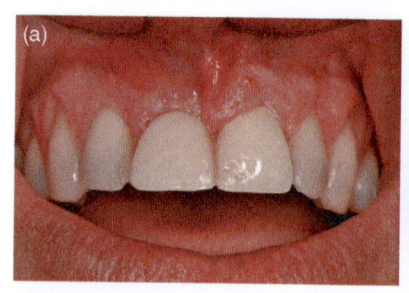

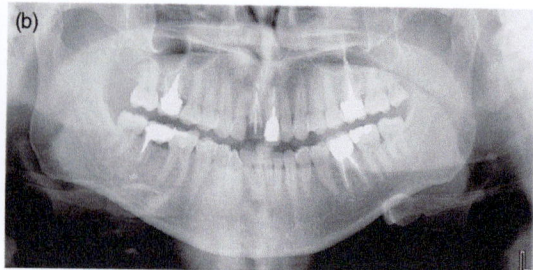

Figure 6.19 Upper right central incisor extracted. Radiographic examination showing fracture of the root.

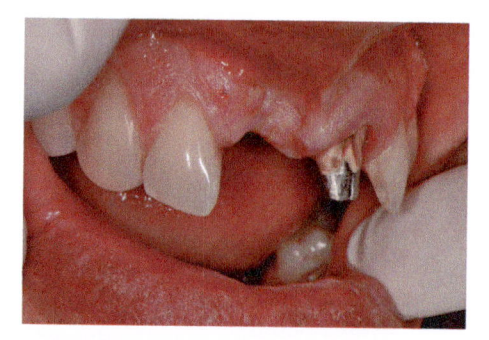

Figure 6.20 Result of the extraction. Loss of the ridge and papillae.

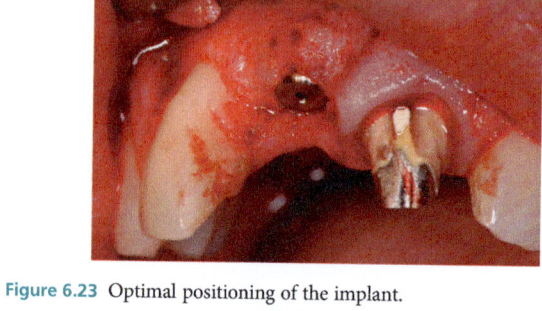

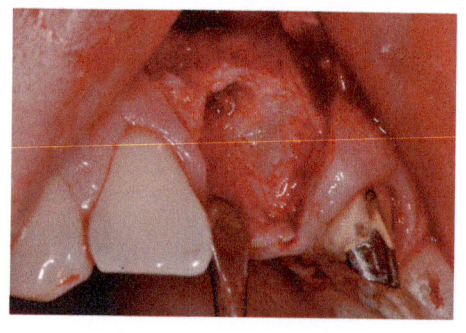

Figure 6.21 Clinical situation. Loss of the labial plate of bone and need for ridge augmentation.

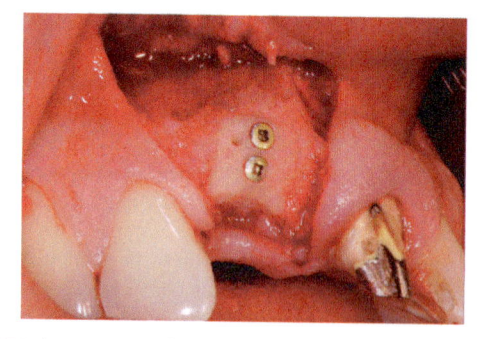

Figure 6.22 An autogenous bone graft is placed, recreating the initial anatomy.

Figure 6.23 Optimal positioning of the implant.

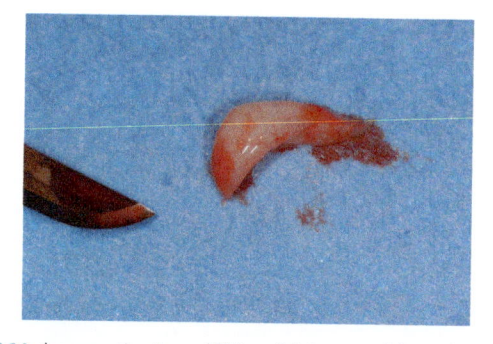

Figure 6.24 A connective tissue (CT) graft is harvested from the tuberosity region and then situated into the desired position.

Thus, the final aesthetic and functional outcome is related to three main factors: the jawbone, the soft tissue, and the design of the prosthetic reconstruction. The replacement of missing teeth is only one part of the treatment, especially in the anterior maxilla. Another part is the replacement of the lost portion of the alveolar process, the covering soft tissue, or both. The re-creation of a normal alveolar contour is an important key to aesthetic success.

Understanding the anterior maxilla classification will guide the clinician to find adequate solutions to obtain consistent and predictable treatment results from a functional and aesthetic point of view.

Precision in implant placement

A straightforward implant placement can be performed without any additional surgery. However, at the time of implant placement, minor hard tissue augmentation may be needed to add support to the peri-implant mucosa. In other situations, soft tissue must be added to enhance the final result and thus facilitate soft tissue maintenance [19, 20].

Both hard and soft tissues must be considered when planning optimal placement of the implants as well as reconstruction of the new papillae. All the different elements have to be perfectly correlated in order to achieve final success [21]:

- hard tissue management,
- soft tissue management,

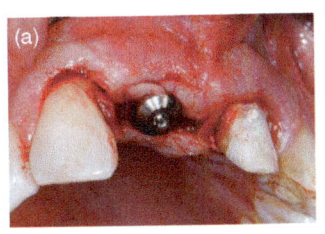

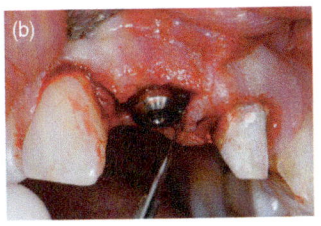

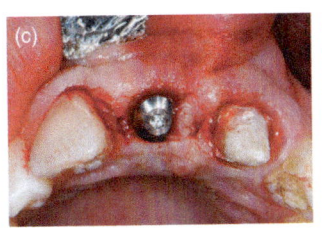

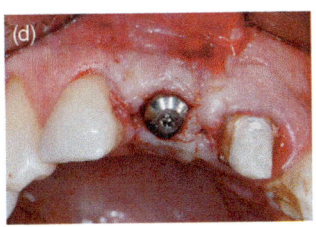

Figure 6.25 (a) Pedicle grafts, papillae regeneration technique (Palacci) allowing the recreation of the lost papillae: pedicle flaps are created on the buccal side of the placed implant and the healing abutment and the blood supply is preserved at the base of both flaps from the intact adjacent gingiva. (b) Distal pedicle flap is flipped to re-create the papilla. (c) Mesial pedicle flap is flipped to form the papilla. (d) Resorbable sutures are placed to secure buccal tissue to the palatal.

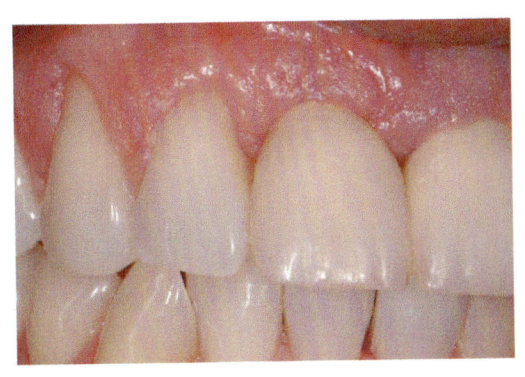

Figure 6.26 Temporary restoration is placed.

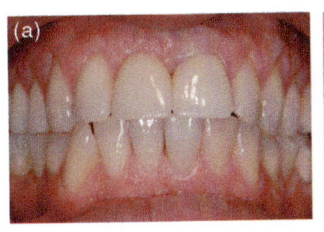

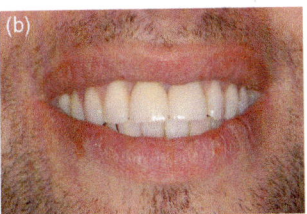

Figure 6.27 Final restoration seven years later: (a) intraoral photograph showing the re-created papillae; (b) extraoral frontal photograph of a patient with a high lip line, showing the re-created papillae as well as the final aesthetic outcome.

- the quality of the prosthetic restoration,
- aesthetic factors.

In addition to all of these emerges the vital concept of precision in implant positioning:

- If the angulation of implants in mesiodistal and buccal-lingual (palatal) directions are optimal, soft tissues will find a way to live, develop, and proliferate between the future prosthetic elements (Figure 6.28).
- The space between two implants must be adequate (7 mm between centers of two implants, 2 mm minimum between two abutments).
- If the implants are too close, no surgical technique will allow the papillae to prosper between the implants. It is obvious that less than 2 mm between abutments will never be enough to ensure sufficient blood supply vertically, meaning that the maximum papilla height will not exceed 2–3 mm above the bone level (Figure 6.29).
- However, if the implants are too far from each other, no papilla will grow between them (Figure 6.30).

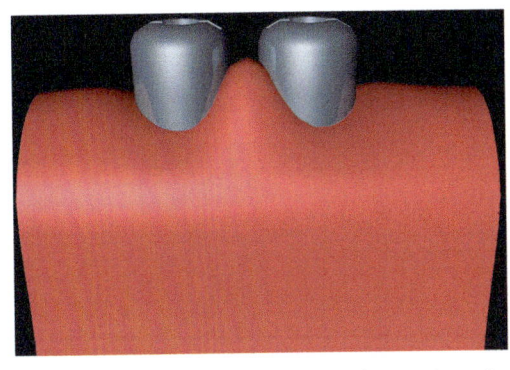

Figure 6.28 Optimal placement between two implants: 7–8 mm from center to center, 2–3 mm from edge to edge of the abutments. The papilla can be present and stable.

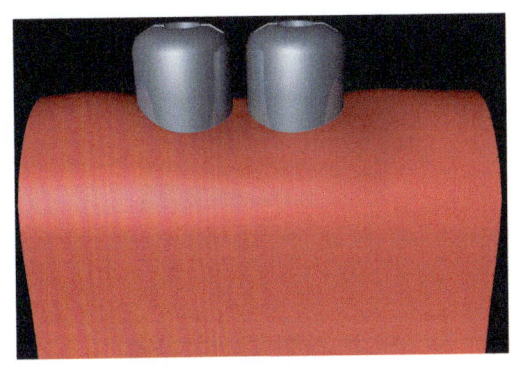

Figure 6.29 Not enough space between two implants: insufficient blood supply resulting in the loss of the papilla as well as hard tissue.

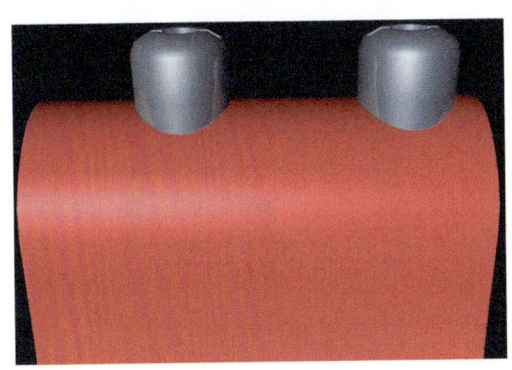

Figure 6.30 More than 4 mm between abutments: no support for the papilla, which will become flat.

- In a similar way, if an implant is placed buccally, a very thin ridge will remain beneath the soft tissues. Knowing that the maximum stress is located at the base of the implant, a labial plate that is too thin may not support the stress, resulting in recession and consequently the loss of the adjacent papillae.

Two implants that are placed in an overly pronounced angulation (one towards the other) will also result in:
- Two convergent crowns and the impossibility for soft tissue to develop between these crowns (Figure 6.31).
- Two divergent crowns with insufficient support for the papillae (Figure 6.32).

In order to understand treatment objectives and the way to achieve them, one should be able to evaluate the clinical situation at the very start of the treatment.

Class IVD

In this situation the main objective is to place implants into the residual bone with or without hard tissue augmentation. We know that, in most of cases, "restitutio ad integrum" will be extremely difficult to be obtained, maybe impossible.

Papillae need hard tissue support to exist and vertical ridge augmentation is one of the most challenging treatment options. A patient should be informed prior to any treatment of the objectives to be reached. Sometimes, it is wise to tell the patient that the best way in this case to obtain an optimal final result it to include prosthetic (acrylic or porcelain) papillae into the prosthetic restoration. The patient, understanding the challenges of problems to be solved, can accept the compromise more easily knowing that without this kind of prosthetic solution he/she will end up with long teeth and black triangles between them. (Figures 6.33 to 6.39).

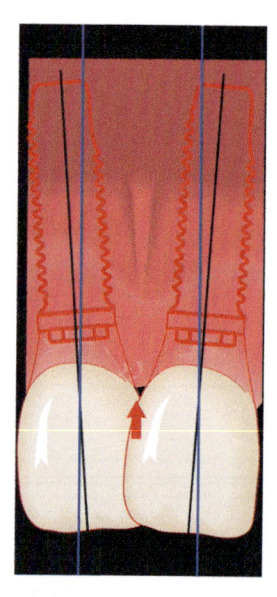

Figure 6.31 If implants are too convergent, the emergence profile will be altered and the papilla is compromised.

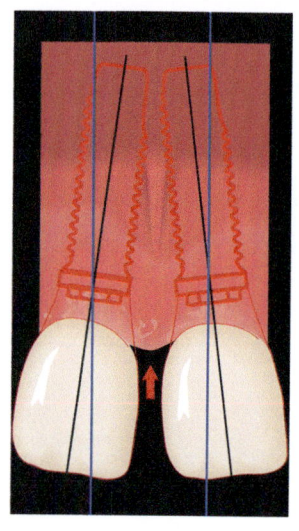

Figure 6.32 Too divergent implants will result in a large embrasure and consequently the loss of the interdental papilla.

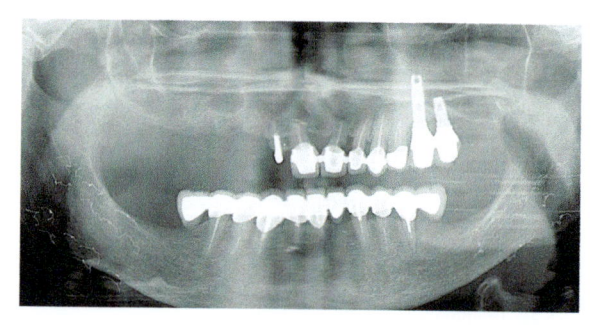

Figure 6.33 Radiographic examination of the edentulous upper ridge area, failing upper incisor, canine and premolars to be extracted, perfectly integrated implants placed several years prior.

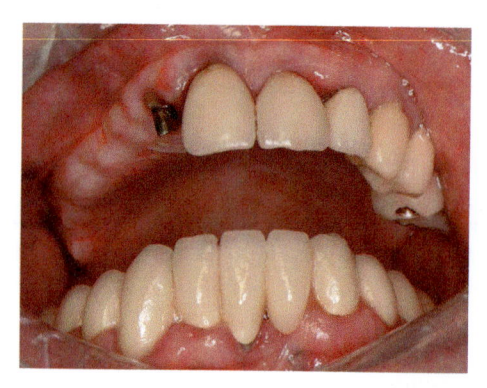

Figure 6.34 Clinical view of the Class IVD in the upper right region seems to be a Class IIIC but bone loss is such that it will become immediately a Class IVD after extraction of these teeth.

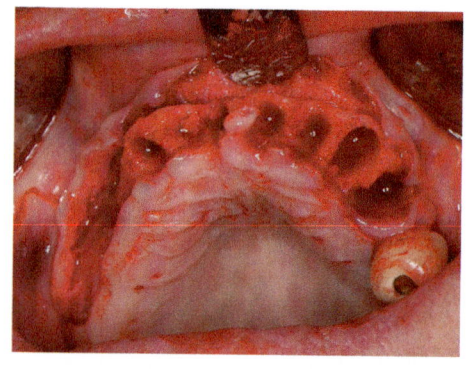

Figure 6.35 Extraction of the interior teeth and preparation of the implant site.

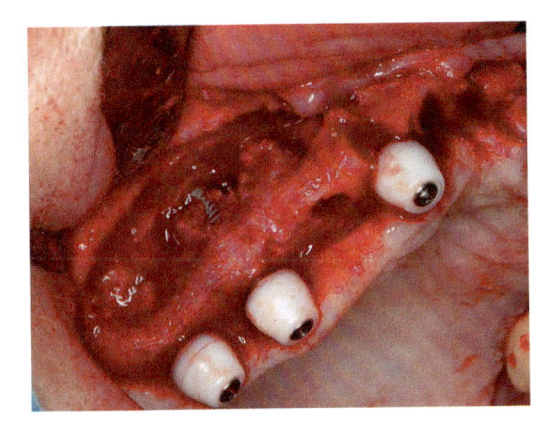

Figure 6.36 Sinus elevation plus implant placement.

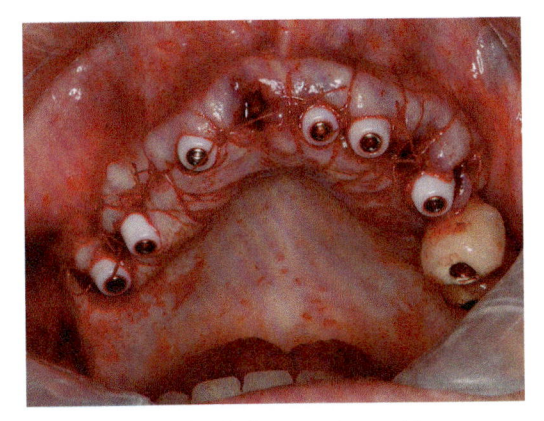

Figure 6.37 Implants are placed, abutments into position.

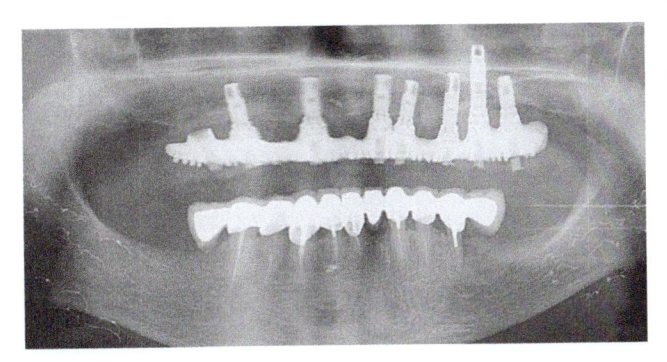

Figure 6.38 Panoramic radiograph of the case.

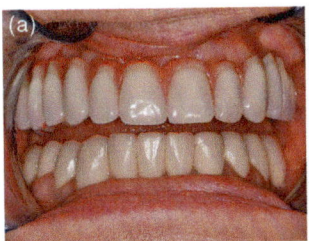

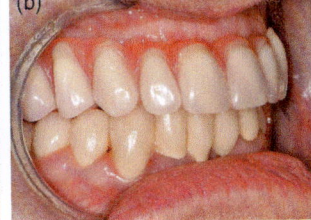

Figure 6.39 (a) Intraoral frontal photograph and (b) intraoral lateral photograph. Note the presence of acrylic (artificial gingiva) included in the restoration to solve functional, esthetic, phonetic, and comfort problems.

Table 6.1 Palacci and Ericsson classification.

	Vertical loss		Horizontal loss
Class I	Intact and healthy papillae	Class A	Intact/slightly reduced buccal tissue
Class II	Limited loss of the papillae less than 50% loss	Class B	Limited loss of the buccal tissue
Class III	Severe loss of the papillae more than 50% loss	Class C	Severe loss of the buccal tissue
Class IV	Absence of papillae (edentulous areas)	Class D	Extensive loss of buccal tissue associated with limited amount of attached mucosa

Discussion

For decades, implant treatment was used to treat edentulous patients where esthetics was not the main goal. Function was recreated by placing fixed anchor bridges with a metallic framework and acrylic teeth mounted on to pink acrylic. The esthetic needs became more obvious with time and after many esthetic failures.

The above-mentioned classification, shown in Table 6.1, gives the clinician the initial diagnostic guideline and also a recommendation for the different treatment sequences needed.

Conclusion

A careful evaluation of the clinical situation has to be done before any implant treatment. The presented classification will help the practitioner to evaluate this situation more precisely in the anterior maxilla or other parts of the jaws and can be a useful guide for the overall treatment with respect to the biological parameters.

References

1. Lekholm U, Zarb GA: Patient selection and preparation. In: Brånemark P-I, Zarb G, Albrektsson T (eds), *Tissue Integrated Prosthesis: Osseointegration in Clinical Dentistry*. Quintessence Books, Chicago, IL, 1985, pp. 199–210.
2. Seibert J, Lindhe J: Esthetics in periodontal therapy. In: Lindhe J, Karring T, Lang NP (eds), *Clinical Periodontology and Implant Dentistry*, 3rd edn. Munksgaard, Copenhagen, 1997, pp. 647–681.
3. Seibert J: Reconstruction of deformed, partially edentulous ridges, using full thickness onlay grafts, II. Prosthetic/periodontal interrelationships. *Compend Contin Educ Dent* 1983;**4**:549–562.
4. Palacci P.: Optimal implant positioning and soft-tissue considerations. *Oral Maxillofac Surg Clin North Am* 1996;**8**:445–452.
5. Olsson M, Lindhe J: Periodontal characteristics in individuals with varying form of the upper central incisors. *J Clin Periodontol* 1991;**18**:78–82.
6. Olsson M, Lindhe J, Marinello CP: On the relationship between crown form and clinical features in the gingiva in adolescents. *J Clin Periodontol* 1993;**20**:570–577.
7. Palacci P, Ericsson I: *Esthetic Implant Dentistry Soft and Hard Tissue Management*. Quintessence Books, Chicago, IL, 2001.
8. Palacci P, Ericsson I, Engstrand P, Rangert B: *Optimal Implant Positioning and Soft Tissue Management for the Brånemark System*. Quintessence Books, Chicago, IL, 1995.
9. Palacci P, Nowzari H: Soft tissue enhancement around dental implants. *Periodontol 2000* 2008;**47**:113–132.
10. Berglundh T, Lindhe J: Dimension of the peri-implant mucosa: biological width revisited. *J Clin Periodontol* 1996: **23**:971–973.
11. Sclar A: *Soft Tissue and Esthetic Considerations in Implant Dentistry*. Quintessence Publishing, Chicago, IL, 2003.
12. Araujo MG, Sukekava F, Wennstrom JL, Lindhe J: Tissue modelling following implant in fresh extraction sockets. *Clin Oral Implants Res* 2006;**17**:615–624.
13. Block M. *Color Atlas of Dental Implant Surgery*, 3rd edn. Saunders, Missouri, 2010, Pp. 255–260.

14 Becker W, Ochsenbein C, Tibbetts L, Becker BE: Alveolar bone anatomic profiles as measured from dry skulls: clinical restorations. *J Clin Periodontol* 1997;24:727–731.
15 Nowzari H, Aalam AA: Mandibular cortical bone graft. Part 2: surgical technique, applications, and morbidity. *Compend Contin Educ Dent* 2007;28:274–280.
16 Palacci P: Soft tissue management and esthetic considerations. In: Brånemark P-I (ed.), *The Osseointegration Book:Ffrom Calvanium to Calcaneum*. Quintessence Publishing, Chicago, IL, 2005, pp. 285–307.
17 Aalam AA, Nowzari H: Mandibular cortical bone grafts. Part 1: anatomy, healing process, and influencing factors. *Compend Contin Educ Dent* 2007;28:206–212.
18 Wennström JL, Bengazi F, Lekholm U: The influence of the masticatory mucosa on the peri-implant soft tissue condition. *Clin Oral Implants Res* 1994;5:1–8.
19 Israelon H, Plemons JM: Dental implants, regenerative techniques, and periodontal plastic surgery to restore maxillary anterior esthetics. *Int J Oral Maxillofac Implants* 1993;8:555–561.
20 Kan JY, Rungcharassaeng K, Umezu K, Kois JC: Dimensions of peri-implant mucosa: an evaluation of maxillary anterior single implants in humans. *J Periodontol* 2003;74:557–562.
21 Sullivan RM: Perspectives on esthetics in implant dentistry. *Compend Contin Educ Dent* 2001;22:685–692.

CHAPTER 7

Alveolar Ridge Augmentation: An Algorithmic Approach

Alan S. Herford, Katina Nguyen, and Ayleen Rojhani
Oral and Maxillofacial Surgery Department, Loma Linda University, Loma Linda, California, USA

Introduction

Loss of teeth is associated with a significant change in the alveolar bone, leading to bone remodeling and loss of bone volume. The most significant change occurs during the first three months following tooth extraction and can continue over time with an additional loss of 11% of volumetric bone over time [1]. A study by Ashman showed that there is an average loss of 40% to 60% of the total bone height and width within the first two to three years [2]. The greatest bone resorption occurs in the horizontal plane, which leads to considerable loss of alveolar width. Patients who desire restoration of their dentition with implants and implant supported prostheses who lack adequate bone may be candidates for bone augmentation procedures. There are a variety of successful techniques that can regenerate new bone such as: guided bone regeneration, the osteoperiosteal split ridge technique, distraction osteogenesis, and block grafting. Aghaloo and Moy [3] performed a systemic review to determine which hard tissue augmentation techniques are the most successful in furnishing bony support for implant placement. They found that maxillary sinus augmentations have long-term success rates, regardless of the type of graft material used, whereas alveolar augmentation techniques may be more technique sensitive and implant survival may be a function of residual bone supporting the implant rather than the grafted bone.

Important characteristics of the defect include the location, geometry, and size of the defect. This information is helpful in determining the preferred technique as well as the location for graft harvest depending on the quantity of graft material needed. Many of these defects have both a hard and soft tissue deficit. It is important to consider the implications of bone augmentation on the surrounding soft tissue, as it may create a defect that affects esthetics.

Patient selection and preparation

The decision to graft is prosthetically driven. It is important to determine what the patient's current condition is and decide on the feasibility of various treatments. The treatment plan should consider whether the patient desires a fixed implant restoration or rather an overdenture fabrication. This has direct consequences on how much bone is required as well as how much interarch space is required for the prosthesis. The prosthetic plan must be in place prior to alveolar grafting.

The most significant complication associated with bone augmentation procedures is infection, which may lead to delayed healing and possibly rejection of the graft or inadequate bone formation. An important factor in selecting patients to undergo this procedure is to make sure that they have excellent oral hygiene, with an attempt at reducing the bacterial load within the oral cavity prior to grafting. Patients should be instructed to avoid tobacco use and any systemic diseases should be well controlled. Patients should also be informed that continued smoking as well as any poorly controlled systemic diseases that are associated with poor wound healing are risk factors that are associated with an increased incidence of complications.

In the evaluation of the patient, a step-wise clinical exam noting the location of the defect as well as the type of defect is necessary to determine the preferred technique and graft material to ensure the best possible outcome [4]. The size of the defect can vary from a localized minimal defect to a more generalized complex defect. Patient stone models and computer guided 3D models may be helpful in the pre-operative planning of the graft and implant placement. Radiographic images using cone-beam CT (CBCT) radiographs for complex defects are often useful in determining the volumetric amount of bone available and missing and what bone augmentation technique will be needed.

The soft tissue should also be evaluated for amount and thickness of keratinized tissue and presence of scar tissue. It may be preferable to correct soft tissue problems prior to grafting if the soft tissue deficit is severe and there is minimal soft tissue to provide coverage for the bone graft.

Types of defects

Defects requiring alveolar augmentation can be categorized based on their characteristics. This will in turn aid in the selection of a technique that has the highest predictability for success. Alveolar defects can present in various shapes and sizes. Defects may be narrow (horizontal deficit) or be deficient in height (vertical). Some patients will present with different types of defects present in the same jaw and treatment should be individualized for each defect (Figure 7.1). Defects that have walls around them generally respond

---

Vertical Alveolar Ridge Augmentation in Implant Dentistry: A Surgical Manual, First Edition. Edited by Len Tolstunov.
© 2016 John Wiley & Sons, Inc. Published 2016 by John Wiley & Sons, Inc.

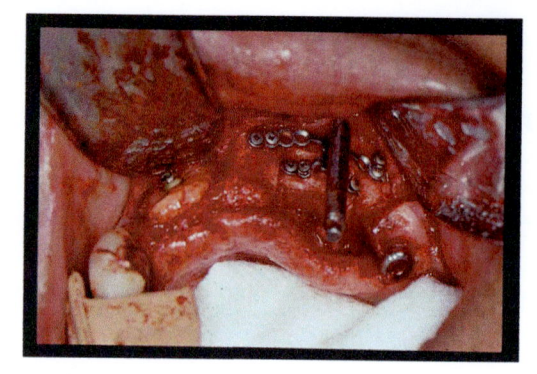

Figure 7.1 Showing two separate techniques. Pictures showing different defects in a patient: vertical that is being corrected with the distraction osteogenesis technique (on the right side of the photograph) and horizontal, with an onlay block graft (on the left side).

Types of procedures

1. Guided bone regeneration

Guided bone regeneration (GBR) is one of the best-documented and widely used procedures for augmenting localized alveolar ridge defects. GBR techniques utilize a particulate graft with an overlying membrane that promotes stabilization of the graft material and protects the healing graft from competing with non-osteogenic cells, like fibroblasts and epithelial cells (Figure 7.6). The membrane may be resorbable or non-resorbable. For horizontal bone augmentations, the use of membranes combined with particulate autogenous bone has led to increased thickness of the alveolar ridge [6, 7]. Vertical augmentations are more technique sensitive and less predictable and for larger, more complex alveolar defects, onlay grafting is likely to be more predictable [8, 9]. GBR with titanium mesh can also be used for localized ridge augmentation [10] (Figures 7.7 and 7.8).

Advantages

The use of either a resorbable or non-resorbable membrane helps prevent the migration of non-osteogenic cells into the graft site, so there is more predictable bone formation. The GBR technique is well documented in the literature and reports a high success rate of 93% in a 12.5-year follow-up study after implant placement [11].

Disadvantages

Instability of the membrane may cause delayed healing and formation of fibrous tissue rather than bone due to the lack of conversion of mesenchymal cells into osteogenic cells.

Collapse of the membrane will lead to inadequate bone formation and possibly fibrous growth. It is necessary to maintain adequate space under the membrane to allow migration of cells and the ingrowth of new blood vessels. Large defects may require support with particulate bone and possibly titanium mesh.

Guided bone regeneration is a well-documented technique that has been in use by surgeons for over two decades and has predictable outcomes. Current research is focused on improving available biocompatible resorbable membranes that can meet the ever-increasing demands of esthetics and the ability to create and enhance alveolar bone.

2. Osteoperiosteal flap ridge-split procedure

The osteoperiosteal flap ridge-split technique is performed for horizontal augmentation of narrow ridges that otherwise would not be suitable for implant placement. This technique consists of splitting the facial or buccal cortical plate from the lingual or palatal and further opening the space with osteotomes [12–14]. This technique may be done anywhere in the mouth, but it is recommended for use in the esthetic zone and posterior mandible. The osteoperiosteal flap ridge-split technique has had a success rate of 98% to 100% according to some studies [15].

Advantages

Fewer disturbances to the osteogenic periosteum allows greater resistance to resorption and remodeling of the grafted site. A major advantage is access to the endosteal marrow, which provides a rich vascular network for acceptance of the new graft. There is improved continuity of the crestal gingivoalveolar form, which is a great advantage when used in esthetic areas.

better to grafting than those that are not contained. The teeth adjacent to the defect should also be evaluated to determine if there is bone loss with exposed root surfaces. It is difficult to predictably regain bone height adjacent to exposed root surfaces of teeth. In some patients it is better to remove the adjacent tooth in order to more predictably graft the area.

The alveolar defect may be present in the maxilla or the mandible (Figures 7.2 and 7.3). The maxilla has less dense bone than the mandible. The bone can also be classified based on the quality of bone (types 1 to 4) [5].

Maxillary alveolar defects can be categorized as being anterior or posterior. In the maxilla the anterior esthetic zone may require augmentation in an anterior and vertical direction because of the pattern of resorption resulting in a Class III relationship with the lower jaw. The posterior maxilla resorbs in a pattern that narrows the maxilla so augmentation will often require lateral augmentation. The position of the maxillary sinuses is another consideration involving the posterior maxilla. The vertical position of the maxilla should be evaluated and a severely resorbed maxilla (severe generalized alveolar resorption) may benefit from inferior and anterior movement (Le Fort I) of the maxillary alveolar process in order to create a better (Class I) maxillomandibular relationship with the lower jaw (Figures 7.4 and 7.5).

The mandible has unique anatomical characteristics that are important to consider when choosing a type of grafting procedure. The defects are categorized as being anterior (between the mental foramen) or posterior to the mental foramen. For posterior deficits, the amount of alveolar resorption and position of the inferior alveolar nerve are important determinants for the type of reconstructive technique. An important question to ask is "How much bone is above the nerve?" If there is only a few millimeters above the nerve then techniques such as a "tunneling" procedure to place a graft just above the residual alveolar ridge may be an option as well as consideration of a guided bone regeneration type of procedure. Care should be undertaken to avoid placing screws that could possibly damage the nerve. Techniques such as block grafts or osteotomies (i.e. distraction, sandwich technique) should be avoided for those cases where the nerve is very close to the crest of the ridge. There are more options for anterior defects because these defects lie between the mental foramen.

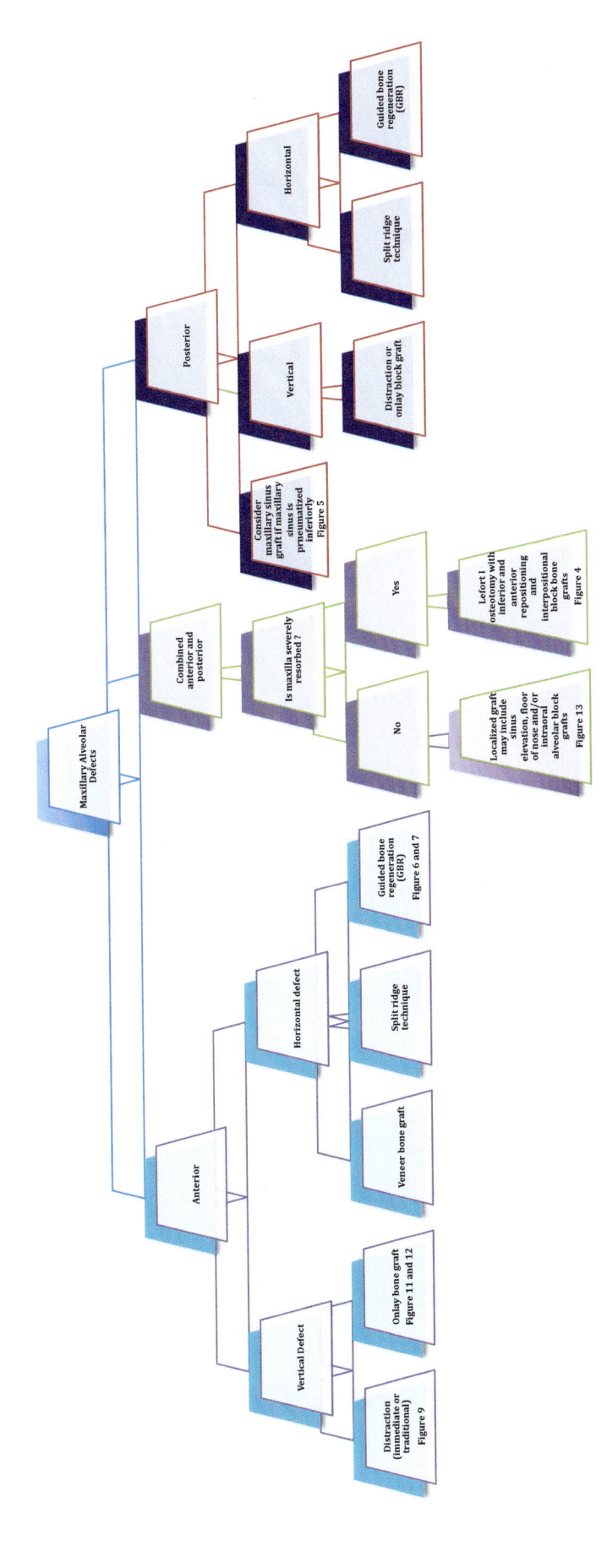

Figure 7.2 Maxillary algorithm of alveolar bone augmentation.

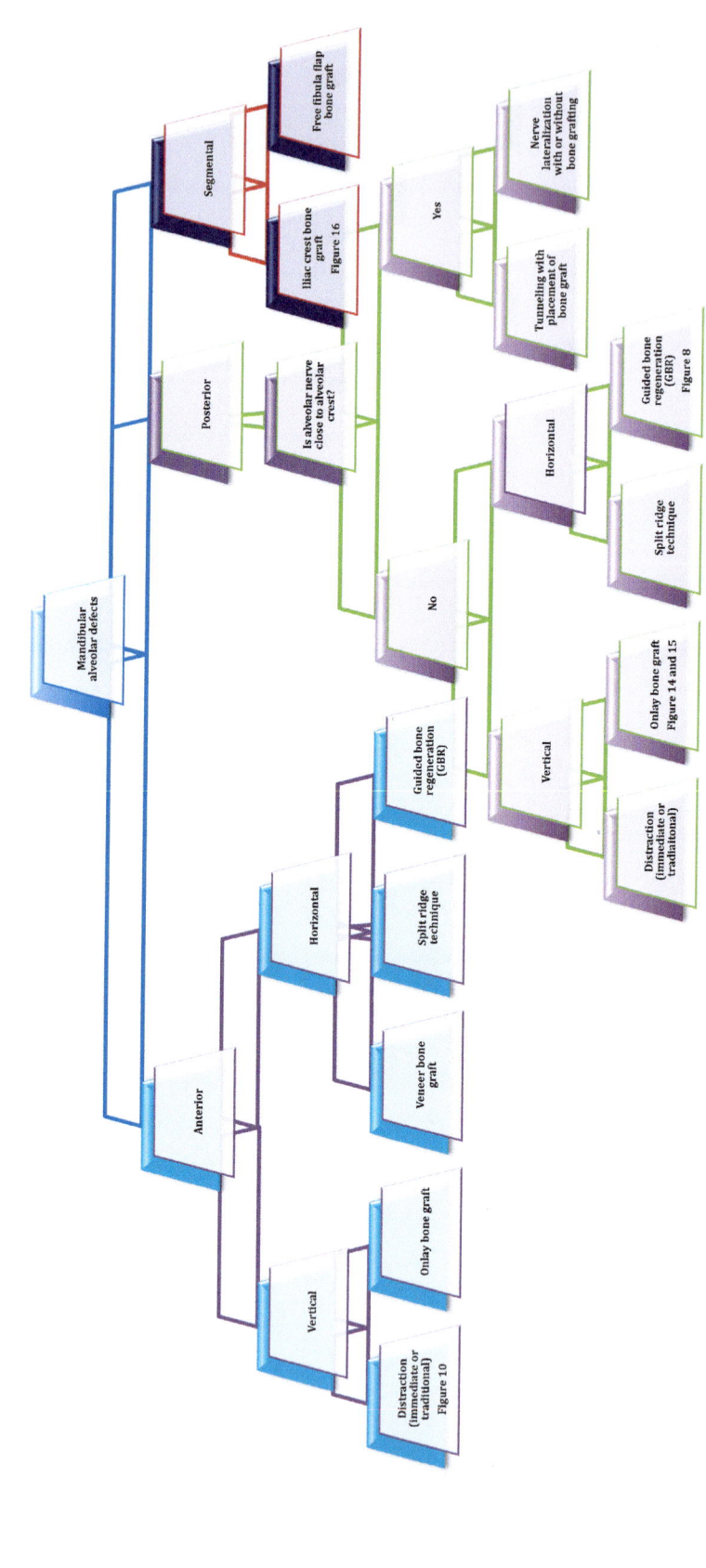

Figure 7.3 Mandibular algorithm of alveolar bone augmentation.

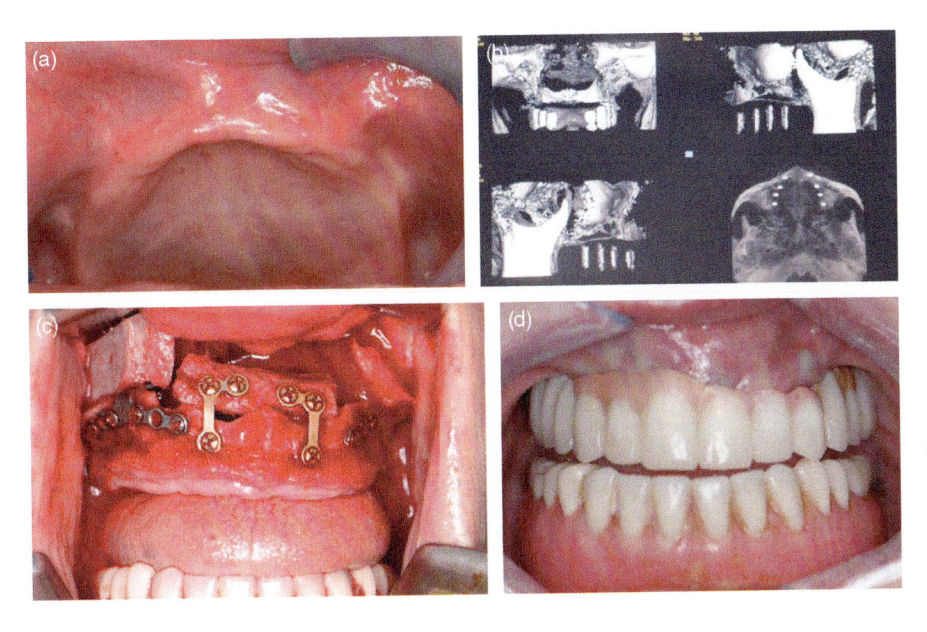

Figure 7.4 Le Fort I osteotomy and interpositional bone grafting: **(a)** severe max atrophy, **(b)** radiograph showing severe bone resorption, **(c)** Le Fort I osteotomy with interpositional bone graft, **(d)** temporary prosthesis in place.

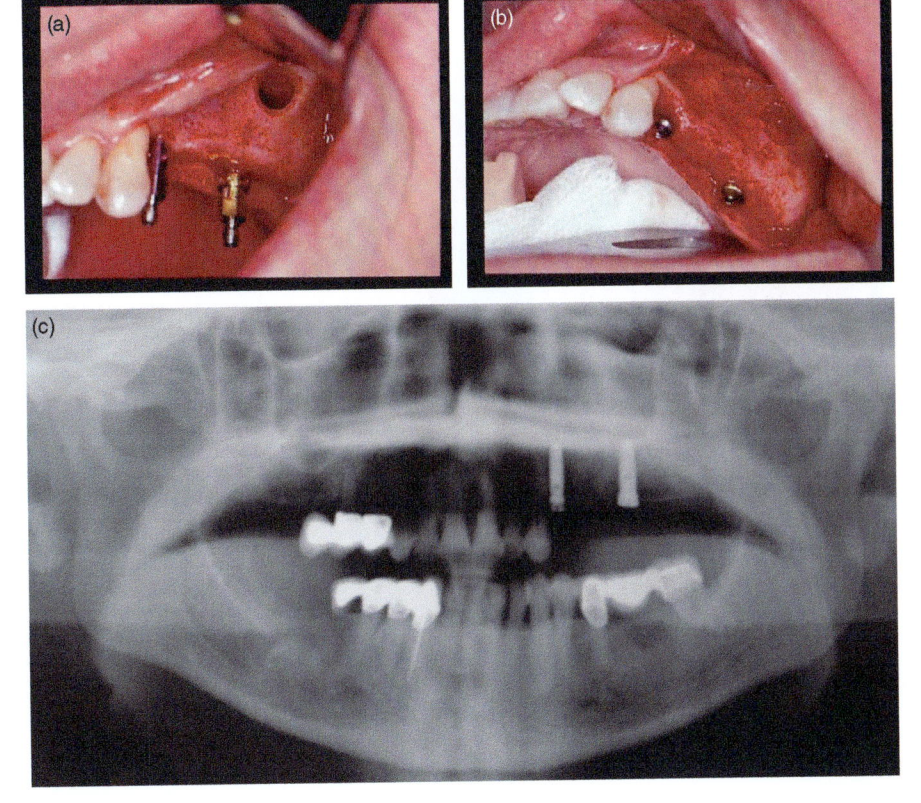

Figure 7.5 Maxillary sinus lift with particulate graft: **(a)** maxillary sinus lift, **(b)** placement of bone graft and implants, **(c)** post-operative radiograph.

Disadvantages
For very thin alveolar ridges this technique is more difficult and is unable to address significant vertical height challenges.

3. Distraction osteogenesis
Distraction osteogenesis (DO) can be used to regenerate missing hard and soft tissue [16, 17] (Figures 7.9 and 7.10). Distraction osteogenesis relies on the body's ability to generate bone as two segments of bone are "distracted" apart. The osteotomies are created and the distraction device is placed. Typically, there is a latency phase of one week were a fibrovascular bridge is formed in the osteotomy site. This provides a template to generate new bone as the segments are distracted apart during the activation phase. Once the desired distraction has occurred, the device is left in place for a period of time. Once consolidation (typically 2 to 6 months) has occurred, the distraction device can be removed and implants can be placed. Chiapasco compared GBR to DO and found that both are equally effective in alveolar bone augmentation for implant placement and further stated that the long-term prognosis of vertical bone gain in DO is more predictable [18].

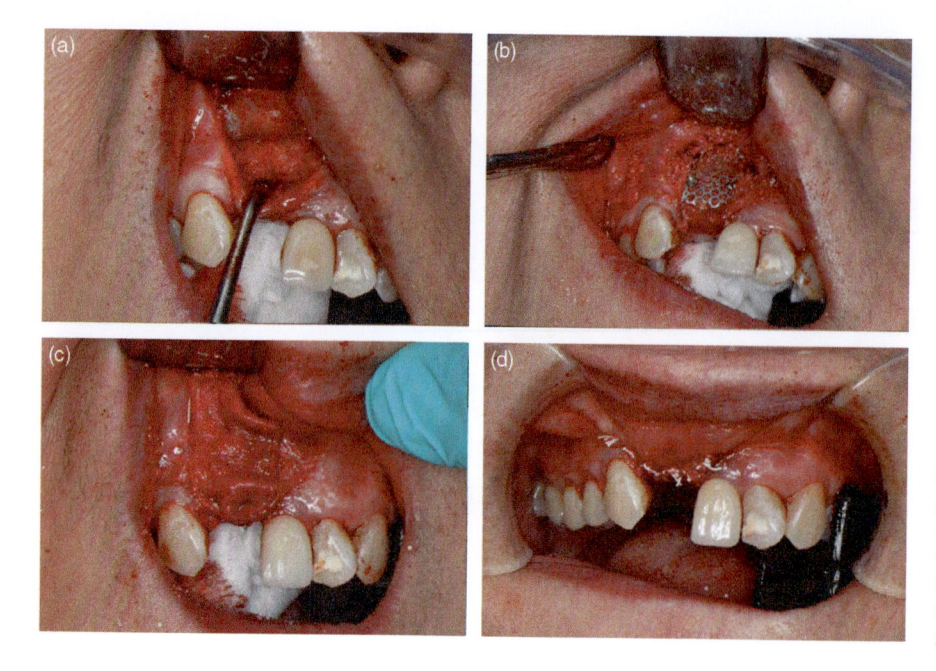

Figure 7.6 Anterior maxilla: localized guided bone regeneration (GBR): (a) localized maxillary anterior defect, (b) particulate graft contained with titanium mesh, (c) placement of collagen membrane over mesh, (d) tension-free closure over graft.

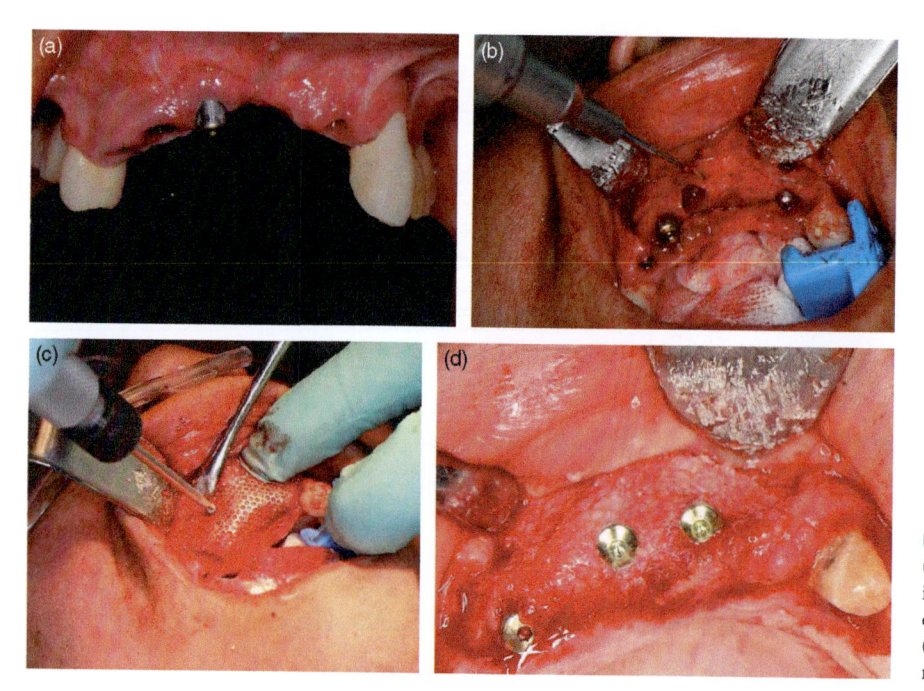

Figure 7.7 Anterior maxilla: GBR: (a) anterior maxillary defect with failing implant, (b) maxillary defect, (c) placement of titanium mesh and particulate graft, (d) placement of titanium implants in reconstructed bone.

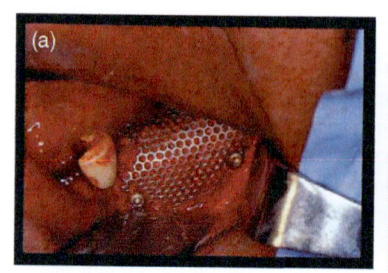

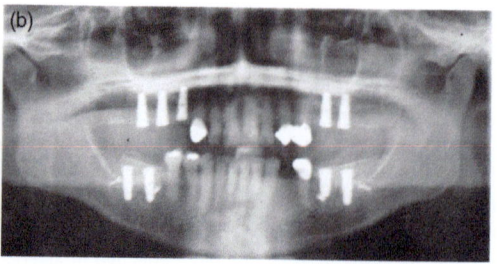

Figure 7.8 Posterior mandible: GBR: (a) titanium mesh and particulate graft, (b) implant placed.

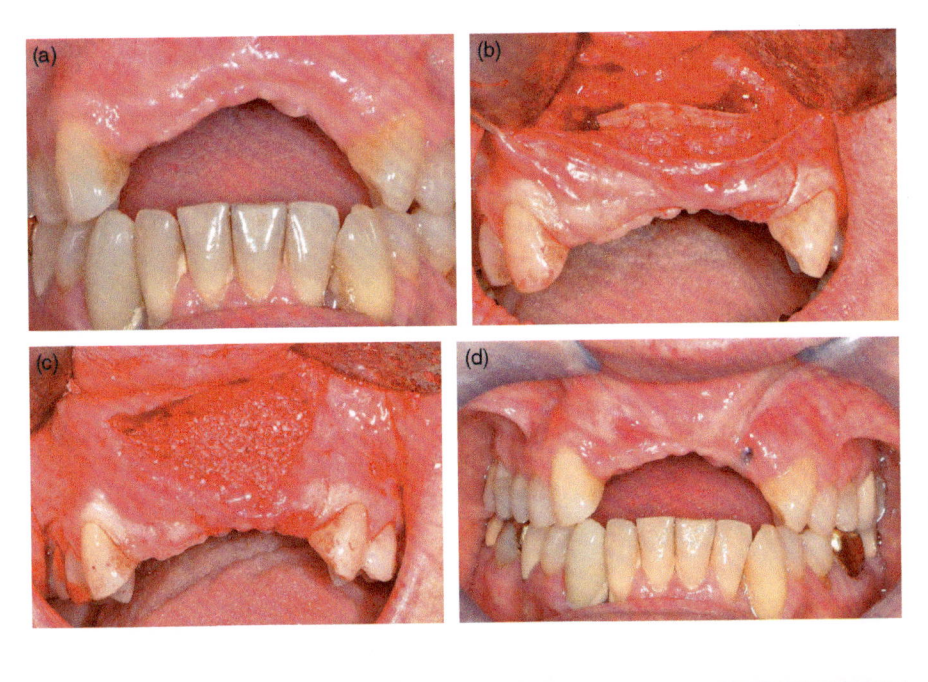

Figure 7.9 Anterior maxilla: immediate (static) distraction or "sandwich technique": (a) maxillary anterior defect, (b) Ramus interpositional graft, (c) Bovine bone graft over osteotomy, (d) post-operative healing.

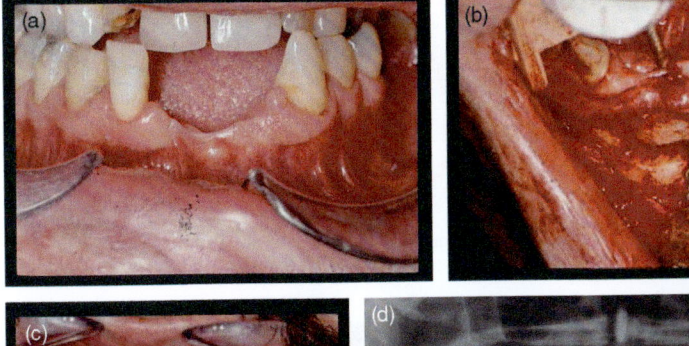

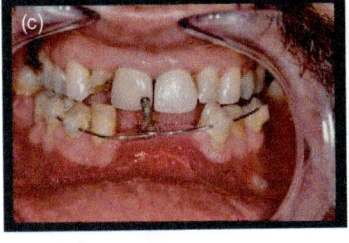

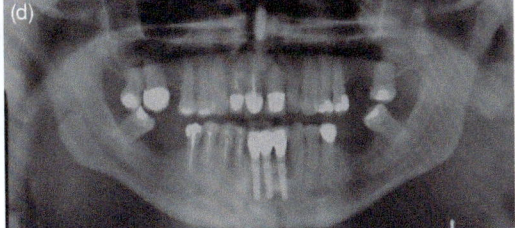

Figure 7.10 Anterior mandible: traditional (dynamic) distraction: (a) anterior mandibular defect, (b) distraction osteogenesis (DO), (c) after DO completion, (d) restored with dental implants.

Advantages

The major advantage of DO is that the gradual traction of the bone transport segment is followed by simultaneous bone osteogenesis and soft tissue regeneration. Distraction osteogenesis is comparable to other techniques for vertical augmentation of bone.

There may be less morbidity with this technique and it does not require a donor site.

Disadvantages

A second surgery to remove the distractor is required.

In a study by Swennen et al. [19] complications occurred in 22% of patients, mostly due to mechanical distractor-related problems and local infections. Infection was seen in 5.8% and device-related problems were present in 7.3% of all patients.

Complications that may resolve spontaneously within six months of the procedure are: temporary inferior alveolar nerve disturbances, pain, trismus, temporary facial nerve palsy, and minor occlusal disturbances. There is also the possibility of localized infection, incorrect vector of distraction, device-related problems, and dehiscence. At times, there may be some technical complications with the device, which may cause device failure that will necessitate another surgery to either remove or replace the device. In cases of device failure, it may cause premature or deficient ossification and/or fracture of the supporting bone [20].

Alternative technique

Immediate (static) distraction or the "sandwich technique" is similar to traditional (dynamic) distraction osteogenesis but the application of the distractor is not necessary [21]. The osteotomy is the same as the traditional alveolar distraction. The transported segment is placed into the desired location and stabilized, usually with titanium mesh and mini screws. This creates a well-defined pocket in which to place a bone graft and can lead to predictable healing. By maintaining the soft tissue attached to the transported segment of bone, the blood supply remains, which is different from placing an onlay block graft and requiring revascularization of the graft along the crest of the alveolus. This may lead to less resorption in this area [18].

4. Onlay block grafting

Bone can be harvested from various sites and used to reconstruct alveolar defects (Figures 7.11 to 7.16). Depending on how block grafts are shaped and used to restore the defect, they may be in the form of inlays, veneers, onlays, or saddle grafts. Ridge defects that have adequate vertical height but are too narrow may be restored with a veneer graft. Deficient alveolar ridges that require both horizontal and vertical augmentation may be restored with a saddle graft. The grafts must have a cortical portion that will allow screws to be placed to prevent the graft from moving during healing. These grafts are revascularized and replaced with host bone. Block grafts take longer to integrate than cancellous bone grafts and a staged surgical approach is more predictable than placing implants in conjunction with the graft. Placing an implant simultaneously with the graft may be considered if there is sufficient basal bone to provide primary stability of the implant without relying on support from the grafted bone [22].

Advantages

Autogenous distant block bone grafts (iliac crest) are excellent to use for many types of augmentation procedures, especially for large vertical defects. These grafts create a source of viable cells and proteins and provide a scaffold for new bone formation, but without antigenicity [1]. Corticocancellous intraoral block bone harvested from the mandibular ramus are reliable grafts with a high rate of

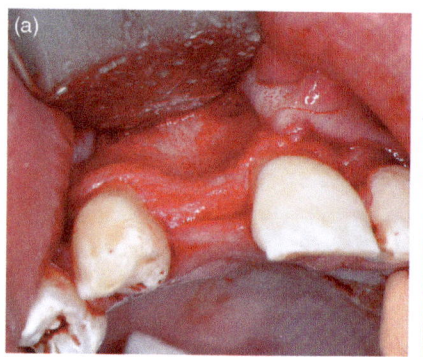

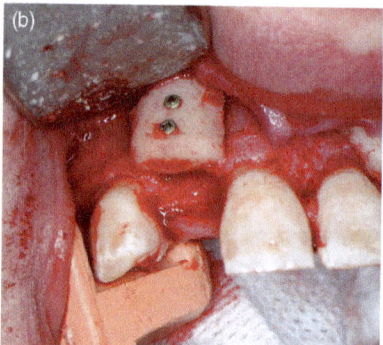

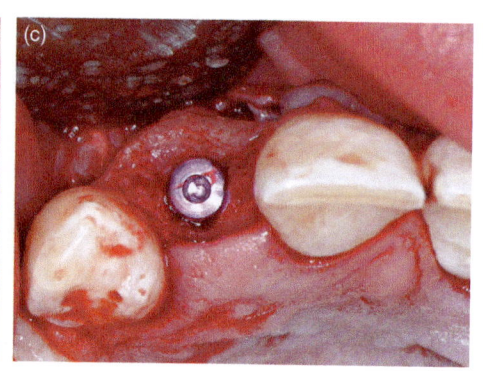

Figure 7.11 Anterior maxillary ramus graft: **(a)** missing congenital lateral incisor, **(b)** placement of ramus veneer graft, **(c)** placement of titanium implant several months later.

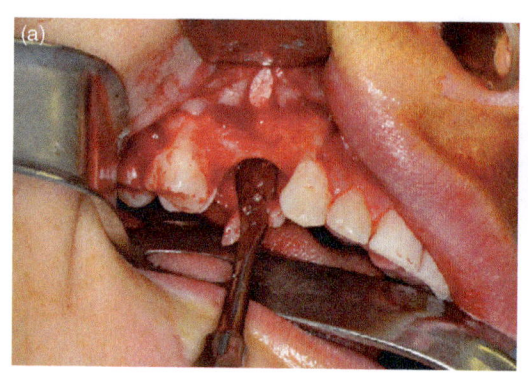

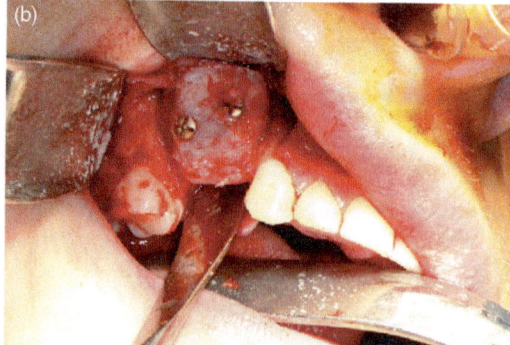

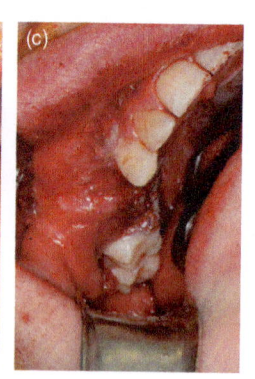

Figure 7.12 Anterior maxillary localized block graft: **(a)** maxillary defect, **(b)** placement of block graft, **(c)** tension-free closure.

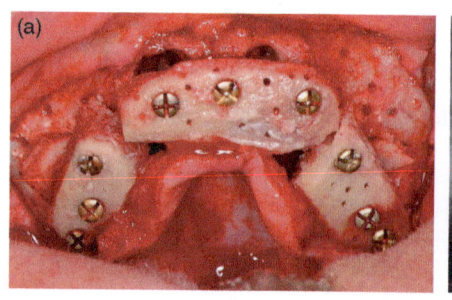

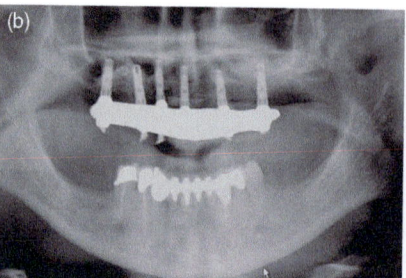

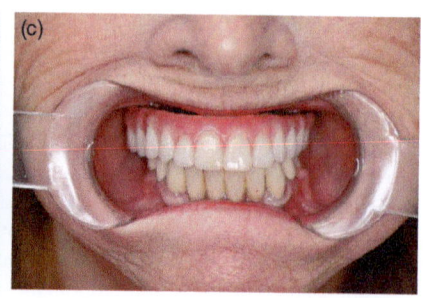

Figure 7.13 Anterior and posterior distant (extraoral) maxillary block grafts: **(a)** iliac crest block grafts, **(b)** radiograph of dental implants, **(c)** dental prosthesis 5 years after grafting.

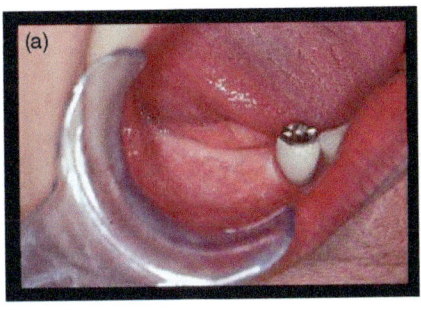

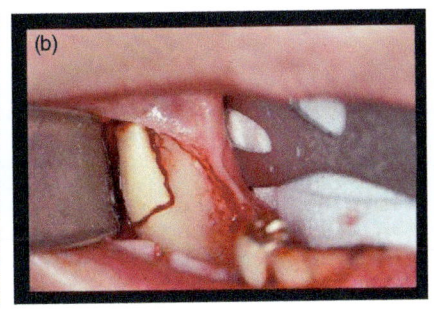

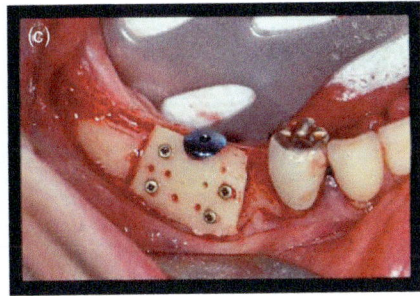

Figure 7.14 Posterior mandible: block graft: (a) mandibular posterior defect, (b) harvest of mandibular ramus graft, (c) graft secured into place.

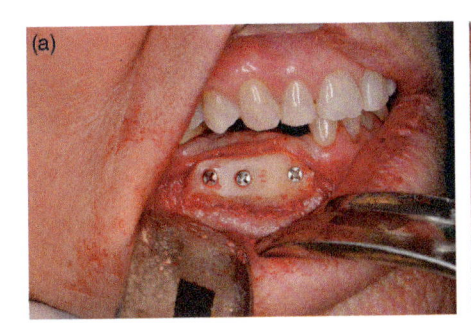

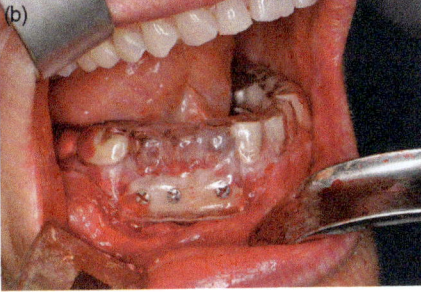

Figure 7.15 Posterior mandible: onlay graft: (a) mandibular posterior defect treated with ramus graft, (b) surgical guide used to aid in placement of block graft.

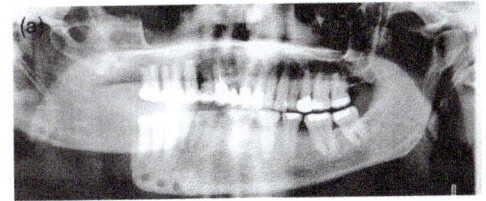

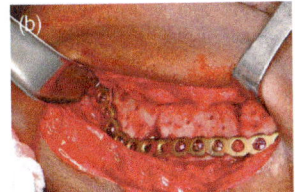

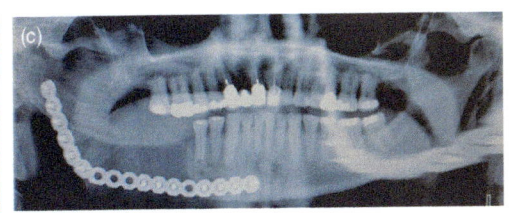

Figure 7.16 Mandibular continuity defect: (a) mandibular continuity defect, (b) iliac crest graft placed, (c) reconstructed mandible.

success for the alveolar reconstruction procedure for horizontal defects but have limited utility for vertical defects [23].

Disadvantages
A secondary donor site is required. There are possible complications associated with the harvest site. These complications are site-specific and may lead to damage to the inferior alveolar nerve or other complications such as gait disturbance, scarring, and infection.

Future possibilities
Autogenous bone remains the most predictable best option for complex alveolar defects. Advances in regeneration such as the incorporation of growth factors, stem cell treatments, virtual surgical planning, and 3D printing hold great promise for improving the way we can treat alveolar defects in the future. These advances may lead to improved outcomes but more studies are necessary to fully evaluate these technologies and their role in alveolar regeneration.

Summary
It is important to develop a treatment plan including the final prosthetic plan prior to performing a graft procedure. Various graft materials including autogenous and non-autogenous grafts are available. There are also various techniques available for alveolar ridge augmentation. The least invasive and the most predictable procedure should be chosen, if possible. For more complex defects, techniques such as block grafts can give predictable results.

References
1. Chiapasco M, Casentini P, Zaniboni M: Bone augmentation procedures in implant dentistry. *Int J Oral Maxillofac Implants* 2009;**24**:237–259.
2. Ashman A1, LoPinto J, Rosenlicht J: Ridge augmentation for immediate post-extraction implants: eight year retrospective study. *Pract Periodontics Aesthet Dent* 1995 Mar;**7**(2):85–94;quiz 95.
3. Aghaloo TL1, Moy PK: Which hard tissue augmentation techniques are the most successful in furnishing bony support for implant placement? *Int J Oral Maxillofac Implants* 2008 Jan–Feb;**23**(1):56.
4. Boyne PJ, Herford AS: An algorithm for reconstruction of alveolar defects before implant placement. *Oral and Maxillofacial Surgery Clinics of North America* 2001;**13**(3):533–542.
5. Lekholm U, Zarb GA: Patient selection and preparation. In: *Osseointegration in Clinical Dentistry*. Quintessence Publishing Company, Chicago, IL, 1985, pp. 199–209.
6. Buser D, Ingimarsson S, Dula K, et al: Long-term stability of osseointegrated implants in augmented bone: a 5-year prospective study in partially edentulous patients. *Int J Periodontics Restorative Dent* 2002;**22**:109.
7. Von Arx T, Buser D: Horizontal ridge augmentation using autogenous block grafts and the guided bone regeneration technique with collagen membranes: a clinical study with 42 patients. *Clin Oral Implants Res* 2006;**17**:359–366.

8. Chiapasco M, Abati S, Romeo E, et al: Clinical outcome of autogenous bone blocks or guided bone regeneration with e-PTFE membranes for the reconstruction of narrow edentulous ridges. *Clin Oral Implants Res* 1999;**10**:278.
9. Simion M, Dahlin C, Blair K, et al: Effect of different microstructures of e-PTFE membranes on bone regeneration and soft tissue response: a histologic study in canine mandible. *Clin Oral Implant Res* 1999;**10**:73.
10. Von Arx T, Walkamm B, Hardt N: Localized ridge augmentation using a micro-titanium mesh: a report on 27 implants followed form 1 to 3 years after functional loading. *Clin Oral Implants Res* 1998;**9**:123.
11. Benic GI, Hämmerle CHF: Horizontal bone augmentation by means of guided bone regeneration. *Periodontol 2000* 2014 Oct;**66**(1):13-40.
12. Kheur M, Gokhale SG, et al: Staged ridge splitting technique for horizontal expansion in mandible: a case report. *J Oral Implantology* 2014;**4**:479-483.
13. Jensen OT, Bell W, Cottam J: Osteoperiosteal flaps and local osteotomies for alveolar reconstruction. *Oral Maxillofac Surg Clin North Am* 2010 Aug;**22**(3):331-346.
14. Jensen OT, et al: Island osteoperiosteal flap for alveolar bone reconstruction. *J Oral Maxillofac Surg* 2010 Mar;**68**(3):539-546.
15. Jensen OT, Ringeman JL, Cottam JR, et al: Orthognatic and osteoperiosteal flap augmentation strategies for maxillary dental implant reconstruction. *Oral Maxillofac Surg Clin North Am* 2011;**23**:301-319.
16. Herford AS: Distraction osteogenesis: a surgical option for restoring missing tissue in the anterior esthetic zone. *J Calif Dent Assoc* 2005;**33**:889-895.
17. Elo JA, Herford AS, Boyne PJ: Implant success in distracted bone versus autogenous gone-grafted sites. *J Oral Implantol* 2009;**35**:181-184.
18. Chiapasco M, Romeo E, Casentini P, et al: Alveolar distraction osteogenesis vs vertical guided bone regeneration for the correction of vertically deficient edentulous ridges: a 1-3 year prospective study on humans. *Clin Oral Implants Res* 2004;**15**:82-95.
19. Swennen G, Schliephake H, Dempf R, Schierle H, Malevez C: Craniofacial distraction osteogenesis: a review of the literature. Part 1: Clinical studies. *Int J Oral Maxillofac Surg* 2001;**30**:89-103.
20. Verlinden CRA, van de Vijfeijken SECM, Jansma EP, Becking AG, Swennen GRJ: Complications of mandibular distraction osteogenesis for congenital deformities: a systematic review of the literature and proposal of a new classification for complications, *International Journal of Oral and Maxillofacial Surgery* 2015 Jan;**44**(1):37-43.
21. Herford AS, Tandon R, Stevens TW, et al: Immediate distraction osteogenesis: the sandwhich technique in combination with rhBMP-2 for anterior maxillary and mandibular defects. *J Craniofac Surg* 2013;**24**:1383-1387.
22. Bell RB, Blakey GH, White RP, et al:. Staged reconstruction of the severely atrophic mandible with autogenous bone graft and endosteal implants. *J Oral Maxillofac Surg* 2002;**60**:1135.
23. Misch CM:. Comparison of intraoral donor sites for onlay grafting prior to implant placement. *J Periodontal Implant Sci* 2014;**44**:33-38.

CHAPTER 8

The Fourth Dimension of 3D Surgical Alveolar Ridge Reconstruction: Bone and Soft Tissue Grafting to Compensate for Dynamic Craniofacial Changes Associated with Aging in Partially Edentulous Patients Influencing Placement Consideration for Osseointegrated Implants

Oded Bahat,[1] Richard Sullivan,[2] Fereidoun Daftary,[3] Ramin Mahallati,[3] and Peter S. Wöhrle[4]

[1]American Board of Periodontology, Beverly Hills, California, USA
[2]Clinical Technologies, Nobel Biocare North America, Yorba Linda, California, USA
[3]Center for Implant and Esthetic Dentistry, Beverly Hills, California, USA
[4]Newport Beach, California, USA

Introduction

It has recently been recognized that changes in the bones and soft tissues of the face are a normal dynamic phenomenon that continues throughout life [1–7]. Some of the changes are similar for the two sexes, and some are not. For example, in a study by Kahn and Shaw of the orbit involving three-dimensional computed tomography of 60 patients who were not edentulous [8], facial changes were demonstrable in all age groups. The changes in the bones of the face appear to begin earlier in female patients [8, 9] (Figure 8.1), although the exact age of onset, along with the magnitude and vectors of the changes, are variable and not predictable. Such three-dimensional changes in the position of teeth and associated hard and soft tissue relative to the static position of dental (oral) implants over the course of time can introduce both esthetic and functional compromises of the original implant in a restoration, with unintended consequences. These problems are discussed herein.

Changes associated with aging

The changes with aging arise from a number of sources. The increasingly common addition of body weight and the impact of gravity and sun exposure are obvious causes of facial change [4, 5]. Less obvious is normal redistribution of fullness as a result of fat atrophy or hypertrophy, alterations that contribute significantly to facial aging [6, 10]. Also important are histologic and microstructure changes such as reduction in skin elasticity [6, 11, 12] and loss of facial bone density [13]. Tooth wear may become prominent as a result of occlusal changes and shifting jaw relations [4, 5].

The numerous age-related changes in the maxilla and mandible can create several important alterations [3, 14–17]. Both bones grow downward and forward such that the face gets larger [4] and there is an increase in facial height both anteriorly and posteriorly, especially in the lower face, with an increase in the mandibular angle [3, 16, 17]. Confusingly, different studies have produced different results. For example, Shaw et al. [18] found that ramus height and mandibular body height both decreased significantly with age in both sexes, whereas the mandibular angle increased significantly. The extent of these changes differs in men and women [4, 19], with the posterior change being greater in men [20]. In males, there is downward growth of the ramus and autorotation of the mandible (Figure 8.2) [14, 15], whereas in females, an increase in the mandibular angle occurs (Figure 8.3) [3, 16, 17].

In both men and women, arch circumference and length decrease [4, 7], and the teeth drift mesially [11, 21], leading to tooth crowding, especially in the mandible [22]. In the sagittal plane of the posterior mandible, bony changes will result in lingual resorption and facial bone deposition. The intermolar distance increases (Figure 8.4) [12, 23–27].

In both sexes, the resorption pattern in the sagittal plane of the maxilla results in *facial (buccal) bone loss* (Figure 8.5) [14, 15]. In a female patient, the anterior maxilla exhibits downward growth with a lingual vector. This may cause earlier implant thread exposure [3, 17, 28]. In the male patient, on the other hand, the anterior maxilla exhibits only vertical downward growth (Figure 8.6a to d) [3, 17, 28]. In both the male and female populations, the orbital spaces enlarge [6, 8] and the chin changes in shape and degree of projection [6].

Several soft-tissue changes also occur with aging. The upper lip length increases [4] and its thickness decreases [19]. Maxillary incisor display declines, whereas mandibular incisor visibility increases as the bone rotates anteriorly in males and posteriorly

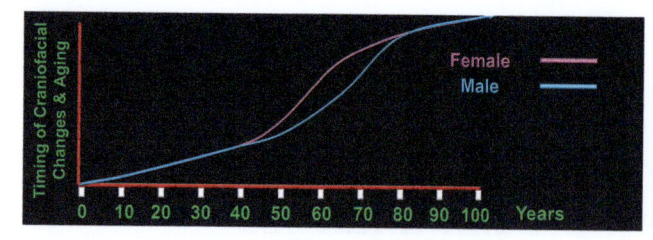

Figure 8.1 Generalized timing of facial and craniofacial aging in males and females. The onset occurs earlier in the female population.

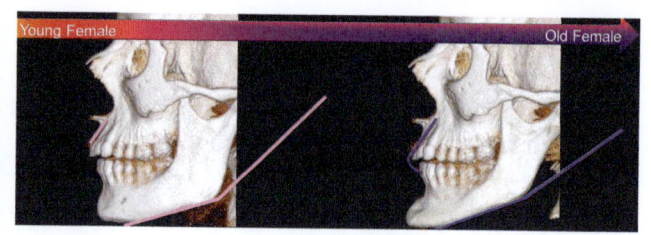

Figure 8.3 Illustrates the general changes in females, including increased mandibular angle and down-growth in lingual vector of the anterior maxilla.

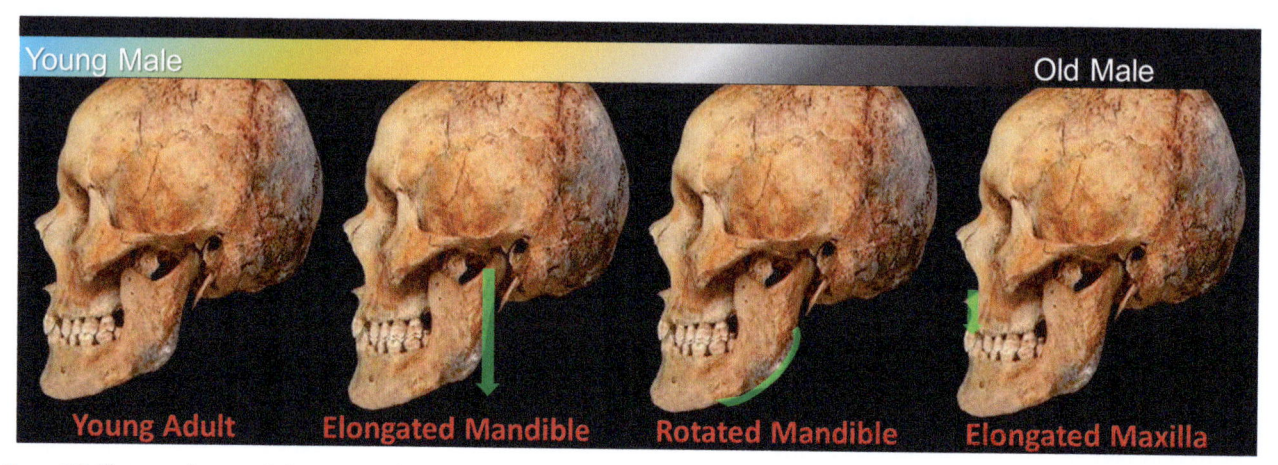

Figure 8.2 Illustrates the general changes in males, including elongation of the ramus, autorotation of the mandible and the down-growth in vector of the anterior maxilla.

in females [17]. The vermilion display of the lip declines, nearly disappearing in the old [6].

These vertical and horizontal changes are more pronounced in patients with short or long faces (Figure 8.7). Whereas all other structures are free to shift in three dimensions as a result, the true position of implants does not change, whereas the relative position of other structures may. Therefore, any implant to be placed in a short or long face may create greater asymmetry secondary to bone changes in the adjacent sites [19, 29, 30].

Figure 8.4 Illustrates increase in intermolar distance with lingual bone resorption and facial apposition.

Implant treatment planning to reduce adverse effects of the aging face

The challenge for treatment planning, therefore, is to consider and anticipate potential changes over time. This will necessitate application of a protocol that is time dependent and that will reduce the future adverse effects of implant placement in an aging face.

Patients can be divided between those who present a high risk and those who present a low risk of significant later craniofacial changes (Table 8.1). The high-risk patient is one with a high smile line and considerable esthetic demands, a short or long face, rapid onset of aging, missing or thin facial or interseptal bone (Figure 8.8), a need for asymmetrical implant placement, thin soft tissue biotype, and highly scalloped soft tissue. The lower-risk patients are those with a low smile line, minimal esthetic expectations, a need for symmetrical implant placement, intact or thick facial and interproximal bone, thick soft tissue

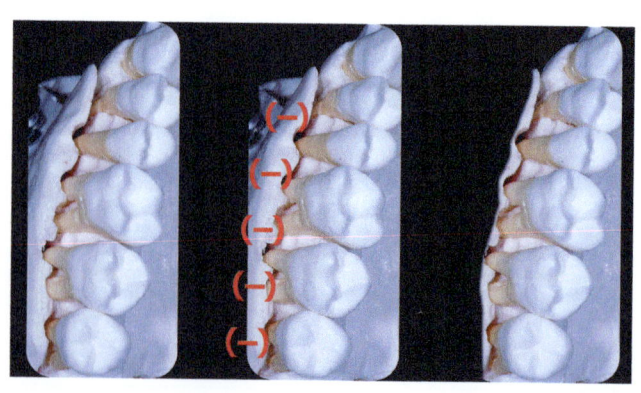

Figure 8.5 Illustrates posterior maxilla with bone resorption on the facial aspect associated with craniofacial aging.

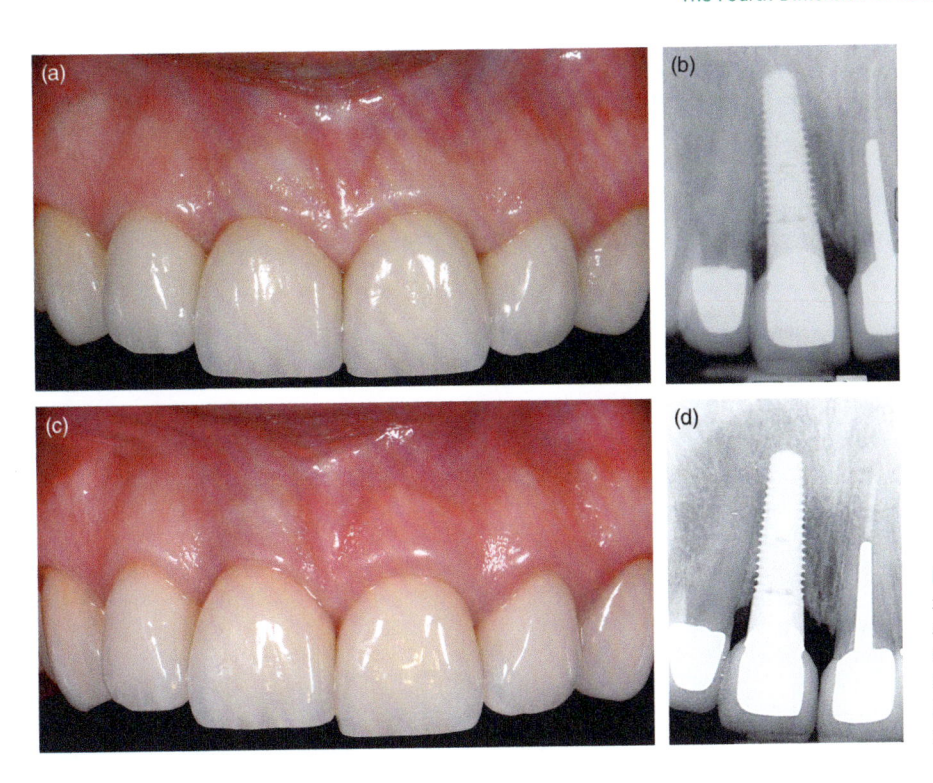

Figure 8.6 Illustrates changes in the anterior maxilla for a male patient aged 35. Images show 9 years post-operative. Continuous down-growth of the maxillary left central incisor with associated structures while the implant position remains the same (as an ankylosed unit).

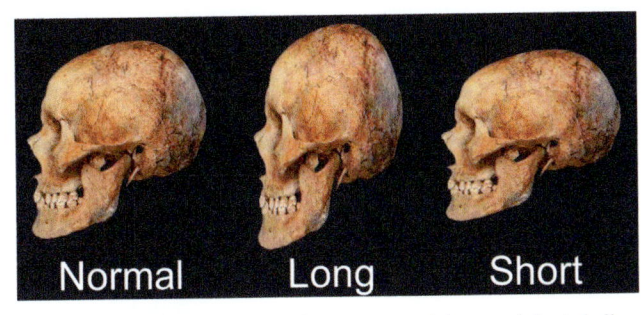

Figure 8.7 Craniofacial variations between normal, long, and short skull anatomy.

biotype, soft tissue coronal to the adjacent dental unit, and flat soft tissue architecture.

The clinical decisions that must be made prior to treatment are described in the Table 8.2. They include selection of an appropriate implant macrostructure and microstructure (Figure 8.9a and b). Rough and smooth surfaces in the coronal third of the implant will react differently to bony changes. Overthinning of the bone and subsequent possible loss may cause an adverse reaction by the soft tissue to a rougher implant surface. A wide-diameter implant will be more susceptible to early exposure and detrimental results in a given ridge dimension. A clinical decision weighing implant strength, loading forces, the age of the patient, and the likelihood of earlier thread exposure is important. Similar decision making is valuable with regard to the apical third of the implant. Sharp threads and cutbacks increase the penetration and its sharpness. However, in areas of a high esthetic demand, where exaggerated vertical discrepancies occur with common thinning of the soft tissue, retrieval of the implant may be necessary. An extensive vertical asymmetry in the esthetic zone cannot be resolved by overextending the incisal

Table 8.1 Algorithm for risk factor.

Reduced risk	High risk
Intact interproximal bone	Compromised blood supply
Intact facial bone	High esthetic demands
Thick soft tissue biotype	Short or long face
Soft tissue coronal to adjacent unit	Facial or interseptal bone missing
Flat soft tissue scallop	Thin biotype
	Highly scalloped periodontium

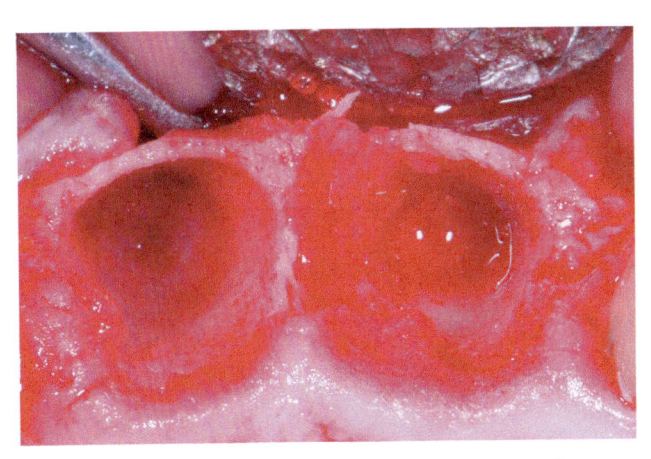

Figure 8.8 Occlusal view of the anterior maxilla after extraction illustrates thin interseptal and buccal bone, which may result in a complete loss of bone subsequent to dynamic changes during aging.

Table 8.2 Clinical decisions to be made.

Asymmetrical placement
Implant diameter
Implant macrostructure
Implant microstructure
Healed site or placement at time of removal of tooth or implant
Immediate versus delayed loading
Hard and soft tissue grafts: staging, approach and biomaterials
Mode of provisionalization

edge of the implant, as the disharmony of the gingival architecture will display unfavorable results. Removal of such an implant with a high penetrating capacity will result in a greater residual defect that will be more difficult to reconstruct and may create a residual defect on adjacent dental units (Figure 8.10).

A treatment plan should be created for modification of the conventional osteotomy in order to accommodate future bone and soft tissue changes. Those directional modifications may necessitate early decisions regarding the need for grafting and the appropriate graft materials. Variation of the conventional osteotomy is clinically challenging and admittedly not always possible. The general intention should be to accommodate future physiologic bony changes without compromising initial implant stability and the long-term esthetic and restorative outcome. This necessitates translation of the point of entry of the osteotomy to allow for increased dimension of bone and soft tissue in the area of highest risk (posterior maxilla and mandible) (Figures 8.11 and 8.12). The influence of craniofacial changes over time for the *posterior maxilla* have been shown to move the buccal plate and associated soft tissue toward the medial/palatal direction. While the necessity of optimal restorative support and emergence profile are a primary objective, sometimes flexibility allows more medial implant placement (Figure 8.11c and d) compared to more lateral placement (Figure 8.11a and b), thereby decreasing risk or at least prolonging any compromise that may be introduced by craniofacial changes over the long term. In the *posterior mandible*, the tendency for movement of bone is from medial to lateral.

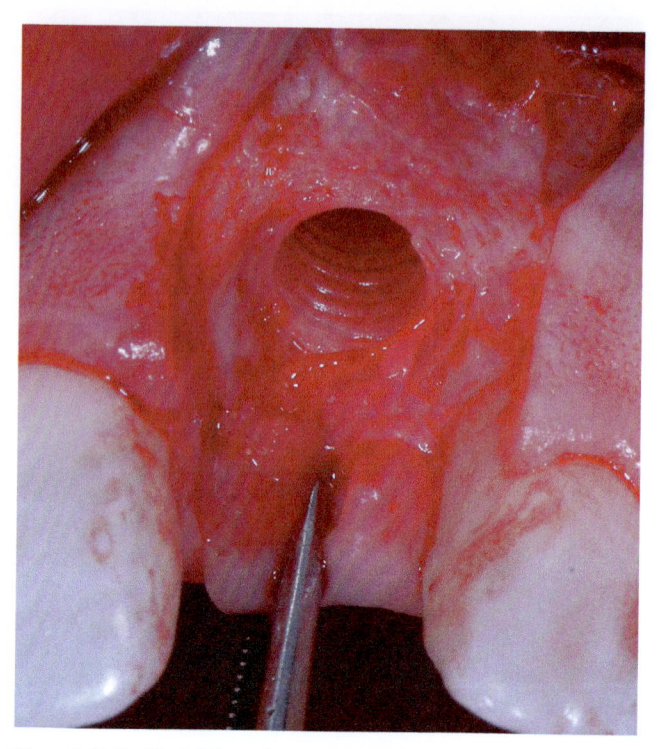

Figure 8.10 Residual defect subsequent to implant removal in the anterior maxilla in a patient with a high smile line. Adjacent anterior maxillary teeth with associate structures in the esthetic zone have continued in a down and lingual vector of movement with age. The implant acted as an ankylosed unit and has not changed its position, eventually residing in the infraocclusion relative to adjacent natural teeth.

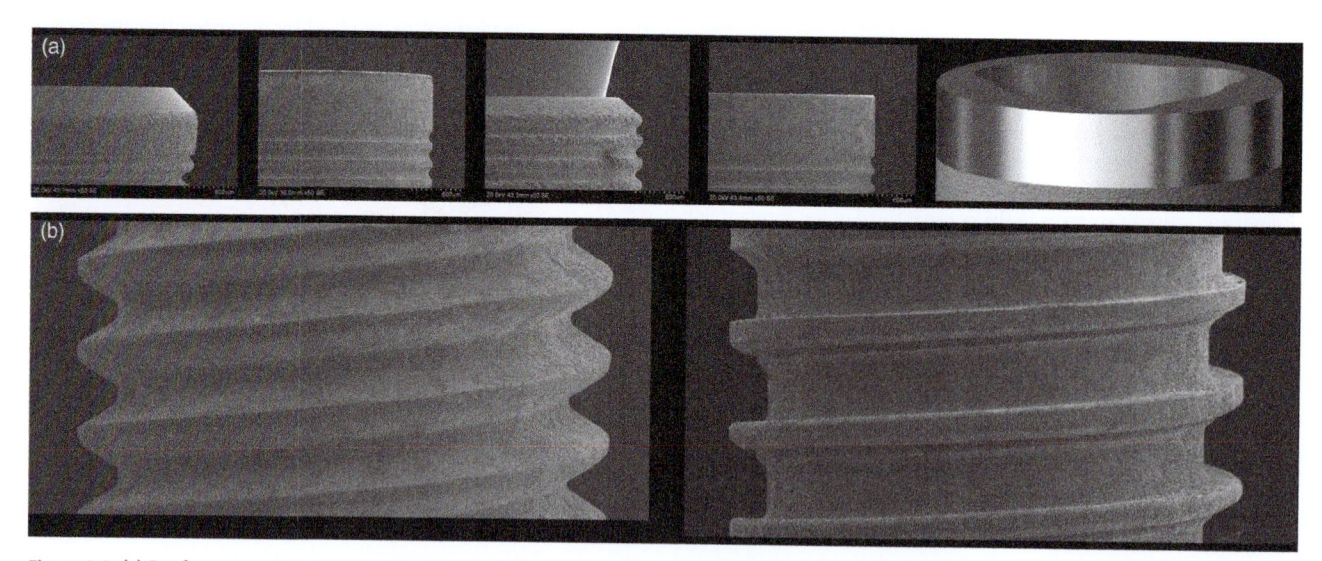

Figure 8.9 (a) Implant macrostructure considerations today include variations in abutment emergence or platform shift as well as the degree and extension of surface texture roughness. (b) Implant thread geometry may be either rounded or squared, its significance is not known to thinning of buccal bone, and potential thread exposure secondary to physiologic bone changes can become a clinical concern for soft tissue.

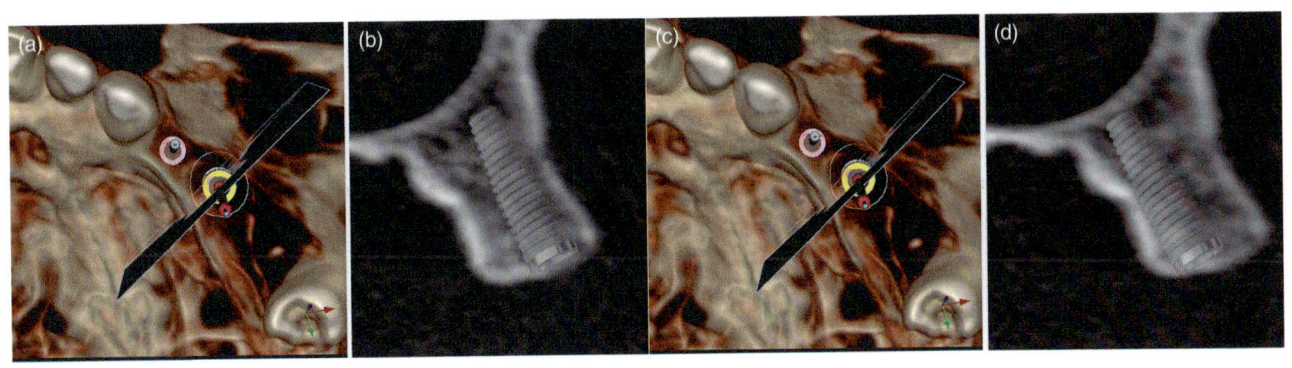

Figure 8.11 The influence of craniofacial changes over time for the posterior maxilla have been shown to move the buccal plate and associated soft tissue toward the medial or lateral direction. While the necessity of optimal restorative support and emergence profile are a primary objective, sometimes flexibility allows more medial implant placement (**c, d**) compared to more lateral placement (**a, b**), thereby decreasing risk or at least prolonging any compromise that may be introduced by craniofacial changes over the long term.

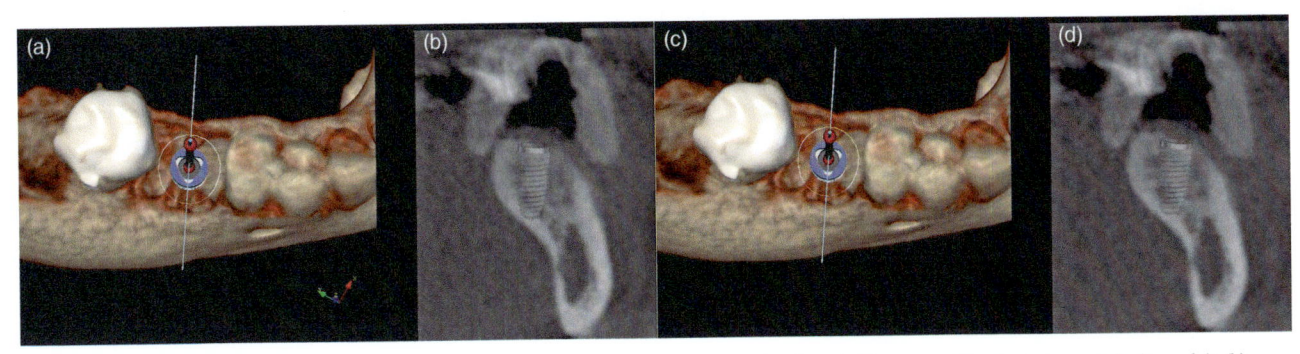

Figure 8.12 In the posterior mandible, the tendency for movement of bone is from medial to lateral. Placement of implants toward the lingual (**a, b**) could result in eventual lingual thread exposure even though restoratively ideal. Positioning the implants in the lower jaw more laterally (**c, d**) while still fulfilling restorative requirements provides an additional safeguard anticipating any craniofacial shifting.

Placement of implants toward the lingual (Figure 8.12a and b) could result in eventual lingual thread exposure, even though restoratively ideal. Positioning the implants in the lower jaw more laterally (Figure 8.12c and d) while still fulfilling restorative requirements provides an additional safeguard anticipating any craniofacial shifting. These modifications may result in thread exposure intraoperatively on the opposite side, which may necessitate grafting.

The selection of grafting material deserves further attention. Once grafting has been successful, the graft will respond in a way similar to the local anatomy, undergoing the same craniofacial changes. Therefore, alteration in grafting techniques and materials may be needed for a single tooth replacement in the anterior zone (Figure 8.13a and b) or a complete reconstruction of a deficient ridge (Figure 8.14a to e). The facial aspect may be at risk of resorption and may benefit from xenografts or allografts as facial layering.

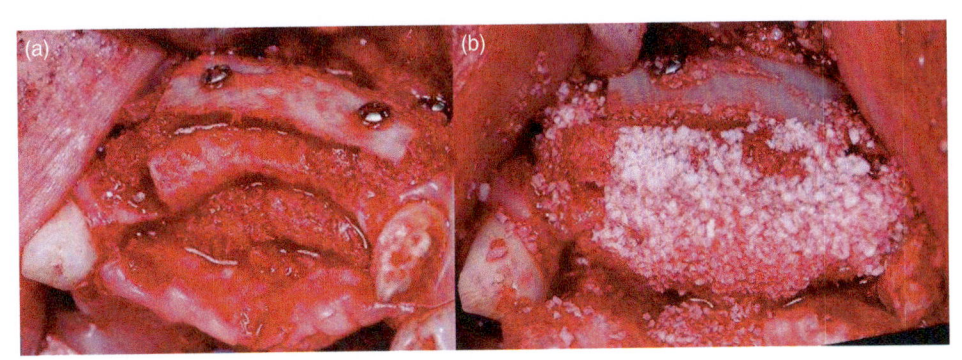

Figure 8.13 (**a**) Facial and lingual grafting with autogenous bone to reconstruct the anterior maxilla. Once vascularization occurs and implants are placed, the graft will respond to craniofacial growth in a similar fashion to the normal alveolus with possible threads exposure. (**b**) Addition of non-resorbable graft material will result in fibrous tissue that may mask exposed threads.

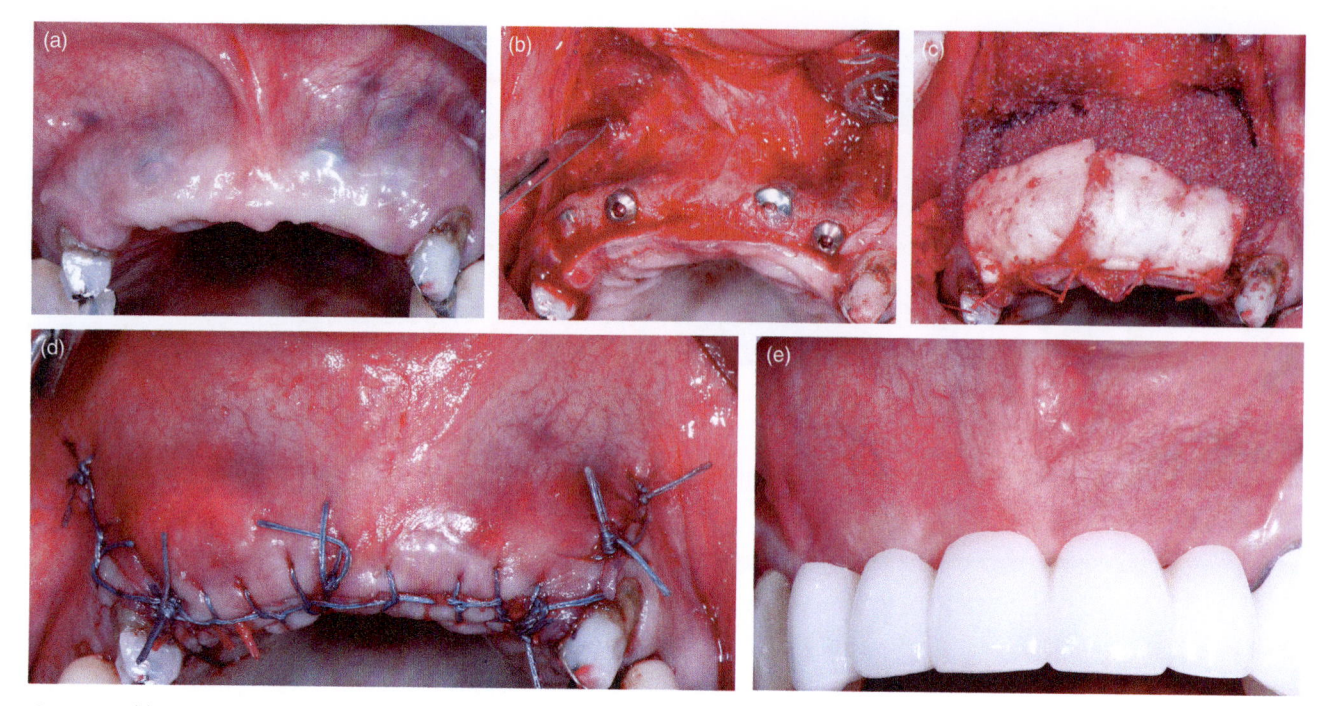

Figure 8.14 (a) Anterior maxilla in an adult female patient showing exposure and thinning of bone and soft tissue over previously placed implants due to down-growth in the lingual vector of the alveolus. (b) Flaps elevated and bone exposed. (c) Grafting crestally with Symbios non-resorbable OsteoGraf LD-300 and overlayed with Biohorizon AlloDerm. The AlloDerm is stabilized with resorbable sutures. (d) Flap advanced and closed primarily. (e) Two months post-operatively. Anterior maxilla reconstructed to compensate for facial resorption.

Summary

Clinical challenges of implant placement in adult patients have not been addressed adequately. Although infraocclusion, open contacts adjacent to implant restorations, thread exposure, and such have been discussed, a systematic approach for pre-treatment and intra-operative changes have to be included in order to compensate for the changes with time. The adult face undergoes normal dynamic physiologic aging, which results in diminished bone volume and structural changes over both teeth and implants. Those cumulative factors cannot be avoided. However, with proper care, its esthetic and functional impact on implant reconstruction can be diminished (Table 8.3).

Table 8.3 Clinical risks and conclusions.

Craniofacial changes continue throughout adult life
Onset differs in the two sexes
Informed consent that takes account of changes with time is necessary
Risks differ among patients (e.g., patients with high smile lines and significant esthetic demands will create greater difficulties)
Pre-operative analysis and protocol should be modified as appropriate
Asymmetrical implant placement creates a higher risk than symmetrical placement
Site recovery is challenging, especially in the esthetic zone

References

1. Behrents RG: *Growth in the Aging Craniofacial Skeleton* [monographs 17 and 18]. University of Michigan, Ann Arbor, MI, 1985.
2. Bishara SE, Treder JE, Jakobsen JR: Facial and dental changes in adulthood. *Am J Orthod Dentofac Orthop* 1994;**106**:175–186.
3. Forsberg CM: Facial morphology and aging: a longitudinal cephalometric investigation in young adults. *Eur J Orthod* 1979;**1**:15–23.
4. Oesterle LJ, Cronin RJ: Adult growth, aging, and the single-tooth implant. *Int J Oral Maxillofac Surg* 2000;**15**:252–260.
5. Albert AM, Ricanek K, Patterson E: A review of the literature on the aging adult skull and face: implications for forensic science research and applications. *Forensic Sci Int* 2007;**172**:1–9.
6. Coleman SR: The anatomy of the aging face: volume loss and changes in 3-dimensional topography. *Aesthet Surg J* 2006; (Suppl): S4–S9.
7. Shaw RB, Katzel EB, Koltz P, et al: Aging of the facial skeleton: aesthetic implications and rejuvenation strategies. *Plast Reconstr Surg* 2011;**127**:374–383.
8. Kahn DM, Shaw RB: Aging of the bony orbit: a three-dimensional computed tomographic study. *Aesthet Surg J* 2008;**28**:258–264.
9. Doual JM, Ferri J, Laude M: The influence of senescence on craniofacial and cervical morphology in humans. *Surg Radiol Anat* 1997;**19**:175–183.
10. Donofrio LM: Fat distribution: a morphologic study of the aging face. *Dermatol Surg* 2000;**26**:1107–1111.
11. Clauser LC, Tieghi R, Galiè M, Carinci F: Structural fat grafting: facial volumetric restoration in complex reconstructive surgery. *J Craniofac Surg* 2011;**22**:1695–1701.
12. Little JW: Volumentric perceptions in midfacial aging with altered priorities for rejuvenation. *Plast Recon Surg* 2000;**105**:252–266.
13. Shaw RB JR, Katzel EB, Koltz PF, et al: Facial bone density: effects of aging and impact on facial rejuvenation. *Aesthet Surg J* 2012;**32**:937–942.
14. Carmichael RP, Sandor GK: Dental implants, growth of the jaws, and determination of skeletal maturity. *Atlas Oral Maxillofac Surg Clin North Am* 2008;**16**:1–9.
15. Enlow DH: *Handbook of Facial Growth*. WB Saunders, Philadelphia, PA, 1990.
16. Tallgren A, Solow B: Age differences in adult dentoalveolar heights. *Eur J Orthod* 1991;**13**:149–156.

17. West KS, McNamara JA: Changes in the craniofacial complex from adolescence to midadulthood: a cephalometric study. *Am J Orthod Dentofac Orthop* 1999;**115**:521–532.
18. Shaw RB, Katzel EB, Koltz PF, et al: Aging of the mandible and its aesthetic implications. *Plast Recon Surg* 2010;**125**:332–342.
19. Bondevik O: Growth changes in the cranial base and the face: a longitudinal cephalometric study of linear and angular changes in adult Norwegians. *Eur J Orthod* 1995;**17**:525–532.
20. Op Heij DG, Opdebeeck H, van Steenberghe D, et al: Facial development, continuous tooth eruption, and mesial drift as compromising factors for implant placement. *Int J Oral Maxillofac Implants* 2006;**21**:867–878.
21. Björk A: Variations in the growth pattern of the human mandible: a longitudinal radiographic study by the implant method. *J Dent Res* 1963;**42**:400–411.
22. Bishara SE, Treder JE, Damon P, Olsen M: Changes in the dental arches and dentition between 25 and 45 years of age. *Angle Orthod* 1996;**66**:417–422.
23. Bondevik O: Changes in occlusion between 23 and 34 years. *Angle Orthod* 1998;**68**:75–80.
24. Enlow DH: The "V" principle. *Am J Orthod* 1984;**85**:96.
25. Enlow DH: A study of the post-natal growth and remodeling of bone. *Am J Anat* 1962;**110**:79–101.
26. Enlow DH: A morphogenetic analysis of facial growth. *Am J Orthod* 1966;**52**:283–299.
27. Enlow DH, Harris DB: A study of the postnatal growth of the human mandible. *Am J Orthod* 1964;**50**:25–50.
28. Sarnas KV, Solow B: Early adult changes in the skeletal and soft-tissue profile. *Eur J Orthod* 1980;**2**:1–12.
29. Opdebeeck H, Bell WH: The short face syndrome. *Am J Orthod* 1978;**73**:499–511.
30. Opdebeeck H, Bell WH, Eisenfeld J, Mishelevich D: Comparative study between the SFS and LFS rotation as a possible morphogenetic mechanism. *Am J Orthod* 1978;**74**:509–521.

SECTION II

Guided Bone Regeneration (GBR) with Particulate Graft for Vertical Alveolar Ridge Defects

CHAPTER 9

Dental Implant Site Development with Particulate Bone Grafts and Guided Bone Regeneration

Flavia Q. Pirih[1] and Paulo M. Camargo[2]

[1]Section of Periodontics, UCLA School of Dentistry, Los Angeles, California, USA
[2]UCLA School of Dentistry, Los Angeles, California, USA

Introduction

Dental implants have revolutionized the provision of dental treatment. The use of dental implants to support restorations allow individuals who would otherwise have to wear poorly retentive and unstable prosthetic appliances to receive fixed restorations or to enjoy removable appliances that are fully functional, therefore enhancing the patient's quality of life [1]. A requirement for the placement of dental implants on the human jaws is the availability of adequate bone volume. Due to the natural bone modeling and remodeling that occurs during healing following tooth extraction, the possibility of placing dental implants can often only be created with the implementation of reconstructive ridge preservation/augmentation procedures, which allow for adequate development of the future implant site. These reconstructive procedures may enable implant fixture installation in positions that satisfies the biological, functional, and esthetic demands of the restoration.

The aim of this chapter is to discuss ridge preservation and augmentation procedures that can be achieved with particulate grafting in implant dentistry. The following topics will be addressed: (1) regenerative material selection, (2) indications for particulate grafting, (3) extraction socket/alveolar ridge preservation, (4) alveolar ridge augmentation, (5) dehiscences/fenestrations around implants, (6) regenerative treatment of peri-implantitis, and (7) management of surgical complications. Three cases will be presented to illustrate the text.

Regenerative material selection

The clinician has several options in terms of graft materials and other devices and agents to treat extraction sockets and atrophic ridges. The first controlled clinical trials that examined the preservation of the dimensions of extraction sockets during tooth extraction utilized guided bone regeneration (GBR), where membranes were the sole treatment devices [2–4]. GBR is a cell exclusion technique where the membrane prevents cells from the soft tissues next to the extraction socket from migrating into the area, thereby preserving the space and allowing time for bone cells to populate the socket space [2]. When used alone, most membranes tend to collapse into the socket space, creating a technical problem for hard tissue regeneration. Bone grafts, when placed in fresh extraction sockets, have the ability to work as a scaffold for osteogenesis, as well as maintaining the space for bone formation during wound healing. Because there are distinct advantages in using GBR and bone grafts, the majority of regenerative procedures in extraction sockets are performed with a combination of a resorbable membrane and a graft material.

Membranes

Several membrane materials have been examined and utilized for GBR in extraction sockets. These devices can be categorized into resorbable and non-resorbable materials. Membrane selection depends on several factors, including biocompatibility, rate of integration/resorption by the host tissue, tolerance to exposure to the oral cavity, cell occlusiveness, physical characteristics such as stiffness and ability to maintain the space and ease of use [5].

Non-resorbable membranes

Non-resorbable membranes, such as expanded polytetrafluoroethylene (e-PTFE) were the first membranes utilized in GBR [2, 4]. Although great results can be achieved with the use of a non-resorbable membrane, a major risk associated with its use is flap dehiscence and membrane exposure to the oral cavity. If an e-PTFE membrane is exposed, it has to be removed, which often results in less than optimal results in bone regeneration [6]. In order to overcome the wound healing problems inherent to non-resorbable membranes, resorbable barriers made of materials that have a higher degree of biocompatibility were developed [7].

Despite the fact that the use of non-resorbable membranes is technique and case sensitive, titanium-reinforced non-resorbable membranes are a suitable option for situations when a large volume of bone needs to be augmented or when vertical bone regeneration is desirable, because they allow for more efficient maintenance of the defect space when compared to resorbable membranes [8, 9].

For cases of intended horizontal bone augmentation and implant placement, a meta-analysis has found that there is no significant difference in the implant survival rate when comparing implant placement with a simultaneous GBR procedure using resorbable or non-resorbable membranes [10]. Additionally, resorbable membranes are much less technique sensitive and

---

Vertical Alveolar Ridge Augmentation in Implant Dentistry: A Surgical Manual, First Edition. Edited by Len Tolstunov.
© 2016 John Wiley & Sons, Inc. Published 2016 by John Wiley & Sons, Inc.

tend to perform well even in cases where they are exposed to the oral cavity environment.

Resorbable membranes

Resorbable membranes can be made of several natural and synthetic materials. The ones made of collagen are the most researched and commonly utilized membranes for GBR [11].

There are several advantages in using resorbable membranes as compared to non-resorbable membranes. There is no need for removal, they are tolerant to intentional or accidental exposure to the oral cavity [6], post-operative complications such as infections are rare, and the overall morbidity is low [12–15].

The potential disadvantages associated with resorbable membranes are limited resistance to collapsing into the bony defect, not being effective space-makers or maintainers [16], variable and potentially excessively fast resorption rate [16], and rapid hydrolyzation in cases of exposure to the oral cavity, which may result in graft exposure, potential infection, and a diminished GBR effect. With these limitations in mind, technology keeps evolving with the goal of providing clinicians with membranes made of materials and configurations that can overcome the above-mentioned problems.

As previously stated, the most commonly used resorbable membranes are made of collagen; however, synthetic resorbable membranes are commercially available as made of polylactic acid, polyglycolic acid [17], polyethyleneglycol [18], polyurethane, and lactide/glycolide copolymers (e.g., polyglactice-910) and calcium sulfate [19]. The main drawback of synthetic resorbable membranes is the increased possibility of inflammatory foreign-body types of reaction [20].

In summary, resorbable membranes are usually adequate for extraction socket regenerative treatment and for alveolar ridge augmentation cases that do not require extensive vertical bone regeneration. As long as the resorbable membrane is well adapted to the surgical area and stable, it should lead to a predictable outcome.

Bone graft materials

Clinical studies have demonstrated that there are additional benefits to combine a bone graft with a membrane when treating extraction sockets or augmenting the alveolar ridge, when compared to using a membrane alone. The selection of a bone graft material depends on its biological and physical properties, rate of resorption, risks associated with post-operative complications, and patient acceptance [21]. Below is a discussion of the advantages and disadvantages of the most common particulate materials utilized for bone regeneration.

With respect to their role in new bone formation, bone graft materials can be classified into osteogenic, osteoinductive, and osteoconductive. These properties should be taken into consideration when selecting a bone graft material for use in the regenerative treatment of extraction sockets and alveolar ridges. A bone graft with osteogenic qualities forms new bone from viable cells contained in the graft itself; one with osteoinductive qualities induces bone formation by cells that are located immediately adjacent to the grafted material, as it basically "attracts" cells with osteogenic potential to the grafted area [22]; finally, a bone graft with osteoconductive qualities simply serves as a scaffold for bone formation, where actual bone formation originates in the host's adjacent bone [23].

Autografts

An autogenous bone graft (autograft) is defined as a graft derived from the individual receiving the graft. Autografts can be obtained from: extraoral and intraoral sources. Extraoral sources include the iliac crest, calvaria, and other bones [24, 25]. Intraoral sources include the maxillary tuberosity, a healed edentulous area, lower retromolar/mandibular ramus, exostoses/tori, as well as other locations. Intraoral sources are a more practical alternative as compared with extraoral donor sites given the morbidity and logistical difficulties associated with donor areas that cannot be accessed through the oral cavity.

The main advantages of autogenous grafts are their osteogenic, osteoinductive and osteoconductive capabilities. Because of these qualities, autogenous grafts are considered by many to be the gold standard for bone regeneration [26]. Even though there may be many advantages to utilizing autogenous grafts, in many instances their disadvantages should be considered, and include limited amount, need for a second surgical site, increased post-operative pain and discomfort, unpredictable rate of graft resorption, and increased surgical and increased recovery time [27, 28].

Allografts

An allograft is defined as a graft from a donor that belongs to the same species as the recipient. Currently used modalities of allografts do not contain viable cells, but have (limited) osteoinductive and osteoconductive properties [29]. The most common types of particulate allogenic graft are cadaveric mineralized freeze-dried bone allografts (FDBAs) and decalcified freeze-dried bone allografts (DFDBAs). These materials are commercially available from tissue banks. Raw materials are obtained from donors who have been screened and tested for contagious diseases. It has been shown that the osteogenic capabilities of allografts are not uniform and may depend on various donor-related factors such as age [30].

Xenografts

A xenograft is as a graft material harvested from an individual of one species and placed on a being of a different species. Xenografts have been shown to have osteoconductive capacities, therefore acting as a scaffold. The bovine mineral bone matrix is comparable to the human bone matrix and its biocompatibility has been demonstrated [31]. Compared to allografts, one of the main advantages of this material is its slower absorption rate because it allows for prolonged space maintenance of the augmented area [32]. Additionally, it has been shown that particles of this modality of graft are incorporated into the new bone matrix. These properties, combined with abundance and ease of use, make it an attractive option for the regenerative treatment of extraction sockets and deficient alveolar ridges. It has also been shown that deproteinized bovine-derived bone mineral is the most commonly used and best documented bone substitute for the treatment of dehiscences and fenestrations around implant fixtures [33].

Alloplasts

Alloplastic materials are bone graft substitutes that are synthetic in nature or that originate from natural mineral materials. These materials include calcium phosphate (tricalcium phosphate, hydroxyapatite and calcium phosphate cement), bioactive glass and other polymers. Also, alloplasts can be found in resorbable and non-resorbable forms [34].

Bone graft selection

An evidence-based choice of bone graft material cannot be easily made. Research has shown that all modalities of bone grafts described above can be successfully used in the regenerative treatment of extraction sockets and deficient alveolar ridges. However, there is no objective data indicating the superiority of one modality of bone graft over another. With the current evidence, graft selection should take into consideration the preference of the clinician, patient beliefs, and acceptance, besides the characteristics of the material and objectives of the surgical procedure.

Indications for particulate bone grafts

Particulate bone grafts can be utilized for alveolar ridge maintenance/socket preservation, healed ridge augmentation, implant dehiscence or fenestration, and bone grafting after implant placement. Particulate grafts usually benefit from their combination with a membrane or barrier for GBR, not only because of its ability to control the cellular dynamics of wound healing but also because such devices aid in the stabilization and containment of the materials that are usually granular in nature. The combination of GBR with a bone graft has been proven to successfully regenerate bone in extraction sockets and ridge defects in animal and human studies [35] and, more importantly, to allow implant placement and survival in the previously augmented areas.

Particulate grafts combined with GBR in ridge preservation prior to implant placement

It is well documented that the alveolar process is influenced by the presence or absence of teeth and that vertical and horizontal bone loss occurs after tooth extraction [36–39]. A systematic review by Tan et al. concluded that horizontal bone loss ranges from 29 to 63% and the vertical bone loss from 11 to 22% six months after tooth extraction [40]. Given that bone loss is inevitable after tooth extraction and that the stability and ideal implant positioning might be compromised by osseous defects, ridge preservation/augmentation are commonly utilized procedures to modify the natural extraction socket healing.

Alveolar ridge/socket preservation

Alveolar ridge/socket preservation procedures aim at minimizing the amount of horizontal and vertical ridge alteration after tooth extraction. Therefore, the main objectives of ridge/socket preservation are the maintenance of the existing soft and hard tissue to optimize functional and esthetic outcomes and also the simplification of subsequent procedures, such as implant placement by eliminating or minimizing the need of subsequent bone augmentation [41]. The survival rate of implants placed on areas that have undergone bone augmentation is similar to the survival rates of implants that were placed in native bone [42, 43].

There are different procedures that aim at alveolar ridge/socket preservation procedures that have been described in the literature. These procedures range from the use of a membrane (for GBR) alone, bone graft alone, or the use of a bone graft material in conjunction with a membrane [44, 45]. In addition, the graft materials examined for such a purpose included those from auto-, allo-, and xenografts, as well as alloplasts [46]. The surgical techniques proposed below take into account the socket morphology after tooth extraction and separate the treatment choices into three groups, depending on the degree of destruction of the buccal bony plate: none or minimal, moderate, and severe.

Alveolar ridge/socket preservation with no or minimal buccal bone destruction

If immediately after tooth extraction that was conducted with minimal trauma, it is confirmed that there is no or minimal buccal bone destruction, preserving the socket is not as challenging and is one of the rare situations that can be treated with a bone graft alone, in the absence of a membrane for GBR. In such cases, the use of a low resorbing particulate bone graft material, such as a deproteinized bovine-derived bone mineral, can be placed into the sockets and sealed with a collagen plug (modified Bio-Col technique) and/or a free gingival graft, which contains the graft during the early phases of soft tissue healing. Such cases, in which extraction is usually dictated by non-restorability of a tooth with intact periodontal support, do not require GBR because the walls of the socket protect the space from invasion by soft tissues [47–49].

Alveolar ridge/socket preservation with moderate buccal bone destruction

If after tooth extraction there is moderate facial bone loss (≥ 2–<5 mm range), the ridge preservation procedure needs to address the possibility of the buccal soft tissues migrating into the socket area. In such cases, a flapless procedure can be employed, with a membrane being shaped like an ice cream cone and adapted against the inner aspect of the buccal bony plate [50]. Following socket-fill with a particulate bone graft material, the top portion of the membrane (ice cream portion of the ice cream cone) is folded over the bone graft so as to obliterate the entrance of the socket, and is then tucked and sutured under the palatal tissue. A collagen plug or a free gingival graft can be placed over the membrane in order to protect it from hydrolyzation that can occur too fast. Any particulate bone graft can be used with this technique, although preference is given to a slow substitution material, such as deproteinized bovine-derived bone.

Alveolar ridge/socket preservation with severe buccal bone destruction

If after tooth extraction there is severe (≥ 5 mm) vertical destruction of the buccal plate, preservation of the socket space becomes more challenging because most of the buccal wall has to be rebuilt. In such cases, a GBR procedure with a resorbable collagen membrane that involves buccal flap elevation and also particulate bone graft should be utilized. Following tooth extraction and elevation of a buccal flap apical to the mucogingival junction, the socket area should be thoroughly debrided. A membrane, usually resorbable, should be trimmed so as to overlap with the bone margins of the buccal defect, is adapted on the outer surface of the buccal plate, and is secured with bone tacks or sutures. Once the membrane is secure, the particulate bone graft material ought to be placed in the socket space. The membrane is tucked under the palatal tissue and can be sutured. A second membrane, slightly smaller than the one that was first utilized, can be placed over it in order to maximize the possibility of an effective GBR effect. Finally, the buccal flap is sutured over the membrane [44] and the clinician has the option of achieving primary flap closure. Cases in which a buccal flap is elevated are amenable for treatment with a non-resorbable membrane such as e-PTFE; primary and sustainable closure of the flap must be ensured during surgery, as any exposure of the non-resorbable membrane to the oral cavity during healing will compromise results.

Alveolar ridge augmentation

Alveolar ridge augmentation can be performed for horizontal, vertical, or combination defects. Although the focus of this book is vertical ridge augmentation, the width of the alveolar ridge is often deficient in 3D bone collapse situations. It is often important to use particulate grafting to improve the alveolar width first, followed by the vertical augmentation. In this chapter we will focus on the applications of particulate bone graft materials for the horizontal bone augmentation, which is a predictable procedure. Vertical augmentation, if needed, can be also done with a particulate or block materials, or other techniques described in this book. It is also done after horizontal augmentation as a second surgical phase in *staged* reconstructive techniques.

In attempting to increase the buccolingual dimension of the alveolar ridge, the clinician may find two distinct situations: horizontal defects within the confines of the alveolar housing, where GBR with a resorbable membrane and combined with bone graft can be utilized; or horizontal defects where the intended degree of augmentation extends beyond (outside) the confines of the alveolar housing, in which GBR with a titanium-reinforced membrane and a bone graft is the most predictable surgical technique.

Horizontal defects within the alveolar housing: GBR with resorbable membranes and particulate bone grafts

If the horizontal ridge augmentation is *within* the confines of the alveolar bone housing, bone augmentation is mostly predictable. In such cases, the use of a resorbable membrane combined with a particulate bone graft material is adequate since the area does not require additional support for space maintenance; the most prominent margin of the bony contour around the periphery of the defect is usually sufficient to prevent the membrane from collapsing. In brief, following buccal flap elevation and defect decortication to maximize blood supply, a resorbable collagen membrane should be secured in place over the outer surface of the buccal bony plate. This is usually accomplished with the use of bone tacking systems. Once the membrane is secure, particulate bone graft material is placed on the defect area under the membrane. The membrane can be sutured to the palatal tissues. A second membrane can be placed over the first one, as described earlier in this chapter, for protection, in case the membrane gets exposed. The buccal flap is advanced and sutured over the membranes; such advancement may require periosteal release in the most apical area of the flap. Care should be exercised to create a tension-free flap, which would minimize the chances of early membrane exposure.

Horizontal defects that require augmentation beyond the existing confines of the alveolar housing: GBR with titanium-reinforced membranes and particulate bone grafts

If horizontal ridge augmentation is needed *outside* the existing confines of the alveolar bone housing, it is imperative that such a component of the intended augmentation space be maintained throughout the healing process. In such situations, GBR with a titanium-reinforced membrane combined with a particulate bone graft can be used. Alternatively, onlay bone grafts (autogenous/allograft), in combination or not with GBR, can be recommended. The utilization of GBR combined with a particulate graft (xenograft) for the above-described purpose is relatively predictable.

The GBR/particulate graft combination technique, when compared to autogenous block grafts, has the advantages of being technically easier and resulting in less morbidity to the patient. Harvesting block grafts can result in several complications, including devitalization of teeth and damage to the inferior alveolar nerve. However, the long-term efficacy of utilizing allograft and xenograft blocks lacks research, and has therefore not been determined.

While the surgical technique used for these procedures is similar to the one employed in cases where a resorbable membrane is used, primary passive and sustainable closure of the flap is essential, as non-resorbable membranes are not tolerant to exposure to the oral cavity. In addition to periosteal release and vertical incisions on the buccal flap, the temporary prosthesis must be extensively alleviated so that no mechanical pressure is placed on the suture line during the early phases of healing.

Indications for particulate grafts in conjunction with implant placement

Often, during implant placement, dehiscences and fenestrations occur. These occurrences are more common on the buccal surfaces of implant fixtures. GBR combined with a particulate graft can be used to regenerate bone in such iatrogenic defects. The technical principles of such procedures are similar to the ones described for regenerative treatment of extraction sockets and deficient alveolar ridges. After implant placement and primarily fixture stability is ensured, decortication of the buccal plate should be performed around the area of the dehiscence or fenestration, as allowable by the anatomy of the area.

Fenestrations are usually treatable with a resorbable membrane for GBR combined with a particulate graft. As long as the bony plate coronal to the fenestration is thick (≥ 2 mm), the implant can be treated in one stage (i.e., connection of a healing abutment) and the regenerative procedure to heal during implant integration. Membrane stabilization may not be easily achievable in such cases and it should be attempted via suturing to the vertical incision. Resorbable bone tacking systems are available for such a purpose.

Dehiscences can be treated in a similar fashion, but implants should be treated in a two-stage fashion, with the fixture being submerged during the osseointegration period. This prevents contamination of the regenerative materials and minimizes the chances for invagination of soft tissues into the area that received GBR/grafting. Stabilization of the membrane is easier in these cases because the implant cover screw may immobilize it, and metal (titanium) bone tacks can be utilized as they can be removed during the implant exposure surgery.

Indications for particulate grafts after implant placement

The most common application of particulate graft material after implant placement is in the treatment of peri-implantitis. Even though the pathogenesis, development, and treatment of peri-implantitis are not well understood, many treatment approaches have been proposed [51] and, as mentioned above, they can involve particulate bone grafts [52–54].

When a regenerative procedure is attempted on an implant that has lost supporting bone due to peri-implantitis, the fixture needs to be debrided and a particulate graft material is placed around the defect, often in combination with a membrane or other barrier, such as calcium sulfate. The use of particulate bone grafts in the treatment of defects initiated by peri-implantitis has been associated with clinical and radiographic improvements [53, 54]; however, gingival recession is commonly observed post-surgically. In an effort to minimize the risk of gingival recession, a soft tissue graft can be performed in conjunction with the use of a particulate bone graft [55, 56].

Management of complications associated with particulate grafts

When using particulate grafts, complications during implant site development and implant placement are not common. However, when complications arise, the most common scenarios are non-resorbable membrane exposure, encapsulation of the particulate graft by soft tissue, and infection.

Membrane exposure

It is clear that, when a non-resorbable membrane becomes exposed to the oral cavity early in the course of healing, the amount of bone augmentation is compromised [57] even in situations where clinical infection does not occur. Should infection occur, the result can be disastrous. Therefore, when a non-resorbable membrane gets exposed, it is prudent to have it removed and the area retreated after soft tissue healing. In addition, in such cases, part or all of the graft material may be lost [6, 15]. Resorbable membranes are once again advantageous as compared to non-resorbable ones, as spontaneous healing usually occurs in cases of flap dehiscence [58, 59].

Encapsulation of particulate grafts and the need for retreatment

There are situations when a ridge preservation or augmentation procedure is performed and portions of the particulate graft material are not incorporated into the bone matrix. This is more common in the coronal aspect of the previously treated area, particularly in extraction socket areas. When facing these situations, the clinician has to make a decision about whether to remove the encapsulated material and proceed with implant placement or remove the encapsulated material, perform a second regenerative procedure, and, at a later time, perform another attempt at implant placement. Fortunately, situations where a significant amount of encapsulated material is present to the point that they make implant placement impossible are not common. Secondary GBR/grafting in conjunction with implant placement in order to regenerate bone in areas where previously encapsulated graft material needs to be removed is often successful.

Infection

The risk of infection in GBR and implant placement is very small. It ranges from 1 to 4.5% [60–62]. Moreover, despite the fact that the use of perioperative antibiotics for bone regenerative procedures and implant placement is advocated by many authors, a study done by Powell et al. concluded that the risk of infection in GBR procedures was 4% (1/25 procedures), the use of a bone graft was not associated with increased risk for infection, and the use of a membrane did not statistically increase the risk of infections. Based on their findings, the authors suggested that the use of antibiotics perioperative may not be beneficial. However, the authors suggested that a larger-scale, controlled clinical study is warranted [62]. A meta-analysis conducted by Chiapasco compared the rate of membrane exposure/infection between non-resorbable and resorbable membranes around 374 peri-implant defects (dehiscences and fenestrations) and concluded that 20% of the non-resorbable membranes had exposure/infection and 14% of them had to be removed, compared to 5% of the resorbable membranes [63]. All together, it appears prudent to prescribe systemic antibiotics in cases where particulate grafts and membranes are used. Such a practice, combined with 0.12% chlorhexidine rinses, should be enforced until the wound is completely closed with soft tissues.

Case 1: Socket preservation

This patient was congenitally missing his maxillary anterior teeth. Some permanent teeth had poor root form. He would like to have dental implants in the upper anterior segment. In preparation to receive implant-supported restorations, the patient was subjected to orthodontic treatment combined with orthognathic surgery.

Clinical examination revealed tooth formation anomalies and partial edentulism. Additionally, a maxillary labial frenum with low attachment was present (Figures 9.1 and 9.2). After clinical and radiographic examination, extraction of the maxillary anterior teeth with socket preservation and subsequent replacement of the missing permanent anterior teeth from canine on one side to canine on the other side with an implant-supported fixed partial denture was recommended.

Extraction of primary canines and incisors on both sides was performed under local anesthesia and with minimal trauma. An intrasulcular incision was made around the teeth, which were carefully luxated with an elevator and extracted with a forceps (Figure 9.3). Sockets were curetted and inspected. As there was no loss of facial bone, socket preservation was performed by filling the alveolus with bovine-derived porous bone mineral to the levels of the surrounding bony walls (Figure 9.4). A collagen plug was placed over the particulate bone graft (Figure 9.5), which was secured in place with 4.0 chromic gut (Figure 9.6). A buccal frenectomy was performed and a free gingival graft delivered to the area where the frenum was attached.

Three months after the extractions and socket preservations, evaluation of the area, for the placement of implants, was conducted. The soft tissue in the edentulous area was clinically healthy (Figures 9.7 and 9.8).

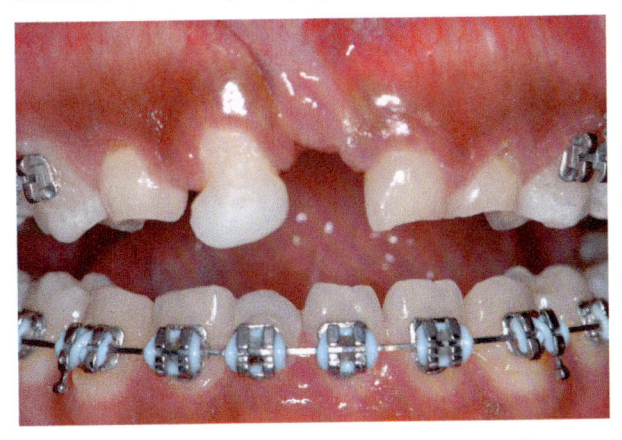

Figure 9.1 Buccal view of the maxillary anterior region, which presented with retained primary canines and incisors on both sides and missing permanent anterior teeth from canine on one side to canine on the other side.

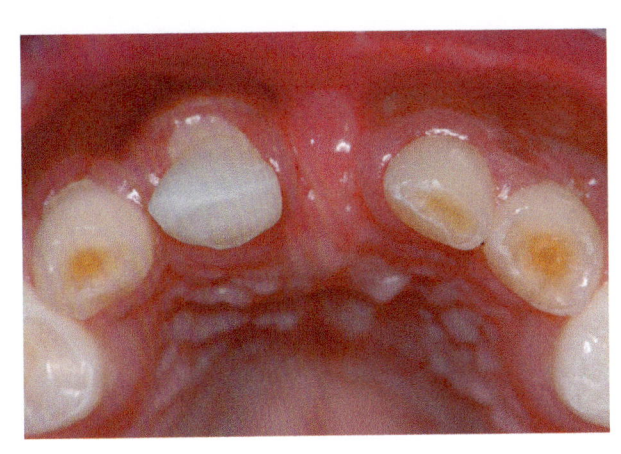

Figure 9.2 Occlusal view of the maxillary anterior region.

(continued)

(continued)

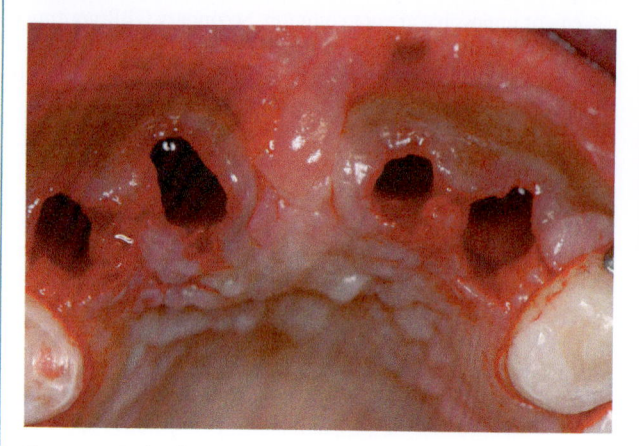

Figure 9.3 Occlusal view of the maxillary anterior region after atraumatic, flapless, teeth extraction.

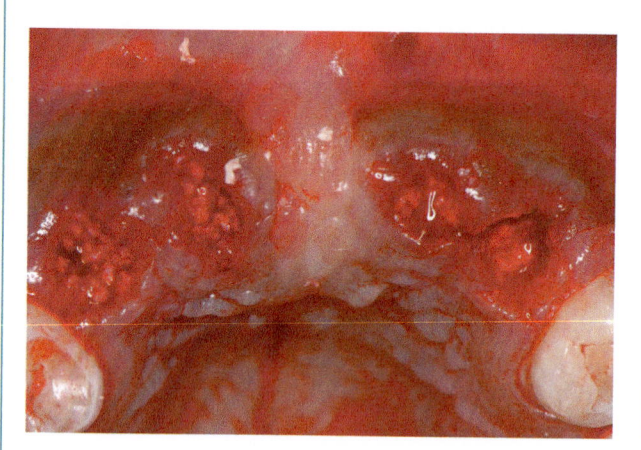

Figure 9.4 Occlusal view of the maxillary anterior region. Extraction sockets were filled with a bovine-derived porous mineral.

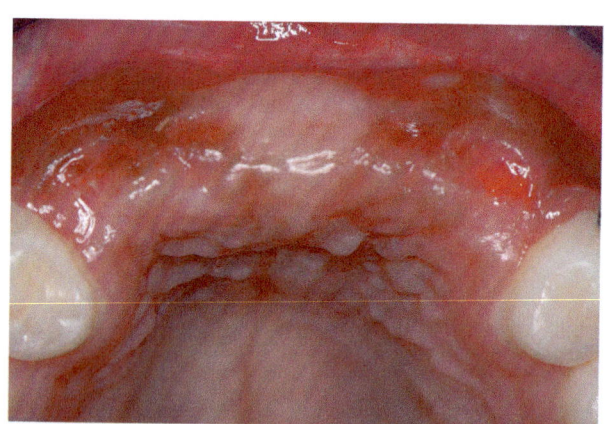

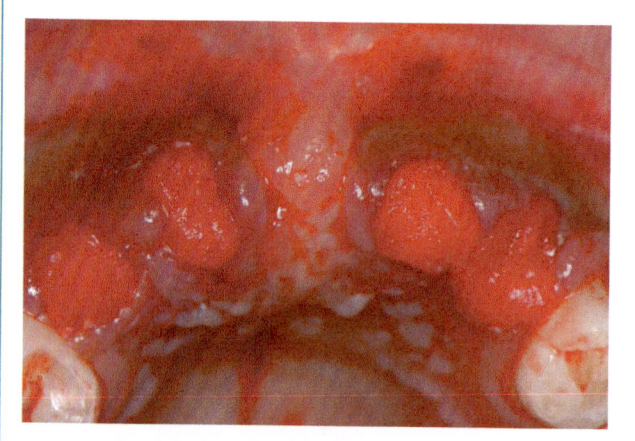

Figure 9.5 Occlusal view of the maxillary anterior region. A collagen plug was placed over the graft material.

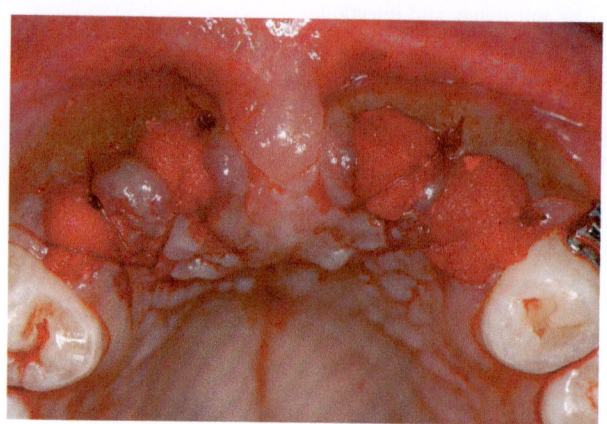

Figure 9.6 Occlusal view of the maxillary anterior region. Chromic gut sutures were placed over the collagen plug.

Figure 9.7 Occlusal view of the maxillary anterior region 3 months after extractions.

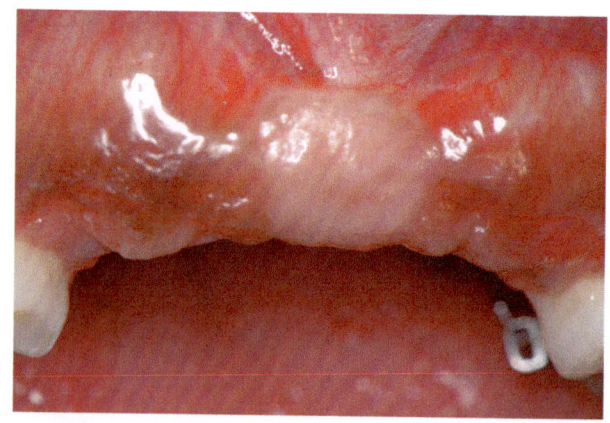

Figure 9.8 Buccal view of the maxillary anterior region 3 months after extractions.

Case 2: Implant fenestration

This patient presented with hopeless maxillary right central incisor and maxillary left lateral incisor. One year after the extractions and socket preservation procedures, the patient presented for another consultation and fabrication of a radiographic stent. Clinical examination of the area revealed horizontal and vertical ridge deficiencies (Figure 9.9). A computerized tomographic scan was performed to determine the amount of vertical and horizontal bone at the future implant sites (Figures 9.10 and 9.11). Given the horizontal and vertical bone present in the areas of the maxillary right central incisor and the maxillary left lateral incisor, a clinical decision was made to place two implants, one on the maxillary right central incisor and one on the maxillary left lateral incisor regions, and perform bone augmentation concomitant with implant installation utilizing a particulate graft and a resorbable membrane.

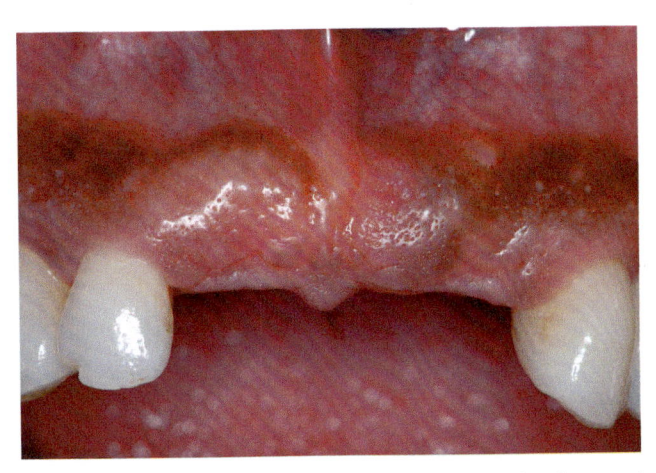

Figure 9.9 Buccal view of the maxillary anterior region, which presented with a concavity apical to the mucogingival junction.

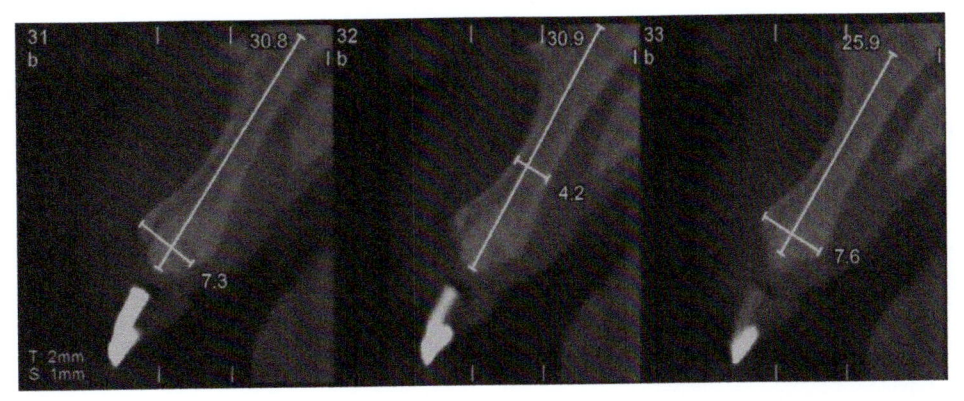

Figure 9.10 Computerized tomographic scan of the maxillary right central incisor area prior to implant placement. The image shows a marker present in the radiographic stent depicting the path of insertion for the implant. Notice the buccal thickness of 4.2 mm.

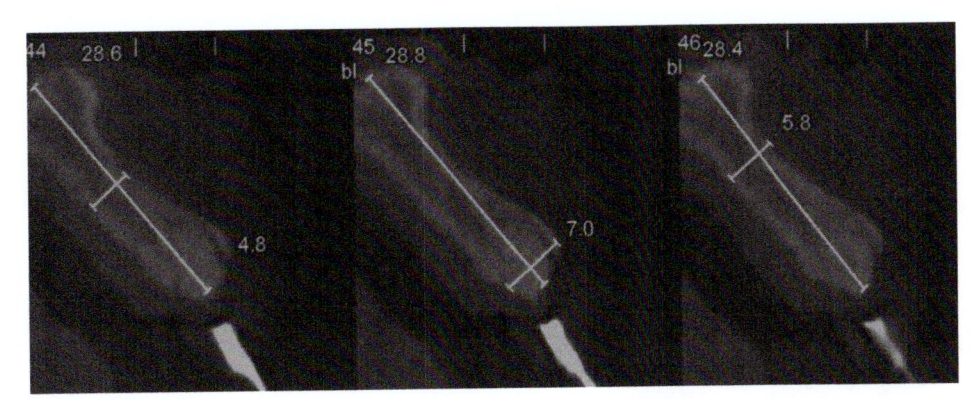

Figure 9.11 Computerized tomographic scan of the maxillary left lateral incisor area prior to implant placement. The image shows a marker present in the radiographic stent depicting the path of insertion for the implant. Notice the buccal thickness of 4.8 mm.

(continued)

(continued)

At the time of implant placement, given that a bone augmentation procedure was going to be necessary, vertical incisions, extending beyond the mucogingival junction, were made at the distobuccal line angle of the maxillary right lateral incisor and at the distobuccal line angle of the maxillary left first bicuspid. A full-thickness flap was elevated. Osteotomies were performed with a surgical guide (Figure 9.12). Two implants (4 mm × 13 mm) were placed. Implants had primary stability and, as expected, fenestrations were present on both implants (approximately 6 mm height × 3 mm wide) (Figure 9.13). A particulate graft, deproteinized bovine bone, was placed on the facial surfaces of both implants (Figure 9.14) and combined with a double layer of resorbable collagen membrane (Figure 9.15). A one-stage approach was adopted, where the healing abutments were installed. The flap was sutured with a non-resorbable material (Figure 9.16). A temporary partial treatment was delivered to the patient at the time of surgery. Nine months after implant placement, an implant-supported bridge was fabricated and delivered (Figures 9.17 to 9.19).

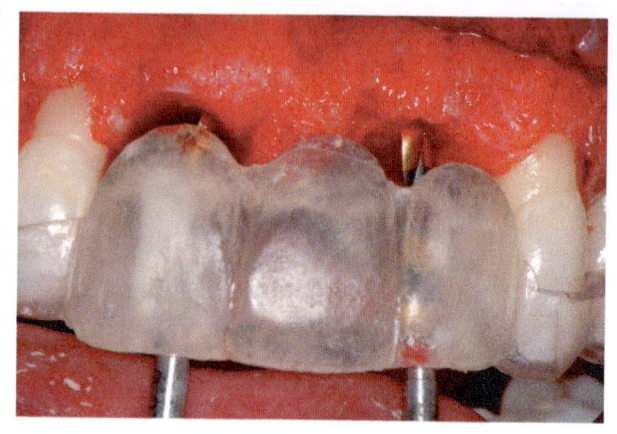

Figure 9.12 Buccal view with surgical guide with the surgical drills in place.

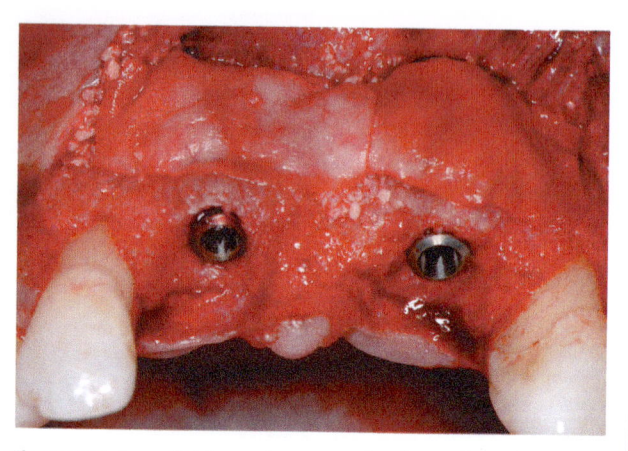

Figure 9.15 A resorbable membrane was placed over the grafted area.

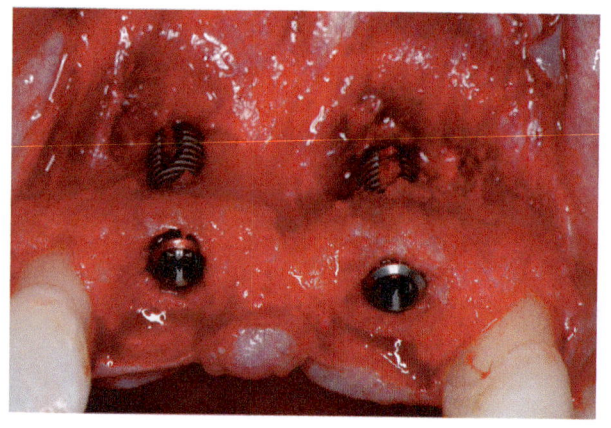

Figure 9.13 Buccal view of implants in place. Notice the fenestration on both implants.

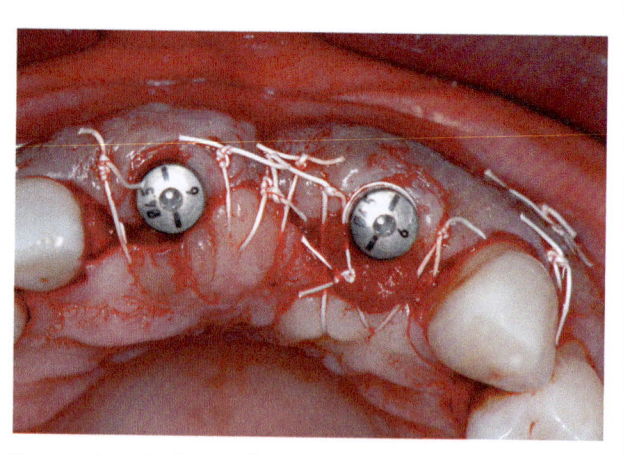

Figure 9.16 Occlusal view of healing abutments and sutured flap.

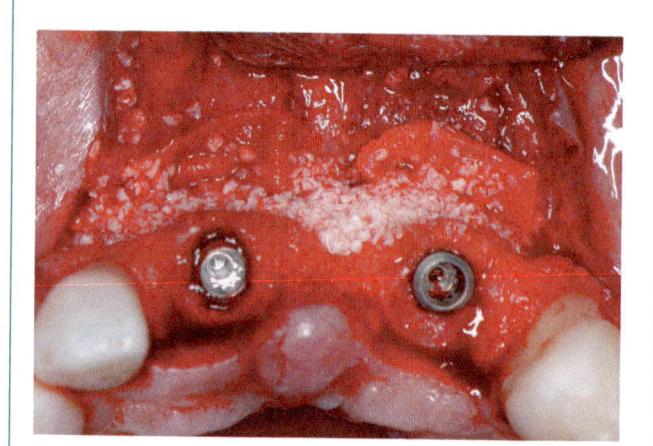

Figure 9.14 Placement of the particulate bone graft.

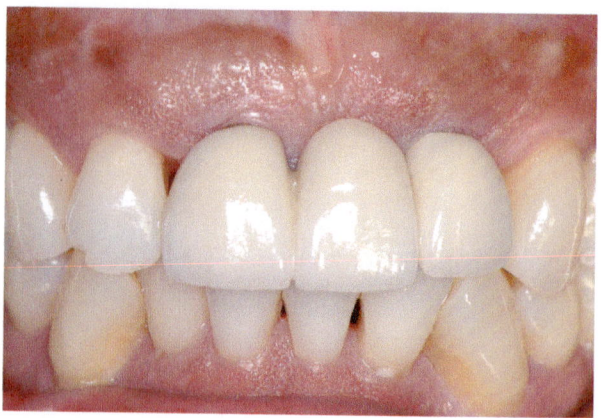

Figure 9.17 Fixed partial denture delivered, 9 months after the implant placement.

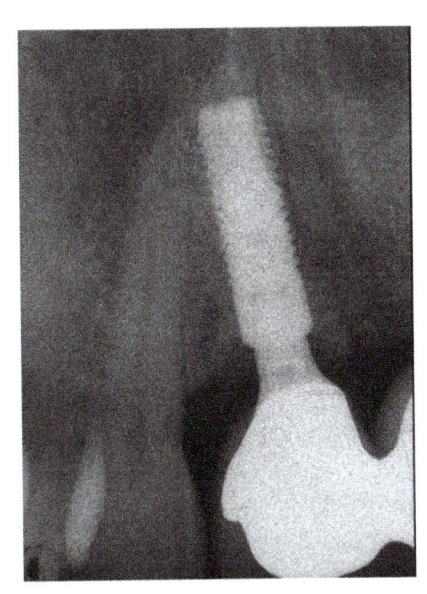

Figure 9.18 Periapical radiograph of the implant on the region of the maxillary right central incisor immediately after the implant-supported bridge was delivered, 9 months after the implant placement.

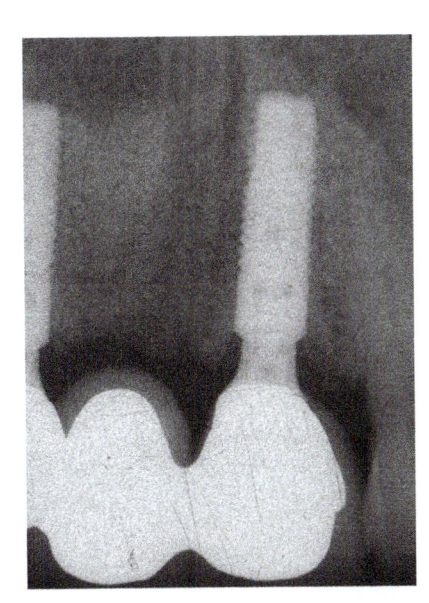

Figure 9.19 Periapical radiograph of the implant on the region of the maxillary left lateral incisor immediately after the implant-supported bridge was delivered, 9 months after the implant placement.

Case 3: Peri-implantitis treatment with bone regeneration

A 60-year-old male needed to have the maxillary right lateral incisor extracted due to fracture and replaced by an implant-supported restoration. The maxillary right lateral incisor was extracted atraumatically; socket preservation was performed with deproteinized bovine bone and allowed to heal. Approximately four months after tooth extraction, an implant was placed on the preserved edentulous site (Figure 9.20). Four months after implant placement, prior to implant restoration, a radiograph was taken and the interproximal bone levels around the implant were found to be similar to the bone levels present at implant placement (Figure 9.21). Two years

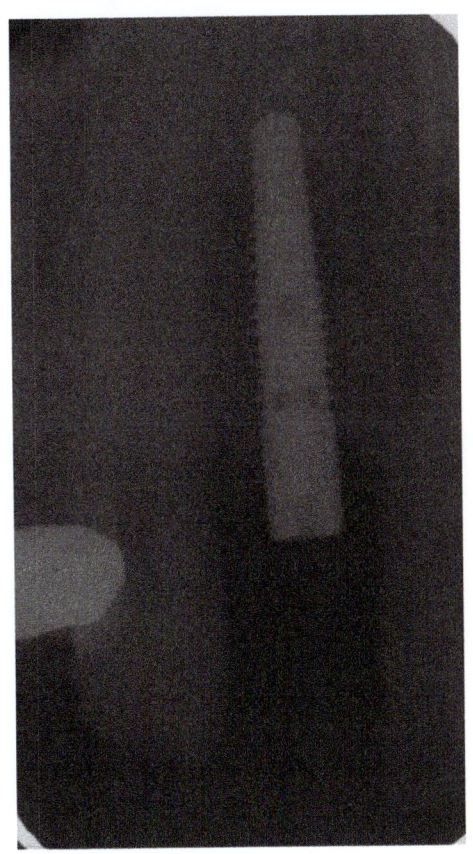

Figure 9.20 Periapical radiograph at the time of the implant placement. Note the interproximal bone level.

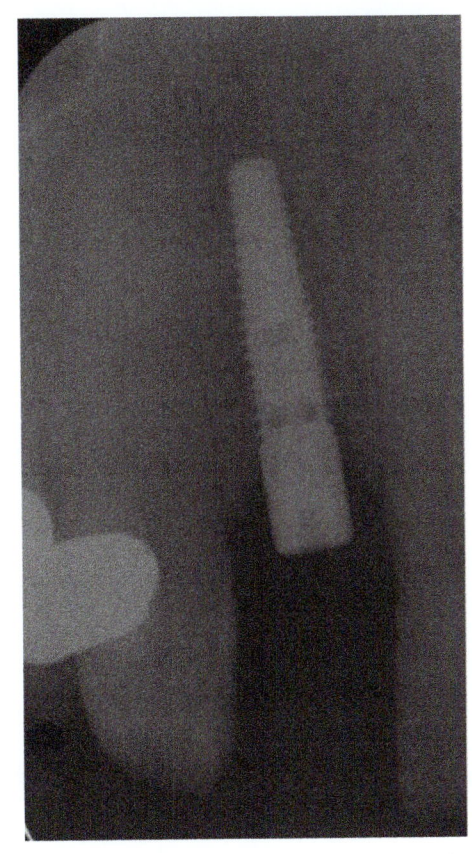

Figure 9.21 Periapical radiograph four months after the implant placement, just prior to implant restoration.

(continued)

90 Guided Bone Regeneration (GBR) with Particulate Graft

(continued)

after implant placement, the patient was seen for a periodic exam. Upon radiographic and clinical evaluation (Figures 9.22 and 9.23), the patient was diagnosed with peri-implantitis. At the time, a decision was made to attempt to regenerate the lost bone around the implant.

To perform the regenerative procedure, two vertical incisions, extending beyond the mucogingival junction, were made at the distobuccal line angle of the maxillary right canine and the mesioobuccal line angle of the maxillary right central incisor. A full-thickness flap was then elevated, the granulomatous tissue was removed, and the implant surface was debrided (Figure 9.24). A particulate bone graft (deproteinized bovine bone) was placed on the defect around the implant fixture (Figure 9.25). A resorbable collagen membrane was adapted over the graft material (Figure 9.26). The flap was sutured over the membrane (Figure 9.27). Six months after surgery, there was partial radiographic bone fill of the defect (Figure 9.28).

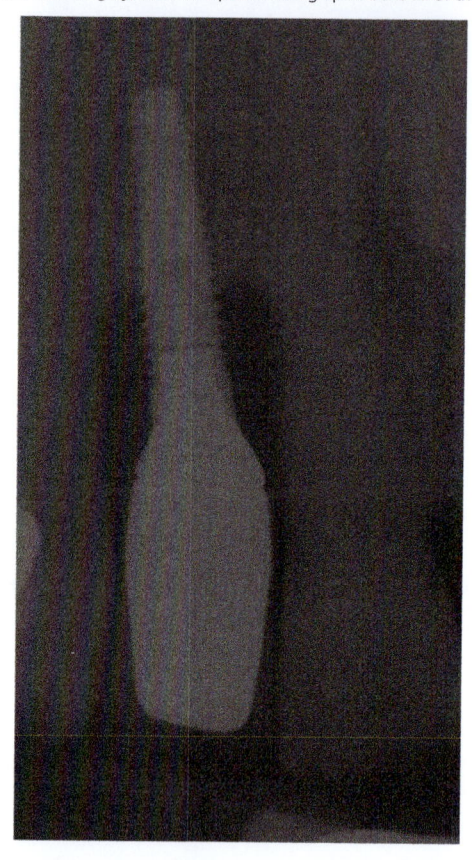

Figure 9.22 Periapical radiograph, two years after the implant placement. Note significant interproximal bone loss.

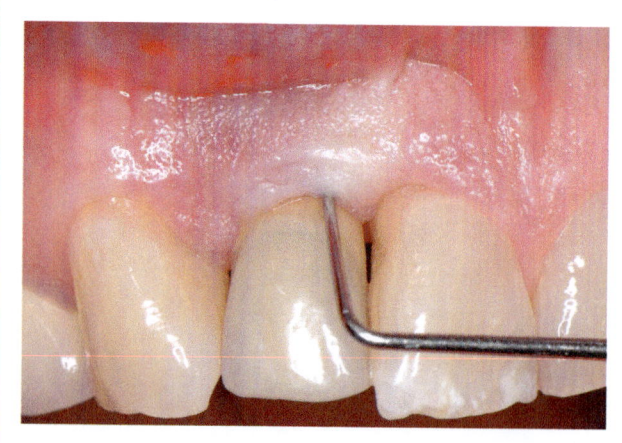

Figure 9.23 Clinical image, two years after the implant placement, indicating an increased pocket depth around the implant fixture.

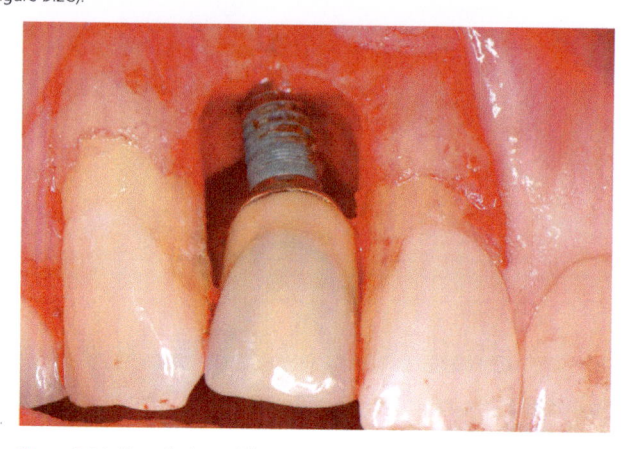

Figure 9.24 Buccal view of the implant after removal of granulomatous tissue.

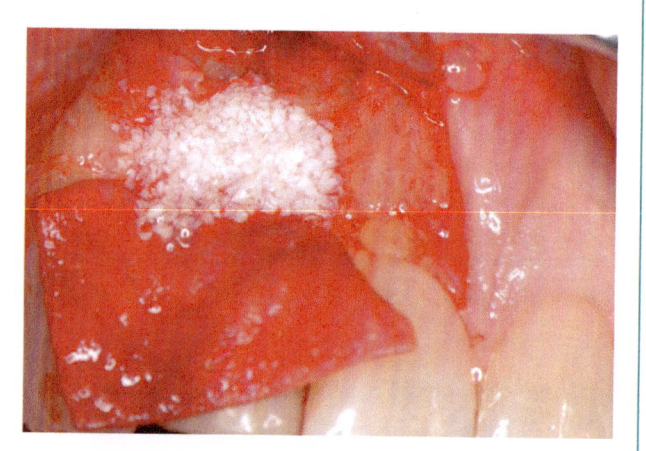

Figure 9.25 Placement of the particulate bone graft.

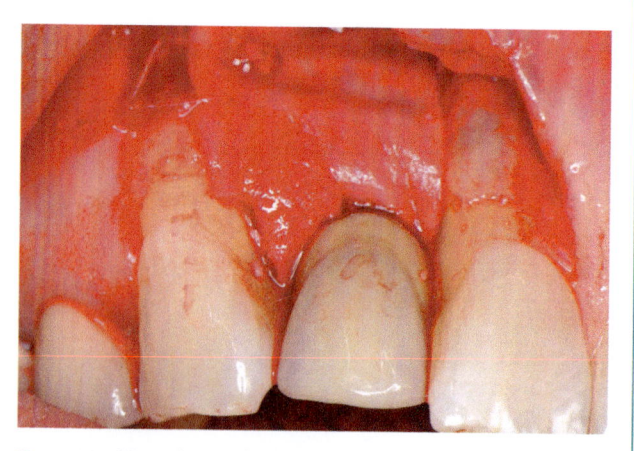

Figure 9.26 View of a resorbable membrane adapted over the grafted area.

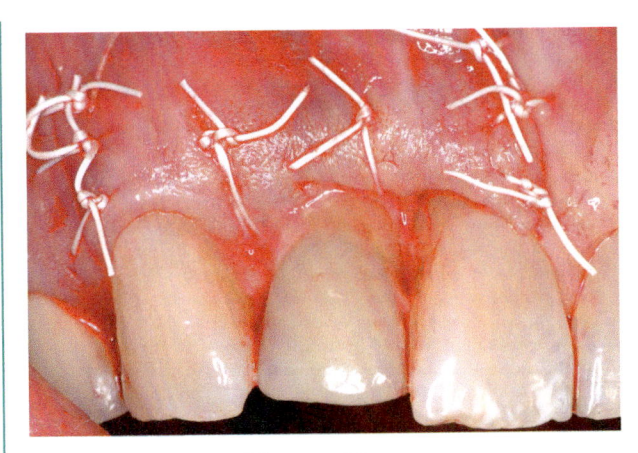

Figure 9.27 Buccal view of the sutured flap.

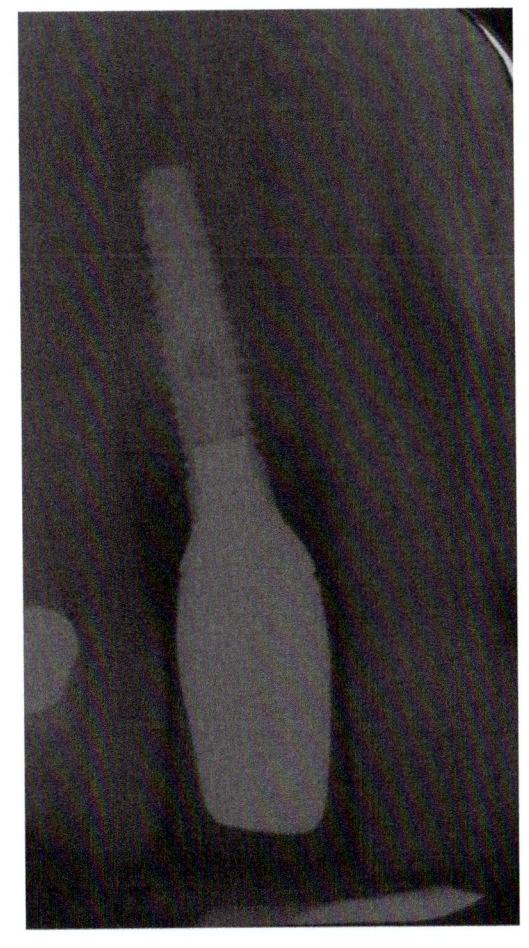

Figure 9.28 Periapical radiograph 6 months after the bone regenerative procedure. Note the improved interproximal bone level.

References

1. Boven GC, Raghoebar GM, Vissink A, Meijer HJ: Improving masticatory performance, bite force, nutritional state and patient's satisfaction with implant overdentures: a systematic review of the literature. *J Oral Rehabil* 2015;**42**(3):220–233. Epub 2014/10/14.
2. Dahlin C, Linde A, Gottlow J, Nyman S: Healing of bone defects by guided tissue regeneration. *Plast Reconstr Surg* 1988;**81**(5):672–676. Epub 1988/05/01.
3. Dahlin C, Gottlow J, Linde A, Nyman S: Healing of maxillary and mandibular bone defects using a membrane technique. An experimental study in monkeys. *Scandinavian Journal of Plastic and Reconstructive Surgery and Hand Surgery/Nordisk Plastikkirurgisk Forening [and] Nordisk Klubb for Handkirurgi* 1990;**24**(1):13–19. Epub 1990/01/01.
4. Dahlin C, Sennerby L, Lekholm U, Linde A, Nyman S: Generation of new bone around titanium implants using a membrane technique: an experimental study in rabbits. *Int J Oral Maxillofac Implants* 1989;**4**(1):19–25. Epub 1989/01/01.
5. Nyman S, Lang NP, Buser D, Bragger U: Bone regeneration adjacent to titanium dental implants using guided tissue regeneration: a report of two cases. *Int J Oral Maxillofac Implants* 1990;**5**(1):9–14. Epub 1990/01/01.
6. Zitzmann NU, Naef R, Scharer P: Resorbable versus nonresorbable membranes in combination with Bio-Oss for guided bone regeneration. *Int J Oral Maxillofac Implants* 1997;**12**(6):844–852. Epub 1998/01/13.
7. Benic GI, Hammerle CH: Horizontal bone augmentation by means of guided bone regeneration. *Periodontol 2000* 2014;**66**(1):13–40. Epub 2014/08/16.
8. Jovanovic SA, Nevins M: Bone formation utilizing titanium-reinforced barrier membranes. *Int J Periodontics Restorative Dent* 1995;**15**(1):56–69. Epub 1995/02/01.
9. Simion M, Jovanovic SA, Trisi P, Scarano A, Piattelli A: Vertical ridge augmentation around dental implants using a membrane technique and autogenous bone or allografts in humans. *Int J Periodontics Restorative Dent* 1998;**18**(1):8–23. Epub 1998/04/29.
10. Jung RE, Fenner N, Hammerle CH, Zitzmann NU: Long-term outcome of implants placed with guided bone regeneration (GBR) using resorbable and non-resorbable membranes after 12–14 years. *Clin Oral Implants Res* 2013;**24**(10):1065–1073. Epub 2012/06/16.
11. Hammerle CH, Jung RE: Bone augmentation by means of barrier membranes. *Periodontol 2000* 2003;**33**:36–53. Epub 2003/09/03.
12. Hurzeler MB, Kohal RJ, Naghshbandi J, Mota LF, Conradt J, Hutmacher D, et al: Evaluation of a new bioresorbable barrier to facilitate guided bone regeneration around exposed implant threads. An experimental study in the monkey. *Int J Oral Maxillofac Surg* 1998;**27**(4):315–320. Epub 1998/08/11.
13. Oh TJ, Meraw SJ, Lee EJ, Giannobile WV, Wang HL: Comparative analysis of collagen membranes for the treatment of implant dehiscence defects. *Clin Oral Implants Res* 2003;**14**(1):80–90. Epub 2003/02/04.
14. Sevor JJ, Meffert RM, Cassingham RJ: Regeneration of dehisced alveolar bone adjacent to endosseous dental implants utilizing a resorbable collagen membrane: clinical and histologic results. *Int J Periodontics Restorative Dent* 1993;**13**(1):71–83. Epub 1993/01/01.
15. Zitzmann NU, Scharer P, Marinello CP: Long-term results of implants treated with guided bone regeneration: a 5-year prospective study. *Int J Oral Maxillofac Implants* 2001;**16**(3):355–366. Epub 2001/07/04.
16. Zellin G, Gritli-Linde A, Linde A: Healing of mandibular defects with different biodegradable and non-biodegradable membranes: an experimental study in rats. *Biomaterials* 1995;**16**(8):601–609. Epub 1995/05/01.
17. Simion M, Misitano U, Gionso L, Salvato A: Treatment of dehiscences and fenestrations around dental implants using resorbable and nonresorbable membranes associated with bone autografts: a comparative clinical study. *Int J Oral Maxillofac Implants* 1997;**12**(2):159–167. Epub 1997/03/01.
18. Wechsler S, Fehr D, Molenberg A, Raeber G, Schense JC, Weber FE: A novel, tissue occlusive poly(ethylene glycol) hydrogel material. *J Biomed Mater Res A* 2008;**85**(2):285–292. Epub 2007/08/11.

19 Sottosanti JS: Calcium sulfate is a safe, resorbable barrier adjunct to implant surgical procedures. *Dental implantology update.* 1993;4(9):69–73. Epub 1993/09/01.
20 von Arx T, Cochran DL, Schenk RK, Buser D: Evaluation of a prototype trilayer membrane (PTLM) for lateral ridge augmentation: an experimental study in the canine mandible. *Int J Oral Maxillofac Surg* 2002;31(2):190–9. Epub 2002/07/10.
21 Schallhorn RG: Present status of osseous grafting procedures. *J Periodontol* 1977;48(9):570–576. Epub 1977/09/01.
22 Narang R, Wells H, Laskin DM: Experimental osteogenesis with demineralized allogeneic bone matrix in extraskeletal sites. *J Oral Maxillofac Surg* 1982;40(3):133–141. Epub 1982/03/01.
23 Misch CE, Misch-Dietsch F: Keys to bone grafting and bone grafting materials. In: Misch CE (ed.), *Contemporary Implant Dentistry*, 3rd edn. Mosby Elsevier, Missouri 2008, pp. 839–869.
24 Schallhorn RG: Eradication of bifurcation defects utilizing frozen autogenous hip marrow implants. *Periodontal Abstracts* 1967;15(3):101–105. Epub 1967/09/01.
25 Schallhorn RG: The use of autogenous hip marrow biopsy implants for bony crater defects. *J Periodontol* 1968;39(3):145–147. Epub 1968/05/01.
26 Simion M, Fontana F: Autogenous and xenogeneic bone grafts for the bone regeneration. A literature review. *Minerva Stomatologica* 2004;53(5):191–206. Epub 2004/07/21.
27 Dragoo MR, Sullivan HC: A clinical and histological evaluation of autogenous iliac bone grafts in humans. I. Wound healing 2 to 8 months. *J Periodontol* 1973;44(10):599–613. Epub 1973/10/01.
28 Rosenberg MM: Reentry of an osseous defect treated by a bone implant after a long duration. *J Periodontol* 1971;42(6):360–363. Epub 1971/06/01.
29 Goldberg VM, Stevenson S: Natural history of autografts and allografts. *Clin Orthop Relat Res* 1987;(225):7–16. Epub 1987/12/01.
30 Schwartz Z, Somers A, Mellonig JT, Carnes DL, Jr. Dean DD, Cochran DL, et al: Ability of commercial demineralized freeze-dried bone allograft to induce new bone formation is dependent on donor age but not gender. *J Periodontol* 1998;69(4):470–478. Epub 1998/06/03.
31 Klinge B, Alberius P, Isaksson S, Jonsson J: Osseous response to implanted natural bone mineral and synthetic hydroxylapatite ceramic in the repair of experimental skull bone defects. *J Oral Maxillofac Surg* 1992;50(3):241–249. Epub 1992/03/01.
32 Jensen SS, Broggini N, Hjorting-Hansen E, Schenk R, Buser D: Bone healing and graft resorption of autograft, anorganic bovine bone and beta-tricalcium phosphate. A histologic and histomorphometric study in the mandibles of minipigs. *Clin Oral Implants Res* 2006;17(3):237–43. Epub 2006/05/05.
33 Jensen SS, Terheyden H: Bone augmentation procedures in localized defects in the alveolar ridge: clinical results with different bone grafts and bone-substitute materials. *Int J Oral Maxillofac Implants* 2009;24(Suppl):218–236. Epub 2009/12/04.
34 Knapp CI, Feuille F, Cochran DL, Mellonig JT: Clinical and histologic evaluation of bone-replacement grafts in the treatment of localized alveolar ridge defects. Part 2: bioactive glass particulate. *Int J Periodontics Restorative Dent* 2003;23(2):129–137. Epub 2003/04/25.
35 Seibert J, Nyman S: Localized ridge augmentation in dogs: a pilot study using membranes and hydroxyapatite. *J Periodontol* 1990;61(3):157–165. Epub 1990/03/01.
36 Schropp L, Wenzel A, Kostopoulos L, Karring T: Bone healing and soft tissue contour changes following single-tooth extraction: a clinical and radiographic 12-month prospective study. *Int J Periodontics Restorative Dent* 2003;23(4):313–323. Epub 2003/09/06.
37 Van der Weijden F, Dell'Acqua F, Slot DE: Alveolar bone dimensional changes of post-extraction sockets in humans: a systematic review. *J Clin Periodontol* 2009;36(12):1048–1058. Epub 2009/11/26.
38 Tallgren A: The continuing reduction of the residual alveolar ridges in complete denture wearers: a mixed-longitudinal study covering 25 years. *J Prosthet Dent* 1972;27(2):120–132. Epub 1972/02/01.
39 Araujo MG, Lindhe J: Ridge alterations following tooth extraction with and without flap elevation: an experimental study in the dog. *Clin Oral Implants Res* 2009;20(6):545–549. Epub 2009/06/12.
40 Tan WL, Wong TL, Wong MC, Lang NP: A systematic review of post-extractional alveolar hard and soft tissue dimensional changes in humans. *Clin Oral Implants Res* 2012;23(Suppl 5):1–21. Epub 2012/01/11.
41 Vignoletti F, Matesanz P, Rodrigo D, Figuero E, Martin C, Sanz M: Surgical protocols for ridge preservation after tooth extraction. A systematic review. *Clin Oral Implants Res* 2012;23(Suppl 5):22–38. Epub 2012/01/11.
42 Hammerle CH, Jung RE, Feloutzis A: A systematic review of the survival of implants in bone sites augmented with barrier membranes (guided bone regeneration) in partially edentulous patients. *J Clin Periodontol* 2002;29(Suppl 3):226–231; discussion 232–233. Epub 2003/06/06.
43 Donos N, Mardas N, Chadha V: Clinical outcomes of implants following lateral bone augmentation: systematic assessment of available options (barrier membranes, bone grafts, split osteotomy). *J Clin Periodontol* 2008;35(8 Suppl):173–202. Epub 2008/09/09.
44 Camargo PM, Lekovic V, Carnio J, Kenney EB: Alveolar bone preservation following tooth extraction: a perspective of clinical trials utilizing osseous grafting and guided bone regeneration. *Oral Maxillofac Surg Clin North Am* 2004;16(1):9–18, v. Epub 2007/12/20.
45 Lekovic V, Camargo PM, Klokkevold PR, Weinlaender M, Kenney EB, Dimitrijevic B, et al: Preservation of alveolar bone in extraction sockets using bioabsorbable membranes. *J Periodontol* 1998;69(9):1044–1049. Epub 1998/10/17.
46 Avila-Ortiz G, Elangovan S, Kramer KW, Blanchette D, Dawson DV: Effect of alveolar ridge preservation after tooth extraction: a systematic review and meta-analysis. *J Dent Res* 2014;93(10):950–958. Epub 2014/06/27.
47 Sclar AG: Strategies for management of single-tooth extraction sites in aesthetic implant therapy. *J Oral Maxillofac Surg* 2004;62(9 Suppl 2):90–105. Epub 2004/08/28.
48 Tal H: Autogenous masticatory mucosal grafts in extraction socket seal procedures: a comparison between sockets grafted with demineralized freeze-dried bone and deproteinized bovine bone mineral. *Clin Oral Implants Res* 1999;10(4):289–296. Epub 1999/11/07.
49 Wang HL, Tsao YP: Mineralized bone allograft-plug socket augmentation: rationale and technique. *Implant Dent* 2007;16(1):33–41. Epub 2007/03/16.
50 Elian N, Cho SC, Froum S, Smith RB, Tarnow DP: A simplified socket classification and repair technique. *Pract Proced Aesthet Dent* 2007;19(2):99–104; quiz 6. Epub 2007/05/12.
51 Romanos G, Ko HH, Froum S, Tarnow D: The use of CO_2 laser in the treatment of peri-implantitis. *Photomed Laser Surg* 2009;27(3):381–386. Epub 2009/07/03.
52 Froum SJ, Froum SH, Rosen PS: Successful management of peri-implantitis with a regenerative approach: a consecutive series of 51 treated implants with 3- to 7.5-year follow-up. *Int J Periodontics Restorative Dent* 2012;32(1):11–20. Epub 2012/01/19.
53 Schwarz F, Sahm N, Bieling K, Becker J: Surgical regenerative treatment of peri-implantitis lesions using a nanocrystalline hydroxyapatite or a natural bone mineral in combination with a collagen membrane: a four-year clinical follow-up report. *J Clin Periodontol* 2009;36(9):807–814. Epub 2009/07/30.
54 Roos-Jansaker AM, Lindahl C, Persson GR, Renvert S: Long-term stability of surgical bone regenerative procedures of peri-implantitis lesions in a prospective case-control study over 3 years. *J Clin Periodontol* 2011;38(6):590–597. Epub 2011/04/15.
55 Schwarz F, John G, Sahm N, Becker J: Combined surgical resective and regenerative therapy for advanced peri-implantitis with concomitant soft tissue volume augmentation: a case report. *Int J Periodontics Restorative Dent* 2014;34(4):489–495. Epub 2014/07/10.
56 Schwarz F, Sahm N, Becker J: Combined surgical therapy of advanced peri-implantitis lesions with concomitant soft tissue volume augmentation. A case series. *Clin Oral Implants Res* 2014;25(1):132–136. Epub 2013/01/29.
57 Machtei EE: The effect of membrane exposure on the outcome of regenerative procedures in humans: a meta-analysis. *J Periodontol* 2001;72(4):512–516. Epub 2001/05/08.
58 Friedmann A, Strietzel FP, Maretzki B, Pitaru S, Bernimoulin JP: Observations on a new collagen barrier membrane in 16 consecutively treated patients. Clinical and histological findings. *J Periodontol* 2001;72(11):1616–1623. Epub 2002/01/05.
59 Friedmann A, Strietzel FP, Maretzki B, Pitaru S, Bernimoulin JP: Histological assessment of augmented jaw bone utilizing a new collagen barrier membrane compared to a standard barrier membrane to protect a granular bone substitute material. *Clin Oral Implants Res* 2002;13(6):587–594. Epub 2003/01/10.
60 Pack PD, Haber J: The incidence of clinical infection after periodontal surgery. A retrospective study. *J Periodontol* 1983;54(7):441–443. Epub 1983/07/01.
61 Gynther GW, Kondell PA, Moberg LE, Heimdahl A: Dental implant installation without antibiotic prophylaxis. *Oral Surg Oral Med Oral Pathol Oral Radiol Endod* 1998;85(5):509–511. Epub 1998/06/10.
62 Powell CA, Mealey BL, Deas DE, McDonnell HT, Moritz AJ: Post-surgical infections: prevalence associated with various periodontal surgical procedures. *J Periodontol* 2005;76(3):329–333. Epub 2005/04/29.
63 Chiapasco M, Zaniboni M: Clinical outcomes of GBR procedures to correct peri-implant dehiscences and fenestrations: a systematic review. *Clin Oral Implants Res* 2009;20(Suppl 4):113–123. Epub 2009/08/12.

CHAPTER 10
Vertical Augmentation of the Alveolar Ridge with Titanium-Reinforced Devices (Protected Bone Regeneration)

Tetsu Takahashi[1] and Kensuke Yamauchi[1,2]

[1]Department of Oral and Maxillofacial Surgery, Tohoku University Graduate School of Dentistry, Sendai, Miyagi, Japan
[2]Dental Implant Center, Tohoku University Hospital, Sendai, Japan

Introduction

Vertical alveolar ridge augmentation remains a challenging procedure for implant placement in atrophic maxilla and mandible. Several bone-augmentation techniques have been introduced, including block bone graft [1, 2], guided bone regeneration (GBR) [3–5], distraction osteogenesis (DO) [6–9], and bone splitting [10–12]. Although an autologous block bone graft is considered to be a "gold standard", one of its disadvantages is bone resorption [13, 14]. GBR with resorbable or non-resorbable membrane is also a versatile procedure. Titanium-reinforced barrier membrane (TR membrane) and especially GBR with a resorbable barrier membrane provide a limited augmentation volume.

Titanium (Ti) mesh has been widely used in oral and maxillofacial surgery for the reconstruction of large and small defects. The use of titanium mesh for the reconstruction of the atrophic alveolus was first introduced by Boyne in 1985 [15]. von Arx et al. established titanium mesh bone augmentation procedure as the TIME technique (autogenous bone grafting combined with titanium mesh stabilization) [16]. The use of titanium mesh is known to have several advantages compared to the other augmentation procedures. Titanium mesh provides superior space maintenance because of its mechanical strength. Titanium mesh well protects graft materials from the pressure of soft tissue cover and also stabilizes the graft materials and facilitates the revascularization of the graft bed [17–20]. Furthermore, the mesh pores are believed to play a critical role in maintaining the blood supply to a graft defect [20].

Titanium mesh device

Several titanium micromesh devices are commercially available. The authors use a 0.1 or 0.2 mm thick commercially pure (CP) titanium mesh plate "M-TAM" (Stryker Leibinger GmbH & Co. KG, USA), a 0.1 or 0.2 mm thick ASTM F-67 (Jeil Medical Co. Ltd., Seoul, South Korea), and a 0.2 mm thick Ultraflex mesh plate (Kyocera Medical Co. Ltd., Osaka, Japan). They also used a 0.4 mm thick "Dynamic mesh plate" (Stryker Leibinger GmbH & Co. KG, USA), while 4 to 6 mm long self-drilling screws (Jeil Medical Co. Ltd., Seoul, South Korea) were used for the stabilization of the titanium mesh plate.

Surgical procedure

All the surgical procedures are usually performed under local anesthesia with/without intravenous sedation, except for cases of severe maxillary and mandibular atrophy. After delivery of local anesthesia, a crestal incision was made followed by two vertical releasing incisions, to form full mucoperiosteal flaps to the labial aspect (Figures 10.1 and 10.2). The full-thickness flap was completely reflected with careful preservation of the periosteum inside the flap. Vital structures, like the mental nerve, facial arteries, and lingual artery, were protected. After elevation of the flaps, the bone should be carefully examined and then the buccal cortical plate is perforated with a round bur by a rolling instrument or by piezoelectric surgical instruments (Figure 10.3). This "decortication" procedure provokes bleeding and infiltration of osteoprogenitor cells from the bone marrow and facilitates revascularization in the grafted material. The autogenous particulate bone chips are harvested from the intraoral, mainly mandibular retromolar, region with a scraper (mx-grafter: Maxilon Laboratories, Inc., Hollis, NH, USA). In the case of an iliac crest bone graft, a curette was used to obtain particulate bone and marrow (PCBM). In some cases, a deproteinized bovine bone matrix (DBBM) (Bio-Oss; Geistlich Pharma, Wolhusen, Switzerland) or beta tricalcium phosphate (β-TCP, OSferion, Olympustermobiomaterial, Japan; particles sized 0.5 to 1.5 mm) combined with an autogenous particulate bone chip was used. A bone graft material was soaked with autologous blood drawn from the vein and was mixed with the autogenous bone chips to form a 50/50 mixed bone graft. A titanium mesh device was sterilized, trimmed, and performed to the basic shape of the defect to be grafted prior to surgery. Adaptation of the titanium mesh during surgery created a defined space between the mesh and the decorticated area that mimicked the shape of the desired ridge to support eventual dental implant placement (Figure 10.4). Bone graft material was placed on the defects (Figure 10.5) and shaped titanium mesh was fixed with 4 or 5 mm long titanium screws (Figure 10.6). After the fixation of the bone graft material and titanium mesh, the surgical field was irrigated with saline and the buccal flap was coronally repositioned with significant apical periosteal undermining.

Vertical Alveolar Ridge Augmentation in Implant Dentistry: A Surgical Manual, First Edition. Edited by Len Tolstunov.
© 2016 John Wiley & Sons, Inc. Published 2016 by John Wiley & Sons, Inc.

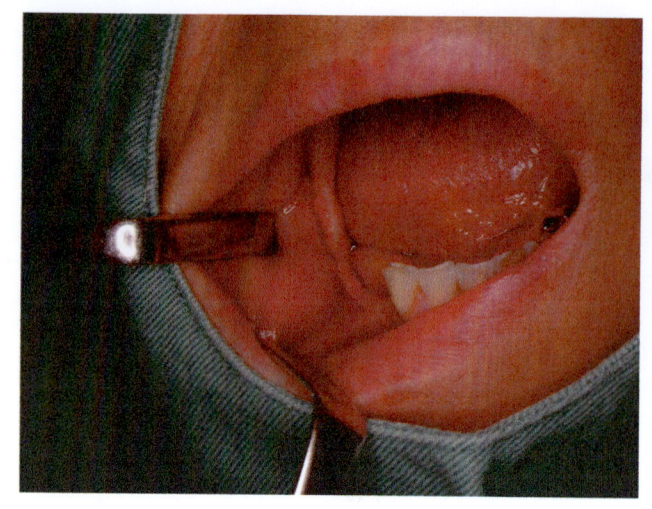

94 Guided Bone Regeneration (GBR) with Particulate Graft

Figure 10.1 Pre-operative intraoral view.

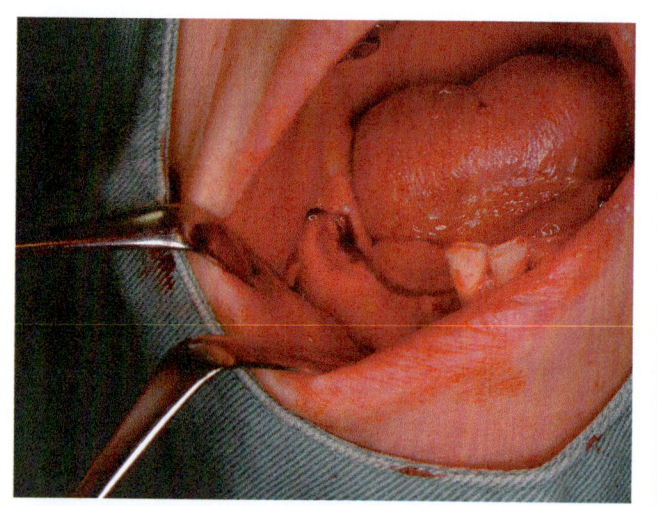

Figure 10.2 A crestal incision was made and the flap was raised.

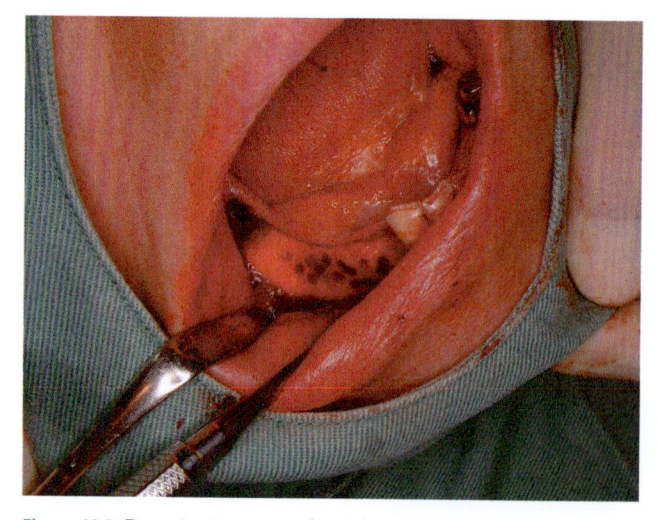

Figure 10.3 Decortication was made on the cortical bone with a round bur.

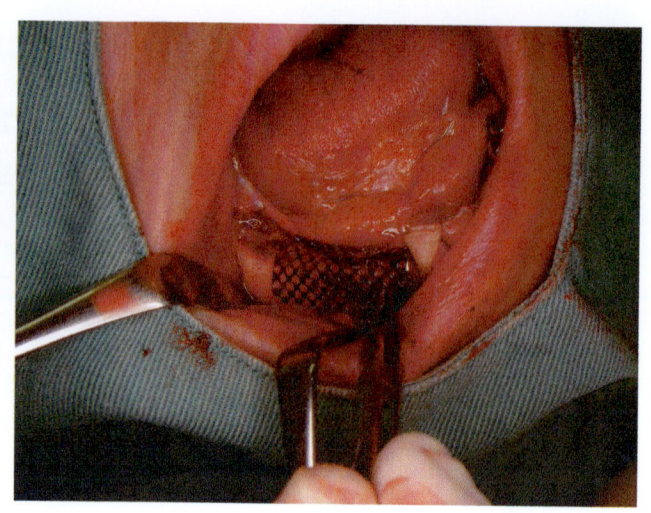

Figure 10.4 Titanium mesh was trimmed and adjusted to the desired shape.

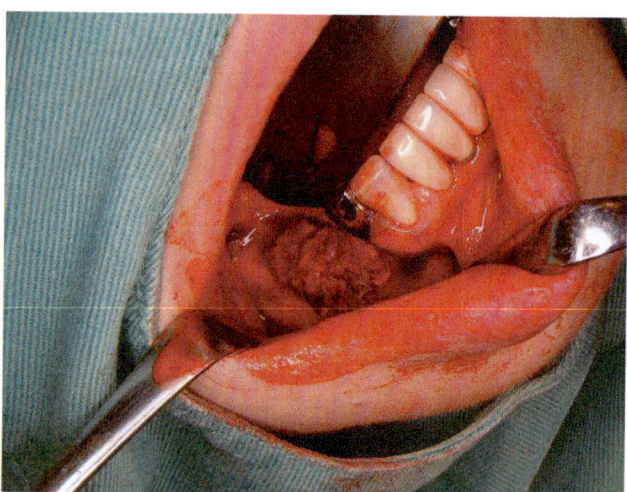

Figure 10.5 Autogenous bone chips harvested from the ipsilateral ramus were placed on the defect.

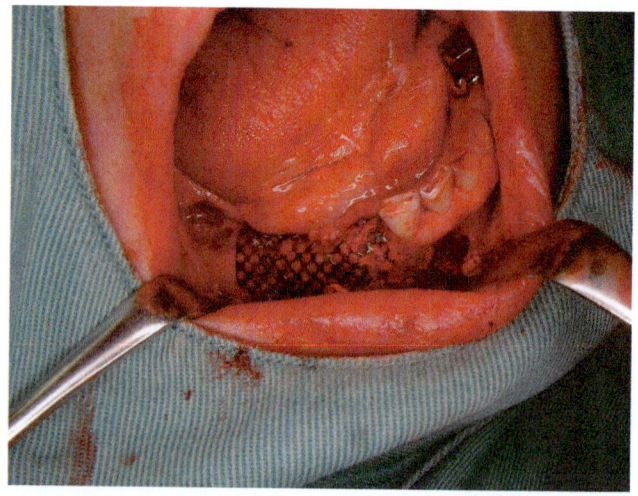

Figure 10.6 Titanium mesh was fixed with titanium 4 mm long screws.

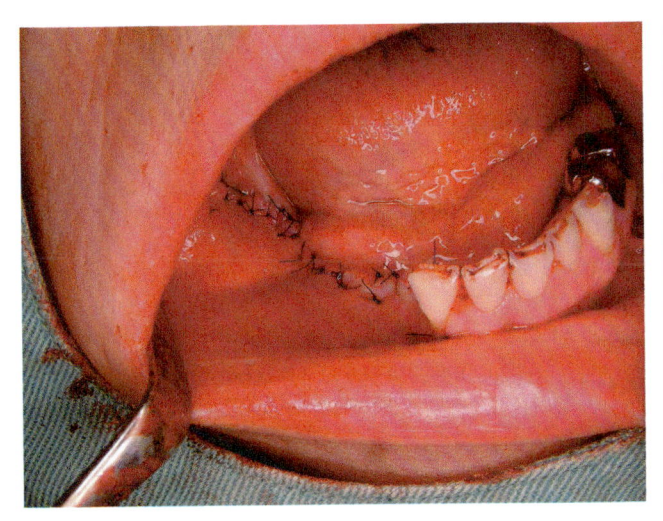

Figure 10.7 The periosteum was released along the facial vestibule to facilitate a tension-free closure of the wound and the flap was sutured by 5-0 nylon in a watertight manner.

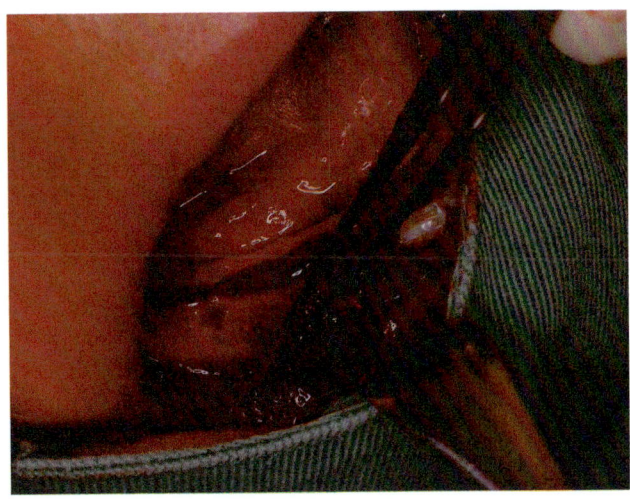

Figure 10.9 The mesh was removed.

Tension-free 5-0 nylon sutures were placed across the incision on the periosteal membrane above the flap in a watertight manner (Figure 10.7). Post-operatively, the patient received broad-spectrum antibiotics for 5–7 days. Corticosteroids were also beneficial to reduce post-operative trismus, swelling, and pain. Extraorally, ice packs were applied to reduce swelling. Patients should preferably take a seated position at rest, and during the first post-operative night, may lie down with the upper part of the body slightly raised. Analgesics are usually required for some days after surgery. Care should be taken not to wear a denture or temporary prosthesis on the grafted area for at least 2 weeks. The sutures are usually removed after 10 days. Approximately 6 months after the surgery, a flap was raised and the Ti mesh was exposed (Figure 10.8). After the removal of titanium screws, mesh was removed (Figures 10.9 and 10.10) and the augmented area should be completely consolidated. After removal of the Ti mesh, dental implants can be placed immediately or later (Figure 10.11).

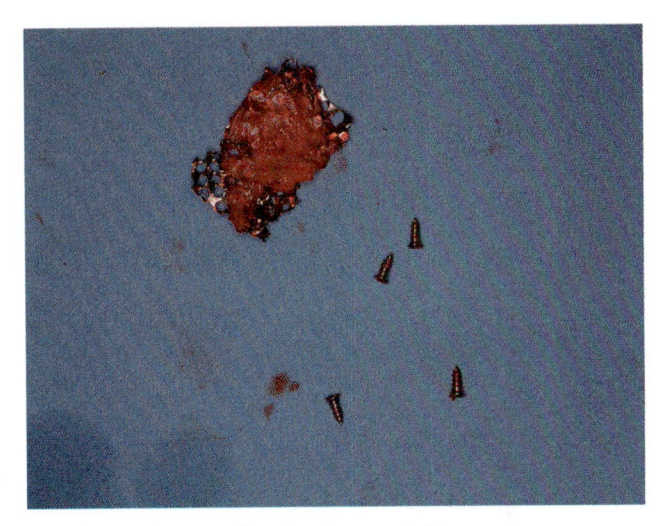

Figure 10.10 The removed mesh and screws. A thin scar tissue was attached to the mesh.

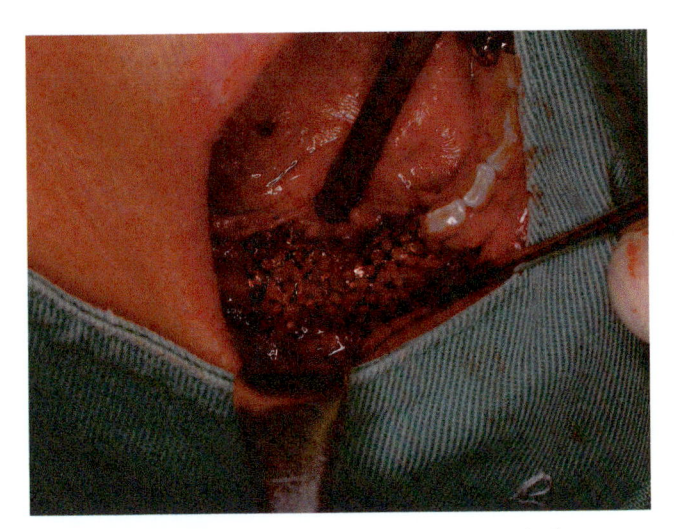

Figure 10.8 Six months after the augmentation procedure, the flap was raised and the mesh was exposed.

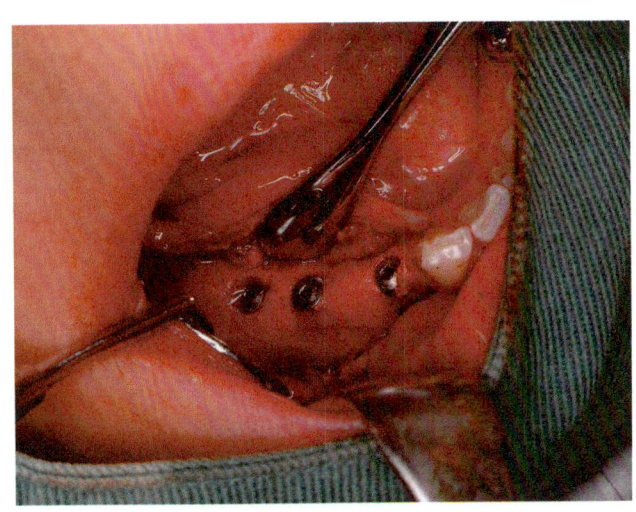

Figure 10.11 Subsequently, dental implants were placed.

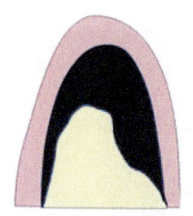

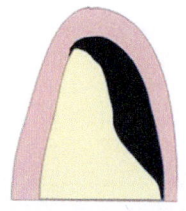

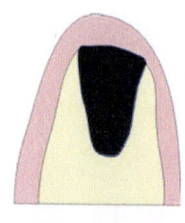

	Horizontal Vertical type (HV)	Horizontal type (H)	Socket type (S)
Horizontal length	4.1 mm (0.5-7.7)	4.2 mm (1.6-7.3)	5.2 mm (4.0-7.5)
Vertical length	6.1 mm (1.7-12.2)	-	10.7 mm (2.1-17.0)

Figure 10.12 Defect type and bone gain (mm). Source: Ikuya et al 2011. Reproduced with permission from Wiley.

Bone quality and quantity of the augmented area by titanium mesh and autogenous particulate bone graft

In our previous study, we evaluated the bone quality and quantity of the augmented area by the titanium mesh–bone graft procedure [21]. We first classified the bone defects according to the shape into three types: complex horizontal–vertical (HV) type, horizontal (H) type, and socket (S) type (Figure 10.12). Fifty bone defects sites were treated with 29 maxillary and 21 mandibular augmentation procedures. The success rate of the titanium mesh–bone graft procedure was 88%. The bone defects were 59% H type in the maxilla and 71% HV in the mandible. The mesh was removed approximately 6 months after the operation. When the titanium mesh was removed, granulation tissue around the titanium mesh without mucosal membrane was observed. We evaluated the augmented bone by a CT scan. Bone qualitative evaluations expressed by the Hounsfield Unit (HU) value were 354 for PCBM from the iliac crest and 599 for intraoral bone grafts. The HU value for the intraoral bone was significantly higher than those of PCBM from the ilium (Table 10.1). The mean horizontal bone gain of augmented area was 4.3 ± 2.0 (SD) mm and the mean vertical bone gain was 8.1 ± 4.8 (SD) mm. For the HV-type defects, the mean horizontal gain was 3.7 ± 2.0 (SD) mm and the mean vertical gain was 5.4 ± 3.4 (SD) mm (Figure 10.13a and b). For the H-type defects, the mean horizontal gain was 3.9 ± 1.9 (SD) mm (Figure 10.14a and b). For the S-type defects, the mean horizontal gain was 5.7 ± 1.4 (SD) mm and the mean vertical gain was 12.4 ± 3.1 (SD) mm (Figures 10.12 and 10.15a and b). The results showed a statistically significant difference between the HV and S types in vertical bone gain ($p < 0.05$); however, no statistically significant difference was observed in horizontal bone gain (ANOVA: $p > 0.05$). The HV-type defect was the most difficult type to augment and the S-type defect had the most efficient bone augmentation.

Table 10.1 Qualitative evaluation of the augmented bone and defect type. Source: Ikuya et al 2011. Reproduced with permission from Wiley.

	Iliac bone N = 5	Intraoral bone N = 16
HU value	392	596

Unpaired t test, $p < 0.05$.

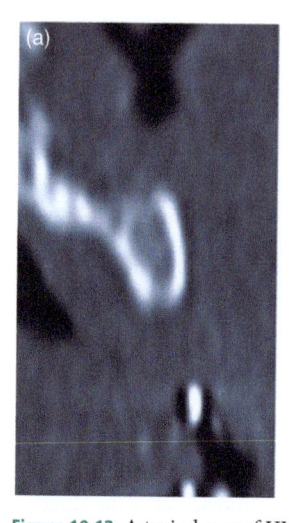

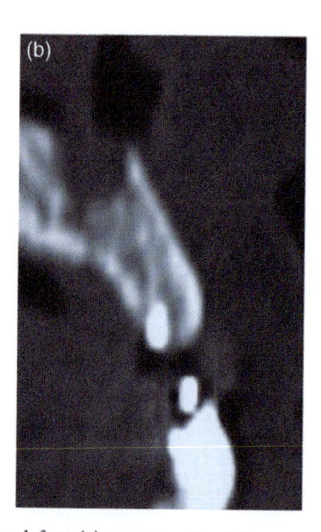

Figure 10.13 A typical case of HV-type defect: **(a)** pre-operative CT scan and **(b)** 6 month post-operative CT scan. The Hounsfield value of the grafted area was 702 (autogenous bone was harvested from the mandibular ramus).

Complications

A major complication of the titanium mesh technique is mesh exposure during the healing period. In our previous study, mesh exposure occurred in 36% of the surgical sites [21], which was a similar rate of mesh exposure to that of the recent report by Her et al.: 26% of the 27 surgical sites [22]. Total bone resorption due to early mesh exposure and infection (4.8%) and partial bone resorption with minor infection (10%) in the authors' previous study was similar to the bone resorption rate by the study of Maiorana et al., where exposure of titanium mesh led to early graft resorption in the exposed area of about 15 to 25% [23]. HV-type bone defect caused more mesh exposure and subsequent bone resorption compared to H-type and S-type defects. This is probably because of the soft tissue condition after surgery. H- and S-type bone defects have relatively more periosteal coverage than the HV-type defect. Moreover, in HV-type bone defects, the tension of the mucosal or periosteal membrane after suturing would be higher than in the other types of defects. These conditions affect adequate blood supply for wound healing. Most of these problems did not influence the implant treatment results even in cases of mesh exposure. Implant treatment was possible in 84% of the surgical sites and the cumulative implant

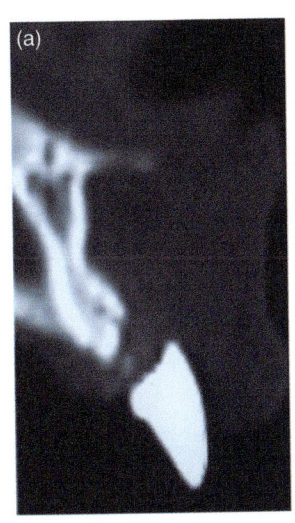

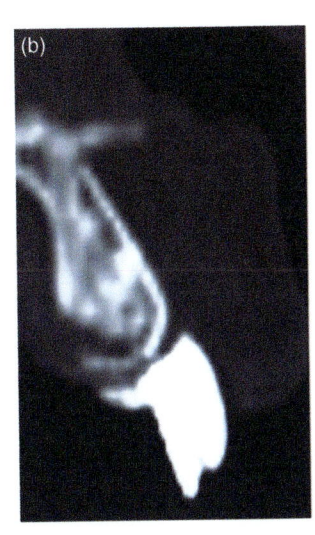

Figure 10.14 A typical case of H-type defect: (a) pre-operative CT scan and (b) 6 month post-operative CT scan. The Hounsfield value of the grafted area was 524.

survival rate was 92.8% by Kaplan–Meier analysis up to 96 months after implant placement [21].

Exposure of non-resorbable membranes, such as e-PTFE and titanium-reinforced e-PTFE is well known to result in infection, which can jeopardize the results [24, 25]. Previous studies have suggested that a barrier membrane can exclude the entrance of blood supply to a grafted defect that can result in a flap dehiscence and membrane exposure [26, 27]. Such non-resorbable membranes must be removed if flap dehiscence and exposure occurs to prevent infection, because exposure in these cases would not heal spontaneously [24]. Conversely, titanium mesh did not appear to affect the final outcome.

When the mesh exposure occurred within a week, we first perform resuturing of the exposed mucosal membrane. When severe infection was recognized on careful observation, the mesh was removed. However, after 1 to 2 weeks' healing, mesh exposure did not directly result in significant bone resorption and the mesh seems to tolerate infection. Even if the mesh is removed because of infection, partial bone necrosis or resorption would occur, and total bone resorption has not been observed [21]. The reason for the difference between the barrier membranes and titanium mesh is unclear, a possible explanation being that titanium mesh allows blood supply exchange from the periosteum to the grafted bone, enabling nutrition of the grafted bone [21].

Indications and timing of implant placement

The titanium mesh–bone graft procedure can be considered a versatile technique and a prerequisite for any bone augmentation procedure. This is due to the strength of graft protection and great plasticity of the titanium mesh, which permits bending, contouring, and adaptation three-dimensionally to any shape. According to the above-mentioned evaluation of the bone gain, a titanium mesh–bone graft is applicable up to 6 mm horizontally and 12 mm vertically. However, the bone gain completely depends on the shape of the defect and soft tissue condition. Table 10.2 shows the current concept of indications of various bone augmentation procedures according to the defect size. Bone gain by the GBR technique using a barrier membrane is within 3–4 mm vertically; therefore, it is used for marginal bone defects such as thread exposure or fenestration-type defects. It can also be applied to a defect up to a 3–4 mm size of the defect. Because of its limitation of durability for space making, simultaneous implant placement is recommended for the GBR technique with resorbable or non-resorbable membranes.

Although an autogenous block bone graft is the first choice of an augmentation procedure in the anterior maxillary region, it is difficult to apply this technique in the posterior maxilla or mandible, where the defect is uneven and complicated specifically when the defects include the extraction socket. In those cases, a titanium mesh–bone graft procedure is the first choice for alveolar ridge augmentation.

For extra large defects beyond 10 mm vertically or a defect with abundant scar tissues, the titanium mesh–bone graft procedure is extremely difficult. Currently alveolar distraction osteogenesis is the only indication for such defects. Although both simultaneous and delayed implant placement is applicable for the titanium mesh–bone graft procedure, the authors prefer delayed implant placement because, when early mesh exposure and subsequent infection occurs, it jeopardize placed implants as well.

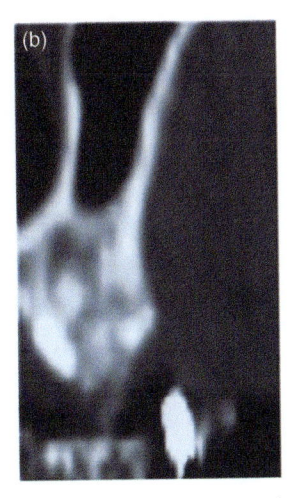

Figure 10.15 A typical case of S-type defect: (a) pre-operative CT scan and (b) 6 month post-operative CT scan. The Hounsfield value of the grafted area was 891.

Table 10.2 Defect size and augmentation procedure.

Defect size	Morphology	Method	Timing of implant placement
Marginal	Thread exposure Fenestration	GBR	Simultaneous
Small (<3–4 mm)	Flat Uneven	Block BG GBR, TIME	Simultaneous/staged
Intermediate (4–7 mm)	Flat Uneven	Block BG, TIME TIME	Staged
Large (<10 mm)	Scar tissue (−) Scar tissue (+)	Block BG, TIME DOG	Staged
Extra large (>10 mm)	Any	DOG	Staged

Case 1: Management of atrophic anterior maxilla

A 60-year-old female presented with a chief compliant of masticatory dysfunction (Figure 10.16). She had been using a removable partial denture for the maxilla and had been suffering from instability of the maxillary denture. A panoramic radiograph showed a severe atrophic anterior maxilla from the right second premolar to the left second premolar because of its extended defect horizontally as well as vertically (Figure 10.17). It was decided to use a titanium mesh–bone graft procedure. A crestal incision was used. The incision was curved toward the line angle of both side molars next to the defect. The subperiosteal dissection was performed with great care to avoid tearing the gingival cuff. As shown in Figure 10.18, the anterior maxillary alveolar ridge showed a knife-edge shape, and vertical deficiency in the anterior region was evident. Furthermore, the incisive foramen was wide open, which made it difficult to place implants. Therefore, nasal floor elevation was performed, and the contents including nerves and vessels in the incisive canal were completely removed to allow bone grafting in the cavity. Decortication was performed using a round bur on the cortical surface of the maxilla (Figure 10.18). Approximately 10 g of PCBM was harvested from the left anterior iliac crest and was placed on the surface of the maxilla, on the nasal floor as well as into the incisive canal (Figure 10.19). Two 0.2 mm thick titanium mesh plates (Jeil Medical Co. Ltd., Seoul, South Korea) were set on the graft materials (Figure 10.20). Once the mesh was in position, it was secured with 5 mm long titanium screws on the facial surface as well as the palatal surface. The periosteum was released along the facial vestibule to facilitate a tension-free closure of the wound. The patient was instructed not to wear any dentures for at least 2 weeks. After two weeks, extensive relief was made for the denture to prevent wound dehiscence, and the patient was instructed to take soft food using the denture minimally in daily life for 2 months. Six months after the graft procedure, a flap was raised, and both Ti mesh devices were exposed (Figure 10.21). After the removal of titanium screws, both mesh devices were removed. Augmented bone was found to be fully consolidated (Figure 10.22). Six 11 mm long dental implants were placed (Figure 10.23). Three months after the implant placement, a bone-anchored prosthesis was fabricated and delivered (Figure 10.24).

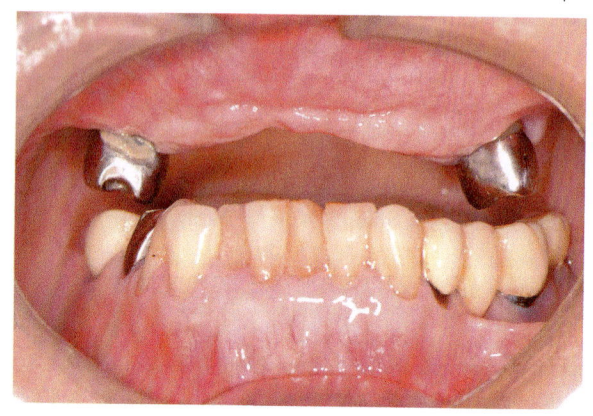

Figure 10.16 Intraoral view of a patient with severe atrophy of the maxilla.

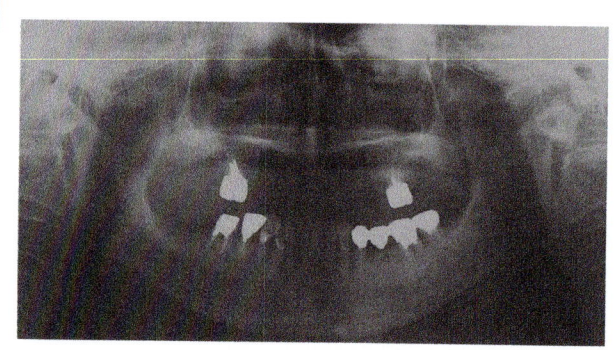

Figure 10.17 Pre-operative panoramic radiograph.

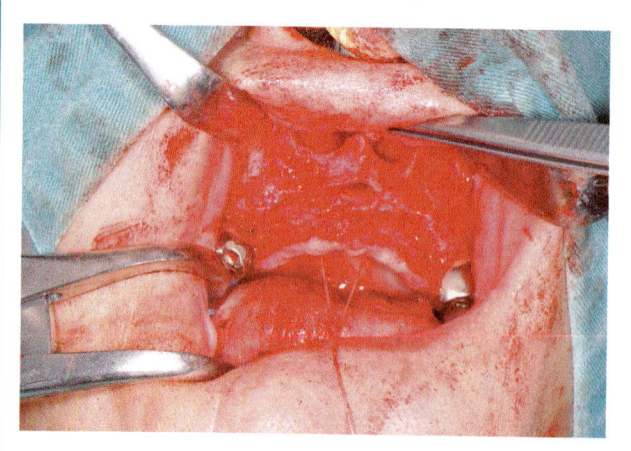

Figure 10.18 Preparation of the recipient site. The incisive foramen was exposed and the content was removed. Nasal floor elevation was also performed.

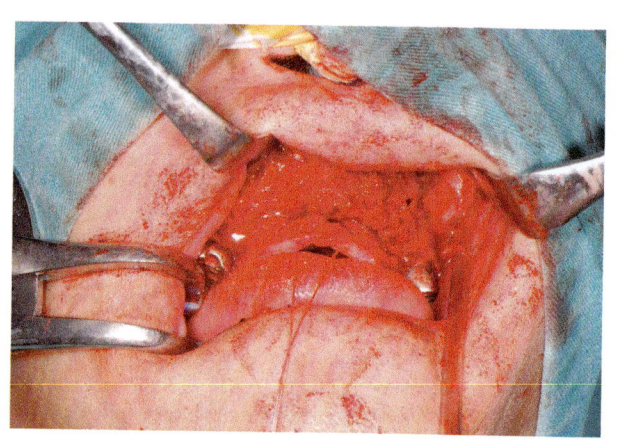

Figure 10.19 PCBM from the iliac crest was placed on the surface of the maxilla, on the nasal floor as well as into the incisive foramen.

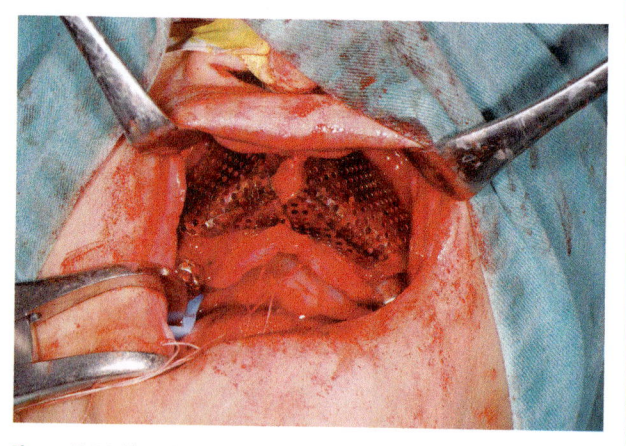

Figure 10.20 Two titanium mesh plates (0.2 mm thick, Jeil Co. Ltd., South Korea) were fixed with titanium screws.

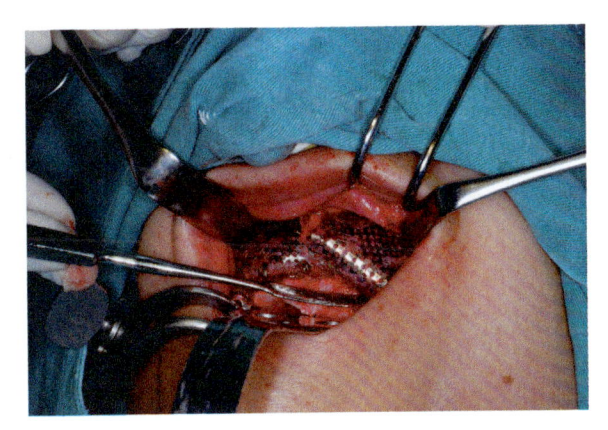

Figure 10.21 Six months after the augmentation procedure, the mesh was exposed and new bone formation was confirmed.

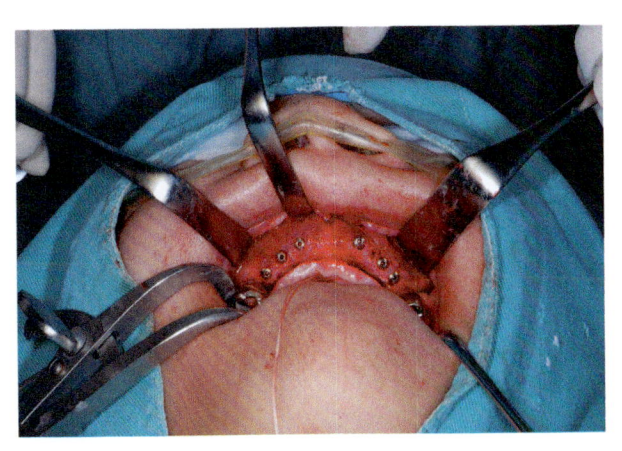

Figure 10.23 Six dental implants were securely placed.

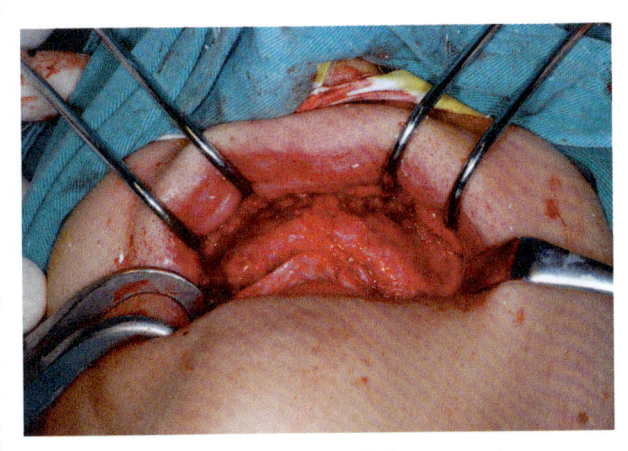

Figure 10.22 After the mesh was removed, the augmented area was completely consolidated.

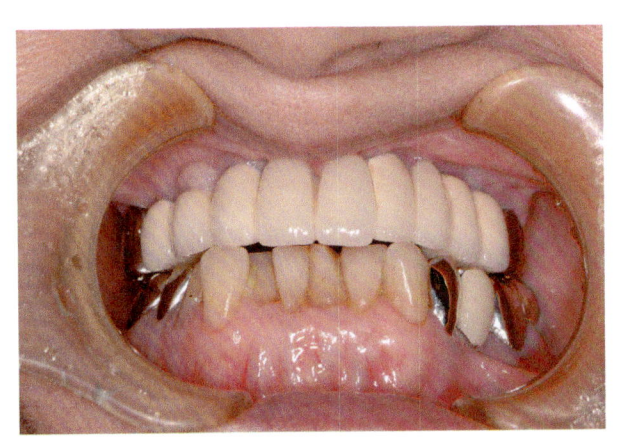

Figure 10.24 Final prosthesis was fabricated.

Case 2: Management of atrophic posterior maxilla (sinus floor elevation combined with alveolar bone augmentation)

Vertical patterns of alveolar bone resorption are known to occur in the posterior maxilla. Whenever there is a greater need for augmentation than simply elevating the sinus floor with an inlay bone graft, horizontal and vertical augmentation of the residual ridge are often necessary. Autogenous bone grafts combined with sinus floor elevation, so-called "inlay–onlay" grafting of the posterior maxilla, is well documented [28]. Sometimes, however, the shape of the residual alveolar ridge is uneven and is difficult to perform onlay bone grafting. In such cases, sinus floor elevation combined with a titanium mesh–bone graft procedure seems to be a viable option for bone augmentation in a severely atrophic posterior maxilla.

This clinical case is of a 57-year-old female referred for treatment of her partially edentulous left maxilla (Figure 10.25). Maxillary left premolars and molars were missing (Figure 10.25). A panoramic radiograph and CT scan revealed a vertical bone deficiency at the molar and premolar sites (Figures 10.26 and 10.27). The sinus floor elevation and inlay grafting were required for implants to be placed. The clinical situation suggested that a horizontal deficiency was also present in the premolar area. Furthermore, vertical alveolar ridge deficiency suggested the crown–root ratio discrepancy even if a sinus floor inlay elevation were to be performed without any vertical onlay grafting. Therefore, the sinus floor elevation combined with titanium mesh for the alveolar ridge augmentation was scheduled.

Surgery was carried out in an outpatient setting under local anesthesia with intravenous sedation. A crestal incision was performed with two vertical releasing incisions. The full thickness flap was raised and the lateral surface of the maxilla was exposed. The bony window was created using a round bur and was removed. The Schneiderian membrane was carefully elevated without membrane perforation (Figure 10.28). Autogenous particulate bone was harvested from the left mandibular ramus using a scraper (mx-grafter: Maxilon Laboratories, Inc., Hollis, NH, USA) (Figure 10.29). A porous beta tricalcium phosphate (β-TCP, Osferion, Olympustermobiomaterial, Japan) was mixed with the same amount of autogenous particulate bone (50/50 mixed bone graft). The 50/50 mixed bone graft material was soaked with autologous blood drawn from the vein, and then used as a graft material. The graft material was placed below the elevated Schneiderian sinus membrane. Furthermore, the remaining graft material was set over the bony window and added laterally as well as coronally (Figure 10.30). Then it was stabilized by a 0.2 mm thick titanium mesh (Jeil Medical Co. Ltd., Seoul, South Korea) and fixed by 5 mm long self-drilling screws (Jeil Medical Co. Ltd., Seoul, South Korea) placed through the buccal bone as well as the

(continued)

(continued)

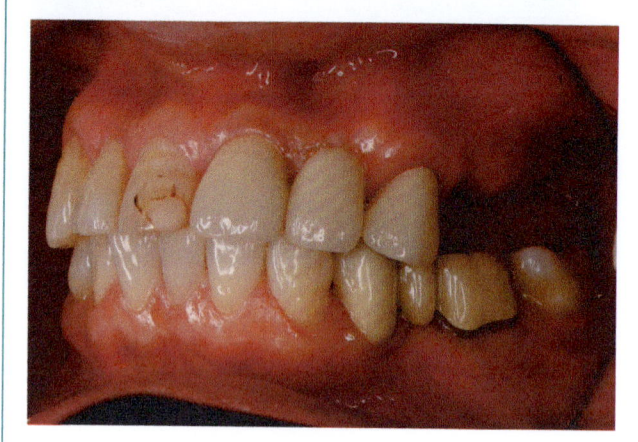

Figure 10.25 Occlusal view of the patient.

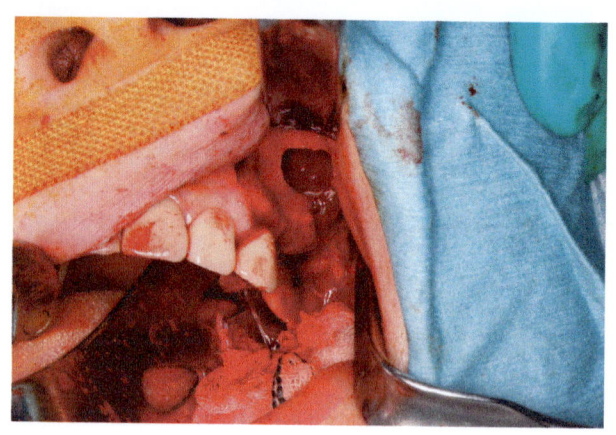

Figure 10.28 Bony window was created and the Schneiderian membrane was elevated.

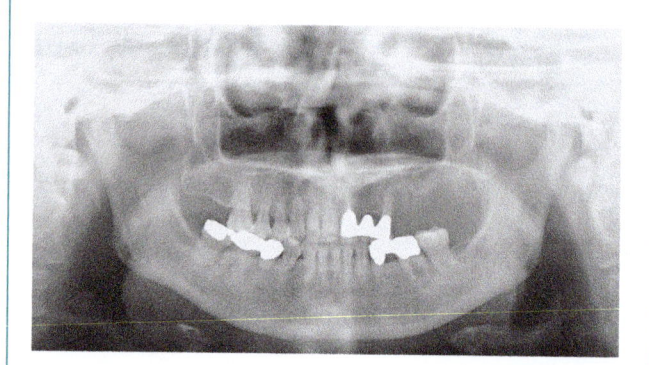

Figure 10.26 A panoramic radiograph showed vertical bone deficiency at the molar and premolar sites.

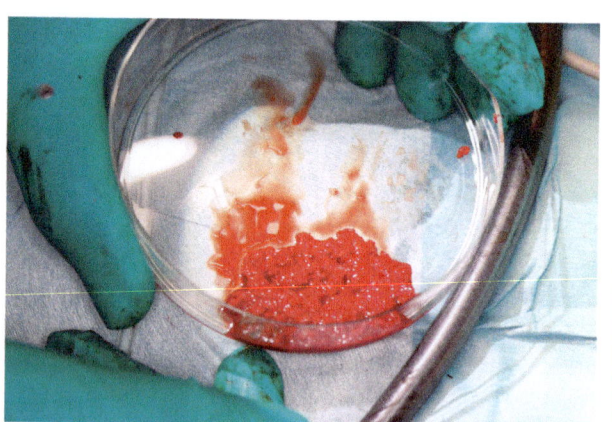

Figure 10.29 Autogenous particulate bone was harvested from the left mandibular ramus.

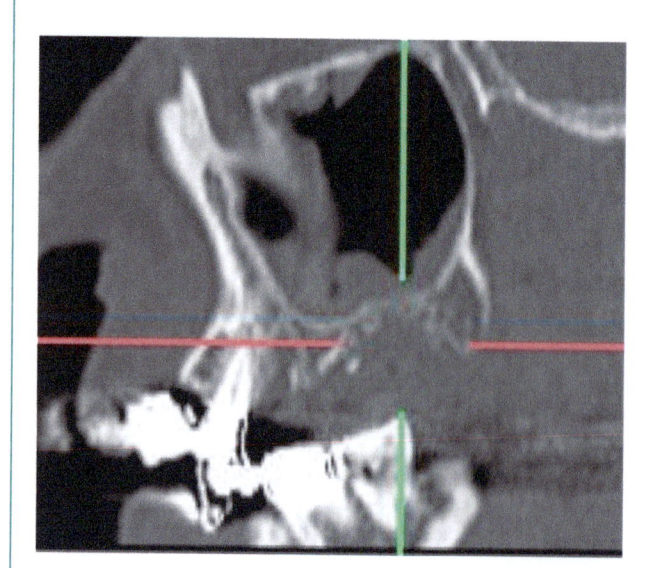

Figure 10.27 CT scan showed vertical bone efficiency at both the sinus floor and alveolar ridge.

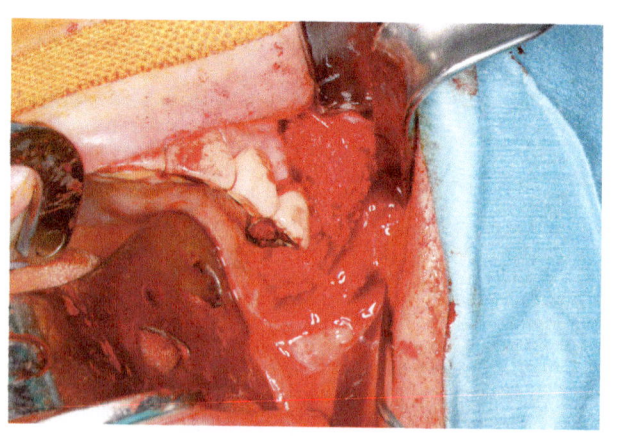

Figure 10.30 Graft material was filled below the Schneiderian membrane and was also set over the bony window.

palatal bone (Figure 10.31). The flap was then mobilized with the aid of periosteal horizontal releasing incisions and closed with a 4-0 nylon suture in a watertight manner.

A post-operative panoramic radiograph demonstrated the ideal vertical height 6 months post-operatively (Figure 10.32). A post-operative CT scan revealed that the vertical bone gain at premolar and molar sites of 9.6 mm (from 8 to 17.6 mm), 14 mm (from 3 to 17 mm), and 12.2 mm (from 2 to 14.2 mm), respectively (Figure 10.33). An ample horizontal width was also obtained for the implant placement in the region. After 6 months of uneventful healing, the second phase of surgery was performed. The flap was raised in the same manner and titanium mesh was removed to expose the reconstructed alveolar crest. The adequate horizontal bone augmentation was achieved (Figure 10.34). Two 3.5 mm × 11 mm and one 4 mm × 11 mm Osseospeed implants (Dentsply IH Co. Ltd., Tokyo, Japan) were placed (Figure 10.35). A three-unit fixed final prosthesis was delivered 3 months later (Figure 10.36). A clinical occlusal view demonstrated the success of the three-dimensional reconstruction.

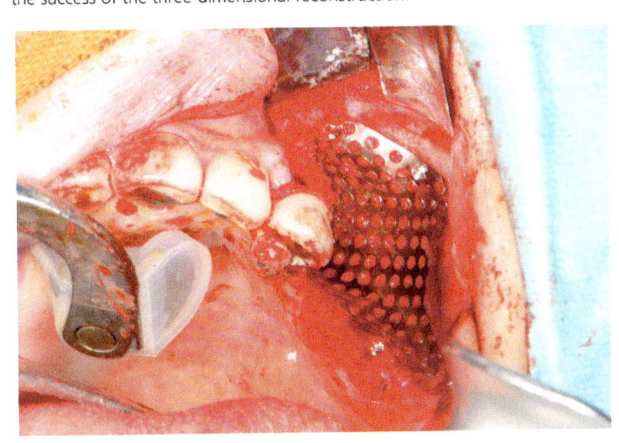

Figure 10.31 A titanium mesh covered the graft material and was fixed with titanium screws.

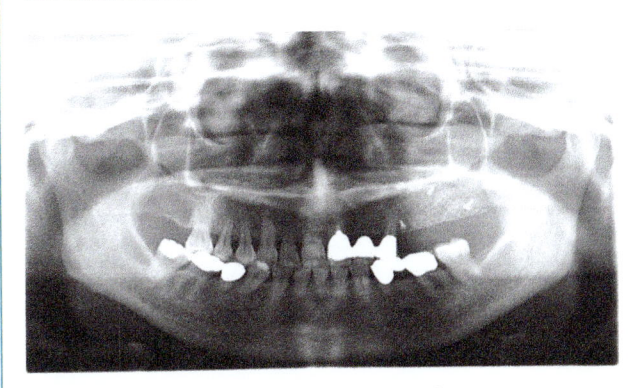

Figure 10.32 Post-operative panoramic radiograph.

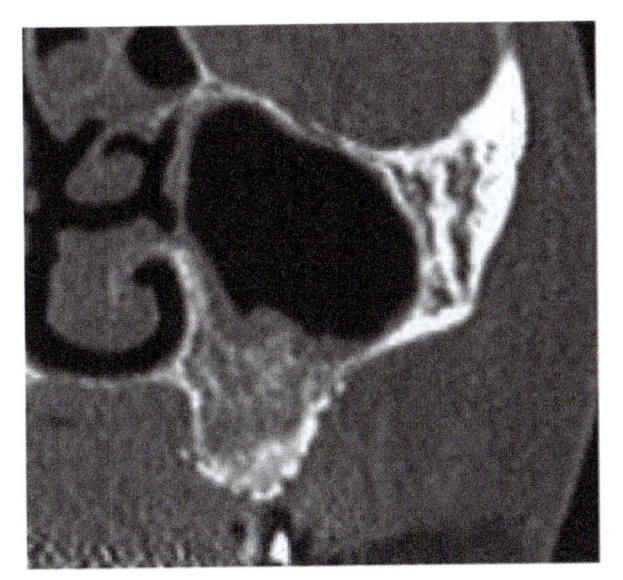

Figure 10.33 Post-operative CT scan showed bone augmentation at the sinus floor as well as at the alveolar ridge.

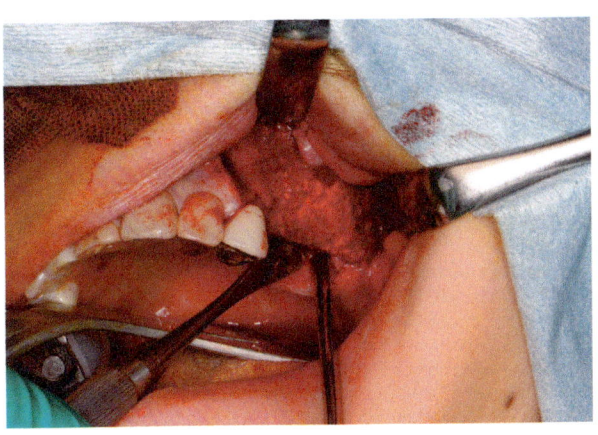

Figure 10.34 After 6 months of the surgical procedure, the titanium mesh was removed; new bone formation was achieved.

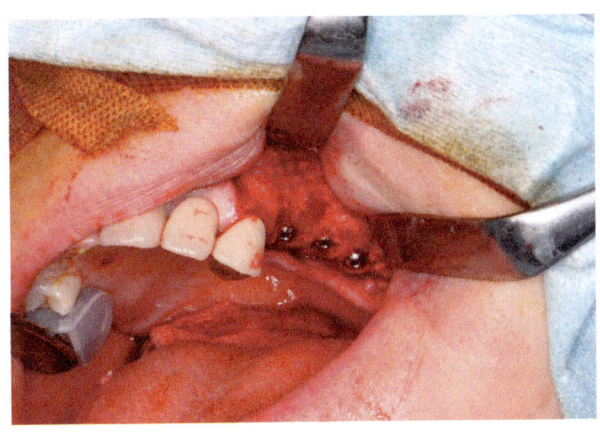

Figure 10.35 Three dental implants were securely placed.

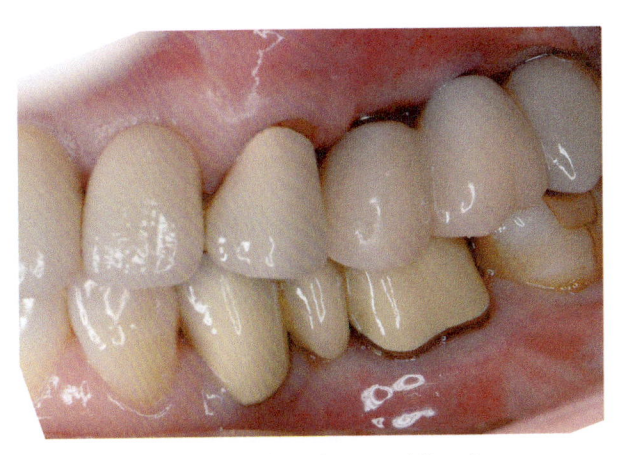

Figure 10.36 A three-unit fixed prosthesis was delivered.

Case 3: Management of severely atrophic edentulous mandible

A 56-year-old man was referred with a chief complaint of ongoing pain at the left posterior mandible during mastication with his removable lower partial denture (Figure 10.37). Approximately 5 years prior most of his teeth were removed because of severe periodontitis. A removable partial denture was fabricated, but he had been suffering from instability of the denture since then. An intraoral clinical view and panoramic radiograph showed a severely atrophic edentulous mandible (Figure 10.38).

Simplant® (Dentsply IH Co. Ltd., Tokyo, Japan) simulation data from the CT scan revealed the extremely atrophic alveolar ridge at both sides of the posterior mandible (Figure 10.39). Specifically, the inferior alveolar nerve seems to be directly exposed beneath the oral mucosa, showing class VI atrophy by Cawood classification. Vertical ridge augmentation at both sides of the mandible was scheduled using the titanium mesh–bone graft procedure. The maximal desired bone gain was 9 mm at the left side, and was 4.5 mm at the right side. Under the general anesthesia, the crestal incision was made from the mandibular second left to second right molar region. Two releasing vertical incisions were made at both ends of the crestal incision. The flap was carefully raised in order not to injure the mental nerves. After the exposure of buccal bone surfaces, the inferior alveolar neurovascular bundle on the left side was directly exposed (Figure 10.40). Approximately 3 g of PCBM was harvested from the left anterior iliac crest. Beta tricalcium phosphate (β-TCP, OSferion, Olympustermobiomaterial, Japan) particles sized 0.5 to 1.5 mm with interconnecting micropores of 5–20 μm were soaked with autologous blood drawn from the vein and was mixed with the autogenous bone chips to form a 50/50 mixed bone graft. After the decortication was performed using a round bur on both sides of the mandible, the 50/50 mixed bone graft materials were placed with 2 g for the right side and 4 g for the left side. The neurovascular bundle was completely covered by the ample amount of graft material. Then, two 0.2 mm thick titanium mesh plates (Dynamic mesh, Stryker & Leibinger GmbH & Co. KG, USA) were placed over the graft materials and were fixed with 1.4 mm wide, 4 mm long titanium screws (Jeil Medical Co. Ltd., Seoul, South Korea) on both sides of the mandible (Figure 10.41). Extreme care was taken to prepare the horizontal releasing incisions and the flap was closed with 4-0 nylon in a watertight manner (Figure 10.42). The patient was instructed not to wear the removable denture for one month. A post-operative clinical course was uneventful. At six months after the augmentation procedure, the mesh was removed. The ideal amount of bone augmentation on both sides of the mandible was achieved. At the left side, the inferior alveolar neurovasucular bundle was completely embedded by newly formed bone and a newly formed inferior alveolar foramen was recognized (Figure 10.43). A CT scan after the removal of the titanium mesh revealed excellent bone regeneration on both sides of the mandible (Figure 10.44a and b). After one month after the removal of the mesh plates, two 4 mm × 11 mm, one 4.5 mm × 11 mm, and one 4.5 mm × 9 mm Tioblast® implants (Dentsply IH Co. Ltd., Tokyo) were placed (Figure 10.45). Finally, bar-clip attachments were made and an implant-supported overdenture-type prosthesis (IOD) was fabricated (Figure 10.46a and b). The patient did not feel any neurosensory disturbance or pain with wearing the IOD and was very satisfied with his treatment.

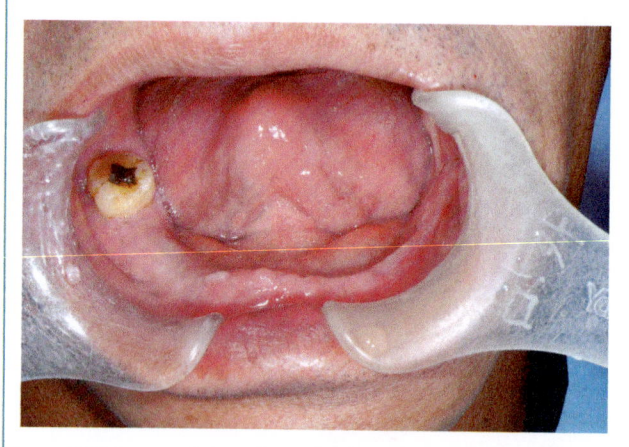

Figure 10.37 Intra-oral view of severely atrophic edentulous mandible.

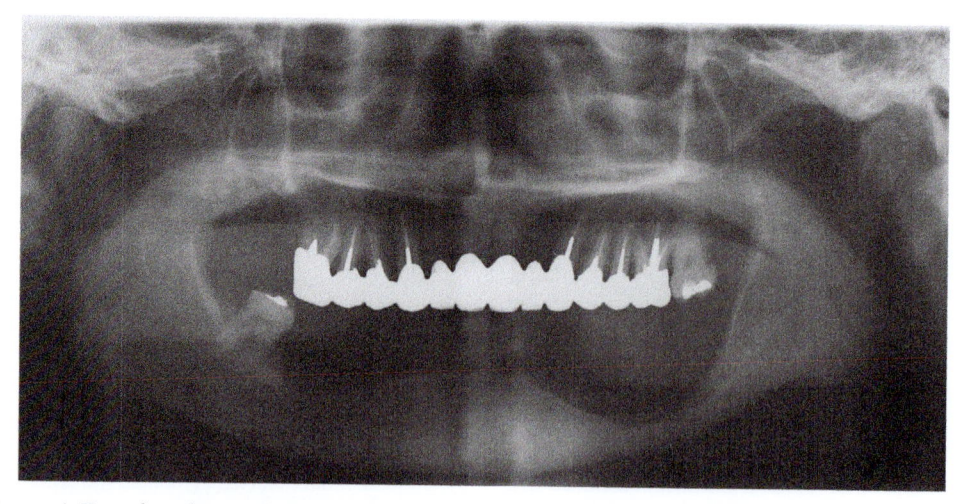

Figure 10.38 Panoramic X-ray showed extremely atrophic edentulous mandible, especially on the left side.

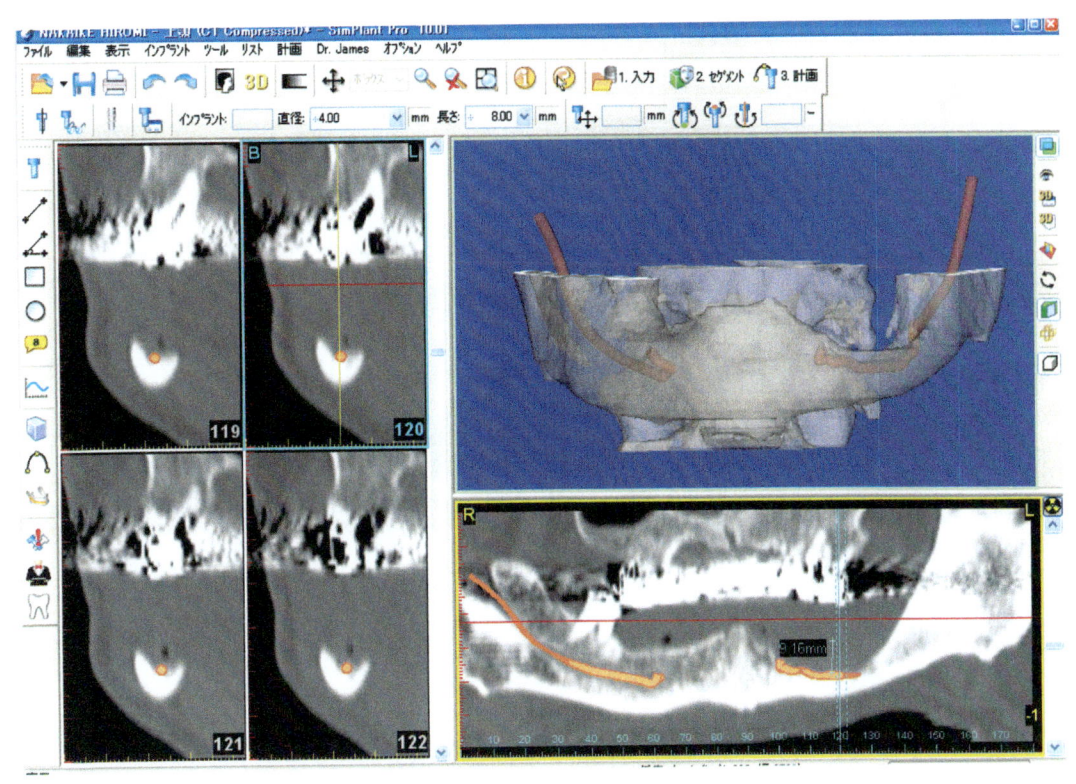

Figure 10.39 Simplant® (Dentsply IH Co. Ltd., Tokyo, Japan) simulation data from a CT scan.

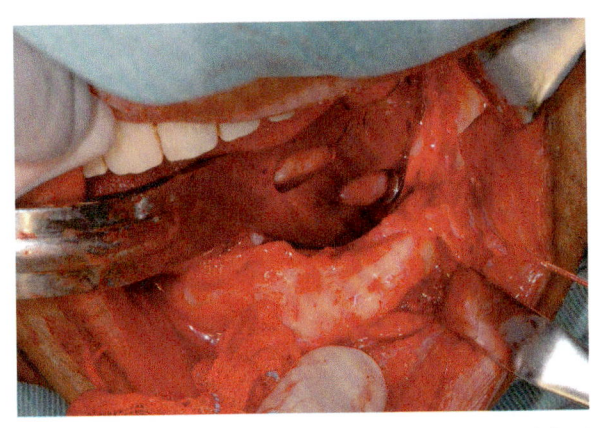

Figure 10.40 The inferior alveolar neurovascular bundle on the left side was directly exposed.

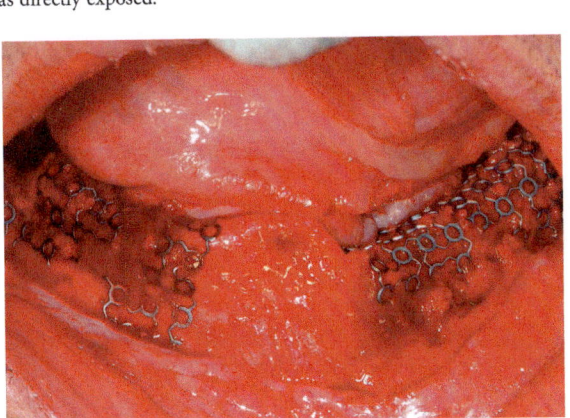

Figure 10.41 Two 0.2 mm thick titanium mesh plates (Dynamic mesh, Stryker & Leibinger GmbH & Co. KG, USA) covered the graft materials and were fixed with 1.4 mm wide, 4 mm long titanium screws.

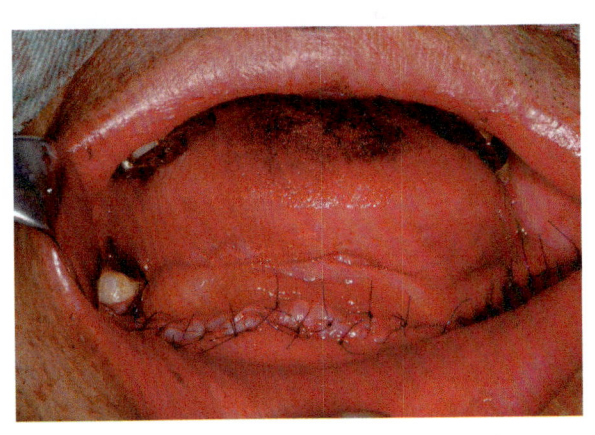

Figure 10.42 The flap was closed with 4-0 nylon in a watertight manner.

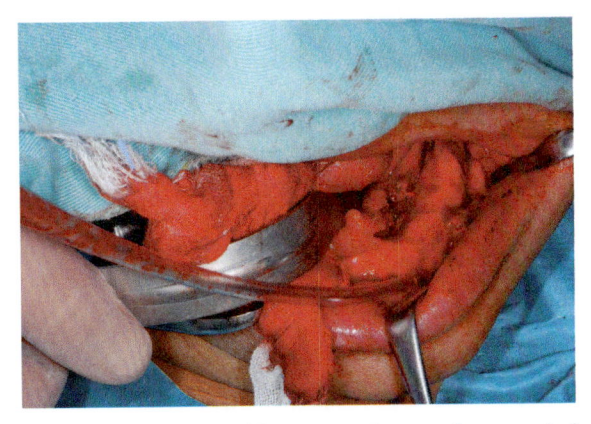

Figure 10.43 Intraoral view of the augmentation area after removal of the titanium mesh. Note that the inferior alveolar neurovasucular bundle was completely embedded by newly formed bone and a newly formed inferior alveolar foramen was recognized at the left side.

(*continued*)

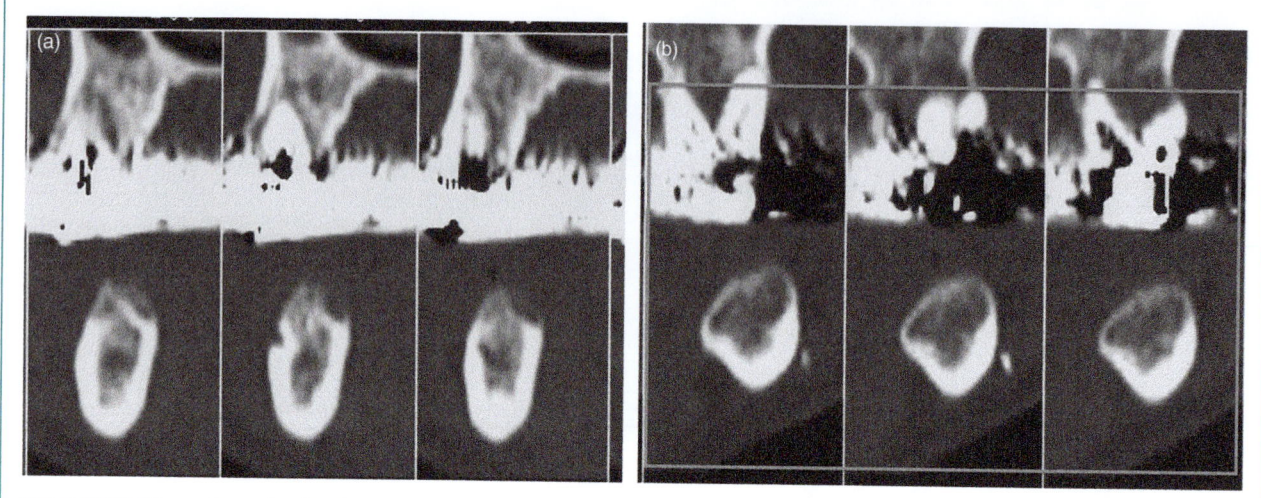

104 Guided Bone Regeneration (GBR) with Particulate Graft

(continued)

Figure 10.44 CT scan 6 months after the augmentation procedure: **(a)** left and **(b)** right.

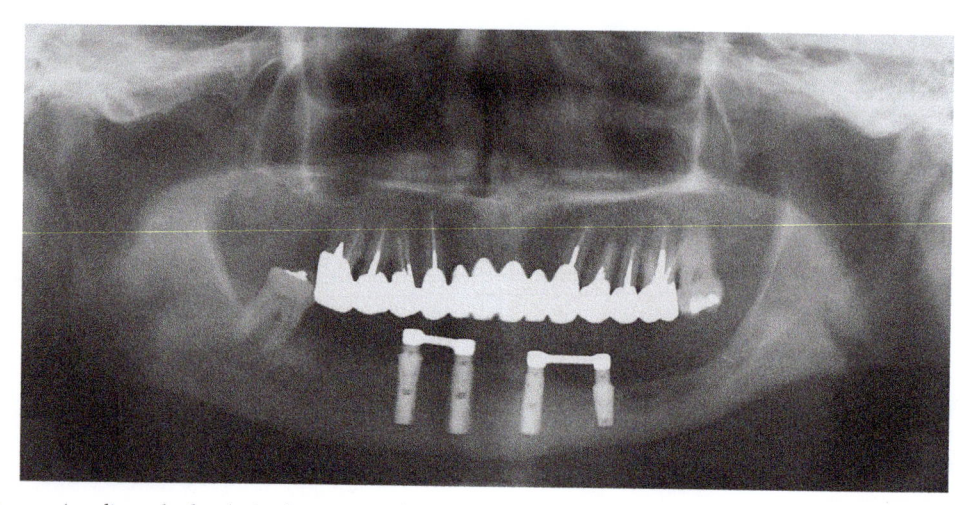

Figure 10.45 Panoramic radiograph after the implant-supported overdenture-type prosthesis was delivered.

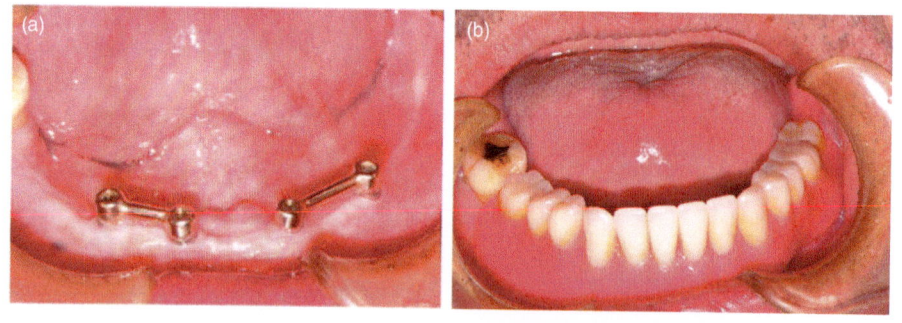

Figure 10.46 Intraoral view of the final IOD prosthesis: **(a)** bur attachment and **(b)** IOD.

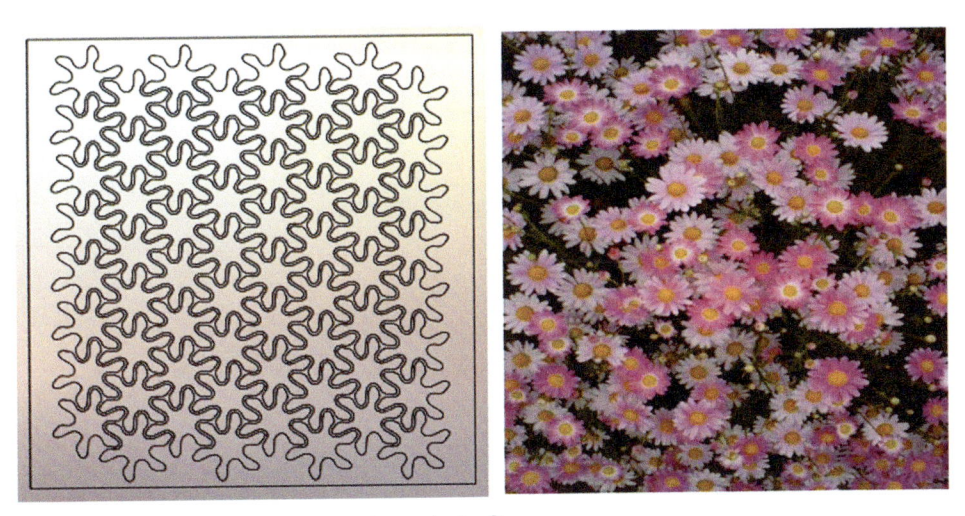

Figure 10.47 The "Margaret flower" like structure of Ultra flex mesh plate®.

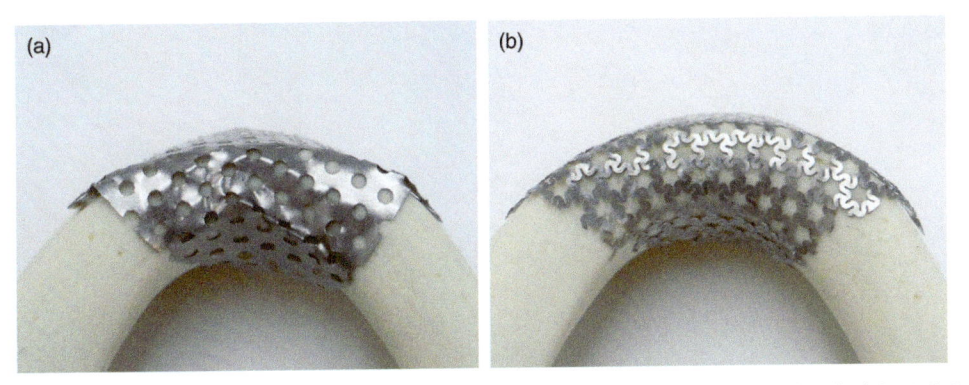

Figure 10.48 A conventional mesh versus Ultra flex mesh plate®: **(a)** 0.1 mm thick conventional mesh plate (Jeil medical Co. Ltd., Seoul, South Korea) and **(b)** 0.1 mm thick Ultra flex mesh plate® (Kyocera Medical Co. Ltd., Osaka, Japan).

Use of a newly developed next generation titanium mesh: Ultraflex mesh plate®

Although commercially available titanium micromesh is flexible and adjustable to many types of the defect, the titanium mesh has to be cut and trimmed and contoured to obtain a desirable shape of the projected alveolar ridge. In the clinical setting, the trimmed edge sometimes can cause an exposure of the mesh and can penetrate through the thin mucoperiosteum. Recently a next-generation titanium mesh, called Ultra flex mesh plate® (Okada Medical Supply Co. Ltd, Tokyo Japan, Olympus Biomaterial Terumo Co. Ltd, Tokyo Japan, and Kyocera Medical Co. Ltd., Osaka, Japan), has been developed. The beauty of this next-generation mesh is its superior flexibility. Ultra flex mesh plate® has a "Margaret-flower" like structure (Figure 10.47a and b). This structure enables the mesh to adjust to any shape and contour, whatever the desired shape of the future alveolar ridge is needed, without any cutting or trimming. As shown in Figure 10.48a, a conventional titanium mesh is adjusted to the curved shape such as the anterior mandibular region, a mesh is twisted, and it is impossible to reproduce the original curved contour without trimming or cutting. However, Ultra flex mesh plate® creates a perfect fitting to the curved structure without any cutting or trimming (Figure 10.48b). This next-generation mesh plate has a great potential to create an ideal contour of the desired shape of a future alveolar ridge.

Case 4: The atrophic edentulous mandible at the right premolar–molar side region

The last clinical case is the atrophic edentulous mandible at the right premolar–molar side region (Figure 10.49). Because of the severe atrophy and proximity to the inferior alveolar canal, implant placement was deemed impossible without bone augmentation (Figure 10.50). Vertical bone augmentation was scheduled using the titanium mesh–bone graft procedure. A vestibular incision was made with two vertical releasing incisions. Great care was taken not to injure the mental foramen and mental nerves. The full thickness flap was raised and bone was exposed (Figure 10.51). Decortication was created with a round bur and piezosurgical electric instrument (VarioSurg, NSK, Tokyo, Japan) (Figure 10.52). Then a 0.2 mm thick Ultra flex mesh plate® was contoured and adjusted to the desired shape of the future alveolar ridge (Figure 10.53). Autogenous particulate bone chips were harvested from the ramus on the ipsilateral side of the mandible. A bone graft material, DBBM (Bio-Oss; Geistlich Pharma, Wolhusen, Switzerland), was soaked with autologous blood drawn from the vein and was mixed with the autogenous bone chips to form a 50/50 mixed bone graft. The 50/50 mixed bone graft material was placed on the defect (Figure 10.54) and a prefabricated Ultra flex mesh plate® was covered on the graft and was fixed with 4 mm long titanium mini screws (Kyocera Medical Co. Ltd., Osaka, Japan) (Figure 10.55). A post-operative CT scan revealed excellent contour formation of the augmented area by the titanium mesh–bone graft procedure (Figures 10.56 and 10.57a and b).

(*continued*)

(continued)

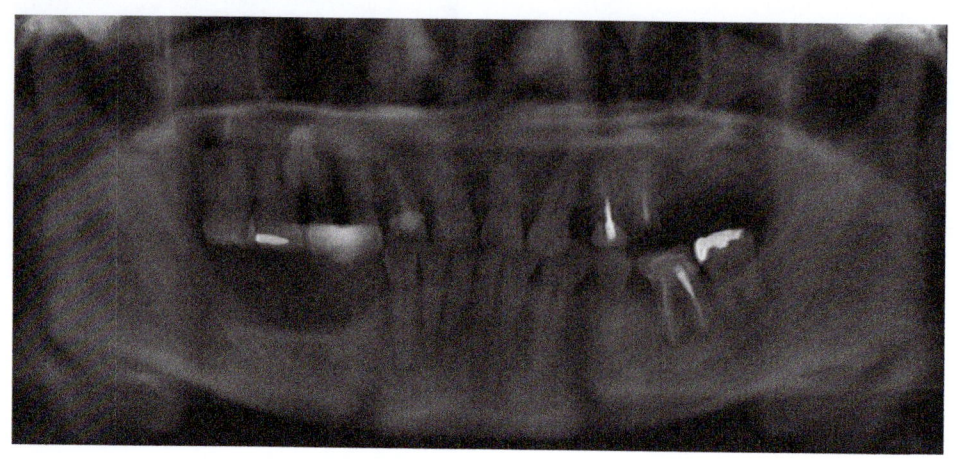

Figure 10.49 Panoramic radiograph of an atrophic edentulous mandible at the right molar region.

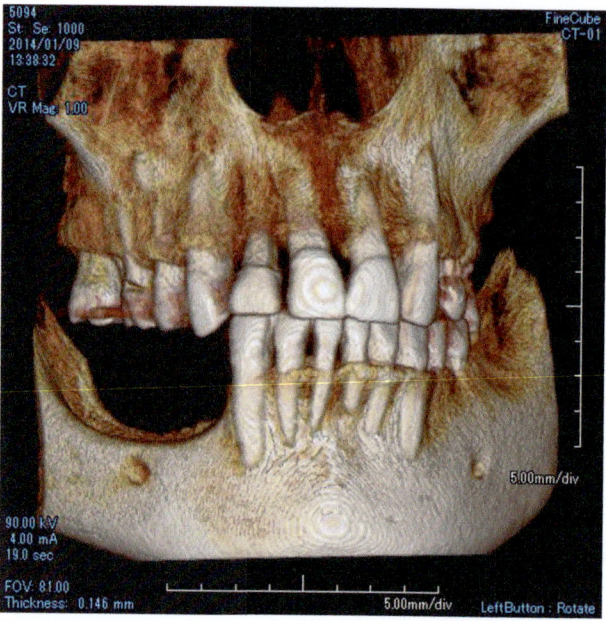

Figure 10.50 A CT scan showed severe atrophy of the right mandibular region.

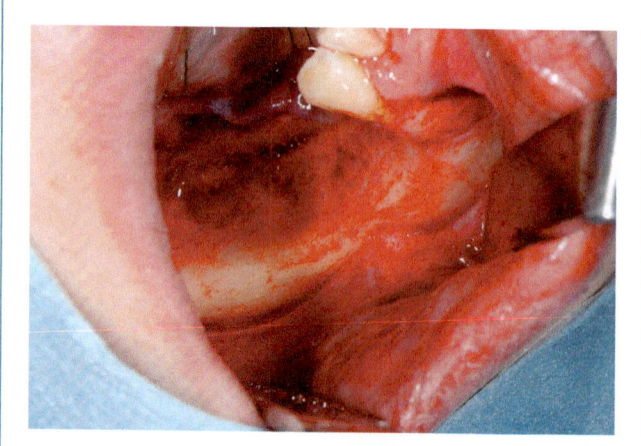

Figure 10.51 Flap was raised not to damage the mental foramen and nerves.

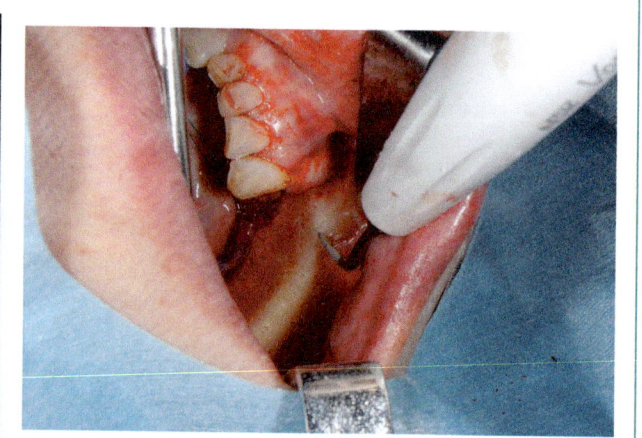

Figure 10.52 Decortication was created by a piezosurgical electric instrument.

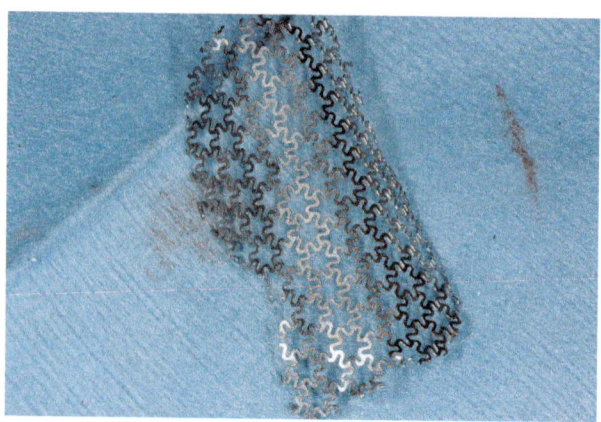

Figure 10.53 A 0.2 mm thick Ultra flex mesh plate® was contoured.

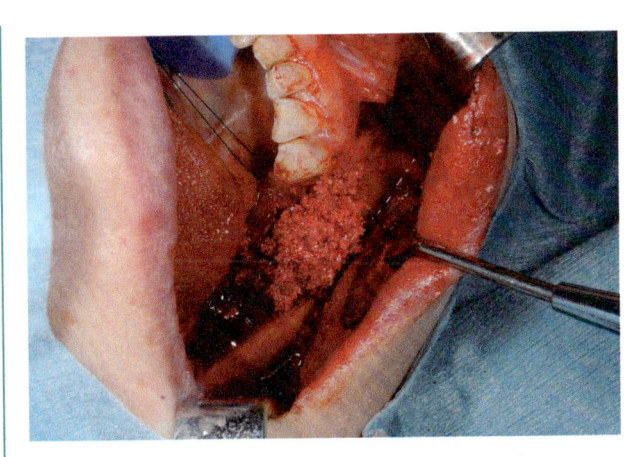

Vertical Augmentation of the Alveolar Ridge with Titanium-Reinforced Devices **107**

Figure 10.54 The bone graft material was placed on the defect.

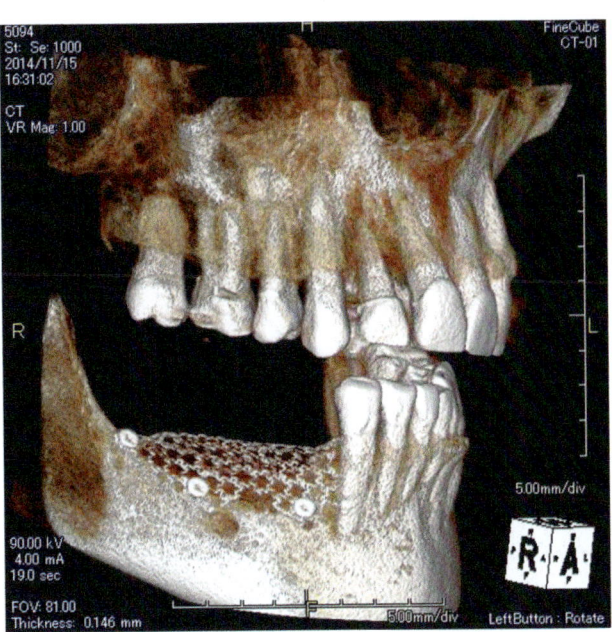

Figure 10.56 A CT scan immediately after the augmentation procedure.

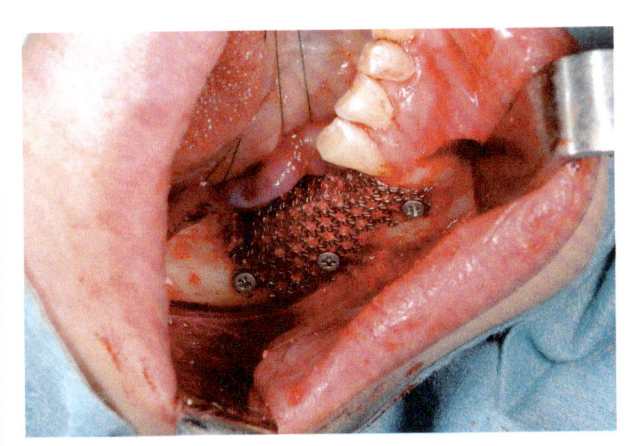

Figure 10.55 The mesh was fixed with mini screws.

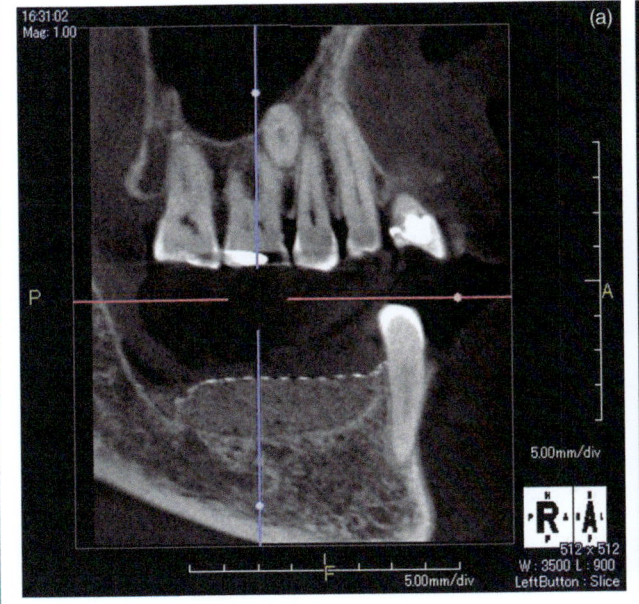

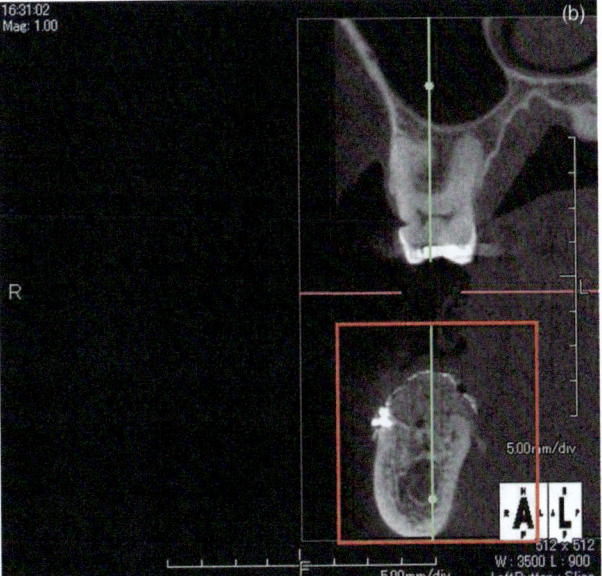

Figure 10.57 ST scans of the grafted area: (a) a panoramic view and (b) a sagittal view.

(continued)

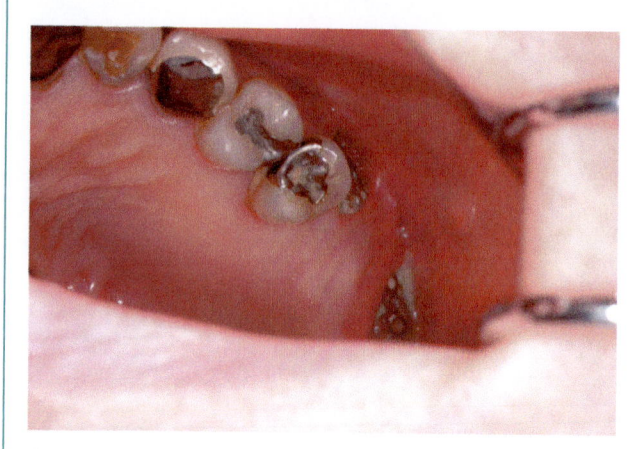

Figure 10.58 A mesh exposure 3 months after the augmentation procedure. No infection was found around the mesh.

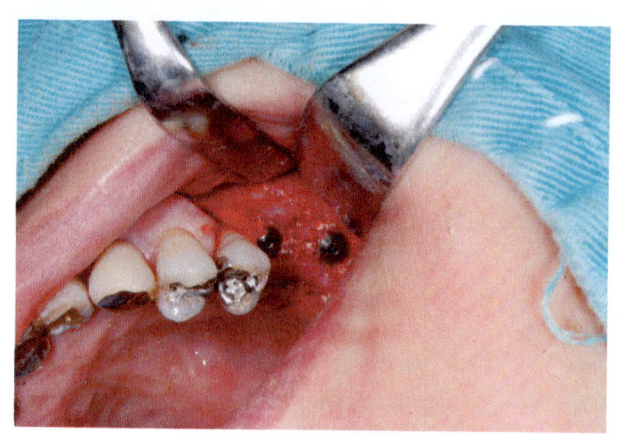

Figure 10.60 Two dental implants were securely placed.

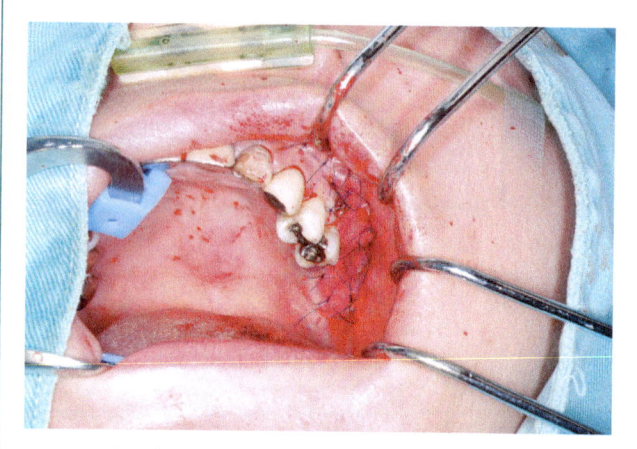

Figure 10.59 A large defect was repaired by suturing the artificial dermal graft "Terdermis®".

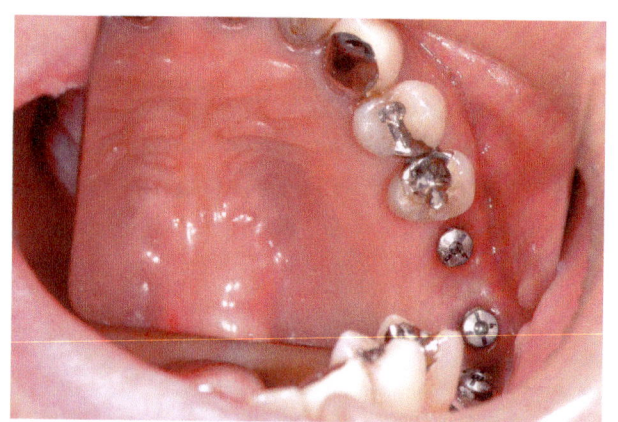

Figure 10.61 After the abutment installation.

Management of the mesh exposure

As mentioned above, a major complication of the titanium mesh–bone graft procedure is mesh exposure during the healing period. Although mesh exposure does not necessarily result in failure of bone augmentation, care should be taken not to develop further bone resorption once a mesh exposure occurred post-operatively. Titanium mesh might not require immediate removal because it does not interfere with blood flow to the underlying tissues owing to the presence of pores within the mesh. The tissue around titanium meshes is frequently observed after the healing period. In the early phase of wound healing, the newly forming immature granulation tissue does not cover the bone graft fully and thus does not allow full protection from exposure and infection. If infection were to occur in the grafted bone at this time, it would result in severe bone resorption. Conversely, after a few weeks of healing, newly formed granulation tissue would cover the bone; therefore, the augmented site can resist infection without severe bone resorption. Once exposure of the mesh occurred, a large defect of the alveolar mucosa might develop after removal of the titanium mesh. In such an occasion, soft tissue management is an essential procedure. Here is a clinical case of the soft tissue management of mesh exposure. Two areas of big circular shaped exposure of the mesh occurred after the titanium mesh–bone graft procedure was performed in a partially edentulous posterior maxilla (Figure 10.58). A sinus floor elevation combined with titanium mesh alveolar bone augmentation was done 3 months prior. No infection of the grafted materials was found and the bone resorption at the mesh-exposed area was minimal. Six months after the graft procedure the mesh was removed and an extended defect of the alveolar mucosa over the grafted area was observed. A granulation tissue was found over the grafted bone area. A large defect was repaired by suturing an artificial dermal graft, "Terdermis®" (Olympus Biomaterial Terumo Co. Ltd., Tokyo, Japan) (Figure 10.58). Finally, implant placement was successfully performed (Figures 10.59, 10.60 and 10.61).

Disadvantages

The main disadvantage of this procedure is the cost and the tendency of the Ti mesh to become exposed during the healing phase. However, as mentioned above, although the risk of exposure is high, the risk of infection remains low. With local wound management, exposure can be tolerated long enough for the graft to mature. Another disadvantage of this procedure is the need for a second surgical intervention to remove the mesh. The mesh removal is sometimes extremely difficult. In fact, some part of the Ti mesh may be left in place, as shown in Figure 10.45. Conversely, if the grafted bone is immature, removal of the mesh may damage some part of the grafted area because the newly formed bone sticks tightly to the mesh while the remaining immature bone comes apart.

Conclusions

The use of titanium mesh devices and autogenous bone combined with graft materials has been a versatile and successful technique for the reconstruction of the atrophic maxilla and mandible. The titanium mesh–bone graft procedure allows adequate three-dimensional augmentation. Although the risk of mesh exposure and subsequent partial bone loss exists, local wound management can help to circumvent this complication and allow the bone graft to mature.

References

1. Triplett RG, Schow SR: Autologous bone grafts and endosseous implants: complementary techniques. *J Oral Maxillofac Surg* 1996;**54**:486–494.
2. Sethi A, Kaus T: Ridge augmentation using mandibular block bone grafts: preliminary results of an ongoing prospective study. *Int J Oral Maxillofac Implants* 2001;**16**:378–388.
3. Buser D, Dula K, Hirt HP, Schenk RK: Lateral ridge augmentation using autografts and barrier membranes: a clinical study with 40 partially edentulous patients. *J Oral Maxillofac Surg* 1996;**54**:420–432.
4. Zitzmann NU, Scharer P, Marinello CP: Long-term results of implants treated with guided bone regeneration: a 5-year prospective study. *Int J Oral Maxillofac Implants* 2001;**16**:355–366.
5. Simion M, Jovanovic SA, Tinti C, Benfenati SP: Long-term evaluation of osseointegrated implants inserted at the time or after vertical ridge augmentation: a retrospective study on 123 implants with 1–5 year follow-up. *Clin Oral Implants Res* 2001;**12**:35–45.
6. Jensen OT, Cockrell R, Kuhlke L, Reed C: Anterior maxillary alveolar distraction osteogenesis: a prospective 5-year clinical study. *Int J Oral Maxillofac Implants* 2002;**17**:52–68.
7. Hidding J, Lazar F, Zöller JE: The vertical distraction of the alveolar bone. *J Craniomaxillofac Surg* 1998;**26**:72–76.
8. Chiapasco M, Romeo E, Casentini P, Rimondini L: Alveolar distraction osteogenesis vs. vertical guided bone regeneration for the correction of vertically deficient edentulous ridges: a 1–3 year prospective study on humans. *Clin Oral Implants Res* 2004;**15**:82–95.
9. Yamauchi K, Takahashi T, Nogami S, Kataoka Y, Miyamoto I, Funaki K: Horizontal alveolar distraction osteogenesis for dental implants: long-term results. *Clin Oral Implants Res* 2013;**24**:563–568.
10. Lustmann J, Lewinstein I: Interpositional bone grafting technique to widen narrow maxillary ridge. *Int J Oral Maxillofac Implants* 1995;**10**:568–577.
11. Sethi A, Kaus T: Maxillary ridge expansion with simultaneous implant placement: 5-year results of an ongoing clinical study. *Int J Oral Maxillofac Implants* 2000;**15**:491–499.
12. Enislidis GE, Wittwer G, Ewers R: Preliminary report on a staged ridge splitting technique for implants placement in the mandible: a technical note. *Int J Oral Maxillofac Implants* 2006;**21**:445–449.
13. Widmark G, Andersson B, Ivanoff CJ: Mandibular bone graft in the anterior maxilla for single-tooth implants. Presentation of surgical method. *Int J Oral Maxillofac Surg* 1997;**26**:106–109.
14. Cordaro L, Amadé DS, Cordaro M: Clinical results of alveolar ridge augmentation with mandibular block bone grafts in partially edentulous patients prior to implant placement. *Clin Oral Implants Res* 2002;**13**:103–111.
15. Boyne PJ, Cole MD, Stringer D, Shafgat JP: A technique osseous restoration of deficient edentulous maxillary ridges. *J Oral Maxillofac Surg* 1985;**43**:87–91.
16. Von Arx T, Hardt N, Wallkamm B: The TIME technique: a new method for localized alveolar ridge augmentation prior to placement of dental implants. *Int J Oral Maxillofac Implants* 1996;**11**:387–394.
17. Louis PJ: Vertical ridge augmentation using titanium mesh. *Oral Maxillofac Surg Clin N Am* 2010;**22**:353–368.
18. Roccuzo M, Ramieri G, Bunino M, Berrone S: Autogenous bone graft alone or associated with titanium mesh for vertical alveolar ridge augmentation: a controlled clinical trial. *Clin Oral Implants Res* 2007;**18**:286–294.
19. Watzinger F, Luksch J, Millesi W: Guided bone regeneration with titanium membranes: a clinical study. *Br J Oral Maxillofac Surg* 2000;**38**:312–315.
20. Weng D, Hürzeler MB, Quiñones CR, Ohlms A, Caffesse RG: Contribution of the periosteum to bone formation in guided bone regeneration. A study in monkeys. *Clin Oral Implants Res* 2000;**11**:546–554.
21. Miyamoto I, Funaki K, Yamauchi K, Kodama T, Takahashi T: Alveolar ridge reconstruction with titanium and autogenous particulate bone graft: computed tomography-based evaluations of augmented bone quality and quantity. *Clin Implant Dent Related Res* 2012;**14**:304–311.
22. Her S, Kang T, Fien MJ: Titanium mesh as an alternative to a membrane for ridge augmentation. *J Oral Maxillofac Surg* 2012;**70**:803–810.
23. Maiorana C, Santoro F, Rabagliati M, Salina S: Evaluation of the use of iliac cancellous bone and anorganic bovine bone in the reconstruction of the atrophic maxilla with titanium mesh: a clinical and histologic investigation. *Int J Oral Maxillofac Implants* 2001;**16**:427–432.
24. Simion M, Baldoni M, Rossi P, Zaffe D: A comparative study of the effectiveness of e-PTFE membranes with and without early exposure during the healing period. *Int J Periodontics Restorative Dent* 1994;**14**:166–180.
25. Zitzmann NU, Naef R, Schärere P: Resorbable versus nonresorbable membrans in combination with Bio-Oss for guided bone regeneration. *Int J Oral Maxillofac Implants* 1997;**12**:844–852.
26. Buser D, Ruskin J, Higginbottom F, Hardwick R, Dahlin C, Schenk RK: Osseointegration of titanium implants in bone regenerated in membrane-protected defects: a histologic study in the canine mandible. *Int J Oral Maxillofac Implants* 1995;**10**:666–681.
27. Park SH, Wang HL: Clinical significance of incision location on guided bone regeneration: human study. *J Periodontol* 2007;**78**:47–51.
28. Cordano L: Combined SFE and horizontal ridge augmentation with autologous block grafts, BCP, and GBR using a staged approach. In: Katsuyama H, Jensen SS (eds.), *ITI Treatment Guide*, vol. 5, *Sinus Floor Elevation Procedures*. Quintessence Publishing, Berlin, 2011, pp. 129–135.

CHAPTER 11

Pedicled Sandwich Plasty (Osteotomy) with Particulate Inlay Graft for Vertical Alveolar Ridge Defects

Rolf Ewers

University Hospital for Cranio Maxillofacial and Oral Surgery, Medical University of Vienna, Vienna, Austria

Bone classification and bone regeneration techniques

In pre-prosthetic surgery, the term augmentation means measures taken to restore lost bone tissue. Augmentation of alveolar bone loss should constitute regeneration (*restitutio ad integrum*) of the tissue being replaced and not simply spatial repair (scar formation) [1]. Osseous and soft tissue surgery should therefore reconstruct both form and function of the desired replacement tissue [2]. The bone is a highly dynamic system that retains its structure through a balance between various influences, which is known as remodelling [3, 4]. On the one hand, osteoclasts resorb old bone; on the other hand, osteoblasts form the new bone matrix [5]. A preponderance of resorbing activity may result in the atrophy of areas of the jaw, which have to be built up again (augmented) before an implant insertion. During remodelling, the recruitment process, the activation of osteoclasts, osteoblasts, and their precursor cells, is dependent on the properties of the microcirculation, which also play a major role in metabolic microregulation [6, 7]. Reconstructive bone graft repair of osseous defects does not always form well-vascularized bone, even when the bone defect is augmented [8]. True regeneration implies that the defect is reconstructed with a viable mineralized tissue that models and remodels as natural bone and is *not* just a mixture of devitalized graft inclusions or scar tissue.

Bone regeneration methods for defect reconstruction can be differentiated according to bone graft vitality, the extent of consolidation, and marginal integration. These aspects can only be verified by late-term biopsy findings to determine the extent of vital mineralization [9]. Since the routine biopsy analysis is impractical, short of invasive procedures to verify graft performance, hard tissue augmentation can be empirically classified based on vascularization of the grafting approach and the likely vitality of the graft. Therefore, it is proposed that earlier classification [10] for bone regeneration techniques in defect reconstruction be differentiated into five classes, according to vascularization or induction of vascularization [2] (Figure 11.1).

- Class I: microanastomosed free bone flaps
- Class II: distraction osteogenesis
- Class III: pedicled segmental osteotomies with a non-vascularized interpositional graft (inlay graft)
- Class IV: bone morphogenetic protein induction grafts (tent-pole situation)
- Class V: non-vascularized bone grafts (onlay graft or GBR)

Distraction osteogenesis

Osteotomized bone that is slowly spread apart in a process termed *callus distraction* leads to osteogenesis, a highly vascularized epigenetic response induced by a morphogenetic protein cascade first described by Ilizarov [11]. The end result is a much more vital bone than is found in typical bone grafts [12, 13]. Distraction osteogenesis forms well-vascularized isotropic bone that takes on the same conformation as the distraction callus [14]. There is little resorption within the distraction zone as long as there is an adequate healing time and torsion and compression are avoided until lamellar bone is formed and remodeled, in about 4 to 6 months [15, 16].

Alveolar distraction is primarily used for enhancement of alveolar height or width with numerous indications. The bone quality is type 2 because of good vascularization. The theory that the distracted bone is always vascularized was confirmed in histological studies. In the alveolar region, we distinguish between vertical and horizontal distraction osteoneogenesis. Two disadvantages of this method, which must be mentioned, are perforation of the mucosa by the distracting device and the patient's discomfort caused by having to wear the distractor for several months. Another disadvantage is the possible dislocation of the bony segment. Furthermore, often the distracted bone shows a watch glass-like shape if distracted too fast, and with less than 8–9 mm of basal bone to begin with, complications or imperfect results are often observed. These are the reasons why we do not frequently use this method. Instead, we prefer vertical and transverse one-step or two-step pedicled (pedunculated) sandwich plasty (osteotomy). Distraction osteogenesis is our option of bone augmentation in cases when, in addition to bone loss, a significant amount of new soft tissue is needed in severe trauma or burn cases.

Vertical pedicled sandwich plasty (PSP)

Because of the excellent blood supply in the stomatognathic system, gradual distraction is not always necessary in the maxilla or mandible.

Vertical Alveolar Ridge Augmentation in Implant Dentistry: A Surgical Manual, First Edition. Edited by Len Tolstunov.
© 2016 John Wiley & Sons, Inc. Published 2016 by John Wiley & Sons, Inc.

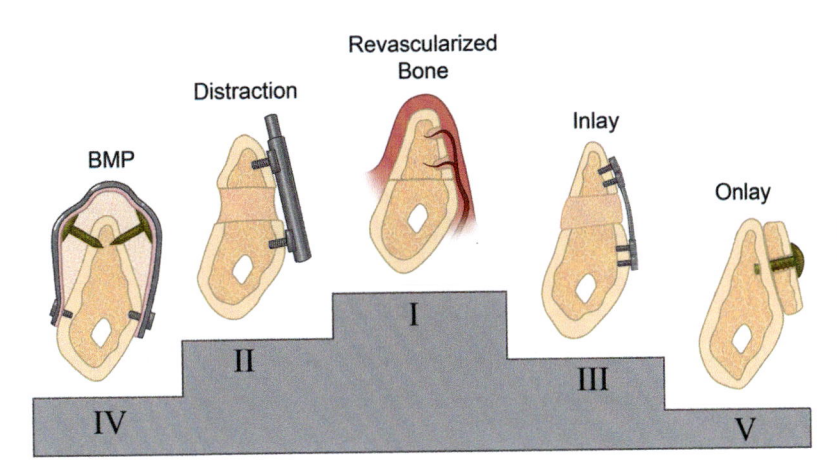

Figure 11.1 Classification of jawbone augmentation techniques. The quality of bone, which is dependent on the vascularization of the graft or the induction of vascularization in native bone, is represented in a form of an "Olympic pedestal": class I: microanastomosed free bone flaps; class II: distraction osteogenesis; class III: pedicled segmental osteotomies; class IV: bone morphogenetic induction grafts; class V: non-vascularized bone grafts.

Alternatively, it has been shown that a pedicled bone segment can be immediately moved up to a distance of 9–10 mm. It can be stabilized with the aid of osteosynthesis plates and screws and an interpositional space can be successfully filled with a particulate graft material [17–23] (Figure 11.2). This method is referred to as the vertical pedicled (pedunculated) sandwich plasty (vertical PSP).

- For the maxilla:
  1 As a special form in a highly atrophied maxilla such as Horseshoe Le Fort I osteotomy [24].
  2 In the anterior region [24].

- For the mandible:
  1 In the posterior mandible.
  2 In the interforaminal edentulous region (Ewers, 2012) [24].

We classify as inlay graft (bone class III) all procedures where particulate bone grafting material, such as autogenous or other types of augmentation material, is used as an interpositional graft and where there is at least two vascularized sources – osteotomized bone surfaces neighbouring the created bone gap. Three sources of vascularization include both osteotomized bone surfaces plus an intact (usually) lingual mucoperiosteum. Vertical PSP (sandwich

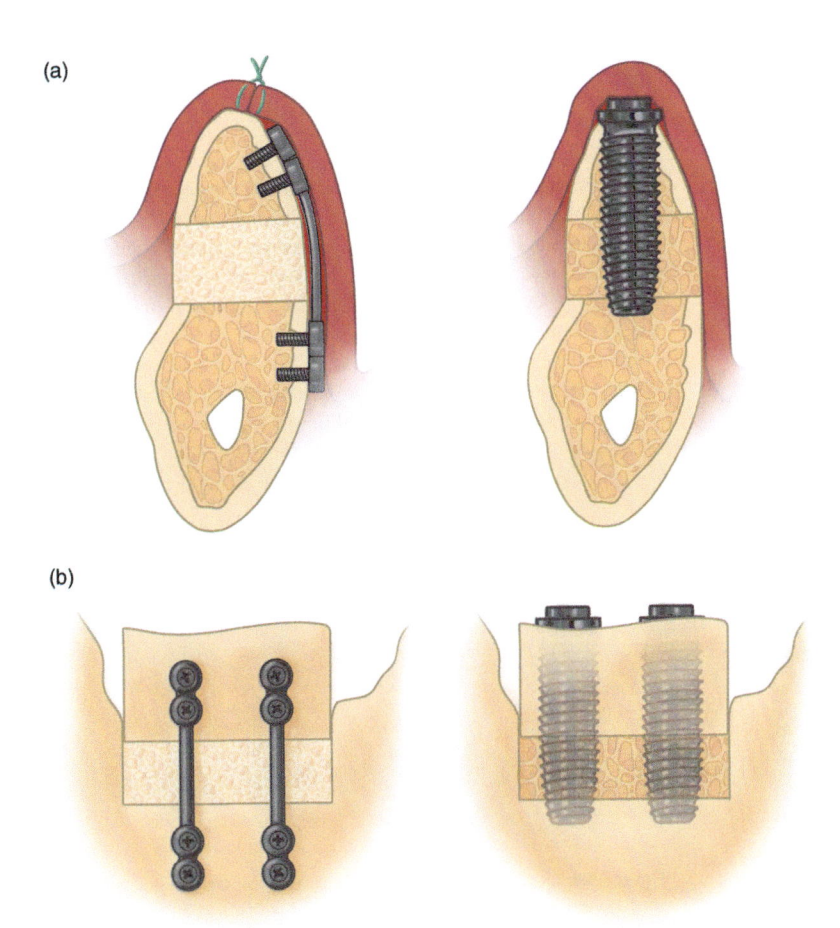

Figure 11.2 Vertical pedicled sandwich plasty (PSP) (sandwich osteotomy) with microplate application (left). Implant placement into healed bone (right). (a) Cross section view. (b) Frontal view.

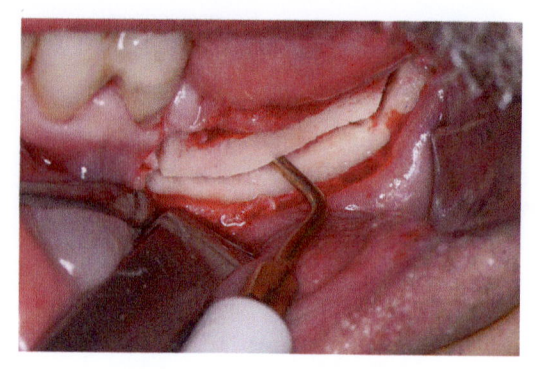

Figure 11.5 Intraoperative situation when performing the box-shaped osteotomy in a vertical pedicled sandwich plasty with a piezosurgical instrument.

osteotomy) and horizontal PSP (ridge split) frequently have all three sources of vascularization.

The following procedures are included in bone class III:
- Ridge preservation through socket fill/graft
- Sinus lift procedures
- Pedicled (pedunculated) sandwich plasties

Clinical example of vertical PSP in the posterior mandible

Compared to distraction osteogenesis (bone class II) when a patient has to have a metal device in the mouth for several months with frequent mucosal perforations, the PSP avoids these complications altogether. However, according to the bone classification relative vascularization, bone class III is positioned at a lower step relatively to bone class II.

Figure 11.3 illustrates the method of vertical pedicled sandwich plasty (PSP) for the posterior mandible. Figures 11.4 to 11.16 demonstrate this method in a 56-year-old patient. A sectional enlargement of the panoramic radiograph reveals that there is not enough vertical bone above the mandibular canal for insertion of implants in the posterior mandible on the left side (Figure 11.4). The incision and osteotomy are the same as for gradual vertical distraction osteogenesis [25]. The mucoperiosteal flap is only detached on the buccal side and dissected away from the alveolar ridge as little as possible (Figure 11.5). When the bone segment is to be mobilized, the mucoperiosteum is carefully detached more and as needed to guarantee preservation of vascularization. This is

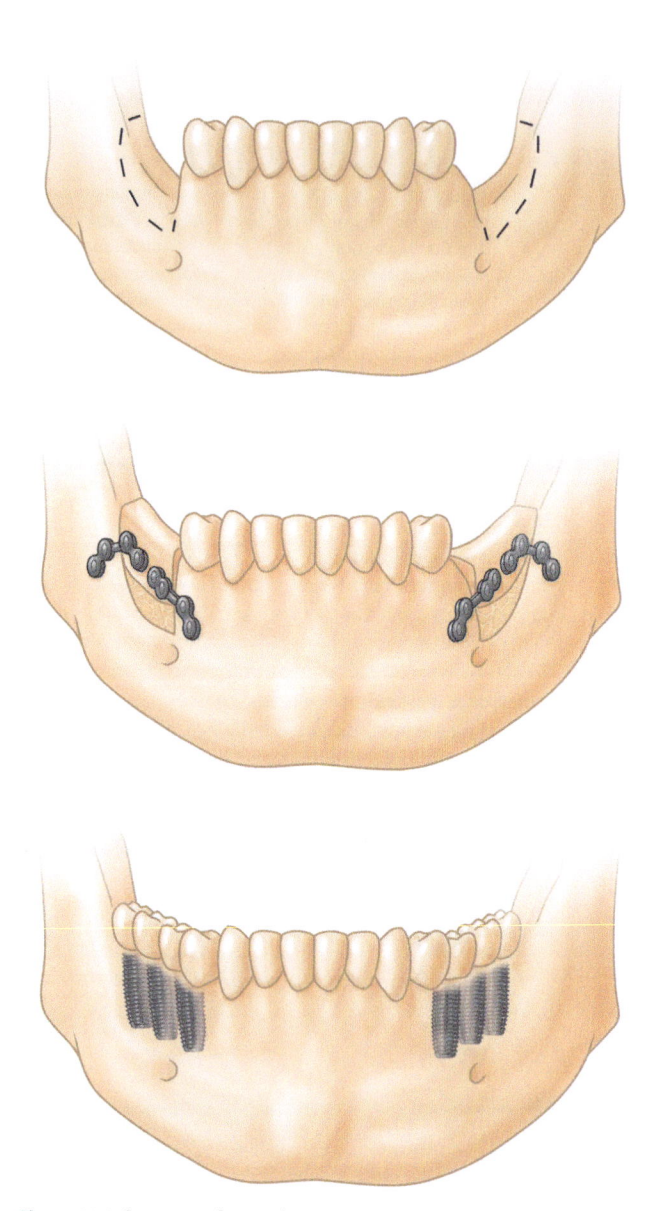

Figure 11.3 Sequence of vertical pedicled sandwich plasty in the posterior mandibular situation.

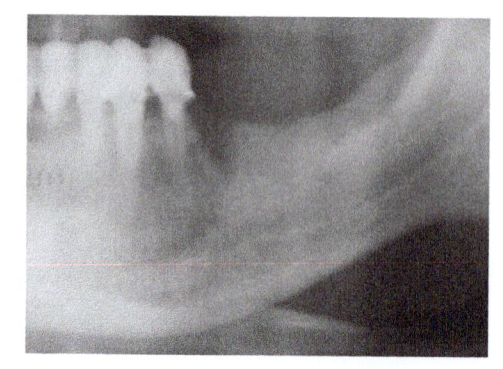

Figure 11.4 Section of the panoramic radiograph showing the left posterior mandible with minimal vertical bone above the mandibular canal (further stages are shown in Figures 11.5 to 11.16).

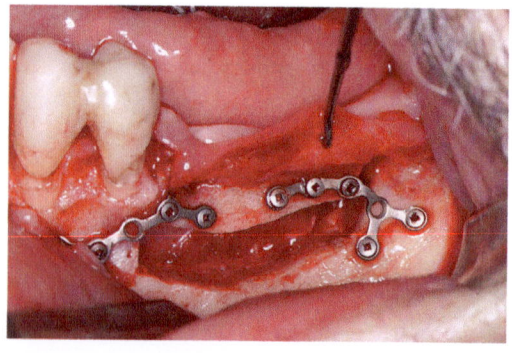

Figure 11.6 Condition after fixation of the osteotomized bone segment moved vertically by approximately 9 mm and with a lingual periosteal–soft tissue pedicle fixed with two microosteosynthesis plates.

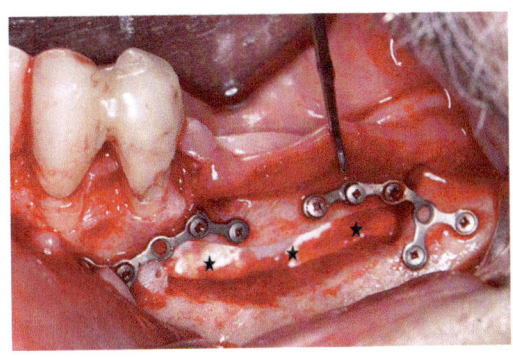

Figure 11.7 Placement of a resorbable collagen membrane on the lingual side (stars) to prevent the augmentation material from displacing.

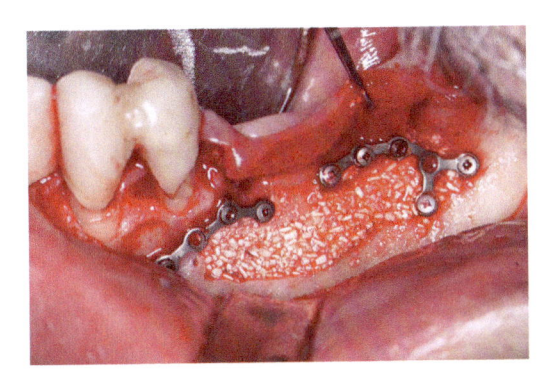

Figure 11.8 The bone gap is filled with algisorb™.

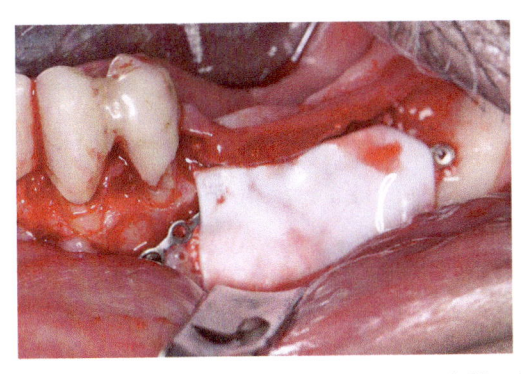

Figure 11.9 The augmented material is covered with a resorbable collagen membrane.

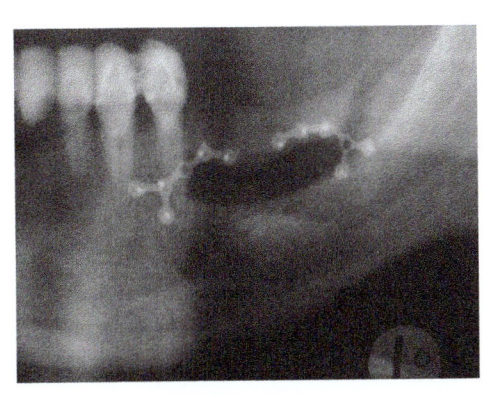

Figure 11.10 Section of the panoramic radiograph immediately after surgery: the algisorb™ is highly porous and therefore has a relatively low radio-opacity.

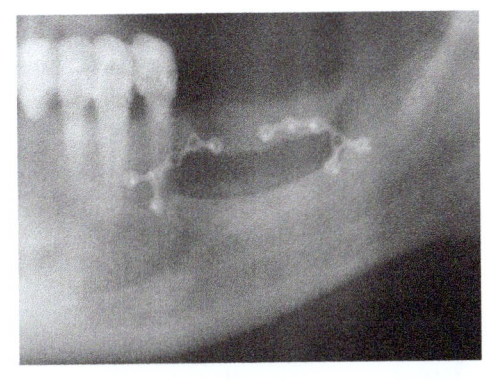

Figure 11.11 Lateral section of the panoramic radiograph two months later with the start of ossification of the algisorb™ augmentation material (with more induced ossification from below than from above).

similar to vertical distraction osteoneogenesis (bone class II). If care is not taken and the periosteum is completely detached, this will create a non-vascularized bone, which corresponds to a bone class V or onlay graft. The osteotomies can be performed either with a Khoury saw or with piezosurgical instruments [26].

In the distraction osteoneogenesis (DO) operation, it is recommended that the bone segment being mobilized first by as much as 9 mm should be checked to see whether it can be moved (distracted). If it can, then it is placed back in intimate proximity and fixated. Then, the distractor is activated a week later. Slow and incremental distraction is accomplished in the following days. In PSP, the transfer disk (bone) can be immediately moved into this mobilized position and secured straight away with micro- or miniosteosynthesis plates and screws (Figure 11.6). After a resorbable membrane is placed on the lingual side (Figure 11.7), the resulting bone gap is filled with algae-derived algisorb™ (a renewable marine red algae product, sold by Osseous Technologies of America, Hamburg, NY, http://www.osseoustech.com) (Figure 11.8) and the augmentation material is covered with a second resorbable membrane (Figure 11.9). A periosteal connective tissue flap is formed on the buccal side and closed in two layers. On the sectional enlargement of the panoramic radiograph, the augmentation material cannot yet be identified immediately post-operatively (Figure 11.10). As the algisorb™ material is highly porous, it produces a less radio-opaque image than highly sintered hydroxyapatite material, which is not very porous. The increasing calcification caused by remodeling the algisorb™ material into newly formed bone is visible on the panoramic radiograph after only 2 months (Figure 11.11). After 3 months, the titanium screws and plates were removed and three 3.0 × 15 mm Xive™ (Dentsply) implants were inserted (Figure 11.12). The panoramic radiograph taken 6 months after implant insertion showed the algisorb™ material to be highly calcified (Figure 11.13). Histological examination of the bone specimen collected during the implant procedure confirms pronounced osteoneogenesis. The partial filling of the pores with newly formed bone and early resorption of the material can be seen on the magnified image (Figure 11.14). The panoramic radiograph taken after 11 years indicated good osseointegration of three implants and complete filling of the former cavity with

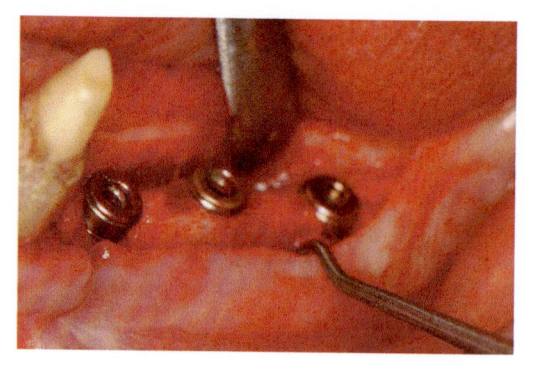

Figure 11.12 Intraoperative situation after removal of fixation plates and insertion of three 3.0 × 15 and × 13 mm Xive (Dentsply) implants.

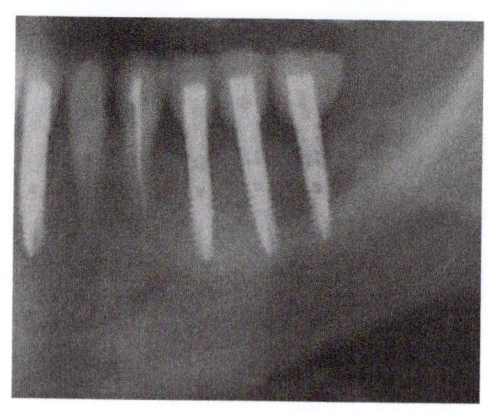

Figure 11.15 Section of the panoramic radiograph after 11 years with unchanged conditions.

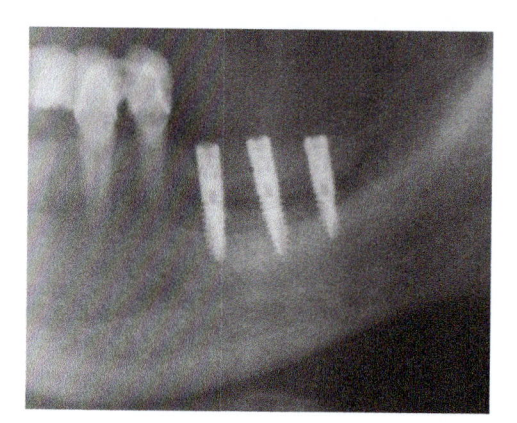

Figure 11.13 Section of the panoramic radiograph 6 months after implant insertion: the osteotomy gap is almost completely filled with newly formed bone.

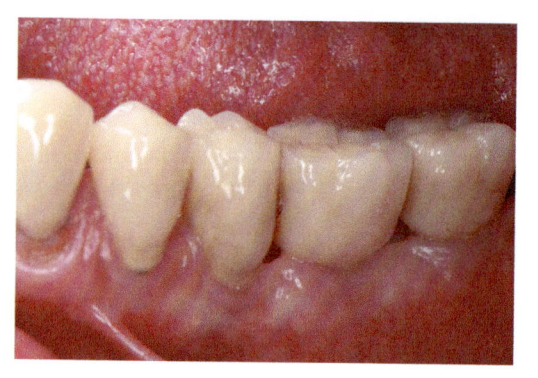

Figure 11.16 Intraoral situation after 11 years with healthy peri-implant mucosa. Prosthetic treatment courtesy of Dr. Fahrenholz, Vienna, Austria. Reproduced with permission from Dr. Fahrenholz.

endogenous bone (Figure 11.15). The clinical examination showed a healthy peri-implant mucosa (Figure 11.16) after 11 years.

Clinical example of vertical PSP in the anterior (interforaminal) mandibular region

Figure 11.17 illustrates the method of vertical pedicled sandwich plasty (PSP) for the anterior mandible. It is demonstrated in a 59-year-old patient (Figures 11.18 to 11.28). After the vestibular incision, the curved osteotomy is performed with either a lengthwise oscillating saw, the Khoury saw, or piezosurgical instruments [26], while sparing the mental nerves (Figure 11.18). The periosteum was not detached from the bone fragment being mobilized. Two osteosynthesis plates with screws were attached to immobilize and fixate the bone fragment. To avoid any dislocation of the augmenting material, a resorbable membrane was placed lingually (Figure 11.19) and, after stabilization with two double Y microplates (Synthes, Inc., West Chester, PA, USA), the resulting cavity was filled with algisorb™ (Figure 11.20). Before closure, the material was covered with resorbable membrane. The panoramic radiographs, the cephalometric radiograph and the reformatted panoramic view showed the gained ridge height (Figures 11.21 to 11.23). Histological examination showed the osteoneogenesis (Figure 11.24a and b). The peri-implant mucosal situation was clinically stable 12 years later (Figure 11.25) and radiographically there was satisfactory osseointegration without crestal bone resorption with a stable implant position without further lingual dislocation (Figures 11.26 and 11.27). The follow-up check after 12 years in

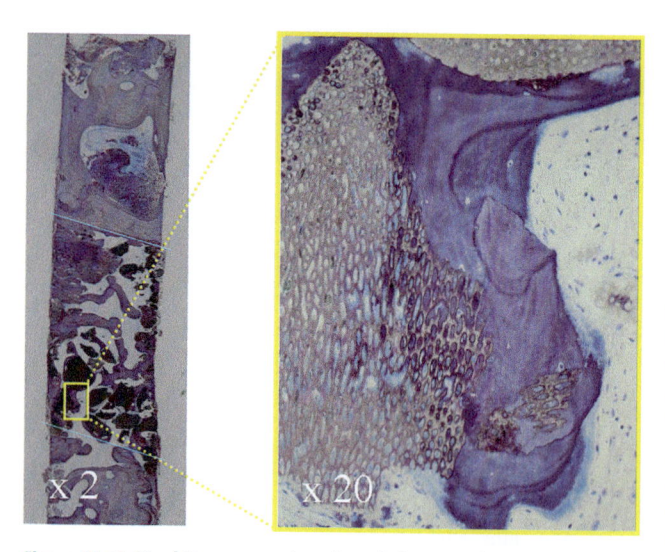

Figure 11.14 Hard tissue ground section of a bone trephine specimen; the overall view under two-fold magnification shows good osteoneogenesis in the area around the algisorb™ augmentation material (turquoise lines indicate the former osteotomy). The yellow box is shown in ×20 sectional magnification on the right side and an algisorb™ granule with bone outside can be seen. In places, the pores are also filled with newly formed bone and resorption is starting in the marginal area. The small algisorb™ fragments are completely surrounded by and also filled with bone.

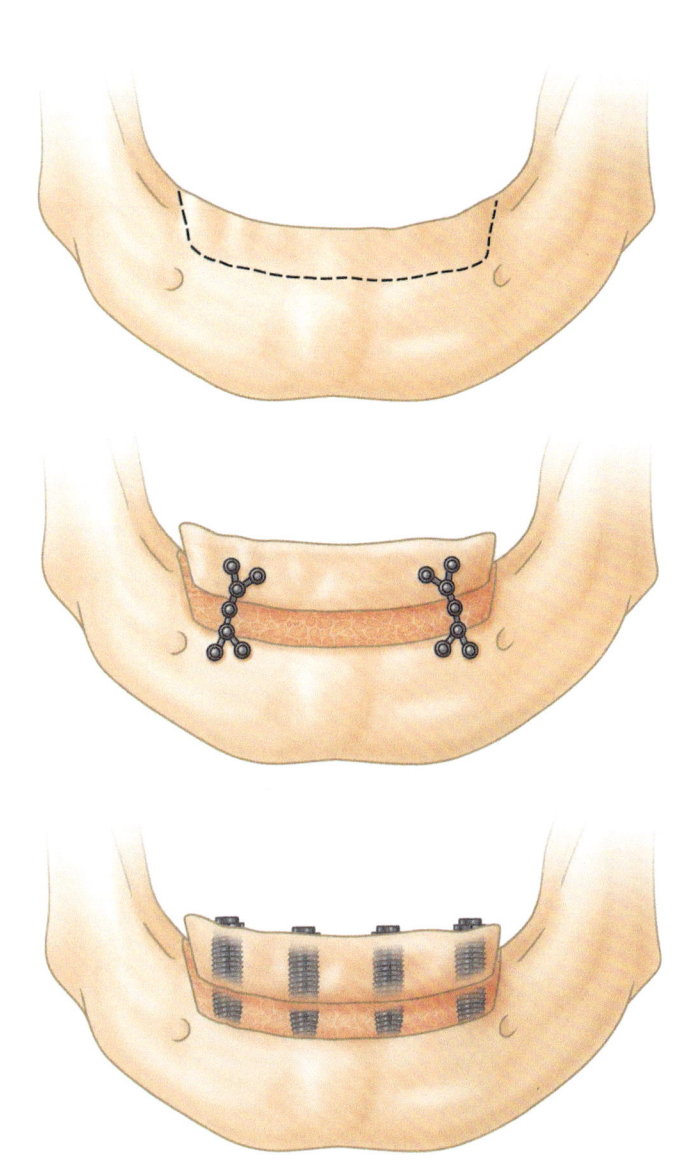

Figure 11.17 Sequence of the vertical pedicled sandwich plasty in the anterior mandible.

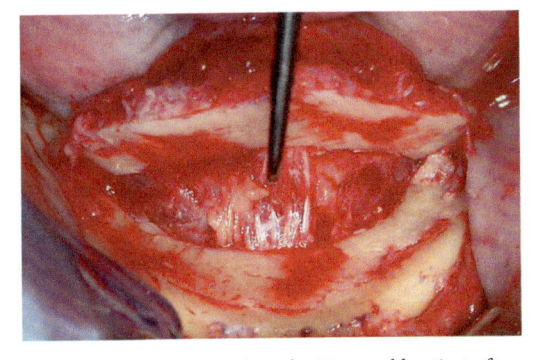

Figure 11.18 Intraoperative situation of a 59-year-old patient after curved osteotomy; the bone segment is elevated with a lingual soft tissue pedicle in the vertical pedicled sandwich plasty (further stages are shown in Figures 11.19 to 11.28).

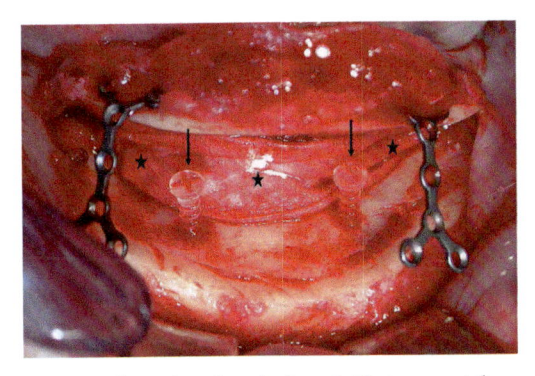

Figure 11.19 Membrane (stars) on the lingual side to prevent the augmentation material from displacing, and the placement of two resorbable miniscrews (black arrows) to prevent the elevated, soft tissue pedicled bone segment from sinking; finally, two microosteosynthesis plates are fixated to the elevated bone segment.

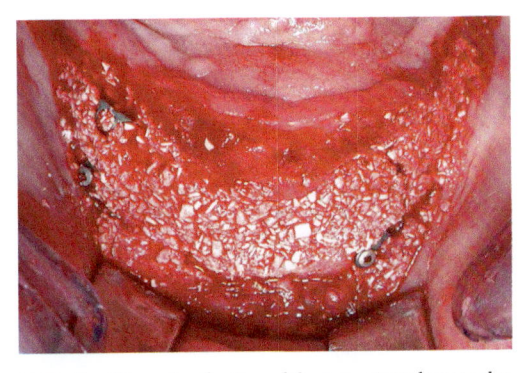

Figure 11.20 Condition after fixation of the two microplates to the vertically separated bone segments and filling the gap with algisorb™.

function showed an esthetically pleasing outcome with a corrected anterior vertical height (Figure 11.28).

Horizontal widening of the alveolar crest (horizontal PSP) (see also Tolstunov, Book I)

To widen the thin alveolar crest horizontally and to enable an implant insertion two principal methods can be used:

(a) Two-step horizontal pedicled (pedunculated) sandwich plasty (PSP)
(b) One-step horizontal pedicled (pedunculated) sandwich plasty (PSP)

(a) Two-step method

In bone splitting, the mucoperiosteal flap is often dissected away so that the appropriate osteotomies can be performed. At the same time, however, this disrupts the blood supply to the bone provided via the periosteum. When the bone segment is then mobilized, the bone is no longer vascularized and actually corresponds to a class V autogenous non vascularized onlay graft [10].

A special form of bone splitting is the two-stage horizontal bone splitting method, in which a preparatory osteotomy is first performed and the final bone splitting with simultaneous insertion of implants takes place at least 28 days later. As this involves creating a pedicled bone graft, this can also be referred to two-step horizontal pedicled sandwich plasty (PSP) and constitutes bone class III

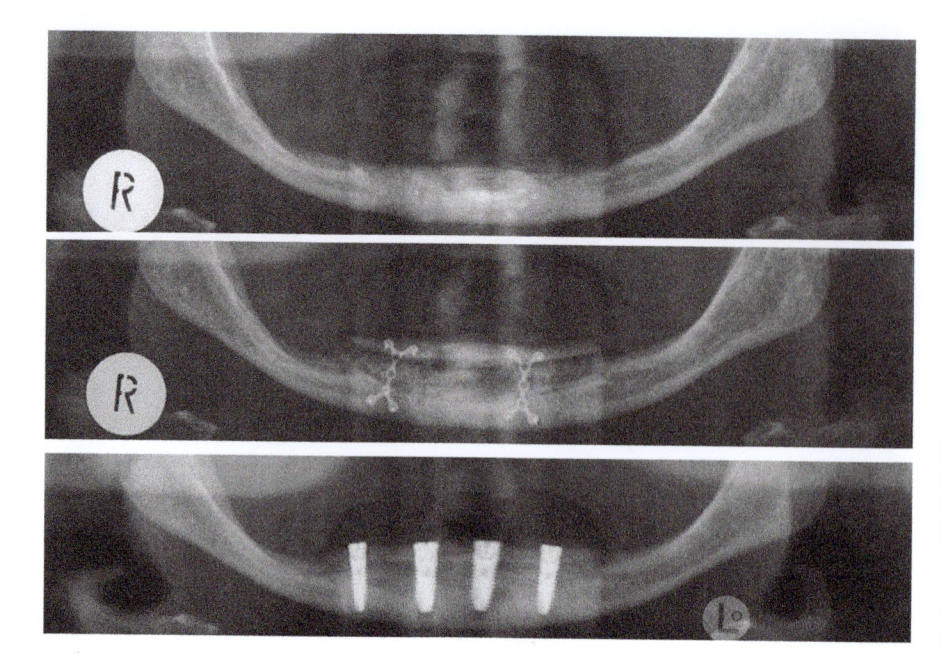

Figure 11.21 Panoramic radiographs pre-operatively (top), after vertical pedicled sandwich plasty (middle) and after plate removal and insertion of four 3.8 and 4.5 × 15 mm Xive (Dentsply) implants 6 months post-operatively (bottom). The augmentation material – algisorb™ – is almost completely ossified.

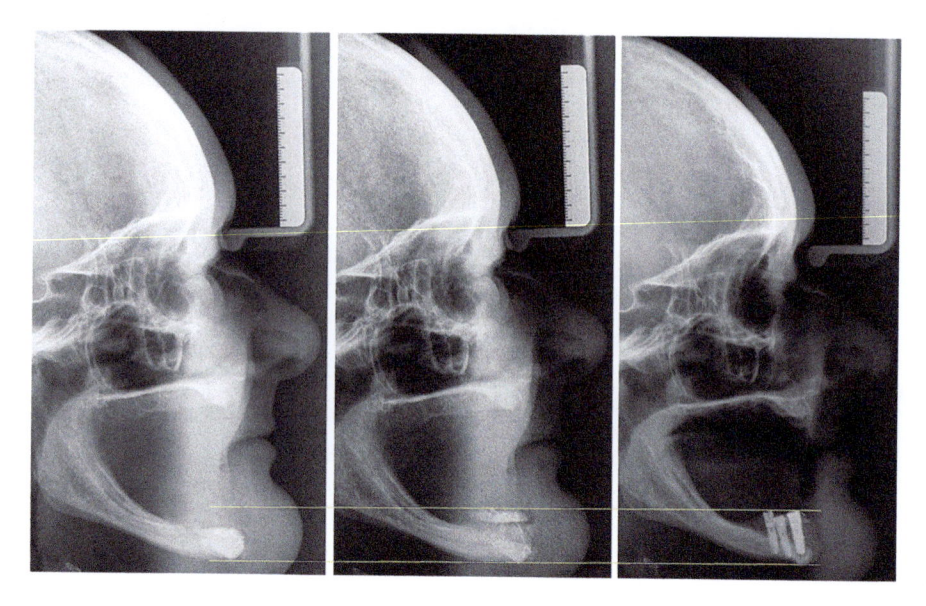

Figure 11.22 Cephalometric radiograph pre-operatively (left), after the vertical pedicled sandwich plasty (middle) and after plate removal and insertion of four implants 6 months later (right). The top yellow line illustrates the increase in bone height.

(Figure 11.29) [10, 27]. This method is usually performed in the mandible where rigid cortical structures exist but can also be performed in the maxilla.

Clinical example of horizontal two-step PSP in the posterior mandible

A 61-year-old patient presented with an edentulous thin (width-deficient) posterior mandible on the left side (Figures 11.30 to 11.32). In the first session, the four osteotomies are performed after the mucoperiosteal flap is opened. The alveolar crest is osteotomized plus two vertical and apical horizontal osteotomies are performed (Figure 11.30). In the second operation 28 days later, the mucoperiosteum is only opened at the crest and the crestal osteotomy is deepened with the Beaver™ knife and then the buccal bone is moved sideways with the chisel (Figure 11.31). After the gap is widened enough, the Xive™ (Dentsply) implants were inserted following the wound closure (Figure 11.32). The bone gap between implants can also be filled with a particulate grafting material of choice. Implants also can be placed at a separate surgical procedure 3–4 months later if an immediate implant stability cannot be achieved at the second step of PSP.

(b) One-step method

For a well-vascularized alveolar crest, bone widening or splitting is possible to be performed in a one-step procedure with a split thickness flap, which does not remove the periosteum from the

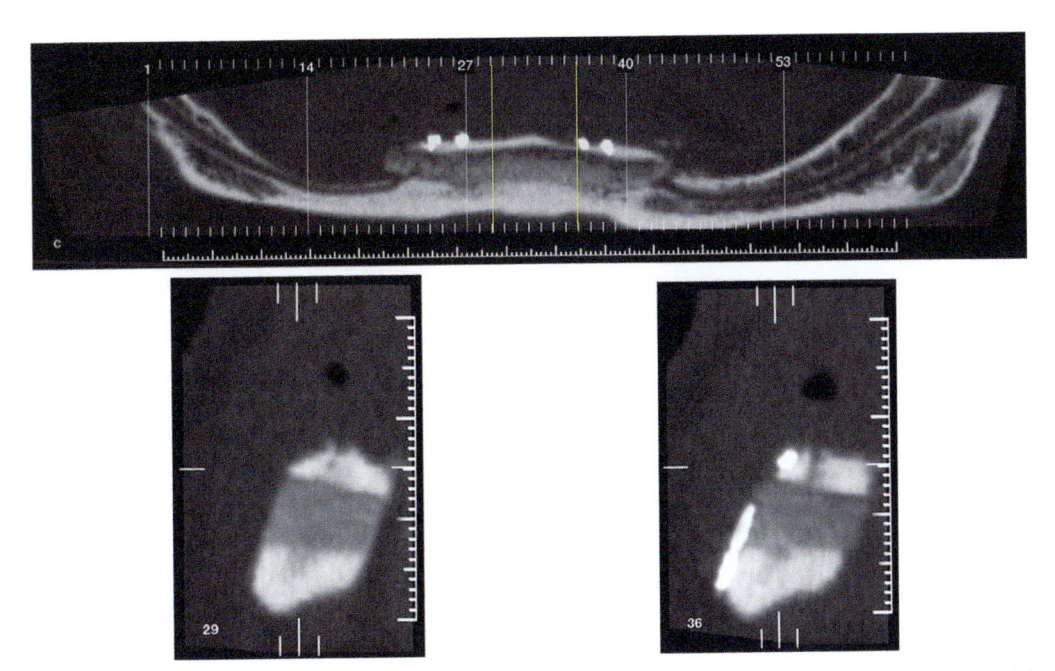

Figure 11.23 Reformatted panoramic view of the post-operative dental computed tomograph with a clearly visible increase in height of the anterior mandibular bone. The reconstructed orthoradial slices 29 and 36 (below) show a 40% increase in vertical bone height and ossified "algae material" – algisorb™.

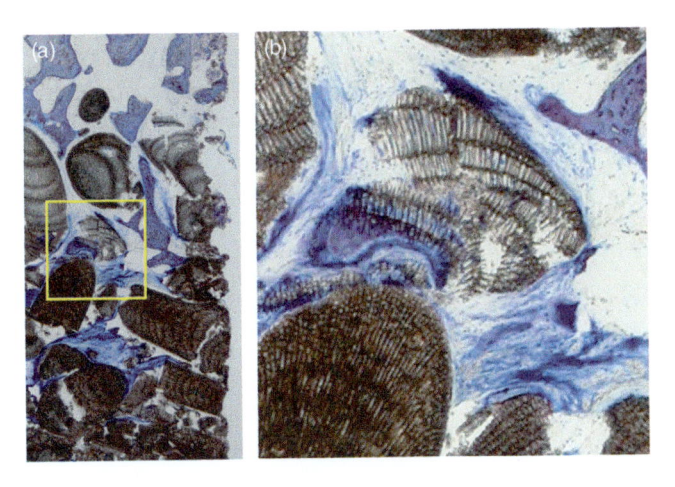

Figure 11.24 (a) Hard tissue ground section of a bone trephine specimen under twofold magnification, showing good osteoneogenesis in the area around the algisorb™ augmentation material. (b) The yellow box is shown in ×20 sectional magnification, where several ossified algisorb™ granules on the outer surface can be seen. The pores are partially filled with newly formed bone. The small algisorb™ fragments are completely surrounded by and filled with bone.

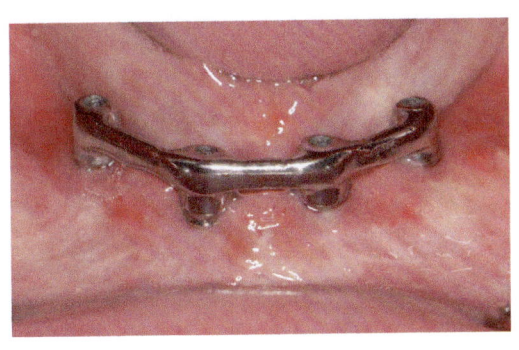

Figure 11.25 Intraoral situation 12 years after prosthetic treatment. Source: Dr. R. Finger, Eggenburg, Austria. Reproduced with permission from Dr. R. Finger.

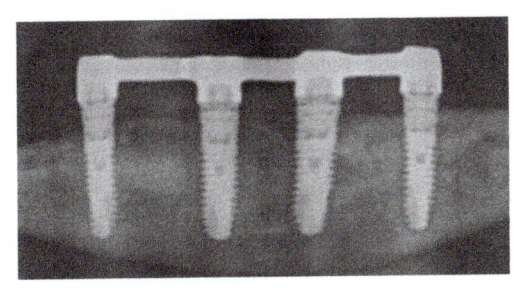

Figure 11.26 Panoramic radiograph 12 years after completion of the prosthetic treatment. The augmentation material algisorb™ is completely ossified and there are only slight signs of peri-implant bone resorption on the left middle Implant.

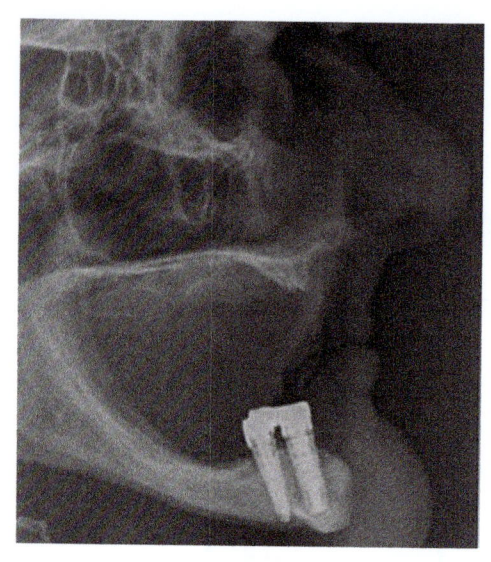

Figure 11.27 Cephalometric radiograph 12 years later with a stable condition and no implant dislocation toward the lingual side. No peri-implant bone resorption is visible.

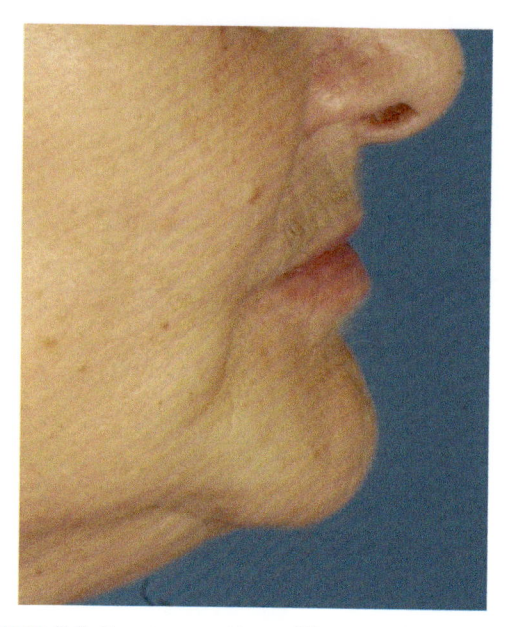

Figure 11.28 Esthetic outcome at 12-year follow-up with harmonious anterior vertical heights.

bone [28–31]. With the split thickness flap and periosteal protection of bone, it has been reported that there is significantly less bone loss [32, 33].

Discussion

In this book, many different methods are shown to enhance or augment bone for better implant applications. Whenever bone is handled, the most important prerequisite for a successful outcome is, in our belief, the vascularization of the bone that is treated. Whenever the vascularization is interrupted, there will be some degree of resorption eventually. All long-term surveillance has proven this observation.

Although the bone quality after distraction osteoneogenesis is possibly better than pedicled sandwich plasty, the PSP is more comforting for the patient, avoiding mucosal perforations of the DO device and functional (mastication) issues related to having a metal device in the mouth for at least three months or longer. These

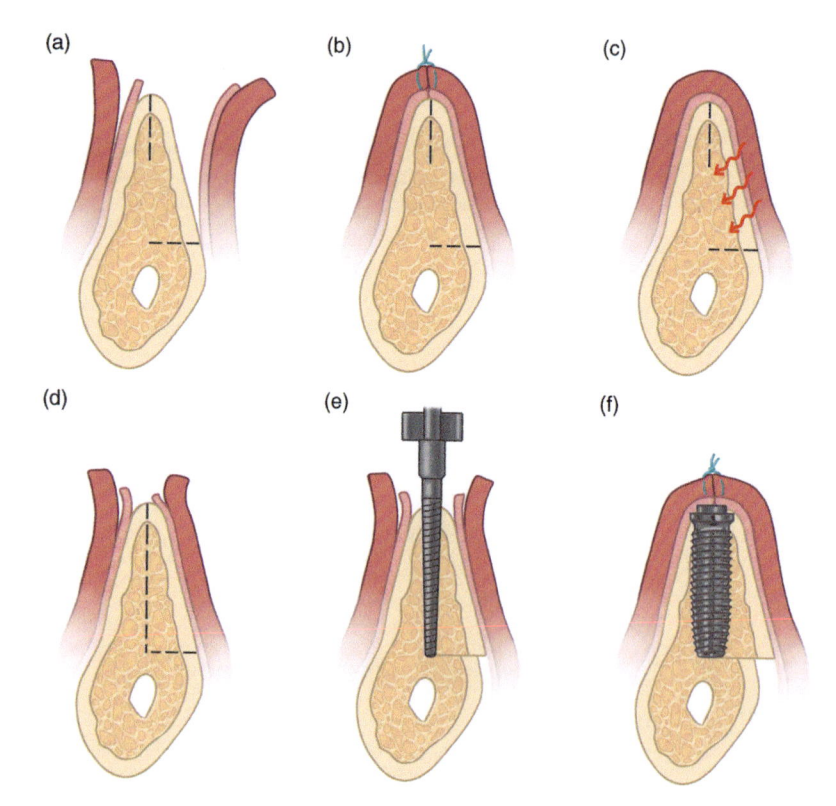

Figure 11.29 Schematic diagram of two-stage horizontal bone spreading (two-step horizontal pedicled sandwich plasty): the first operation (a to c) takes place 4 weeks before the second (d to f). (**a**) After raising the buccal mucoperiosteal flap, the apical, crestal, and both vertical osteotomies are performed. (**b**) The mucoperiosteal flap is folded back and primarily sutured. (**c**) During the healing period, the bone to be mobilized is being revascularized. (**d**) Four weeks after the osteotomy, the mucoperiosteal flap is opened only crestally to avoid jeopardizing revascularization of the buccal bone. (**e**) The bone is slowly driven apart with a double-sided scalpel followed by a chisel and extension screw so that the implant drill hole can be made. (**f**) The implant is inserted and the mucoperiosteal flap is folded back with primary closure.

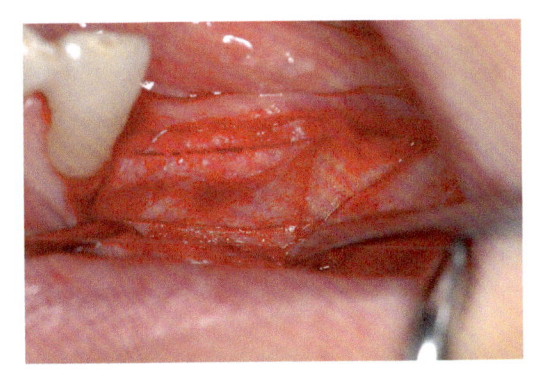

Figure 11.30 All four osteotomies are performed in a 61-year-old patient (further stages are shown in Figures 11.31 and 11.32).

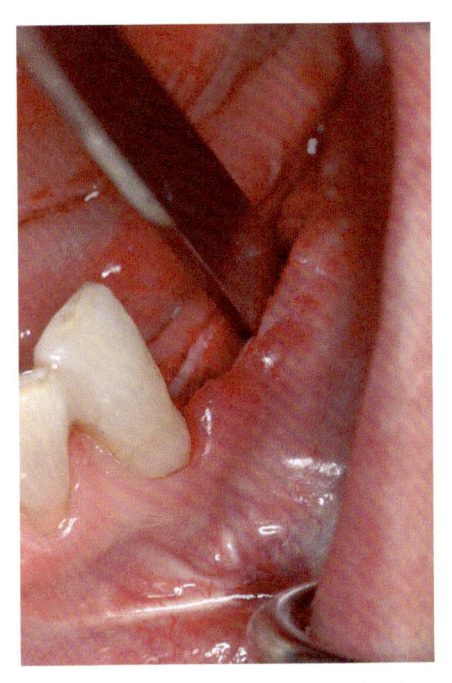

Figure 11.31 Widening of the osteotomy with a chisel and moving the buccal cortical bone horizontally (buccally).

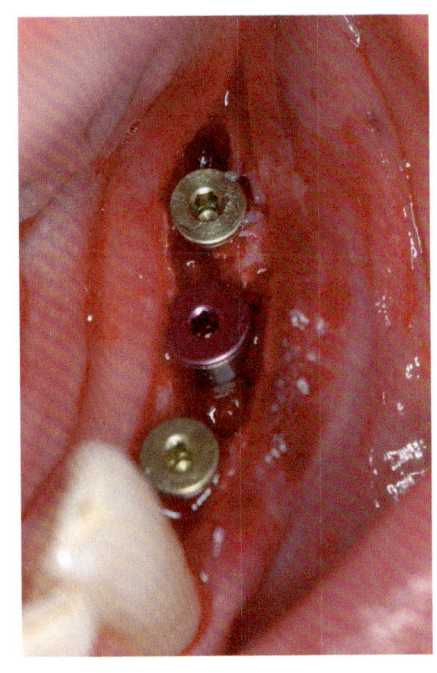

Figure 11.32 After insertion of three Xive™ implants.

results demonstrate similar success of both techniques with more patients' compliance of the PSP procedure.

References

1. Jensen O: Dentoalveolar modification by osteoperiosteal flaps. In: Fonseca RJ, Turvey TA, Marciani RD (eds.), *Oral and Maxillofacial Surgery*, vol. 1, 2nd edn. Saunders, Philadelphia, PA, 2008, pp. 471–478.
2. Ewers R, Tomasetti B, Ghali GE, Jensen OT: A new biologic classification of bone augmentation. In: Jensen OT (ed.), *The Osteoperiostal Flap*. Quintessenz Publ. Co., Chicago, IL, 2010, pp. 19–42.
3. Rauch F, Travers R, Glorieux FH: Intracortical remodeling during human bone development: a histomorphometric study. *Bone* 2007;**40**:274–280.
4. Schopper C, Moser D: Biomaterials and bone repair. In: Ewers R, Lambrecht JT (eds.), *Oral Implants - Bioactivating Concepts*. Quintessenz Publ. Co., Chicago, IL, 2012, pp. 35–40.
5. Probst A, Spiegel HU: Cellular mechanisms of bone repair. *J Invest Surg* 1997;**10**:77–86.
6. Leunig M, Yuan F, Berk DA, Gerweck LE, Jain RK: Angiogenesis and growth of isografted bone: quantitative *in vivo* assay in nude mice. *Lab Invest* 1994;**71**:300–307.
7. Hansen-Algenstaedt N, Joscheck C, Wolfram L, Schaefer C, Muller I, Bottcher A: Sequential changes in vessel formation and micro-vascular function during repair. *Acta Orthop* 2006;**77**:429–439.
8. Aghaloo TL, Moy PK: Which hard tissue augmentation techniques are the most successful in furnishing bony support for implant placement? *Int J Oral Maxillofac Implants* 2007;**22**(Suppl):49–70 [erratum 2008;**23**:56].
9. Ewers R, Goriwoda W, Schopper C, Moser D, Spassova E: Histologic findings at augmented bone areas supplied with two different bone substitute materials combined with sinus floor lifting. Report of one case. *Clin Oral Implants Res* 2004;**15**:96–100.
10. Ewers R: Implant surgery. In: Lambrecht JT (ed.), *Oral and Implant Surgery - Principles and Procedures*, Quintessence Publ. Co., Chicago, IL, 2009, pp. 273–420.
11. Illizarov GA, Deviatov AA: Surgical lengthening of the skin with simultaneous correction of deformities. *Ortop Travmatol Protez* 1969 Mar;**30**(3):32–37.
12. Michieli S, Miotti B: Lengthening of mandibular body by gradual surgical-orthodontic distraction. *J Oral Surg* 1977;**35**:187–192.
13. Block M: Biologic basis of alveolar distraction osteogenesis. In: Jensen OT (ed.), *Alveolar Distraction Osteogenesis*. Quintessence Publ. Co., Chicago, IL, 2002, pp. 17–28.
14. Kojimoto H, Yasui N, Goto T, Matsuda S, Shimomura Y: Bone lengthening in rabbits by callus distraction. The role of periosteum and endosteum. *J Bone Joint Surg Br* 1988;**70**:543–549.
15. Guerrero C: Intraoral distraction osteogenesis. In: Fonseca RJ, Turvey TA, Marciani RD (eds.), *Oral and Maxillofacial Surgery*, vol. 3, 2nd edn. Saunders, Philadelphia, PA, 2008, pp. 338–363.
16. Donath K, Breuner G: A method for the study of undecalcified bones and teeth with attached soft tissues. The Säge-Schliff (sawing and grinding) technique. *J Oral Pathol* 1982 Aug;**11**(4):318–326.
17. Schettler D: Sandwich technic with cartilage transplant for raising the alveolar process in the lower jaw. *Fortschr Kiefer Gesichtschir* 1976;**20**:61–63.
18. Schettler D, Holtermann W: Clinical and experimental results of a sandwich-technique for mandibular alveolar ridge augmentation. *J Maxillofac Surg* 1977 Sep;**5**(3):199–202.
19. Ewers R, Fock N, Millesi-Schobel G, Enislidis G. Pedicled sandwich plasty: a variation on alveolar distraction for vertical augmentation of the atrophic mandible. *Br J Oral Maxillofac Surg* 2004;**42**:445–447.
20. Ewers R, Schicho K, Truppe M, Seemann R, Reichwein A, Figl M: Computer aided navigation in dental implantology: 7 years of clinical experience. *J Oral Maxillofac Surg* 2004;**62**:329–334.

21 Enislidis G, Ewers R: Vertical augmentation of atrophic mandibles-pedicled sandwich-plasty or distraction osteogenesis? *Br J Oral Maxillofac Surg* 2005;**43**:439.
22 Jensen OT, Kuhlke L, Bedard JF, White D: Alveolar segmental sandwich osteotomy for anterior maxillary vertical augmentation prior to implant placement. *J Oral Maxillofac Surg* 2006;**64**:997.
23 Jensen OT: Alveolar segmental "sandwich" osteotomies for posterior edentulous mandibular sites for dental implants. *J Oral Maxillofac Surg* 2006;**64**:471–475.
24 Ewers R: Bone standard clinical situations. In: Ewers R, Lambrecht JT (eds.), *Oral Implants – Bioactivating Concepts*. Quintessenz Publ. Co., Chicago, IL, 2012, pp. 225–383.
25 Millesi-Schobel G, Millesi W, Glaser C, Watzinger F, Klug C, Ewers R: The L-shaped osteotomy for vertical callus distraction in the molar region of the mandible: a technical note. *J Cranio Maxillofac Surg* 2000;**28**:176–180.
26 Vercellotti, T: *Essentials in Piezosurgery: Clinical Advantages in Dentistry*. Quintessence Publ. Co., Chicago, IL, 2009, pp. 1–136.
27 Enislidis G, Ewers R: Vertical augmentation of atrophic mandibles–pedicled sandwich-plasty or distraction osteo-genesis? *Br J Oral Maxillofac Surg* 2005;**43**:439.
28 Scipioni A, Bruschi GB, Calesini G: The edentulous ridge expansion technique: a five-year study. *Int J Periodontics Restorative Dent* 1994 Oct;**14**(5):451–459.
29 Rahpeyma A, Khajehahmadi S, Hosseini VR: Lateral ridge split and immediate implant placement in moderately resorbed alveolar ridges: How much is the added width? *Dent Res J (Isfahan)* 2013 Sep;**10**(5):602–608.
30 Agrawal D, Gupta AS, Newaskar V, Gupta A, Garg S, Jain D: Narrow ridge management with ridge splitting with piezotome for implant placement: report of 2 cases. *J Indian Prosthodont Soc* 2014 Sep;**14**(3):305–309. doi: 10.1007/s13191-012-0216-8. Epub 2012 Nov 25.
31 Khairnar MS, Khairnar D, Bakshi K: Modified ridge splitting and bone expansion osteotomy for placement of dental implant in esthetic zone. *Contemp Clin Dent* 2014 Jan;**5**(1):110–114. doi: 10.4103/0976-237X.128684.
32 Mounir M, Beheiri G, El-Beialy W: Assessment of marginal bone loss using full thickness versus partial thickness flaps for alveolar ridge splitting and immediate implant placement in the anterior maxilla. *Int J Oral Maxillofac Surg* 2014 Jun;**24**: ii, S0901-5027(14)00215-X. doi: 10.1016/j.ijom.2014.05.021 [Epub ahead of print].
33 Seemann R, Perisanidis C, Traxler H, Ewers R: Split-thickness flap with a semicircular punched-ridge pedicled periosteal flap for implant restoration in highly atrophic patients: a technical note. *The International Journal of Oral and Maxillofacial Implants* 2014;**29**:e10–12.

CHAPTER 12

Piezoelectric Surgery for Atrophic Mandible: Vertical Ridge Augmentation with Sandwich Osteotomy Technique and Interpositional Allograft

Dong-Seok Sohn
Department of Oral and Maxillofacial Surgery, Daegu Catholic University, School of Medicine, Daegu, Korea

Introduction

Bone resorption of the alveolar ridge is an unavoidable biologic process of bone remodeling after removal of teeth from hopeless decay or a periodontal condition. In order to restore the edentulous arch with an esthetic and functional implant-supported prosthesis, ridge augmentation surgery such as guided bone regeneration (GBR) or an autogenous block bone graft (ABBG) is often necessary prior to or at the time of implant placement surgery. For the edentulous mandible, there are many different methods to augment the resorbed alveolar ridge [1–5]. In this chapter, we will describe a piezoelectric approach for the vertical alveolar ridge augmentation of the edentulous mandible utilizing the sandwich osteotomy technique.

Among many methods, a pedicled or interpositional alveolar bone graft and the sandwich bone augmentation have shown successful results for the moderately resorbed mandibular ridge. Harle [6] was the first clinician to report visor osteotomy for atrophic mandibular ridge augmentation. Harle sectioned the alveolar bone sagittally between mental foramina and elevated the lingual alveolar bone. He then fixed bone segments with a wire. Many clinicians since have modified the sandwich bone augmentation technique. Schetteler [7] split the atrophic alveolar ridge and added graft material. Peterson and Slade [8] reported a modified Harle visor osteotomy. There have been many other sandwich bone augmentation techniques reported in the literature.

The sandwich technique minimizes bone necrosis by supplying vascularization to the graft and elevated bone fragment from the lingual periosteum without interruption. Furthermore, unlike the distraction osteogenesis technique, it has less patient discomfort from the surgery and does not require high cost associated with the purchase of a distractor device. While in the past the method was mainly used to enhance retention of dentures, it is currently used to augment alveolar ridges for implant placement.

Piezoelectric bone surgery is the preferred technique for sandwich osteotomy since it is kind to surrounding tissues such as the lingual periosteum, mental nerves, and buccal mucosa during the cutting process. Piezoelectric osteotomy cuts bone with precision and minimizes the bleeding from the procedure. The sandwich technique is a simple procedure that does not require a donor site as compared to autogenous block bone graft surgery [9, 10].

Piezoelectric surgical devices have long been used in medical and dental applications [11–15]. These devices use ultrasonic energy generated by vibrations that ultrasonic waves produce at frequencies above the audible range (above 20 000 Hz). Hard tissue surgery requires frequencies of 20 000–30 000 Hz whereas soft tissue surgery and other diagnostic procedures such as procedures for tumors, pregnancy (ultrasonography and echography), and lithotripsy require higher frequencies. Piezoelectric surgery uses piezoelectric effects, and was first described by Jacques and Pierre Curie (1880) for osteotomy [16]. The advantages of piezoelectric surgical instruments, compared to other osteotomy instruments, are (1) micrometric bone cut, (2) selective cut, (3) cavitation effect, and (4) reduced noise [4, 13].

1 Micrometric cut. Micrometric cut reduces undesired bone cutting and cuts the bone surface clean with the desired shape.
2 Selective cut. While soft tissue cutting requires at least a frequency of 50 000 Hz, an ultrasonic device uses frequencies of 20 000–30 000 Hz for selective cutting of hard tissues. The piezoelectric device minimizes the damage to vital structures such as surrounding nerves, blood vessels, and soft tissues.
3 Cavitation effect. The ultrasonic vibrations cause decompression of the air around the insert tip resulting in the cavitation effect. By cavitation of the surgical coolant – saline – the liquid not only reduces the heat in the surgical site but also cleanses the area and allows visibility of the site.
4 Reduced surgical noise. Compared to conventional rotary instruments, the piezoelectric device produced much less noise during osteotomy so patients feel more comfortable than using conventional surgical devices.

Vertical Alveolar Ridge Augmentation in Implant Dentistry: A Surgical Manual, First Edition. Edited by Len Tolstunov.
© 2016 John Wiley & Sons, Inc. Published 2016 by John Wiley & Sons, Inc.

Case Report 1: Piezoelectric sandwich technique with interpositional bone graft for vertical augmentation of severely atrophic *posterior* mandibular alveolar ridge

A 56-year-old man was referred to our university clinic from a private practice. Extensive vertical alveolar bone loss was found due to a failed guided bone regeneration surgery and ailing condition of existing dental implants in the left quadrant of the mandible (Figures 12.1 to 12.3).

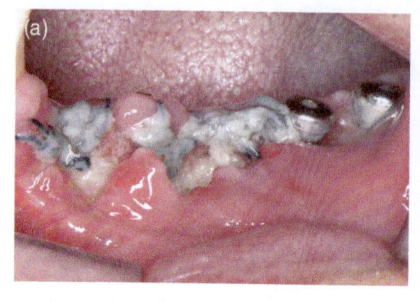

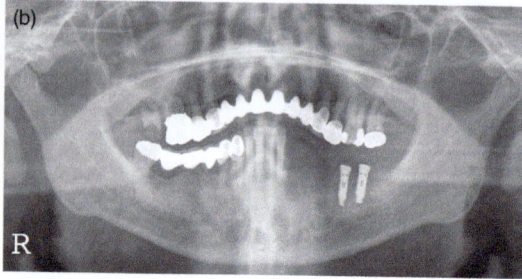

Figure 12.1 Failure of mandibular bone graft 10 days after its placement.

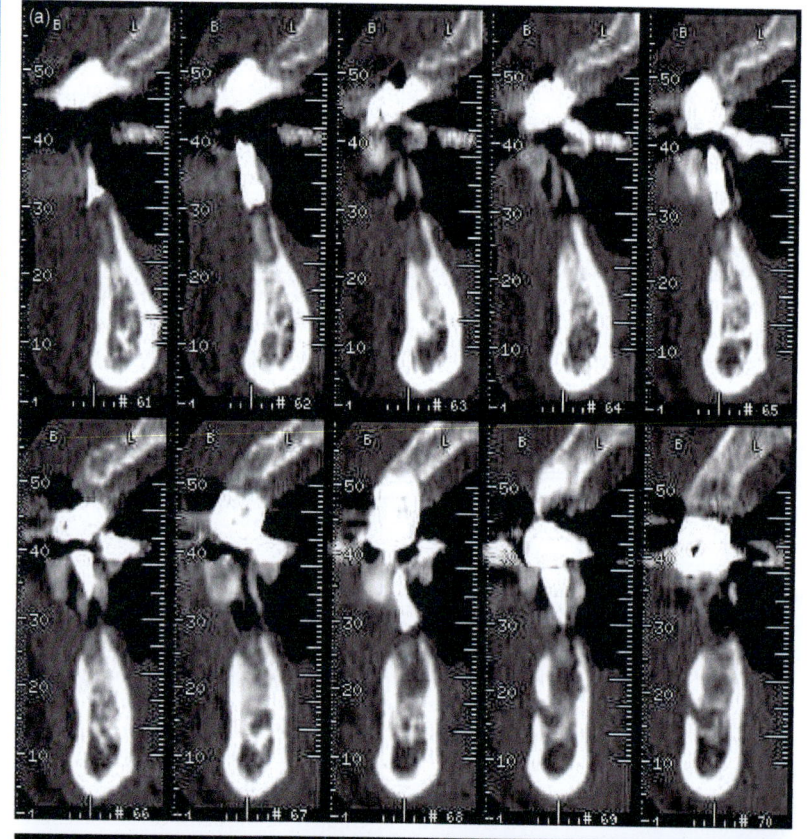

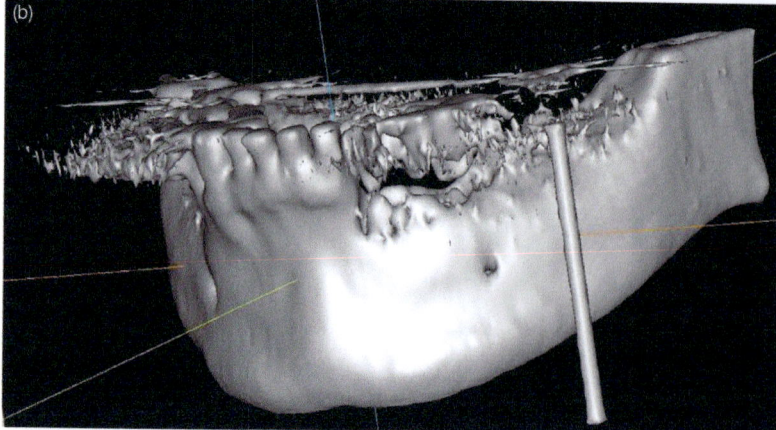

Figure 12.2 Computed tomogram shows vertical and horizontal bone defect in the mandibular left canine and the premolar area.

Piezoelectric Surgery for Atrophic Mandible | **123**

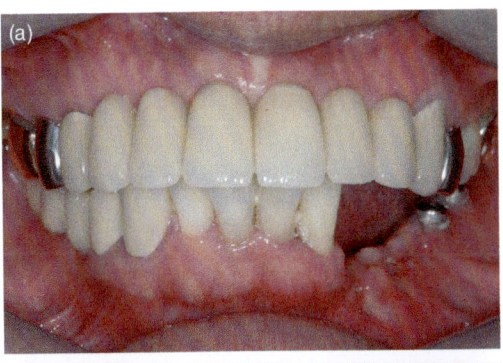

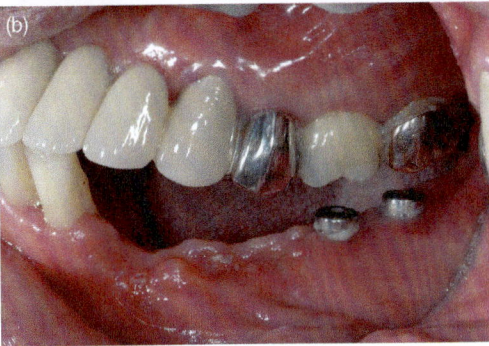

Figure 12.3 Four weeks after the initial bone graft surgery, the clinical view shows vertical bone defects in the edentulous alveolar ridge.

Reconstructive surgery was performed under local anesthesia. A vestibular incision was made in the left mandibular premolar and molar area. The full thickness buccal flap was reflected and the edentulous alveolar bone exposed (Figure 12.4). Mucoperiosteal dissection was not performed toward the alveolar crest or on the lingual side to preserve an adequate blood supply to the bone segment to be osteotomized. One horizontal osteotomy about 5 mm above the inferior alveolar nerve and two slightly divergent vertical osteotomies were performed through the thickness of the alveolar ridge with the piezoelectric device (SurgyBone®, Silfradent srl, Sofia, Italy), paying special attention to keeping the lingual periosteum intact (Figure 12.5). After completion of all three osteotomies, a segmented bone fragment was elevated up to 6 mm by placing a chisel in the osteotomy line (Figure 12.6). The lifted bone segment was then stabilized to the basal bone with an L-shaped microplate and screws (Jeil Corp., Seoul, Korea) (Figure 12.7).

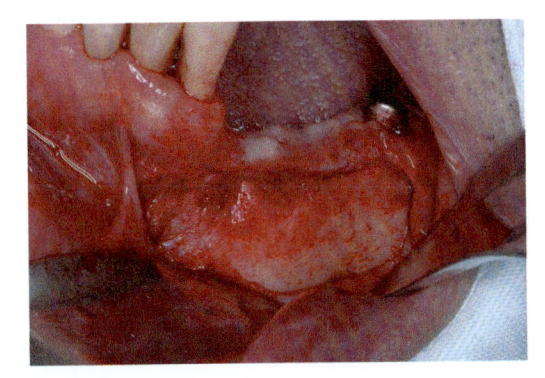

Figure 12.4 Surgery: buccal full thickness flap was raised to expose buccal wall of mandibular body at the edentulous area.

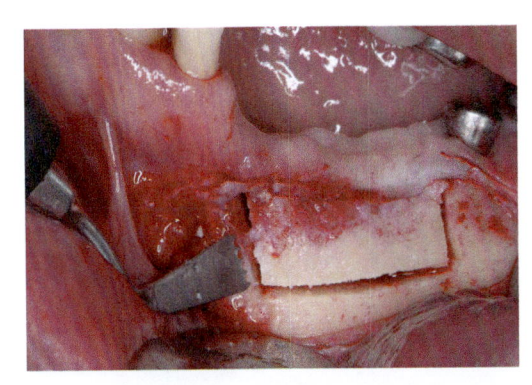

Figure 12.5 Horizontal osteotomy was done 5 mm superior to the inferior alveolar nerve using a piezoelectric saw insert. Anterior vertical osteotomy was made posterior to the lateral incisor and posterior vertical osteotomy was made in front of the previously placed implant. All three osteotomies were connected. All the osteotomies should be done through the lingual cortical bone for easy separation of the crestal segment from the mandibular body. The piezoelectric saw cuts only hard tissue and is protective to soft tissue, like the lingual periosteum and mucosa. The damage to the lingual mucosa reduces blood supply to the crestal segment, which results in bone resorption or bone necrosis.

(continued)

(*Continued*)

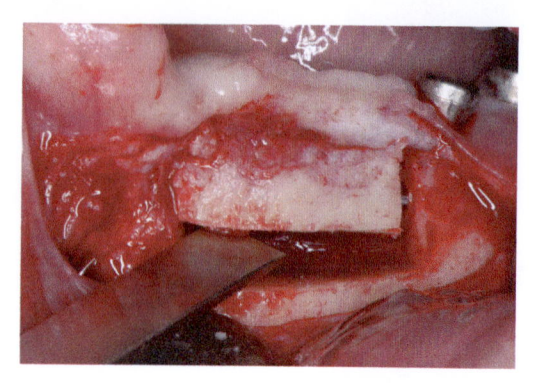

Figure 12.6 Crestal bone segment is being separated from the mandibular body by inserting a chisel osteotome and moved upward.

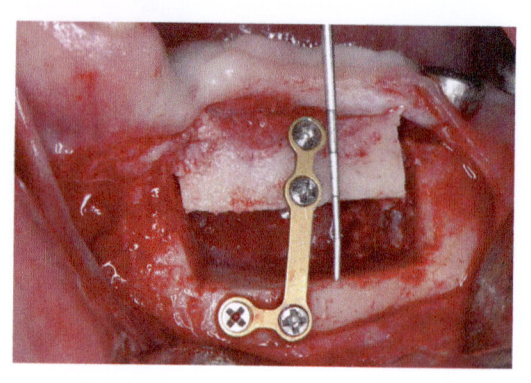

Figure 12.7 Crestal bone segment is moved about 6 mm superiorly and fixated with the micro bone plate. If a bone plate is used to stabilize the crestal bony segment, the resorption of bone is minimized later.

Two bone allografts (OrthoBlast II®, IsoTis OrthoBiologics, Inc., California, USA and Tutoplast® cancellous microchips, Tutogen Medical Inc., Neunkirchem am Brand, Germany, analogous to Puros® in the USA) were placed into the created space between the basal bone and the elevated bone fragment and a resorbable collagen membrane (Tutogen Pericardium®, Tutogen Medical GmbH, Neunkirchem am Brand, Germany) was placed over the graft particles (Figures 12.8 to 12.11). After four weeks, one of two existing implants at the molar site was removed due to failed osseointegration (Figure 12.12). A healing period of four months was allowed.

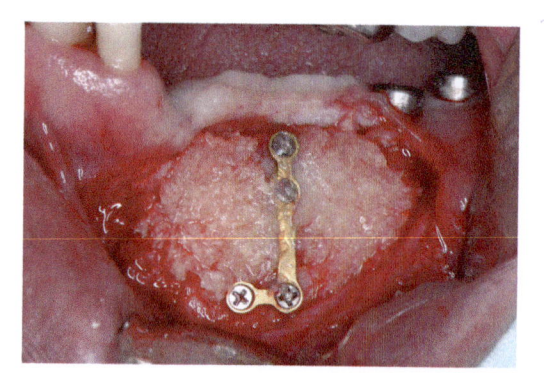

Figure 12.8 Gel conditioned bone (Orthoblast II®) and mineral allograft (Tutoplast cancellous microchip®) were mixed and grafted in the gap between the crestal segment and the basal bone.

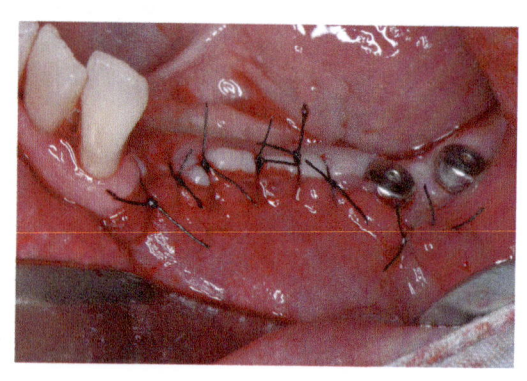

Figure 12.10 Suture without tension was placed.

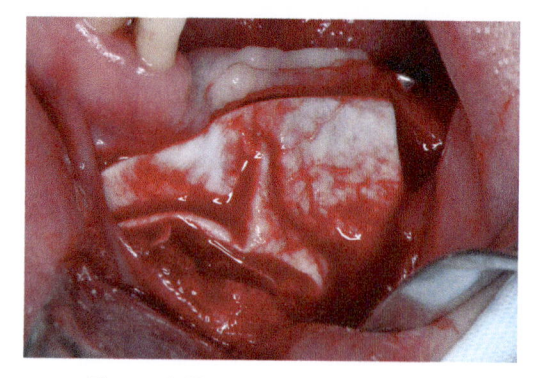

Figure 12.9 The resorbable membrane (Tutoplast Pericardium®) was used to cover the grafted site.

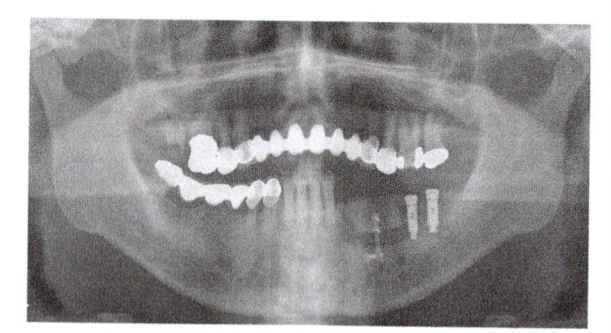

Figure 12.11 Postoperative radiograph showed favorable vertical bone augmentation.

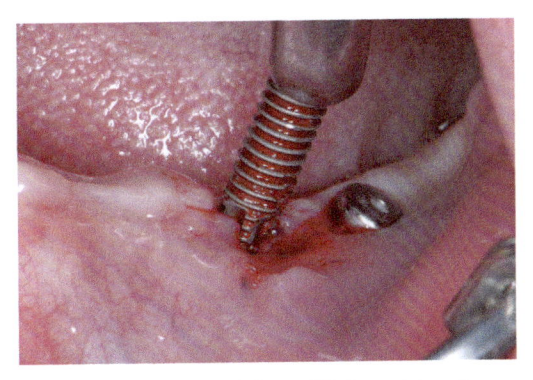

Figure 12.12 After 4 weeks, the implant at the molar site was removed due to failed osseointegration.

The next surgical procedure consisted of a bone biopsy of the grafted area, removal of the fixation plate, and simultaneous placement of three additional implants (two 14 mm and one 11 mm in length, Ankylos®, Friadent GmbH, Mannheim, Germany) (Figures 12.13 to 12.15). A gel conditioned allograft (Orthoblast II®) was grafted over the exposed anterior implant and then a resorbable membrane (Tutogen, Pericardium®) was used to cover the grafted bone site (Figure 12.16). In order to gain attached keratinized gingiva around implant sites, an apically repositioned flap was prepared and a thin palatal strip of tissue was obtained and fixated with sutures to the recipient site at the same time. A tissue adhesive cyanoacrylate was also used (Figures 12.17 and 12.18).

After six months of healing period, an implant-supported prosthesis consisting of two ceramic bridges was constructed and cemented (Figure 12.19). A periapical radiograph showed stability of the alveolar bone after 6 months in function (Figure 12.20a). By the time of writing, an implant-supported prosthesis has been well functioning over a 7-year follow-up period (Figure 12.20b).

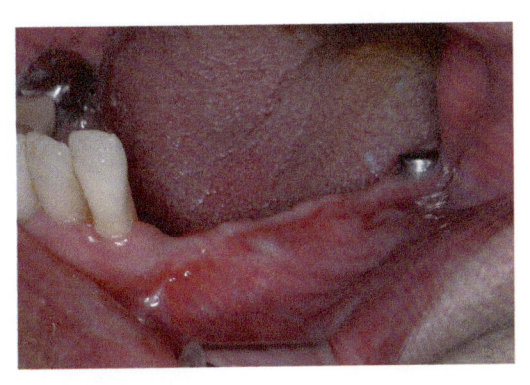

Figure 12.13 After 4 months, the vertically improved alveolar ridge was observed.

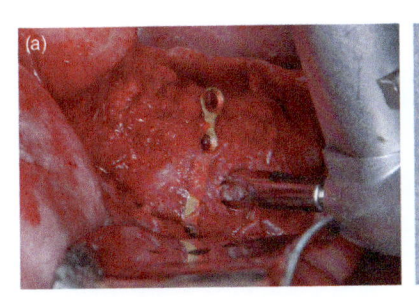

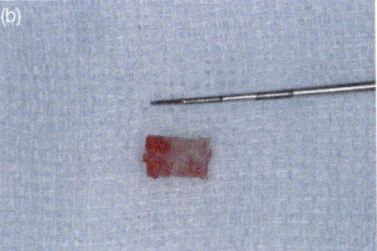

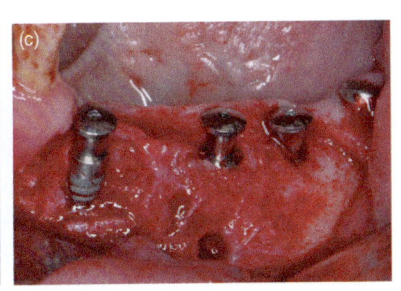

Figure 12.14 The augmented bone was exposed and biopsy was done to evaluate new bone formation in the gap.

(continued)

(Continued)

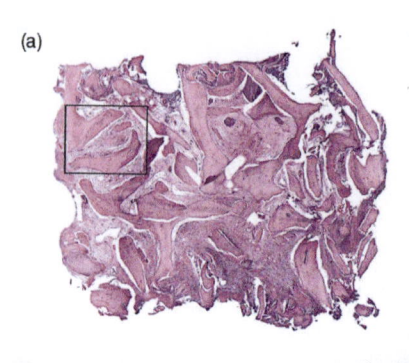

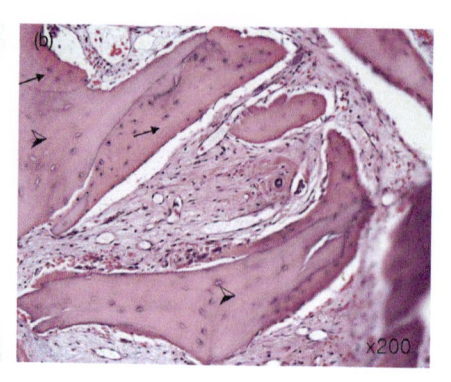

Figure 12.15 New bone formation (arrows) is seen along the bone graft (arrowheads) without inflammatory or foreign body reaction. The percentage of total bone volume was 37.4%.

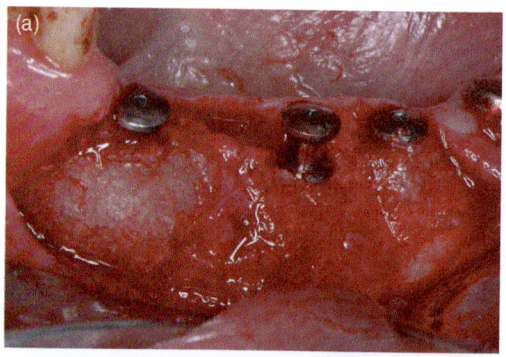

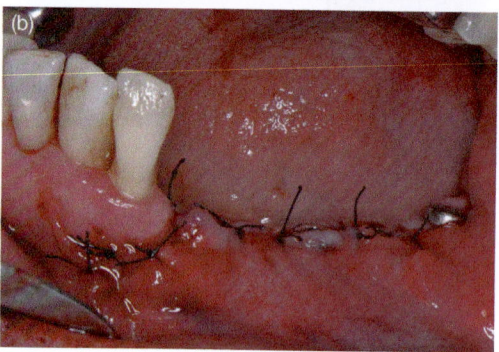

Figure 12.16 Bone plate was removed and three implants (Ankylos®) were placed and connected with healing abutments as the single-stage implant procedure. Orthoblast II® was grafted over the exposed implant and a resorbable membrane was used to cover the grafted bone site. Note the lack of the attached gingiva.

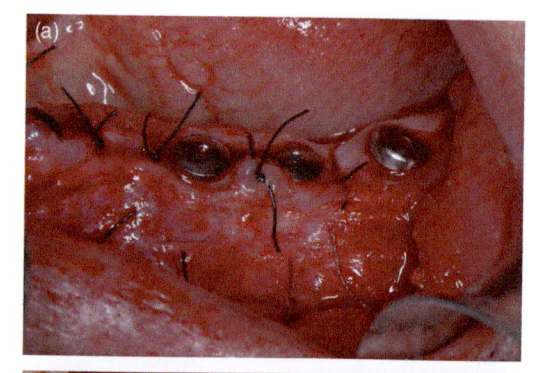

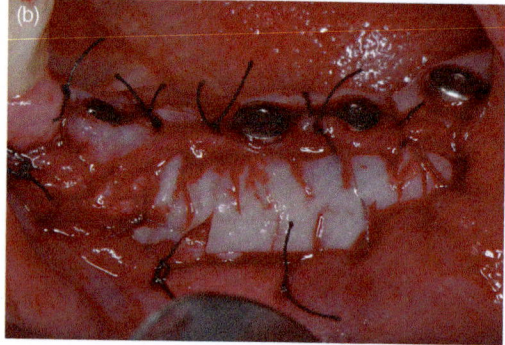

Figure 12.17 Apically repositioned flap was prepared and harvested thin palatal tissue from the palate was grafted to the recipient site and fixated with suture and a tissue adhesive.

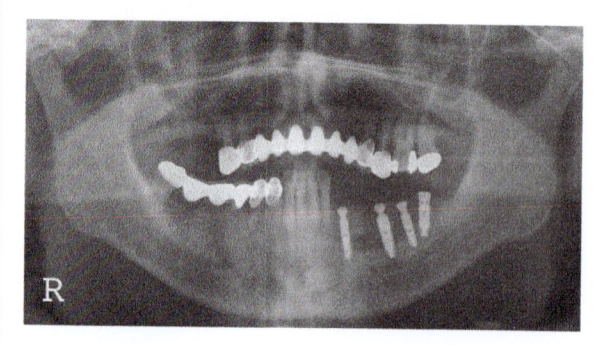

Figure 12.18 Panoramic radiograph showing implants placed into the augmented bone.

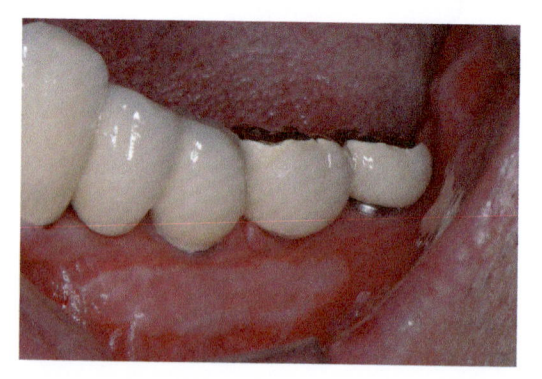

Figure 12.19 Final restoration was cemented after 5 months of healing.

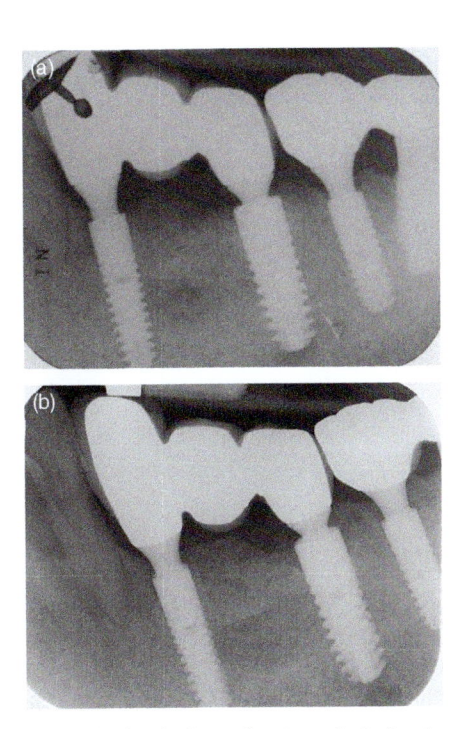

Figure 12.20 Periapical radiograph showing stability of the alveolar bone after 6 months in function and 7 years in function.

Case Report 2: Piezoelectric sandwich technique with interpositional bone graft for vertical augmentation of severely atrophic *anterior* mandibular alveolar ridge

A 45-year-old woman presented with a complaint of poor esthetics resulting from the loss of her anterior mandibular teeth 25 years prior. She had no significant medical history. Clinical examination revealed extensive vertical (about 10 mm) and horizontal atrophy of the anterior mandible and a slight overeruption of maxillary anterior teeth with dental class III malocclusion (Figure 12.21). Because of the insufficient height and width of the mandibular edentulous residual bone, ridge augmentation was required before placement of dental implants.

Various surgical treatment plans, their potential outcomes, benefits, and complications, were analyzed and explained to the patient. An intraoral autogenous block bone graft was not indicated because of limited stock of the donor bone available in the patient's symphyseal area (less than 6 mm of bone height for augmentation). Alveolar bone reconstruction using the distractor osteogenesis technique was ruled out because of its high cost and discomfort for patient during the healing period. Therefore, application of the sandwich osteotomy technique was planned. The patient accepted the plan and agreed to have a piezoelectric sandwich osteotomy with an interpositional bone allograft.

Surgery was performed under local anesthesia. Ceftriaxone (1 g, IV) was administered 1 hour prior to surgery. After a horizontal incision in the vestibule, the mucoperiosteal tissue was carefully dissected to visually expose the underlying bone. No mucoperiosteal dissection was performed toward the alveolar crest or the lingual side to preserve an adequate blood supply to the bone segment to be osteotomized. Two divergent vertical and one horizontal osteotomies were made using a piezoelectric saw (Surgybone, Silfradent srl, Sofia, Italy) without injury of the lingual periosteum (Figures 12.22 and 12.23). After all osteotomies were made, the mobility of the anterior segment was tested. The osteotomized segment was then raised in the coronal direction by about 10 mm to leave a space for the interpositional bone graft, sparing the lingual periosteum from any sharp instruments, like chisels and osteotomes. The mobile bone segment was fixated with a titanium osteosynthesis microplate (Jeil Corp., Seoul, Korea) and microscrews (Jeil Corp., Seoul, Korea) to provide rigid scaffolding for the interpositional bone graft (Figure 12.24a). The interpositional bone graft was the mineral allograft matrix (Ortho-Blast II®, IsoTis OrthoBiologics Inc., CA), which was placed into the created bone space (Figure 12.24b). After releasing the vestibular periosteum, the primary closure was obtained with the cytoplast CS-05 sutures (Osteogenics Biomedical Inc., TX) (Figure 12.25). The post-operative radiograph demonstrated that the sandwich osteotomy technique was successful (Figure 12.26). Antibiotic coverage in this case consisted of amoxicillin (750 mg, three times a day) and naproxen (825 mg, three times a day) for 7 days. The sutures were removed 14 days after the procedure.

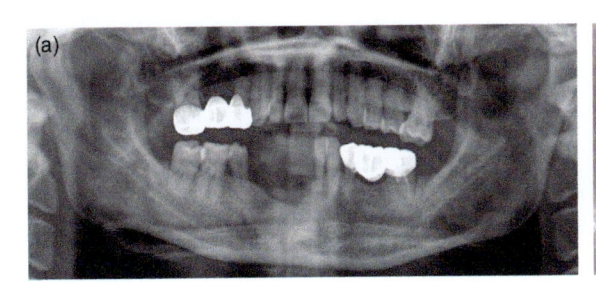

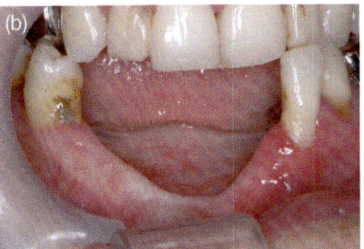

Figure 12.21 Pre-operative panoramic radiograph and intraoral view showing severe atrophy of anterior mandibular bone.

(continued)

(Continued)

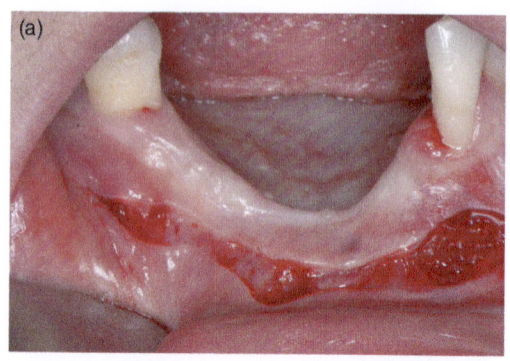

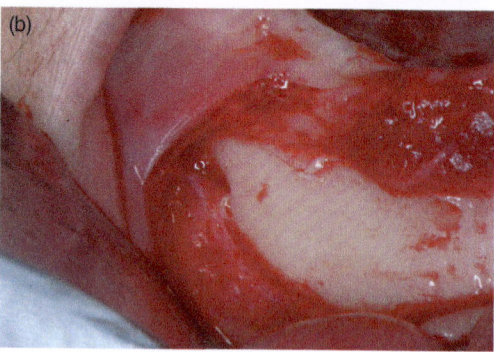

Figure 12.22 An incision in the vestibular mucosa was performed to maximize blood supply to the segmental bone. Bilateral mental nerves were exposed and vertical osteotomy was made at least 5 mm anterior to the mental nerve at each site.

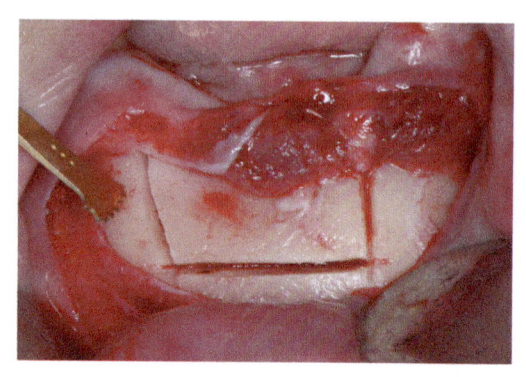

Figure 12.23 Horizontal osteotomy and two vertical osteotomies made by the piezoelectric saw insert were connected. After complete osteotomy, including the lingual cortex, the bone segment was separated with a chisel osteotome.

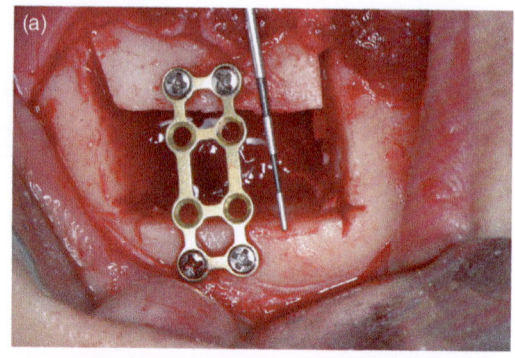

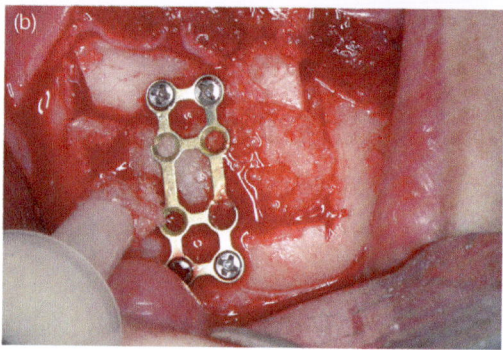

Figure 12.24 The segmental bone was moved upward about 10 mm and fixated using a micro bone plate. This bone plate prevented the segmental bone from moving inferiorly. The gap between the segmental bone and the basal bone was filled with the gel-conditioned allograft (Orthoblast II).

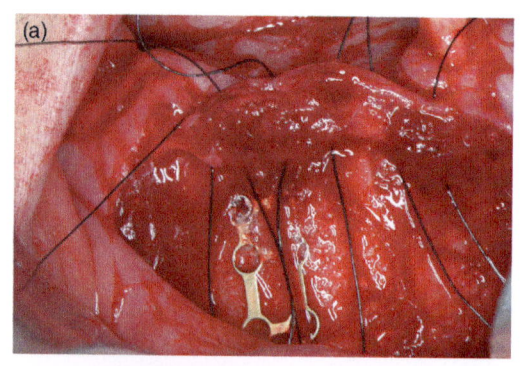

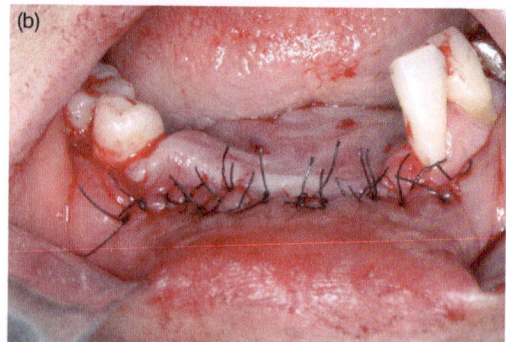

Figure 12.25 The mentalis muscle was sutured to the labial mucosa using three suspension sutures to prevent chin sagging. The mucosa then was closed completely with an interrupted suture.

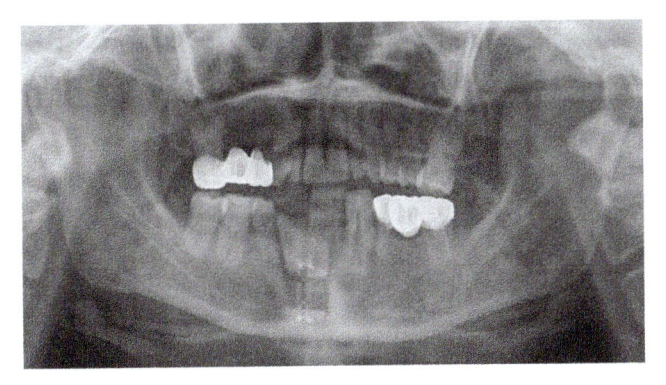

Figure 12.26 Post-operative radiograph showed favorable vertical bone augmentation.

After 6 weeks of healing, vestibuloplasty was performed to regain the lost vestibular space and attached keratinized gingiva on the augmented alveolar ridge (Figure 12.27). The microplate was removed 6 months later and bone biopsy was performed on the augmented bone region for histologic evaluation with hematoxylin and eosin staining (Figures 12.28 and 12.29). The histologic result of bone biopsy showed the well-formed new bone and some grafted bone tissue bridged by new lamellar bone. There was no active resorption of grafted bone or replacement by new bone. The fibrovascular marrow did not contain mature hematopoietic components and showed no inflammatory or foreign body reactions (Figure 12.30).

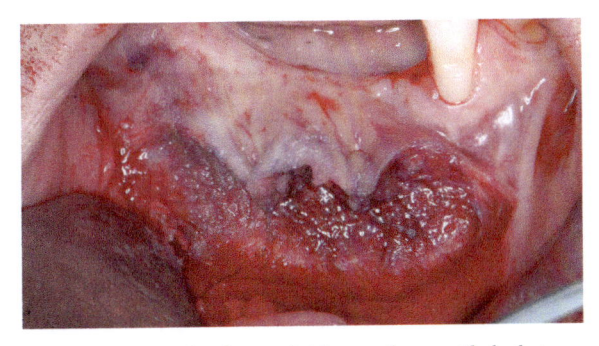

Figure 12.27 Six weeks after sandwich procedure, vestibuloplasty was performed to restore the vestibular space.

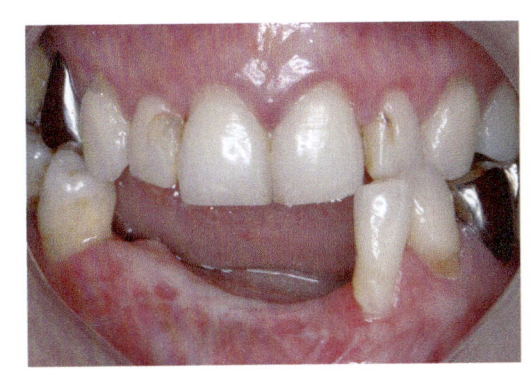

Figure 12.28 After 6 months of healing, the intraoral view showed vertical ridge improvement of the anterior mandible.

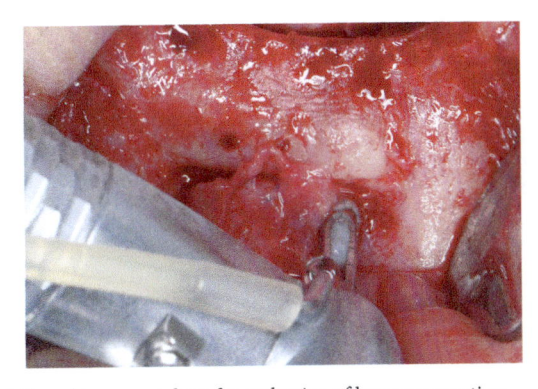

Figure 12.29 The bone plate was removed. Bone biopsy was done for evaluation of bone regeneration.

(continued)

(Continued)

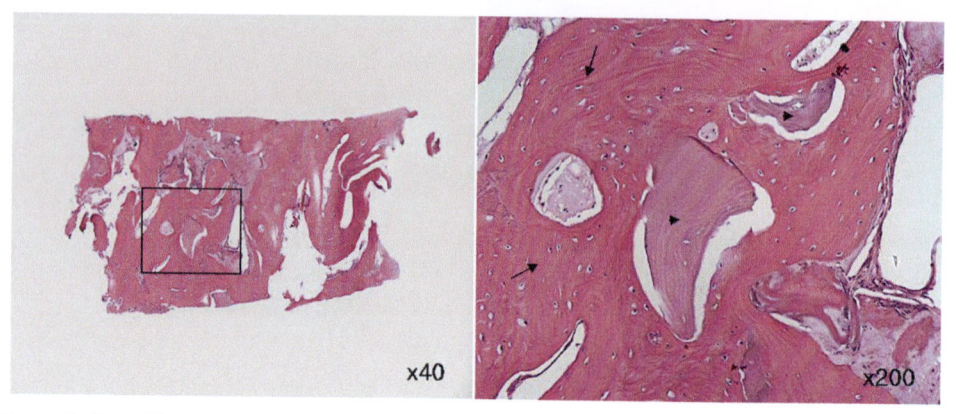

Figure 12.30 Active newly formed bone (arrows) was observed around the grafted bone particles (arrowheads).

Three dental implants (BioHorizons, One-piece 3.0, BioHorizons Inc., Birmingham, AL, USA) were placed simultaneously according to the surgical stent for both mandibular lateral incisors and right canine regions (Figure 12.31). The bovine bone (OCS-B, NIBEC Corp., Seoul, Korea) mixed with fibrin adhesive (Greenplast, Green Cross Co., Yon-gin, Korea) was grafted to add an additional contour to the augmented ridge (Figure 12.32). A temporary implant-supported fixed prosthesis was used for immediate provisionalization (Figure 12.33). A final fixed prosthesis was delivered 5 months later (Figure 12.34a). A stable bone height was confirmed on a radiograph (Figure 12.34b). By the time of writing, an implant-supported prosthesis had been well functioning over an 8-year follow-up period (Figures 12.35).

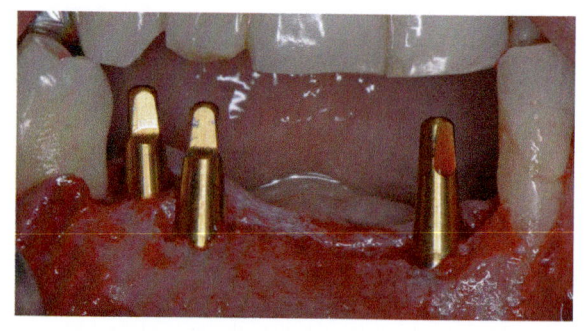

Figure 12.31 One-piece three BioHorizons implants were placed. Note the favorable vertical augmentation but thin alveolar bone around the implants.

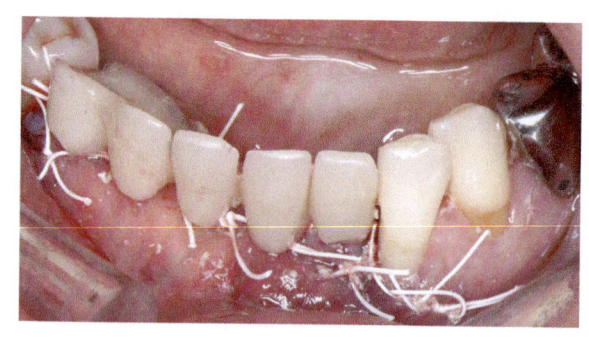

Figure 12.33 An immediate mandibular temporary prosthesis was placed.

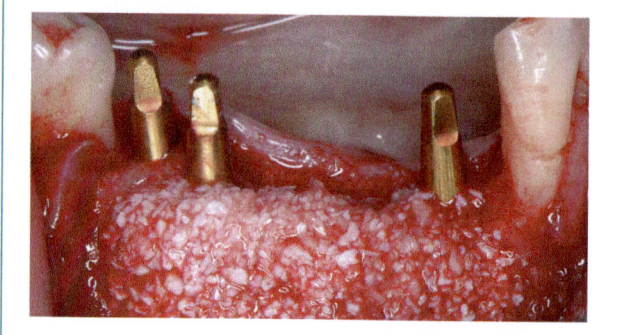

Figure 12.32 An additional bovine bone was grafted for the horizontal augmentation.

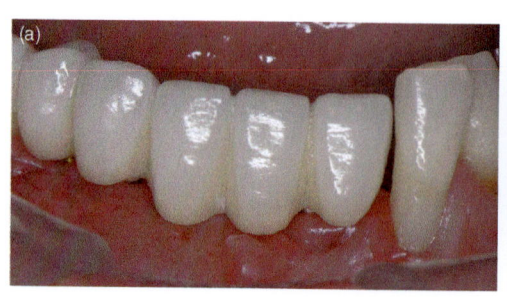

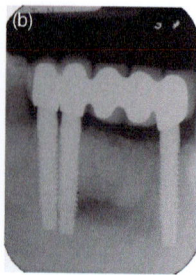

Figure 12.34 Final (three-implant-supported five-unit ceramic) restoration was delivered after 5 months of healing: clinical and radiographic presentation.

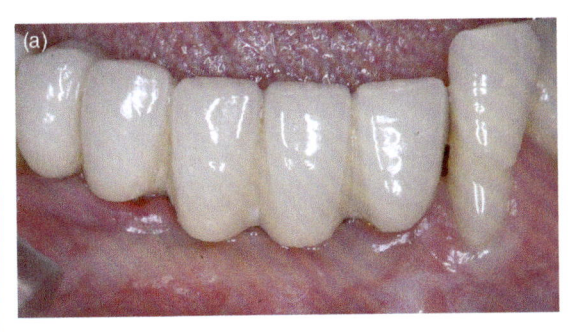

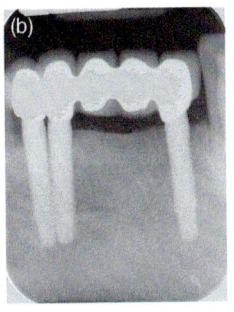

Figure 12.35 Eight years of function: note the stable marginal bone level around implants: clinical and radiographic presentation.

Discussion

It is important that clinicians try to obtain adequate bone height above the inferior alveolar nerve for placing implants without nerve damage in the posterior mandible, as well as to achieve a successful osseointegration of dental implants. Since Harle [6] first reported the use of visor osteotomy to augment the atrophic mandible, a lot of clinicians have modified and developed pedicled or interpositional grafts since the late 1970s [17–20]. In the past, these methods have been used to increase retention of conventional removable prostheses (dentures), but recently they have been used for alveolar augmentation for placement of dental implants.

Politi and Robiony [18] stated that the alveolar sandwich osteotomy had the advantage of guaranteeing a greater vascular supply to the inlay graft than to an onlay graft. That is why it might be less subject to resorption. Jensen et al. [19] also commented that the distraction osteogenesis approach could lead to the same result, but advocated sandwich osteotomy due to its simplicity and bone height correction, which could be as small as 3 to 6 mm of vertical movement. Egbert et al. [20] have reported that the inferior alveolar nerve is located more lingually in many atrophic mandibles and there is also often an insufficient space to make a sandwich osteotomy without damaging the nerve. Jensen [21] stated that many patients had some degree of *transient* paresthesia post-surgically, the longest lasting six weeks, and that the paresthesia was likely to be related to flap retraction of the mental nerve.

For a successful sandwich osteotomy, an atraumatic surgical technique is crucial. Preservation of soft tissue and the lingual periosteal blood supply can be accomplished through osteotomy using a piezoelectric device. Moon et al. [22] and Sohn et al. [23] reported the advantages of piezoelectric bone surgery for precise control of osteotomy in order to reduce trauma to the inferior alveolar nerve and soft tissue during the procedure. No neurosensory disturbances were found in all cases. The lingual periosteum and flap should be maintained intact for optimization of the blood supply to the segmented bone [22, 23].

The piezoelectric surgical device does not cause soft-tissue laceration or burn during osteotomy. It makes micrometric bone cuts, resulting in precise and easily controlled osteotomies with minimal bone loss. Piezoelectric sandwich osteotomy is applicable in extensive alveolar ridge defects, resulting in an increase in alveolar bone height and allowing long-term stability of the augmented alveolar ridge.

Although sandwich osteotomy can be a solution to achieve a reconstruction of severe alveolar ridge deficiency, stability over time is not clear. Choi et al. [24], studying the sandwich osteotomy with interpositional allograft in the atrophic anterior mandible, reported some resorption in the crestal bone height of 1.5 mm (18%) to 3.0 mm (28%) after 3 months. A fixation between the basal bone and mobile bone segment was not used in their study. However, Jensen [21] reported 4 to 8 mm of vertical bone gain in moderate posterior mandibular atrophy cases using an autograft with no bone resorption, except in one patient (1 mm loss at a 2-year follow-up). In the moderately deficient anterior maxilla, the vertical bone gain was between 3 and 6 mm using a particulate autograft with no significant bone resorption at the time of implant placement. Bone resorption of about 1 mm was noticed at most implant sites over a 5-year follow-up period [25]. Sohn et al. [23] in their study demonstrated that less resorption of segmented bone was seen in the fixation cases than in the non-fixation cases. This group also indicated that using the sandwich technique, up to 10 mm of vertical alveolar augmentation can be obtained in the anterior mandible, and a 5–6-year follow-up indicates favorable stability of the augmented bone over time.

The use of an autogenous bone graft is considered a gold standard for bone augmentation [22, 26]. However, there are many problems associated with harvesting an adequate quantity of autogenous bone. It requires a second donor site, causing increases in surgical time and surgical costs, and possible complications at the donor site [27, 28]. The availability of suitable biomaterials to be used as bone replacements that facilitate bone regeneration can potentially eliminate the need for an additional surgical site. Extensive new bone formation by utilizing allografts in bone defects has been reported by various researchers [29–32]. Mineral allograft materials inserted between basal and segmented bone showed favorable new bone formation at 6 months in these studies. A histologic analysis of the bone at the light microscopic level also showed the incorporation of grafted bone particles between formed new bone, serving as a scaffold for new bone formation.

Conclusion

The piezoelectric sandwich alveolar bone augmentation is a relatively simple and predictable surgical procedure for both clinicians and patients. It does not require a donor site and can be applied for vertical alveolar ridge augmentation of moderate-to-severe bone defects prior to implant placement.

References

1 Misch CM, Misch CE, Resnik RR, et al: Reconstruction of maxillary alveolar defects with mandibular symphysis grafts for dental implants; a preliminary procedural report. *Int J Oral Maxillofac Implants* 1992;7:360–366.

2 Jensen OT: Distraction osteogenesis and its use with dental implants. *Dent Implantol* 1999;10:33–36.

3. Maiorana C, Santoro F, Rabagliati M, et al: Evaluation of the use of iliac cancellous bone and anorganic bovine bone in the reconstruction of the atrophic maxilla with titanium mesh: a clinical and histologic investigation. *Int J Oral Maxillofac Implants* 2001;16:427–432.
4. Sohn DS: Piezoelectric block bone graft in severely atrophic posterior maxilla with simultaneous implant placement. *Dent Success* 2003;10:1208–1213.
5. Lee HJ, Ahn MR, Sohn DS: Piezoelectric distraction osteogenesis in the atrophic maxillary anterior area: a case report. *Implant Dent* 2007;16:227–234.
6. Harle F: Visor osteotomy to increase the absolute height of the atrophied mandible. A preliminary report. *J Maxillofac Surg* 1975 Dec;3(4):257–260.
7. Schettler D: Sandwich technique with cartilage transplant for raising the alveolar process in the lower jaw. *Fortschr Kiefer Gesichtschir* 1976;20:61–63.
8. Peterson LJ, Slade EW Jr: Mandibular ridge augmentation by a modified visor osteotomy: a preliminary report. *J Oral Surg* 1977;35(12):999–1004.
9. Vercellotti T: Technological characteristics and clinical indications of piezoelectric bone surgery. *Minerva Stomatol* 2004;53(5):207–214.
10. Sohn DS, Ahn MR., Lee WH, et al: Piezoelectric osteotomy for intraoral harvesting of bone blocks. *Int J Periodontics Restorative Dent* 2007;27(2):127–131.
11. Horton JE, Tarpley TM Jr, Jacoway JR: Clinical applications of ultrasonic instrumentation in the surgical removal of bone. *Oral Surg Oral Med Oral Pathol* 1981;51:236–242.
12. Torrella F, Pitarch J, Cabanes G, Anitua E: Ultrasonic osteotomy for the surgical approach of the maxillary sinus: a technical note. *Int J Oral Maxillofac Implants* 1998;13:697–700.
13. Vercellotti T: Piezoelectric surgery in implantology: a case report – a new piezoelectric ridge expansion technique. *Int J Periodontics Restorative Dent* 2000;4:359–365.
14. Vercellotti T, De Paoli S, Nevins M: The piezoelectric bony window osteotomy and sinus floor elevation: introduction of a new technique for simplification of the sinus augmentation procedure. *Int J Periodontics Restorative Dent* 2001;21:561–567.
15. Sohn DS, Ahn MR, Jang BY: Sinus bone graft using piezoelectric surgery. *Implantology* 2003;7:48–55.
16. Curie J, Curie P: Contractions et dilatations produites par des tensions dans les cristaux hémièdres à faces inclinées. *CR Acad Sci Gen* 1880;93:1137–1140.
17. Bell WH, Buckles RL: Correction of the atrophic alveolar ridge by interpositional bone grafting: a progress report. *J Oral Surg* 1978;36(9):693–700.
18. Politi M, Robiony M: Localized alveolar sandwich osteotomy for vertical augmentation of the anterior maxilla. *J Oral Maxillofac Surg* 1999;57(11):1380–1382.
19. Jensen OT, Kuhlke L, Bedard JF, et al: Alveolar segmental sandwich osteotomy for anterior maxillary vertical augmentation prior to implant placement. *J Oral Maxillofac Surg* 2006;64:290–296.
20. Egbert M, Stoelinga PJ, Blijdorp PA, et al: The "three-piece" osteotomy and interpositional bone graft for augmentation of the atrophic mandible. *J Oral and Maxillofac Surg* 1986;44(9):680–687.
21. Jensen OT: Alveolar segmental "sandwich" osteotomies for posterior edentulous mandibular sites for dental implants. *J Oral Maxillofac Surg* 2006;64(3):471–475.
22. Moon JW, Choi BJ, Lee WH, An KM, Sohn DS: Reconstruction of atrophic anterior mandible using piezoelectric sandwich osteotomy: a case report. *Implant Dent* 2009;18(3):195–202.
23. Sohn DS, Shin HI, Ahn MR, Lee JS: Piezoelectric vertical bone augmentation using the sandwich technique in an atrophic mandible and histomorphometric analysis of mineral allografts: case report series. *Int J Periodontics Restorative Dent* 2010;30(4):383–391.
24. Choi BH, Lee SH, Huh JY, et al: Use of the sandwich osteotomy plus an interpositional allograft for vertical augmentation of the alveolar ridge. *J Craniomaxillofac Surg* 2004;32:51–54.
25. Jensen OT, Kuhlke L, Bedard JF, et al: Alveolar segmental sandwich osteotomy for anterior maxillary vertical augmentation prior to implant placement. *J Oral Maxillofac Surg* 2006;64:290–296.
26. Boyne PJ, James RA: Grafting of the maxillary sinus floor with autogenous marrow and bone. *J Oral Surg* 1980;38:613–616.
27. Wood RM, Moore DL: Grafting of the maxillary sinus with intraorally harvested autogenous bone prior to implant placement. *Int J Oral Maxillofac Implants* 1988;3:209–214.
28. Kalk WW, Raqhoebar GM, Jansma J, et al: Morbidity from iliac crest bone harvesting. *J Oral Maxillofac Surg* 1996;54:1424–1429; discussion, 1430.
29. Shin HI, Sohn DS: A method of sealing perforated sinus membrane and histologic finding of bone substitutes: a case report. *Implant Dent* 2005;14:328–333.
30. Callan DP, Salkeld SL, Scarborough N. Histologic analysis of implant sites after grafting with demineralized bone matrix putty and sheets. *Implant Dent* 2000;9:36–44.
31. Babbush CA: Histologic evaluation of human biopsies after dental augmentation with demineralized bone matrix putty. *Implant Dent* 2003;12:325–332.
32. Froum SJ, Tarnow DP, Wallace SS, et al: The use of a mineralized allograft for sinus augmentation: an interim histological case report from a prospective clinical study. *Compend Contin Educ Dent* 2005;26(4):259–260, 262–264, 266–268.

SECTION III

Subantral Grafting (Sinus Lift) for Vertical Ridge Augmentation in the Posterior Maxilla

CHAPTER 13

Implant Diagnosis and Treatment Planning for the Posterior Edentulous Maxilla

Douglas E. Kendrick

Department of Oral and Maxillofacial Surgery, The University of Iowa Hospitals and Clinics, Iowa City, Iowa, USA

Introduction

The placement of dental implants in the posterior maxilla has often been problematic. Minimal bone volume for implant placement can be due to pneumatization of the maxillary sinus or resorption of the alveolar ridge from tooth loss or periodontal disease. Areas that have been edentulous for several years may present with only a few millimeters or less of bone. These patients require a maxillary sinus lift procedure in order to have adequate bone for implant placement.

History of the sinus lift

The maxillary sinus (antrum of Highmore) was likely to have been first identified by ancient Egyptians [1]. Leonardo da Vinci was the first to illustrate and write about the maxillary sinus in the fifteenth century AD. However, the British surgeon and anatomist, Nathaniel Highmore, was the first to describe the maxillary sinus in detail in 1651. The sinus was originally named after Highmore (antrum of Highmore) due to his illustrations and writings (the drawings of da Vinci were not discovered until 1901). George Caldwell, an American physician, and Henry Luc, a French laryngologist, first described accessing the maxillary sinus by a window in the lateral maxillary wall, and a modification of this approach is used to approach the maxillary sinus for sinus bone grafting (Caldwell–Luc procedure).

Hilt Tatum first described a lateral sinus window approach to elevation of the sinus membrane and placement of grafting material along the sinus floor to increase alveolar bone height [2]. Boyne and James were the first to publish on sinus lift procedures and described using the Caldwell–Luc approach to graft the maxillary sinus floor with autogenous bone, which was used for increasing alveolar ridge bulk prior to ridge reduction to increase interarch distance for removable prosthetics [3]. Several surgeons have published variations in surgical techniques and the use of different graft materials. Summers introduced the crestal sinus lift approach, also known as the indirect sinus lift, in 1994 [4]. Although some of the technology used to perform these procedures have improved, the general surgical approaches have remained relatively unchanged as they were originally described.

Anatomy, development, histology, and physiology of the maxillary sinus

The two maxillary bones are fused in the midline along the palatal sutures. The maxilla forms the upper jaw, anterior hard palate, nasal floor, lateral nasal walls, and inferior orbit. The maxilla also contains the maxillary dentition and contributes to a majority of the maxillary sinus. The lateral maxillary wall is relatively smooth between the canine eminence anteriorly to the zygomatic process posteriorly. The dentate maxilla has prominences associated with the roots of the maxillary teeth; however, the edentulous maxilla often loses these prominences over time.

The maxillary sinus is the largest of the four pairs of paranasal sinuses and is formed by the maxilla, zygomatic bone, palatine bone, sphenoid bone, and inferior concha. The sinus is pyramidal in shape with its base toward the lateral nose and apex toward the zygoma (Figure 13.1). The four walls are the anterior (lateral) maxillary wall, posterior maxillary wall, roof (floor of the orbit), and floor (alveolar process of the maxilla). The maxillary sinus drains into the lateral nasal wall via the maxillary ostium into the semilunar hiatus of the middle meatus. The ostium is found high on the medial aspect of the sinus approximately 35 mm superior to the floor of the maxillary sinus [5]. Patency of the ostium in the osteomeatal complex (OMC) is very important for the health of the maxillary sinus (Figure 13.2). Lack of patency of the OMC prior to sinus lift surgery can be a relative contraindication for the surgery. Reestablishing the OMC patency by endoscopic sinus debridement can lead to improvement of the sinus condition and ability to proceed with the direct (lateral) sinus lift procedure and bone grafting.

Arterial blood supply to the maxillary sinus is via the facial artery and branches of the maxillary artery (infraorbital, posterior superior alveolar, and greater palatine arteries) [6]. Venous drainage is via the sphenopalatine vein, facial vein, and pterygoid plexus. Innervation to the maxillary sinus is from the anterior superior alveolar, middle superior alveolar, posterior superior alveolar, infraorbital, and greater palatine nerves. Lymphatic drainage is via the submandibular, deep cervical, and retropharyngeal lymph nodes.

The maxilla develops from the first branchial arch, which is also called the mandibular arch. Ossification of the maxilla begins during the seventh week *in utero*. The maxillary sinuses develop

---

Vertical Alveolar Ridge Augmentation in Implant Dentistry: A Surgical Manual, First Edition. Edited by Len Tolstunov.
© 2016 John Wiley & Sons, Inc. Published 2016 by John Wiley & Sons, Inc.

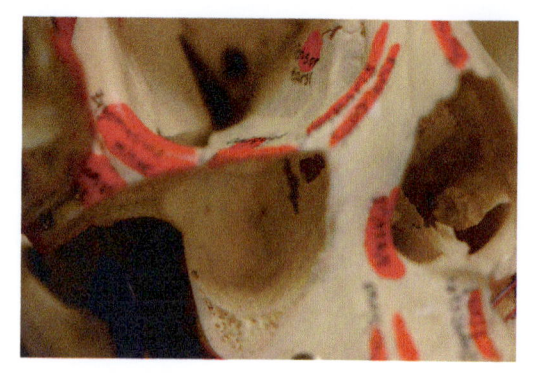

Figure 13.1 Skull demonstrating right maxillary sinus anatomy.

in the 16th week of fetal life as a small portion of the mucous membrane of the lateral nasal wall invaginates into the body of the maxilla. The sinus develops from a tube-like structure at birth and expands to its pyramidal shape at adulthood. The length, width, and height of the maxillary sinus at birth are 7 mm, 4 mm, and 4 mm, respectively [7]. Enlargement of the maxillary sinus occurs via pneumatization – bone resorption on the internal surface of the maxilla and bone deposition on the external surface of the maxilla. An increase in size is also associated with the eruption of the permanent teeth and associated pneumatization of the alveolus. The sinus slowly enlarges throughout life and can extend between roots of the maxillary teeth. Pneumatization is primarily over the first and second molars but can extend as far anteriorly as the canine (Figures 13.3 and 13.4). Pneumatization may cause the bone to completely disappear and lead to direct contact between the sinus membrane and the periodontal ligament of the remaining posterior maxillary teeth. When teeth are lost in the posterior maxilla, the sinus will expand into the area of tooth loss. The average volume of the adult maxillary sinus is 15 ml and the dimensions range from 25 to 35 mm mediolaterally, 36 to 45 mm vertically, and 38 to 45 mm anteroposteriorly [6]. The internal surface of the sinus can be relatively smooth or septa can be present within the sinus. These septa may be single or multiple and are found in up to 37% of patients when evaluated on CT examination [8, 9].

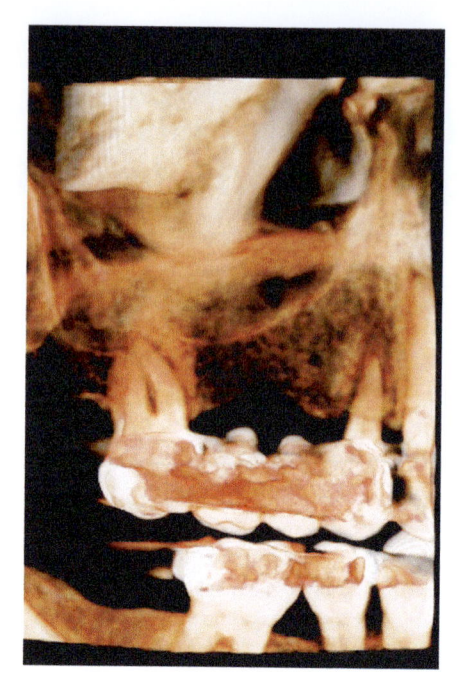

Figure 13.3 CBCT 3D showing pneumatization of the maxillary sinus following tooth loss.

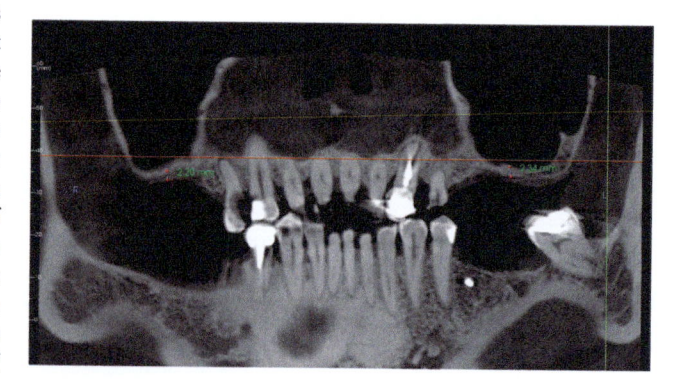

Figure 13.4 Panoramic reconstruction from a CBCT showing pneumatization of the maxillary sinus following tooth loss.

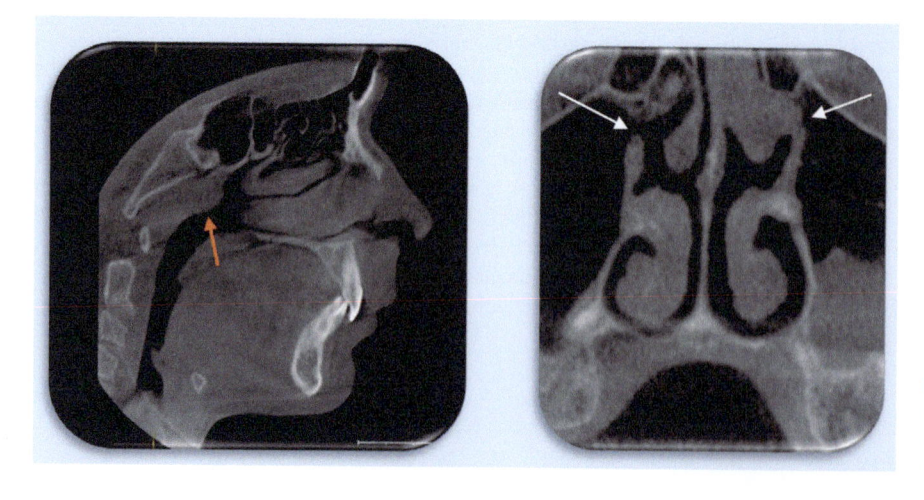

Figure 13.2 Cone beam computed tomography (CBCT) sagittal and coronal images demonstrating patency of the ostium or osteomeatal complex (OMC).

A thin sinus membrane, known as the Schneiderian membrane, lines the maxillary sinus and is composed of epithelium, subepithelial connective tissue (lamina propria), and periosteum. The sinus membrane is approximately 1 mm in thickness or less in a healthy sinus [6,10,11]. The epithelium is composed of respiratory epithelium, which is primarily pseudostratified columnar ciliated cells. The cilia lining the sinus move debris, microorganisms, and mucous toward the maxillary ostium at a rate of approximately 6 mm per minute [12]. Goblet cells are also present, which produce mucin. The subepithelial connective tissue contains collagen, vasculature, myoepithelium, and mixed serous and mucous glands.

The functions of the sinuses are not completely understood but may have developed to decrease the weight of the facial bones, increase resonance of the voice, absorb energy during trauma to the face, humidify and heat inhaled air, and for immunologic defense.

Biological basis of the sinus lift

Healthy teeth without periodontal disease help to maintain the bulk of bone in the alveolus. The loss of teeth in the posterior maxilla and the resultant loss of function and loading on the alveolar bone lead to resorption. The majority of the resorption occurs along the buccal portion of the alveolar ridge. This is due to the thin buccal plate and loosely organized underlying trabecular bone with low density (type 3 and 4 bone) [13]. The resorption of the buccal aspect of the alveolus causes the center of the residual alveolar crest to be located more palatally [14]. As previously discussed, the maxillary sinus is also resorbing the residual alveolus from the floor of the sinus as the alveolar ridge undergoes resorption. This dual resorption often leaves the posterior maxillary ridge with very thin bone, especially in a patient with an edentulous area that has been present for several years.

Osseointegration is partly dependent on primary stability. The posterior maxilla has the least dense bone in the oral cavity, which makes it the most difficult area to obtain primary stability for dental endosseous root-form implants. This decreased density causes decreased bone to implant contact and strain patterns that are spread farther apically on the implant as compared to dense bone [15, 16]. Appropriate bone volume and bone density must be present in the posterior maxilla in order to withstand high occlusal forces, which are greater in the posterior quadrants of the alveolar arches where the main function of mastication occurs. The force generated in the posterior region may be five times greater than in the anterior, with a maximum of 1378 to 1723 Pa in the molar region [17, 18]. Poor bone quality and insufficient implant length may lead to implant failure when the implants are loaded. The use of 4.0 mm diameter or greater implants are recommended as well as implants at least 10 mm in length to aid in disbursement of forces and primary stability of the implant [14]. Increasing the number of implants to allow for one implant per tooth and splinting implants together through a fixed partial denture (implant bridge) are recommended to decrease strain on the implants. This is especially true in patients with parafunctional habits. Due to the high occlusal forces and poor bone quality, the surgeon needs to optimize all aspects of treatment planning and surgery in order for implants to be successful.

The goal of sinus grafting is to restore the resorbed maxillary ridge to allow implant placement. Consolidation of the graft material with the native bone is required for implants to be stable and successful. Consolidation requires an adequate blood supply and osteogenic cells, which are both derived primarily from the periosteum [19, 20]. Careful soft tissue handling is required since 70 to 100% of the alveolar blood supply is from the periosteum [20]. Blood vessels grow into the bone graft material during graft consolidation, which is triggered by cell mediators from platelets, macrophages, and osteogenic cells [19]. Osteoblasts begin to lay down new, immature bone. This bone is then remodeled and replaced by mature, lamellar bone. Many factors may delay bone graft consolidation including the use of non-autogenous graft material, osteoporosis, diabetes, chemotherapy, decreased alveolar bone height, sinus perforation, smoking, and alcohol use.

Autogenous bone is the gold standard for bone grafting, as it is osteoconductive, osteoinductive, and provides osteogenic cells. Many intraoral and extraoral sites are available to harvest autogenous bone. Grafting of the maxillary sinus floor with autogenous bone is intended for use in pneumatized sinuses, previously failed grafts, and during simultaneous lateral ridge augmentation. The use of autogenous bone alone or mixed with xenograft may decrease healing time after sinus grafting [21]. However, sinuses grafted with autogenous bone alone have been found to resorb faster than those augmented with xenograft material [19]. Good results have been seen with the combination of autogenous bone with bovine xenograft [21]. This combination allows for the graft to have increased healing properties from the autograft with the decreased amount of resorption due to the xenograft. Platelet-rich fibrin, recombinant human bone morphogenic protein 2 (rhBMP-2), and fibrin glue have also been used in sinus lift procedures with good results.

Indications

Grafting of the maxillary sinus is indicated when the surgeon feels there is insufficient bone between the maxillary alveolus and sinus. Excessive pneumatization or excessive bone loss from periodontal disease or during extraction may necessitate sinus grafting. Alveolar height less than 10 mm is often an indication for sinus lift surgery via the crestal (indirect) approach and less than 5 mm via the lateral (direct) approach. Sinus lift procedures are indicated for single tooth implant, multiple tooth implants, and the completely edentulous maxilla.

Contraindications

Contraindications for sinus lift procedures include poor oral hygiene, insufficient space for dental restoration, severe parafunctional habits, dental infection, drug or alcohol abuse, untreated acute or chronic sinusitis, anticoagulation or antiplatelet medications use, neoplasms, local cysts, radiation therapy, poorly controlled systemic disease, and immune compromise. Increased risks are associated with smoking and active periodontal disease [10].

The failure rate of implants in smokers is two to three times greater than that of non-smokers [10]. Smokers have a failure rate of bone grafts placed in the posterior maxilla that is approximately 10% greater than that of a non-smoker [22]. Smoking decreases ciliary function, the immune response of the sinus, and increases the risk of sinusitis. Smoking also decreases the blood supply to the graft site and inhibits wound healing. Bone density has also been found to be two to six times less than normal in chronic smokers [22]. It is wise to advise the patient to avoid smoking 2 to 4 weeks prior to surgery and 4 to 6 weeks after surgery to allow adequate healing of the graft site. When comparing diabetics who are well controlled or moderately controlled (hemoglobin A_{1c} < 7 and 7–9%, respectively)

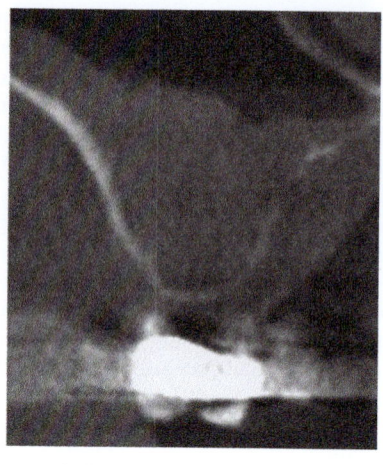

Figure 13.5 Sinus pathology seen on the CBCT cross-sectional image.

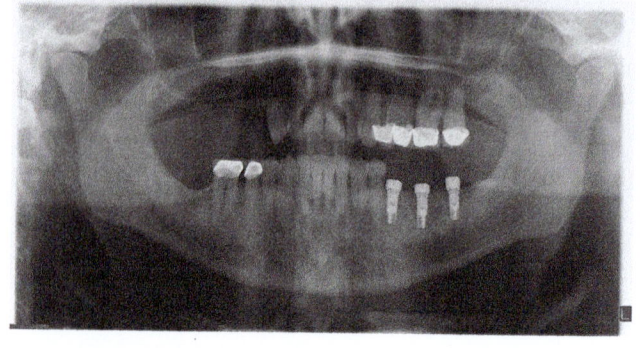

Figure 13.6 Panoramic radiograph showing pneumatized right maxillary sinus and decreased vertical height of the residual alveolus.

to non-diabetic patients, both sets of patients had similar implant success rates of 97.2% versus 98.8%, respectively [23].

Any reversible contraindications should be addressed prior to surgery. Any dental component should be addressed. All sinus pathology should be treated medically or surgically as indicated (Figure 13.5). Any systemic disease should be controlled. Medication modification may be required for patients taking anticoagulants. Failure to identify and treat a compromised host or compromised sinus may exacerbate any sinus disease that is already present.

Diagnosis and treatment planning

Appropriate diagnosis and treatment planning require coordination with the implant surgeon and restorative dentist. The surgeon must obtain the patient's medical, surgical, dental, and social histories. Physical examination should evaluate the patient's overall health as well as the dentition and periodontal structures for health. The alveolar ridge and edentulous space should be evaluated for appropriate dimensions to facilitate an implant and restoration. Diagnostic imaging should be obtained including photographs, periapical radiographs, panoramic radiographs, and computerized tomography (CT).

Radiographic imaging is used to evaluate the vertical and horizontal bone, the presence of pathology, and the need for grafting procedures. Panoramic and periapical radiographs are often used as imaging modalities in an initial evaluation of a site for a sinus lift procedure (Figure 13.6). Cone beam computed tomography (CBCT) is a modern imaging tool to evaluate the health and morphology of the maxillary sinus in three dimensions [24] (Figures 13.2 to 13.5 and 13.7). The use of CBCT has allowed for an in-office option with decreased cost and radiation exposure to the patient. Appropriate imaging of the sinus is needed to determine patency of the osteomeatal complex (OMC), sinus health, and sinus topography. The panoramic radiograph, cone beam CT, and intraoral photograph shown in Figures 13.6 to 13.8 demonstrate pneumatization of the sinus and atrophy of the alveolar bone.

Mounted diagnostic casts aid in treatment planning by allowing evaluation of the occlusion, creating a diagnostic wax-up, and fabrication of surgical guides, if needed. Figures 13.9 and 13.10 are examples of a diagnostic wax-up and a surgical guide. Placement

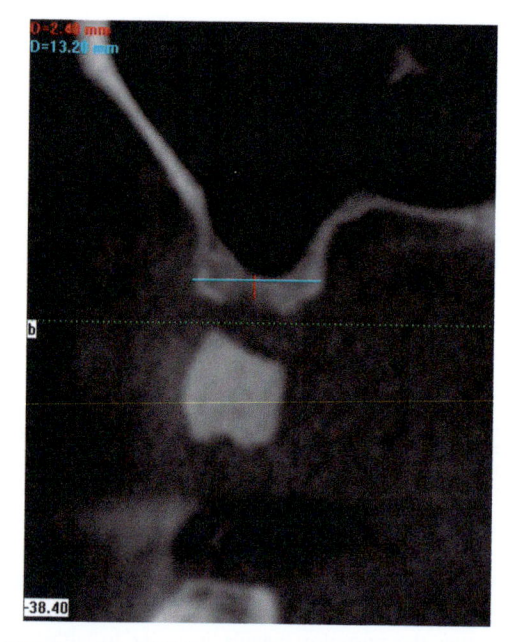

Figure 13.7 Cone beam CT showing pneumatized maxillary sinus and decreased vertical height of the residual alveolus.

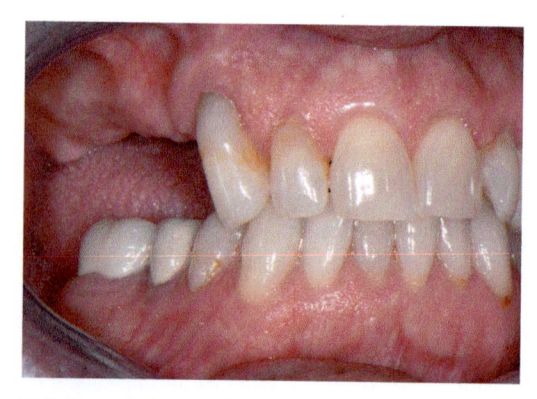

Figure 13.8 Intraoral photograph showing edentulous resorbed area of the right maxilla.

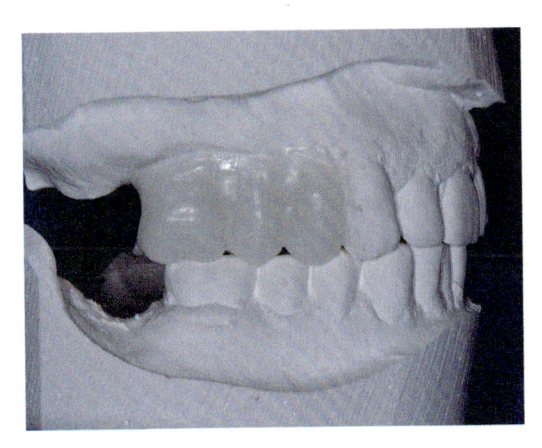

Figure 13.9 Diagnostic wax-up.

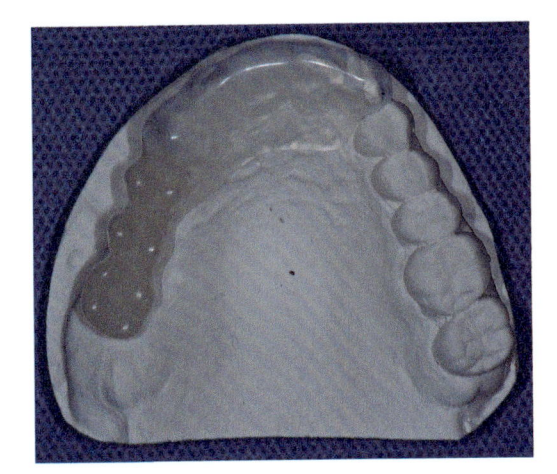

Figure 13.10 Surgical stent.

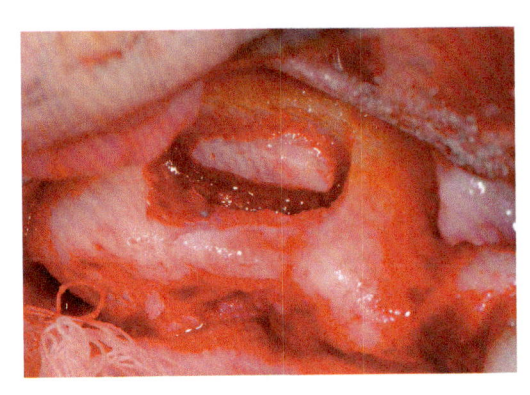

Figure 13.11 Lateral window osteotomy.

of implants should be based on the planned restoration. Due to the poor bone quality of the posterior maxilla, one implant is usually placed at each missing tooth site [25]. Cantilevers should be avoided, also due to the poor bone quality [26]. Alternatives to sinus lift procedures include a shorter implant, a fixed partial denture if a tooth is present posteriorly to the edentulous space, or a removal partial denture. The patient's expectations and goals of treatment are evaluated. The cost and length of treatment should be discussed with the patient as the treatment course can take over a year and be costly.

Lateral window technique (lateral or direct sinus lift)

The modified Caldwell–Luc approach is used to access the maxillary sinus. An incision is made originating from the mid-crestal region or slightly palatal. Anterior and posterior vertical releases are made away from the proposed osteotomy site in case the osteotomy needs to be enlarged and to avoid having a wound margin over the graft area. The vertical releases are flared so the base of the flap is wider than the apex of the flap. A full-thickness mucoperiosteal flap is then reflected to expose the lateral maxillary wall. An oval or round osteotomy is then used with a round diamond bur or piezoelectric instrument until the sinus membrane is encountered. The bony window can be obliterated, removed, or pushed into the sinus during membrane elevation. A curved instrument, such as a sinus curette, is used to gently reflect the sinus membrane. The membrane must be elevated from the sinus floor, but must also extend anteriorly, posteriorly, and medially to allow for adequate space for the graft material. The sinus floor is then grafted with the surgeon's choice of grafting material. The recommended amount of graft material to be placed is often between 2 and 5 ml depending on the extent of the edentulous area and amount of required implants to prevent overfilling and membrane necrosis [27]. If implants are placed at the same time as the graft, the graft material can be placed, especially on the medial aspect of the site, prior to placement of the implants. The bony window is then often covered with a resorbable collagen membrane and sutured to obtain primary closure. Figures 13.11 to 13.14 depict the lateral window technique and placement of a particulate bone graft. In some cases and based on the operator's preference, the outlined bone window is completely removed prior to membrane lift and sometimes it is elevated into the sinus.

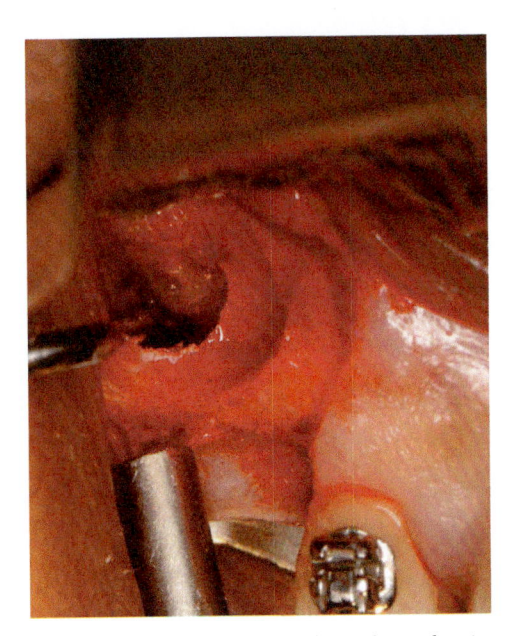

Figure 13.12 Lateral window osteotomy with membrane elevation.

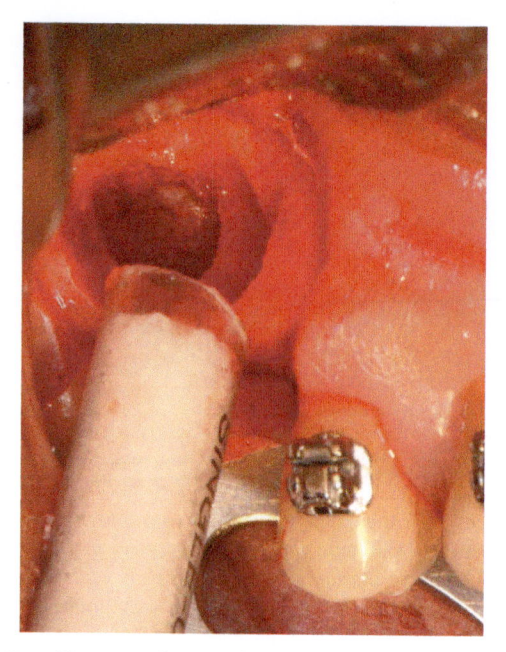

Figure 13.13 Placement of a particulate bone graft.

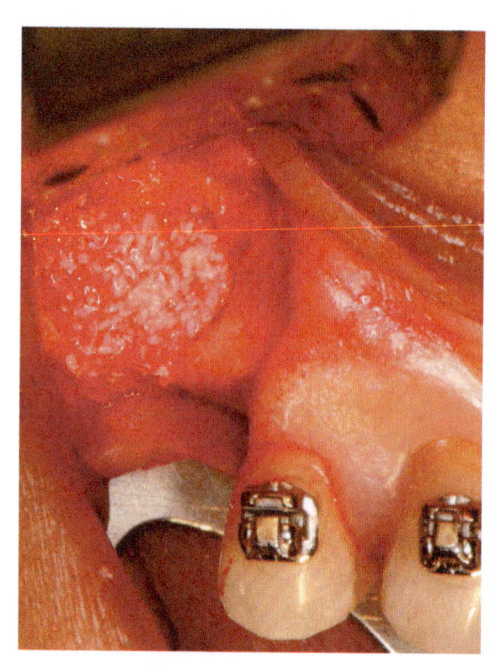

Figure 13.14 Particulate bone graft in place.

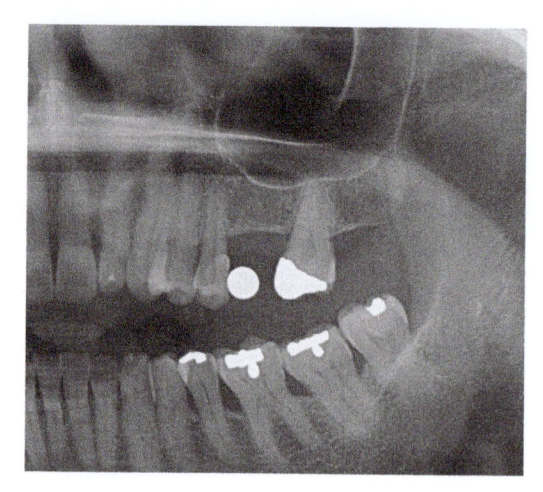

Figure 13.15 Panoramic radiograph in preparation for a crestal sinus lift with osteotomes (Summer's technique).

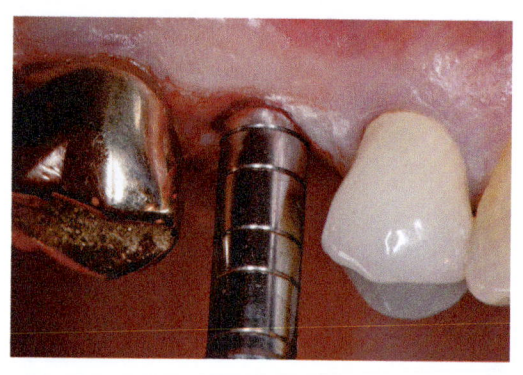

Figure 13.16 Clinical photo with an osteotome being used for a crestal sinus lift.

Crestal approach (crestal or indirect sinus lift)

The crestal approach was developed to achieve an indirect sinus lift using osteotomes in areas where there is at least 4 to 5 mm of bone height [4]; 3 to 7 mm of vertical augmentation along the sinus floor can be obtained [28, 29]. The crestal approach procedure is less invasive than the lateral window approach and has a much lower complication rate with minimal risk of Schneiderian membrane perforation when surgical protocols are followed [30].

The procedure begins with a crestal incision over the proposed site with reflection of the mucoperiosteal flap buccally and palatally to have access to the alveolar crest. Large areas of exposure are not required. The surgeon can then use specifically designed sinus osteotomes in increasing diameter to create an osteotomy. The surgeon stabilizes the sinus osteotome while the assistant uses the mallet to gently tap on to the osteotome as the bone tunnel develops. If the smallest sinus osteotome is unable to penetrate the cortical bone, a drill may be used to initiate the osteotomy. A pilot drill can be used to create an implant osteotomy 2 mm short of the sinus floor and is followed by the use of the sinus osteotomes. The displacement and compaction of bone occurs peripherally around the osteotome, but also apically toward the sinus membrane as bone is cleaved from the walls of the osteotomy and pushed toward the apex (Figures 13.15 and 13.16). This leads to elimination of the bone barrier and displacement of the sinus membrane superiorly and into the sinus. Bone from the pilot drill and xenograft material can then be gently packed into the osteotomy using the sinus osteotomes to further elevate the membrane and allow for increased augmentation of the sinus floor. The surgeon should be gentle with the mallet to advance no more than 1 mm apically with each strike of the mallet to avoid membrane perforation. The osteotomes must be placed at the same angle during the procedure to avoid creating an oval osteotomy instead of a round osteotomy. Irrigation is not required. Pre-operative and intraoperative radiographs with a depth gauge help to guide the surgeon on the appropriate depth of the osteotomy.

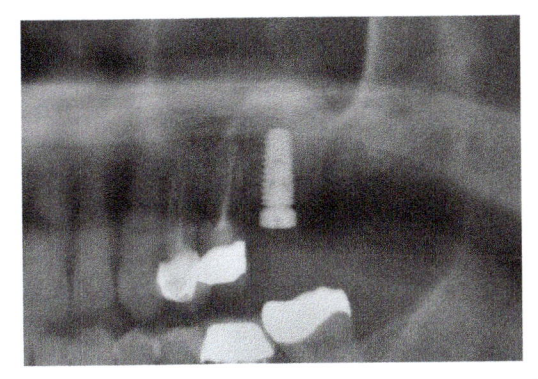

Figure 13.17 Post-operative panoramic radiograph showing the implant placed simultaneously with a crestal sinus lift and increased bone height.

Placement of implants can be performed after the indirect sinus lift is completed (Figure 13.17). The osteotomy should be undersized when compared to the diameter of the proposed implant. Primary stability must be achieved in order to place implants. This approach to the sinus lift usually requires approximately 5 mm of crestal bone height present for a 10 mm dental root-form implant [30].

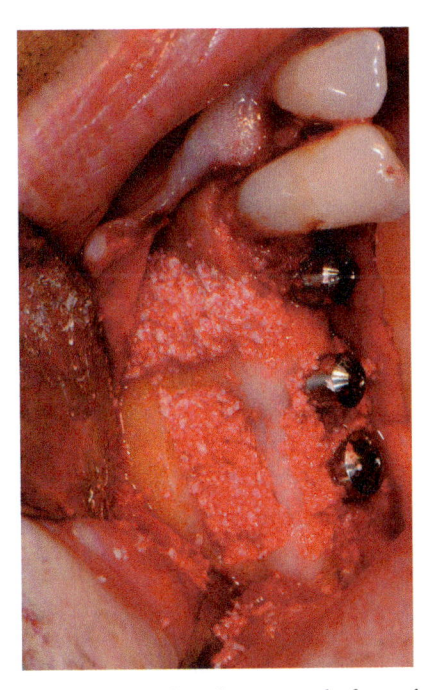

Figure 13.18 Simultaneous implant placement at the first molar and first and second premolar sites and buccal ridge augmentation.

Simultaneous versus delayed implant placement

The surgeon has three options for implant placement and grafting of the maxillary sinus: two-stage lateral sinus augmentation, one-stage lateral sinus augmentation with simultaneous implant placement, and a one-stage osteotome technique with simultaneous implant placement. Table 13.1 shows the advantages and disadvantages of each procedure [31].

The choice to place implants simultaneously with sinus lift procedures or during a second surgery mainly depends on the quantity and quality of the residual alveolar bone. In general, 4 to 5 mm is considered the minimal amount of vertical bone height needed for simultaneous sinus grafting and implant placement [31]. Some surgeons have had success placing simultaneous implants in ridges with less alveolar height. The key for implant success is to obtain primary stability to allow for initiation of osseointegration. Figure 13.18 demonstrates implants placed simultaneously during a lateral window sinus lift procedure.

Guidelines that are based on the vertical height of the residual alveolar ridge can be used as described by Achong and Block [31]. If the alveolar bone height is less than 3 mm, a two-stage procedure consisting of lateral sinus augmentation, 6 months of consolidation, implant placement, 4 months of integration, and restoration of implants should be used. If the alveolar bone height is 3 to 4 mm, a one-stage procedure consisting of lateral sinus augmentation, simultaneous implant placement, 6 months of integration, and restoration of implants should be used. If there is 5 mm or greater of alveolar bone height, a one-stage procedure consisting of indirect sinus lift with osteotomes, implant placement, 6 months of integration, and implant restoration should be used. These are only guidelines and each surgeon has their own protocols based on their own surgical skills and experience.

Delayed implants are used when there is minimal height of native bone in the maxilla and are more successful when compared to implants placed simultaneously [31]. However, some studies have reported similar success rates. In general, it is recommended that sites with very thin bone (less than 3 mm) be treated with delayed implant placement. Delaying implant placement for greater than 8 months has been shown to result in a better success rate (97%) than implants placed with a delay of 4 to 8 months (84%) [32].

Simultaneous indirect implant placement with sinus lift osteotomes via the crestal approach is a very successful procedure. A multicenter study including nine surgeons from eight institutions

Table 13.1 Advantages and disadvantages of different sinus grafting techniques: one-stage lateral antrostomy: implant placed simultaneously with *lateral* sinus lift; two-stage lateral antrostomy: implant placed several months after *lateral* sinus lift; one-stage osteotome technique: implant is usually placed at the time of *crestal* sinus lift.

Technique	Advantages	Disadvantages
Two-stage lateral antrostomy technique (less than 3 mm of bone)	Augmented site has increased bone density Controlled sinus elevation over a broad area	Increased surgical time Longer treatment time Increased risk of sinus membrane perforation
One-stage lateral antrostomy technique (3–4 mm of bone present)	Reduced treatment period	May be difficult to obtain primary stability Technically difficult Increased risk of implant failure
One-stage osteotome technique (bone is above 4–5 mm)	Less invasive Reduced treatment period Shorter healing time More confined area of augmentation	No visibility of membrane Amount of elevation and augmentation is limited

placed 174 implants in 101 patients using the crestal approach [33]. Bone height was found to increase 1 to 7 mm after augmentation. Implants placed using this technique had a success rate of 85.7% in areas of 4 mm or less of bone height and a success rate of 96% in areas of 5 mm or more of bone height. There was no difference in the amount of increased bone height when comparing the different types of graft materials that were used for augmentation. Other studies have shown success rates from 92 to 97% for simultaneous implant placement after indirect sinus lifts when the initial bone height was at least 5 mm [31, 34]. If bone was less than 4 mm in height or less, the procedure was less successful with rates from 73 to 86% [32, 35]. The use of tapered implants appears to compress the crestal bone and aid in obtaining primary stability, unlike non-tapered implants.

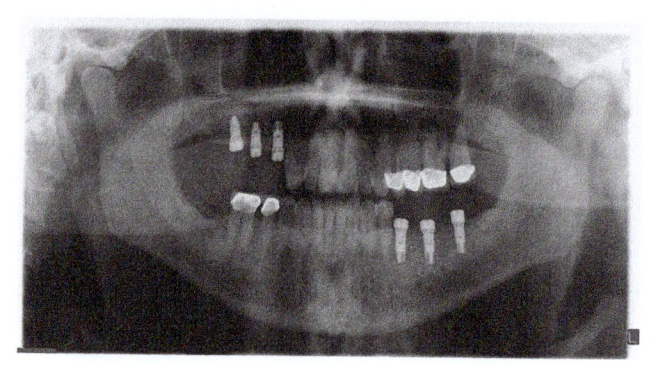

Figure 13.19 Post-operative panoramic radiograph showing implant fixtures and sinus graft.

Sinus lift at the time of tooth removal

The maxillary sinus is often pneumatized between the roots of the maxillary teeth. There may be minimal bone remaining in the extraction site once the tooth is removed. This area will often require augmentation and sinus elevation.

If there is a sufficient amount of inter-radicular bone (4 to 5 mm), then this area can be used to elevate the sinus membrane while being intruded into the maxillary sinus. A small chisel osteotome or a trephine is used to fracture the central portion of the inter-radicular bone. A blunt, round osteotome can then be used to gently intrude the bone fragment superiorly, thus elevating the sinus floor. This procedure can be used to elevate the membrane approximately 5 mm [35]. Although placement of a particulate bone graft is not necessary, placement of the graft with a membrane may aid in preventing resorption of the buccal plate. The area is allowed to heal for 4 to 6 months prior to implant placement. If there is still insufficient bone for implant placement, an additional osteotome technique for an indirect sinus lift can be used if additional vertical height of bone is needed.

Post-operative care

Post-operatively, the patient is informed to avoid hard foods and try to chew on the contralateral side. Patients are given strict sinus precautions and informed to avoid blowing their nose and sneezing. If the patient must sneeze, the mouth should be opened to decrease the amount of pressure in the sinuses. Other activities to avoid are swimming, strenuous exercise, diving, and changing altitude (flying, mountain hiking). The patient may experience pain, swelling, and ecchymosis. Ice can be placed on the face to decrease post-operative edema. The patient should also keep the head elevated for 2 to 3 days to decrease edema. A small amount of bleeding is common and subsides with gentle gauze pressure. A one-week course of antibiotics (amoxicillin 500 mg three times daily or clindamycin 300 mg three times daily) should be prescribed.

Post-operative imaging can be obtained in the form of a panoramic radiograph or CT to confirm the correct placement and volume of the bone graft. Figures 13.19 and 13.20 show a post-operative panoramic radiograph and cone beam CT, respectively, after simultaneous sinus lift/bone graft and implant placement. Radiographic imaging should also be obtained prior to implant restoration. Figure 13.21 shows the final restoration of maxillary implants and the radiopaque uniform sinus bone graft material that was placed 8 months prior.

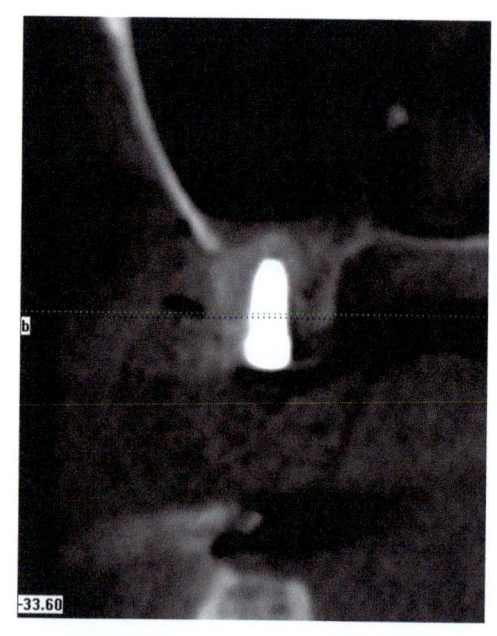

Figure 13.20 Post-operative CBCT scan showing implant fixture at the first molar site and sinus graft.

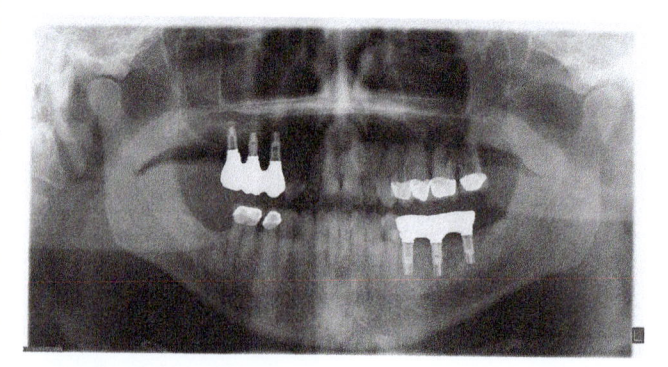

Figure 13.21 Three-unit fixed partial denture (an implant bridge) to restore the maxillary right first molar and first and second premolar sites placed 8 months post-operatively. The radiopaque sinus bone graft material can be visualized in the sinus.

References

1. Mavrodi A, Paraskeva G: Evolution of the paranasal sinuses' anatomy through the ages. *Anat Cell Biol* 2013;**46**:235–238.
2. Tatum H Jr: Maxillary and sinus implant reconstruction. *Dent Clin North Am* 1986;**30**:207.
3. Boyne PJ, James RA: Grafting of the maxillary sinus floor with autogenous marrow and bone. *J Oral Surg* 1980;**38**:613–616.
4. Summers RB: A new concept in maxillary implant surgery: the osteotome technique. *Compend Contin Educ Dent* 1994;**15**:152.
5. Zinner ID, Shapiro HJ, Gold SD: Sinus graft complications. Problem solving. *NY State Dental J* 2008;**74**:40–43.
6. Cauwenberge PV, Sys L, De Belder T, et al: Anatomy and physiology of the nose and paranasal sinuses. *Immunol Allergy Clin N Am* 2004;**24**:1–17.
7. Ogle OE, Weinstock RJ, Friedman E: Surgical anatomy of the nasal cavity and paranasal sinuses. *Oral Maxillofacial Surg Clin N Am* 2012;**24**:155–166.
8. Velasquez-Plata D, Hovey LR, Peach CC, et al: Maxillary sinus septa: a 3-dimensional computerized tomographic scan analysis. *Int J Oral Maxillofac Implants* 2002:**17**:854–860.
9. Park YB, Jeon HS, Shim JS, et al: Analysis of the anatomy of the maxillary sinus septum using 3-dimensional computed tomography. *J Oral Maxillofac Surg* 2011;**69**:1070–1078.
10. Fugazzotto P, Melnick PR, Al-Sabbagh M: Complications when augmenting the posterior maxilla. *Dent Clin N Am* 2015;**59**;97–130.
11. Morgensen E, Tos M: Quantitative histology of the maxillary sinus. *Rhinology* 1977;**15**:129.
12. Tiwana, PS, Kushner GM, Haug, RH: Maxillary sinus augmentation. *Dent Clin N Am* 2006;**50**:409–424.
13. Ulm CW, Solar P, Gsellmann B, et al: The edentulous maxillary alveolar process in the region of the maxillary sinus – a study of the physical dimension. *Int J Oral Maxillofac Surg* 1995;**24**:279–282.
14. Misch, CE, Chiapasco M, Jensen OT: Indications for and classification of sinus bone grafts, Chapter 4. In: Jensen OT (ed.), *The Sinus Bone Graft*, 2nd edn. Quintessence Publishing Co., Chicago, IL, 2006, pp. 41–51.
15. Misch CE: Density of bone: effect on treatment plans, surgical approach, healing and progressive loading. *Int J Oral Implantol* 1990;**6**:23–31.
16. Misch CE: Bone density. In: Misch CE (ed.), *Contemporary Implant Dentistry*, 2nd edn. Mosby, St. Louis, MI, 1999, pp. 329–343.
17. Scott I, Ash MM Jr: A six-channel intra-oral transmitter for measuring occlusal forces. *J Prosthet Dent* 1966;**16**:56.
18. Anderson DJ: Measurements of stress in mastication. *J Dent Res* 1958;**35**:644–671.
19. Watzek G, Furst G, Gruber, R: Biologic basis of sinus grafting, Chapter 2. In: Jensen OT (ed.), *The Sinus Bone Graft*, 2nd edn. Quintessence Publishing Co., Chicago, IL, 2006, pp. 13–26.
20. Chanavaz M: Anatomy and histophysiology of the periosteum: quantification of the periosteal blood supply to the adjacent bone with 85Sr and gamma spectrometry. *J Oral Implantol* 1995;**21**:214–219.
21. Misch, CM: Maxillofacial donor sites for sinus floor and alveolar econstruction, Chapter 11. In: Jensen OT (ed.), *The Sinus Bone Graft*, 2nd edn. Quintessence Publishing Co., Chicago, IL, 2006, pp. 129–145.
22. Chiapasco M, Rosenlicht JL, Ruggiero SL, et al: Contraindications for sinus graft procedures, Chapter 8. In: Jensen OT (ed.), *The Sinus Bone Graft*, 2nd edn. Quintessence Publishing Co., Chicago, IL, 2006, pp. 87–101.
23. Tawil G, Younan R, Azar P, et al: Conventional and advanced implant treatment in the type II diabetic patient: surgical protocol and long-term clinical results. *Int J Oral Maxillofac Implants* 2008;**23**:744–752.
24. Regev E, Smith RA, Perrott DH, et al: Maxillary sinus complications related to endosseous implants. *Int J Oral Maxillofac Implants* 1995;**10**(4):451–461.
25. Zinner AD, Small SA, Landa LS: Prosthetic management of the sinus graft patient, Chapter 7. In: Jensen OT (ed.), *The Sinus Bone Graft*, 2nd edn. Quintessence Publishing Co., Chicago, IL, 2006, pp. 75–85.
26. Small SA, Zinner ID, Panno FV, et al: Augmenting the maxillary sinus for implants: report of 27 patients. *Int J Oral Maxillofac Implants* 1993;**8**:843–848.
27. Ardekian, L, Efrat OP, Mactei EE, et al: The clinical significance of sinus membrane perforation during augmentation of the maxillary sinus. *J Oral Maxillofac Surg* 2006;**64**:277–282.
28. Komarnyckyi OG, London RM: Osteotome single-stage dental implant placement with and without sinus elevation: a clinical report. *Int J Oral Maxillofac Implants* 1998;**13**:799–804.
29. Moy PK, Lundgren S, Holmes RE: Maxillary sinus augmentation: histomorphometric analysis of graft materials for sinus floor augmentation. *J Oral Maxillofac Surg* 1993;**13**:799–804.
30. Summers RB: Osteotome technique for site development and sinus floor augmentation, Chapter 22. In: Jensen OT (ed.), *The Sinus Bone Graft*, 2nd edn. Quintessence Publishing Co., Chicago, IL, 2006, pp. 263–272.
31. Achong RM, Block MS: Sinus floor augmentation: simultaneous versus delayed implant placement, Chapter 5. In: Jensen OT (ed.), *The Sinus Bone Graft*, 2nd edn. Quintessence Publishing Co., Chicago, IL, 2006, pp. 53–66.
32. Jensen OT, Shulman LB, Block MS, et al: Report of the Sinus Consensus Conference of 1996. *Int J Oral Maxillofac Implants* 1998;**13**(Suppl):11–45.
33. Rosen PS, Summers R, Mellado RJ, et al: The bone added osteotome sinus floor elevation technique: multicenter retrospective of consecutively treated patients. *Int J Oral Maxillofac Implants* 1999;**14**:853–858.
34. Wallace SS, Froum SJ: Effect of maxillary sinus augmentation on the survival of endosseous dental implants. *A systematic review. Ann Periodontal* 2003;**8**:328–343.
35. Fugazzotto P, Jensen OT: Sinus floor augmentation at the time of tooth removal, Chapter 6. In: Jensen OT (ed.), *The Sinus Bone Graft*, 2nd edn. Quintessence Publishing Co., Chicago, IL, 2006, pp. 67–74.

CHAPTER 14

Crestal Sinus Floor Elevation: Osteotome Technique

Michael Beckley[1] and Len Tolstunov[2]

[1]Department of Oral and Maxillofacial Surgery, University of the Pacific, Arthur A. Dugoni School of Dentistry Private Practice, Oral and Maxillofacial Surgery, Livermore, California, USA

[2]Department of Oral and Maxillofacial Surgery, University of California San Francisco, School of Dentistry, University of the Pacific, Arthur A. Dugoni School of Dentistry Private Practice, Oral and Maxillofacial Surgery, San Francisco, California, USA

Introduction

Implant placement in the posterior maxilla is often a challenge due to sinus expansion or pneumatization after loss of posterior maxillary teeth. There are many ways to elevate the sinus and augment the bone vertically in posterior maxilla. This chapter will describe the crestal or indirect (transalveolar) sinus floor elevation technique using special osteotomes. This technique can be used either in edentulous sites as a transalveolar sinus floor elevation with bone grafting and immediate implant placement or in the dentate region as a trans-socket sinus floor elevation with bone grafting and, usually, delayed implant placement. Below is the description of both techniques.

Crestal sinus floor elevation, grafting, and implant placement using the osteotome technique

Adequate bone volume is required for successful implant placement and osseointegration. The quantity of bone in the posterior maxilla is often inadequate for implant placement due to the position and size of the maxillary sinus. Crestal sinus floor elevation is a simple and predictable technique to increase vertical bone height and increase alveolar width in the posterior maxilla. This technique can be utilized to place implants with or without bone grafting. A variation of this technique can be employed at the time of tooth extraction. Grafting and, occasionally, implant placement can be combined with crestal sinus floor elevation at the time of tooth extraction [1].

History

In 1986, H. Tatum [2] described the first technique for transalveolar maxillary sinus lift and subsequent placement of implants. In 1994, R.B. Summers [3] developed a technique utilizing modified osteotomes to compact bone laterally and apically in the maxillary sinus with residual bone heights of 5–6 mm (Figure 14.1). A success rate of 96% was reported at 5 years with 143 titanium plasma sprayed (TPS) implants placed in 46 patients. Implants placed in sites that have been augmented with crestal sinus elevation have success rates ranging from 92 to 97% [4].

Indications and contraindications

Prior to surgery the patient's medical history should be reviewed. There are very few absolute contraindications to crestal sinus elevation. Common systemic contraindications include the following conditions when presented in an uncontrolled state: hypertension, diabetes mellitus, thyroid disease, and adrenal disease. Other conditions can include coagulopathies, immunocompromised diseases, substance abuse, neoplastic disease, early or late pregnancy, and untreated mental illness. In general, patients with well-controlled chronic diseases are candidates for sinus elevation and grafting. Anatomic and local contraindications include: acute sinusitis, non-patent osteomeatal complex, residual bone height less than 4 mm, prior radiation therapy, and incomplete craniofacial growth.

Ideally, acute or chronic sinusitis should be resolved prior to surgery. This may not be possible in all situations. However, if there is any doubt about the patency of the osteomeatal complex, treatment should be postponed until the sinus disease is treated. ENT (ear, nose, and throat) consultation may be needed in these cases.

Applied surgical anatomy

Sinus means "pocket" in Latin. The maxillary sinus is usually the largest of the paranasal sinuses. The average height of the adult maxillary sinus is 33 mm, width 23 mm, and 34 mm from anterior to posterior. The second premolar and first and second molars are the teeth most often in proximity to the sinus and often the cause of odontogenic sinusitis. The relationship of the floor of the sinus to teeth is variable. The tooth roots may be covered in bone or project into the sinus with little or no bone covering them. Ridges and septa are common and may partition the sinus into two compartments. These may pose challenges when elevating and grafting the sinus floor. Pre-operative three-dimensional imaging can be helpful in identifying septa and ridges (Figure 14.2). The innervation and blood supply is from the posterior superior alveolar, infraorbital, and anterior superior alveolar arteries and nerves. The maxillary sinus is very small until the secondary dentition appears and develops its final form after the eruption of permanent dentition [5]. After tooth removal and with aging, the sinus may enlarge or become more pneumatized [6].

Vertical Alveolar Ridge Augmentation in Implant Dentistry: A Surgical Manual, First Edition. Edited by Len Tolstunov.
© 2016 John Wiley & Sons, Inc. Published 2016 by John Wiley & Sons, Inc.

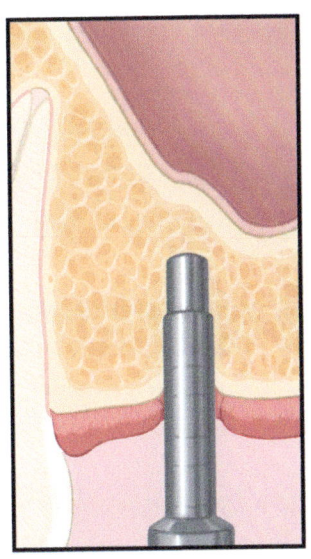

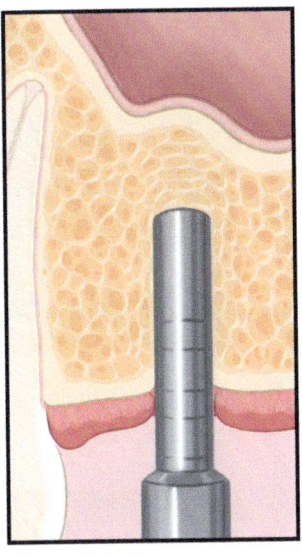

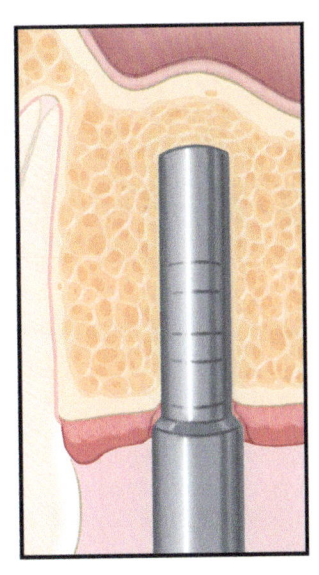

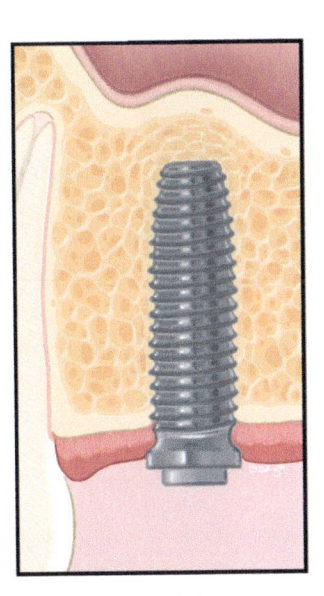

Figure 14.1 An illustration demonstrating the subantral maxillary alveolar bone that is compressed apically and laterally with progressively larger osteotomes. After the osteotomy has been prepared, the implant is placed.

The ostium of the maxillary sinus deserves particular attention because a patent ostium is necessary for a healthy sinus. The ostium is located in the superior part of the medial wall of the sinus and opens into the middle meatus, draining into the nasal cavity through the ethmoid infundibulum. The location of the osteomeatal complex (OMC) does not allow for gravity-dependent sinus drainage. Drainage of the maxillary sinus is primarily through the mucociliary action. The sinus is lined with pseudostratified ciliated columnar epithelium with many goblet cells and an underlying connective tissue layer with many mucous glands. The lining of the sinus is commonly referred as the Schneiderian membrane [7, 8]. A correlation between Schneiderian membrane thickness and gingival phenotype has been reported [9].

Graft sources

Grafting is often combined with crestal floor elevation. Many biologic and synthetic materials have been used for sinus grafting. Graft sources can be divided into the following categories:

- Autogenous bone (intraoral, extraoral sites)
- Allografts (human cadaveric)
- Xenografts (bovine, equine, porcine)
- Biomimetics (bone morphogenetic protein, others)

Bone graft physiology is beyond the scope of this chapter. It is important to note that at this time no particular graft material has demonstrated clinical superiority in sinus grafting [10].

Crestal (indirect or transalveolar) sinus floor elevation with implant placement

Crestal sinus floor elevation can be performed with local anesthesia or local anesthesia combined with intravenous sedation. Currently, there is no standard of care for pre-operative imaging prior to sinus elevation, grafting, and implant placement. Decisions regarding pre-operative imaging should be patient specific and based on the clinician's experience. The available scientific evidence supports antibiotic administration prior to bone grafting and implant surgery. Antibiotics in the penicillin family are commonly used [11–13]. Clindamycin is a good alternative in patients with a penicillin allergy. Whether a course of post-operative antibiotics should be administered is controversial.

The following case illustrates crestal sinus floor elevation with immediate implant placement to replace a missing right maxillary second premolar. A cone beam computed tomography (CBCT) scan demonstrated the distance of 7 mm to the sinus floor (Figure 14.2).

Figure 14.2 Cone beam computed tomographic (CBCT) image of alveolar bone of the edentulous right maxillary second premolar.

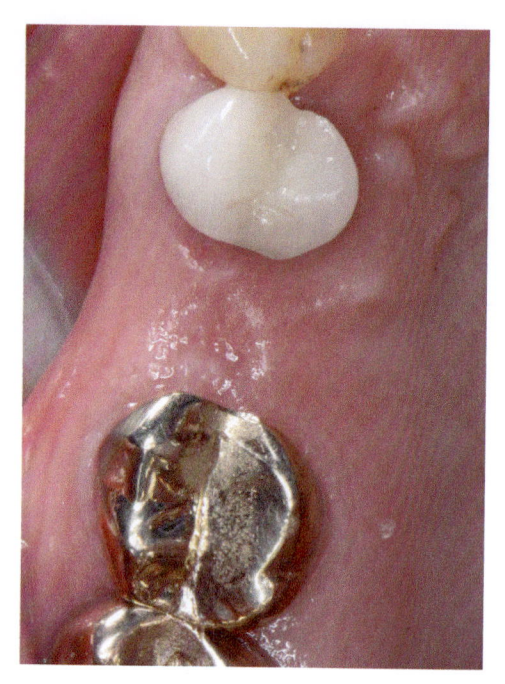

Figure 14.3 This pre-operative clinical image shows the edentulous right maxillary second premolar site.

We planned to place an implant of 13 mm length after crestal sinus floor elevation, thus lifting the sinus floor almost two times that of the native bone that was present. After the surgical site was confirmed (Figure 14.3), a small incision with reflection of the full-thickness mucoperiosteal flap or a punch hole of the occlusal soft tissue can be made to expose the alveolar crest. The authors prefer to hold the osteotome and mallet while the assistant retracts the soft tissue (Figure 14.4). It is important to advance the osteotome slowly and with control to avoid inadvertent perforation of the sinus floor and Schneiderian membrane or damage to adjacent teeth. The goal is to move the alveolar bone apically into the sinus and condense it circumferentially. After each osteotome is advanced to the predetermined depth, the next larger osteotome is placed. Each osteotome usually has markings that help to determine the depth and advancement of the instrument. It should also be correlated to the implant length. The final osteotome should be smaller in diameter than the implant to be placed (Figure 14.5). This allows for adequate primary stabilization. Primary implant stability is important for implant success. The next step is implant placement (Figure 14.6). Small corrections in the axial inclination of the implant can be made during implant placement, when indicated. Often a particular bone graft should be placed into the osteotomy prior to or after an implant placement. If adequate torque is achieved, a healing abutment can be placed at the same time (Figure 14.7). If insertion torque is low, the

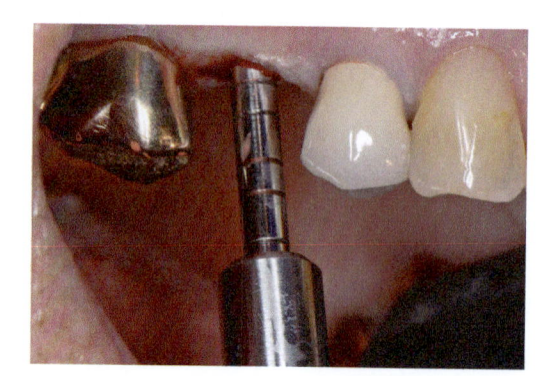

Figure 14.4 The initial osteotome is placed and tapped to a predetermined depth based on the pre-operative image.

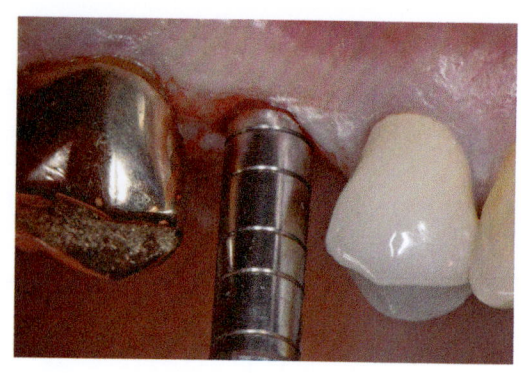

Figure 14.5 The final osteotome diameter is less than that of the implant to be placed. This facilitates initial implant stability.

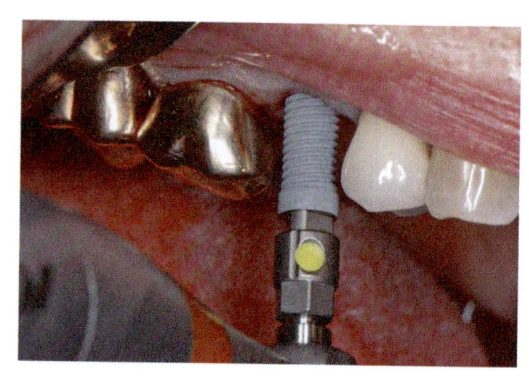

Figure 14.6 A 4.0 mm × 13 mm implant is placed after the final osteotomy is completed.

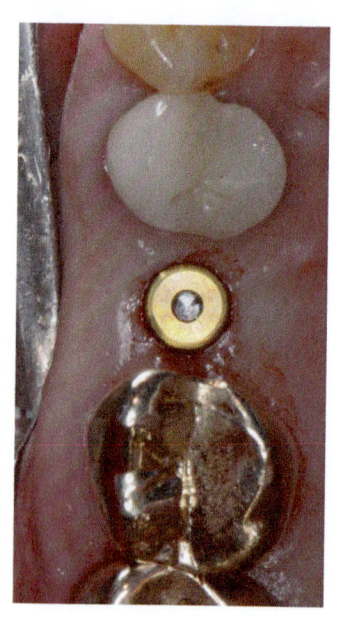

Figure 14.7 Implant healing abutment in place.

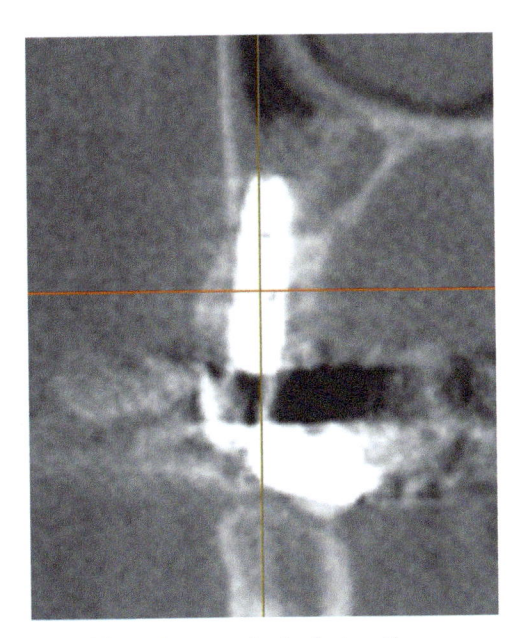

Figure 14.8 CBCT scan demonstrating implant position.

implant can be left submerged after cover screw placement. A postoperative CBCT image demonstrates the position of the premolar implant and its relation to the maxillary sinus (Figure 14.8).

Trans-socket sinus floor elevation with bone grafting after extraction

This is a useful technique to elevate the sinus floor with simultaneous bone grafting at the time of an atraumatic tooth removal. The key concept to making this a successful procedure is preserving the bony socket and, especially, the buccal and interseptal bone. Buccal bone preservation optimizes the grafting procedure and contributes to the success of bone preservation and optimal implant insertion. The interseptal bone can have two purposes in these cases. One purpose relates to it as an internal strut of autogenous (native) bone inside the socket, which helps the bone grafting procedure by compartmentalizing the socket. It has to be stable enough to accomplish this goal. Thicker interseptal bone is preferred and trans-socket sinus elevation is accomplished by careful elevation of the sinus floor mainly through the mesial and distal buccal root sockets. Preservation of the interseptal socket bone is advised during the sinus lift.

The second purpose is to use the interseptal bone as a channel former (a compressing tool) for sinus elevation, similar to a crestal sinus floor elevation described above (Figure 14.9). In this case, the septal bone in the middle of the socket will be pushed superiorly with the residual alveolar bone below the sinus floor by osteotomes to lift it. In both cases, an atraumatic extraction of a tooth by using periotomes and the tooth sectioning technique helps to prevent buccal plate fracture and removal of the interseptal bone.

The following case demonstrates this technique after removal of a failing left maxillary first molar. Pre-operative radiographs help planning the surgery by measuring the distance from the alveolar crest around the tooth and tooth furcation to the sinus floor (Figure 14.10). Once the tooth is atraumatically removed, preserving the buccal and interseptal bone (Figure 14.11), modified

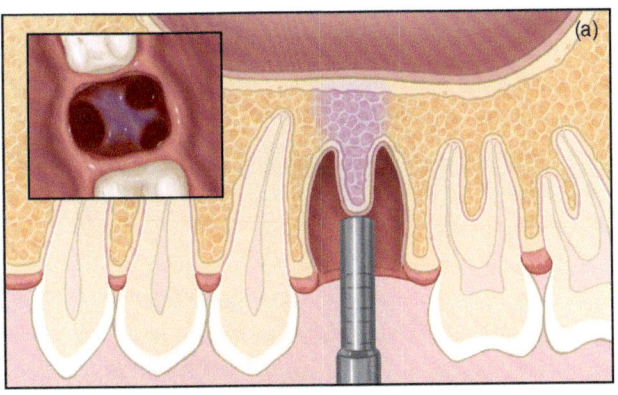

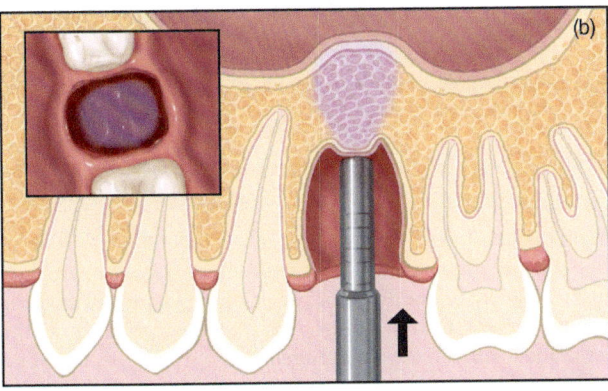

Figure 14.9 (a) Trans-socket sinus floor elevation technique that often utilizes the interseptal bone of a fresh extraction socket as a transport segment for sinus floor elevation similar to a crestal sinus floor elevation approach used in the edentulous regions: the inter-radicular (interseptal) bone here is about to be displaced apically by osteotomes. (b) Trans-socket sinus floor elevation technique where the inter-radicular (interseptal) bone is displaced apically "forcing" elevation of the Schneiderian membrane. The combined newly formed alveolar height consists of the periapical (peri-socket) bone height plus a height of the modified socket (that is also grafted). In the majority of cases, this new height is sufficient for an implant placement 4 to 6 months later.

osteotomes are used to elevate the sinus floor (Figure 14.12a). It is important to control the apical displacement of the osteotome (depth) by using the markings on the instrument (Figure 14.12b). It is also important to control the force applied to the osteotome

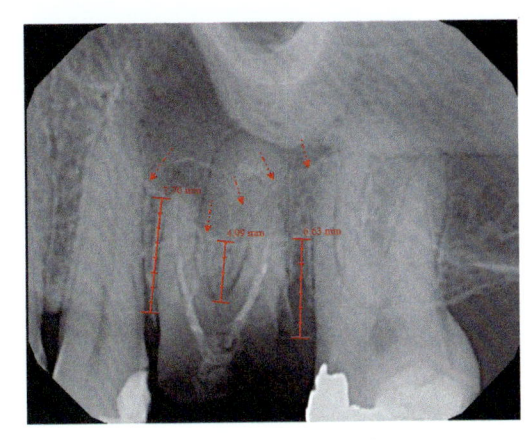

Figure 14.10 Failing left maxillary first molar with measurements to help in planning the crestal sinus lift.

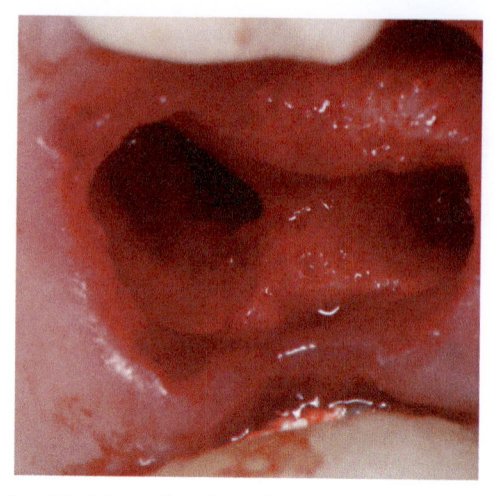

Figure 14.11 The left maxillary first molar was sectioned and the interseptal bone remains intact.

proceed with bone grafting (Figure 14.13a to e). Occasionally, the interseptal bone will need to be sectioned with a small burr or gently fractured so that it can be elevated superiorly.

After the sinus floor has been in-fractured, displaced, and elevated, the vertically enlarged socket is grafted with a bone graft material of the surgeon's choice (Figures 14.14 to 14.16). The surgical site is then closed. Closure may be accomplished with primary closure (less common) or secondary closure after placement of a barrier membrane to contain the graft with 4-0 chromic gut or silk (Figure 14.13e). Early post-operative radiographs can be taken to confirm sinus elevation and graft placement (Figure 14.17). The implant can be placed three to six months later (Figure 14.18). Reliable sinus floor elevation, ideally, should show "rebuilt" stable bone above apices of inserted endosseous implants ("snow capped peaks" effect) on a follow-up radiograph 6+ months later (Figure 14.19).

In some rare situations, tooth extraction, trans-socket sinus elevation, bone grafting, and implant placement can be done at the same time. The opportunity to combine these procedures is dependent on achieving proper implant orientation and primary implant stability.

(Figure 14.12c and d). Too much force will result in perforation of the Schneiderian membrane. This can compromise the bone grafting that follows. In case of a small (pinpoint) perforation of the sinus membrane (less than 4–5 mm), it is possible to close/cover the perforation with a collagen membrane (collagen plug or tape) and

Complications

Serious complications after crestal sinus floor elevation are rare. Potential complications include sinus infection, implant failure, implant displacement into the sinus, graft failure, sinus perforation,

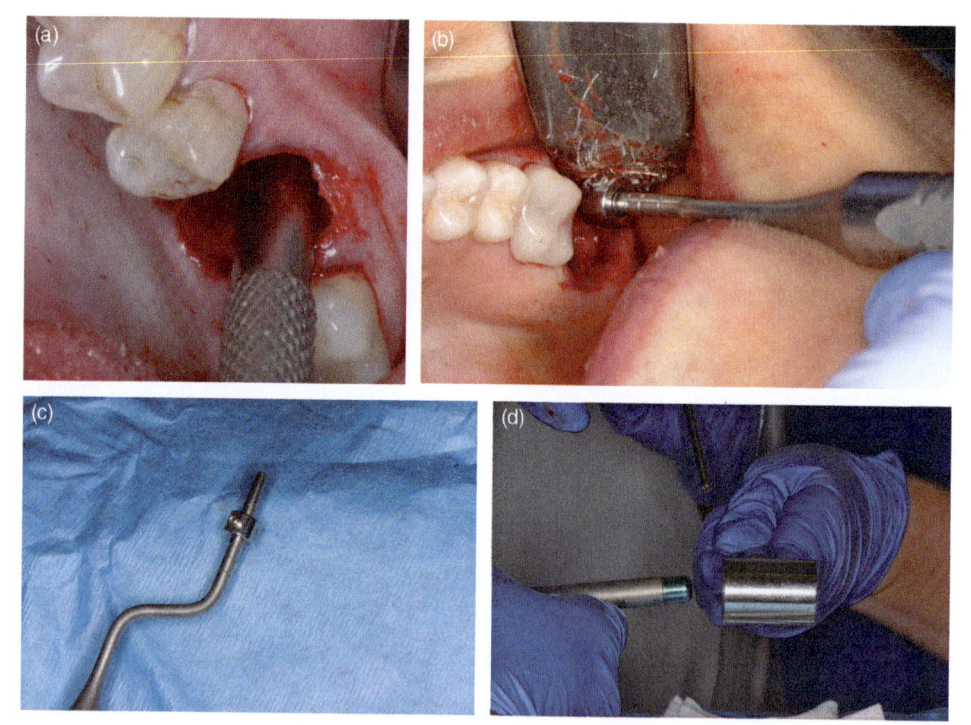

Figure 14.12 (a) Intraoral intraoperative photograph of the post-extraction trans-socket sinus floor elevation technique with a modified straight or curved cup osteotome strategically placed inside the socket for a careful tapping of the existing peri-socket bone apically towards the sinus floor. (b) Intraoral intraoperative photograph of the post-extraction trans-socket sinus floor elevation technique with a modified curved osteotome. It is important to control the apical displacement of the osteotome (depth) by using the markings on the instrument. Pre-operative measurement of the vertical bone between the sinus floor and the socket is very helpful in this sinus lift approach, (c) Example of a curved sinus osteotome that can be used for a trans-socket sinus floor elevation technique, (d) It is important to control the force applied to the osteotome by gentle and controlled tapping of the osteotome with a mallet.

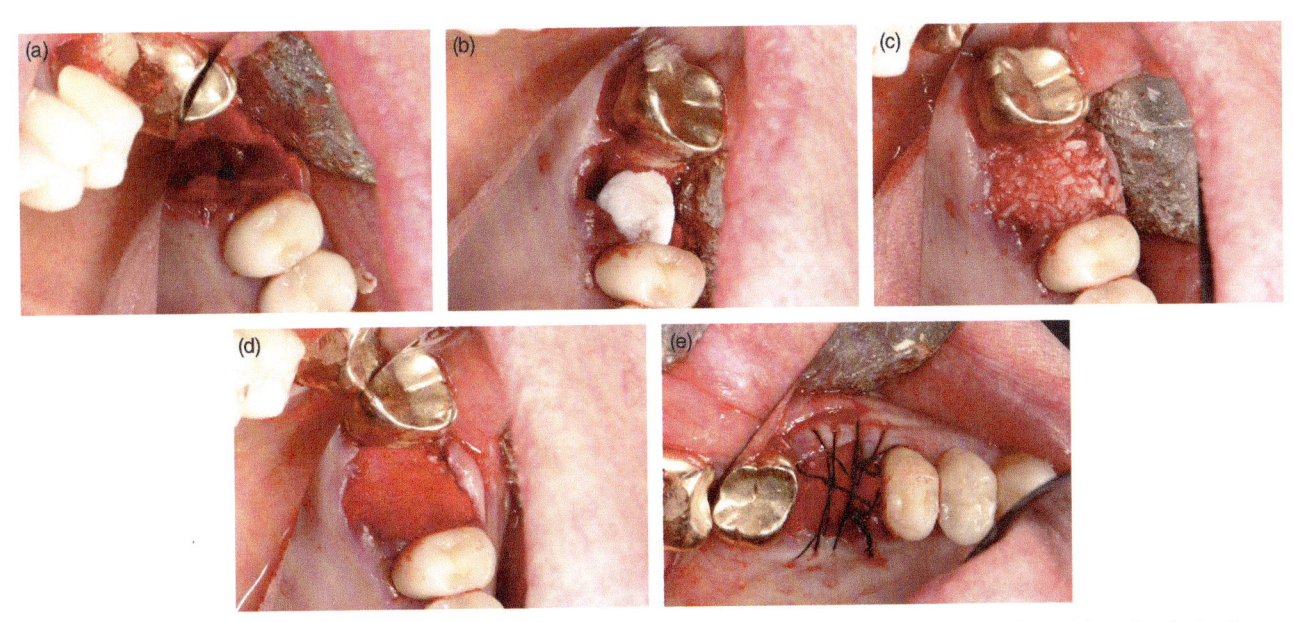

Figure 14.13 Management of a pinpoint perforation during trans-socket sinus floor elevation. (a) Periodic check of the floor of the socket during the tapping/elevation is mandatory for early discovery of the sinus membrane perforation. Pinpoint perforation (less than 4 mm) is seen in this intraoperative clinical photograph. (b) Use of a collagen plug is one of many choices of "membrane" to cover the pinpoint sinus perforation. (c) After a collagen plug, bone grafting material can be loosely placed into the socket. (d) After bone grafting material, a collagen or GTR membrane can be used to isolate the graft from the oral environment similar to any ridge preservation technique, (e) Use of a collagen plug to close the perforation, then socket bone grafting, followed by a collagen or GTR membrane, and, finally, silk sutures for closure, encouraging healing by secondary intention.

and buccal plate fracture. Another infrequent complication of osteotome use in the head region is vertigo secondary to otolith displacement, which can result in benign paroxysmal positional vertigo (BPPV) [14, 15]. If the condition does not improve, an Epley maneuver (head exercises) may need to be performed to "reposition" the stones.

A recent meta-analysis, which included 3092 implants placed from 25 studies, calculated the implant failure rate utilizing osteotome-mediated sinus floor elevation to be 3.85% [16].

Conclusion

Crestal (indirect) or transalveolar sinus lift is a predictable and minimally invasive technique for subantral maxillary sinus augmentation. This technique is routinely and successfully performed in the edentulous posterior maxillary region with simultaneous implant insertion, but can also be implemented at the time of

Figure 14.14 Interseptal bone and socket after trans-socket sinus floor elevation.

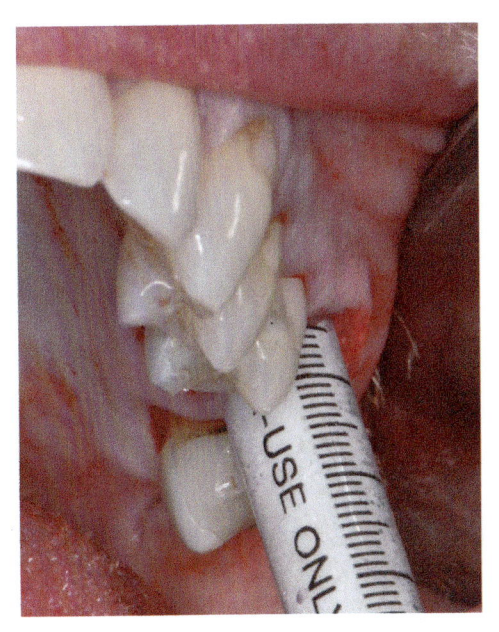

Figure 14.15 Bone graft is being placed into the socket after sinus floor elevation.

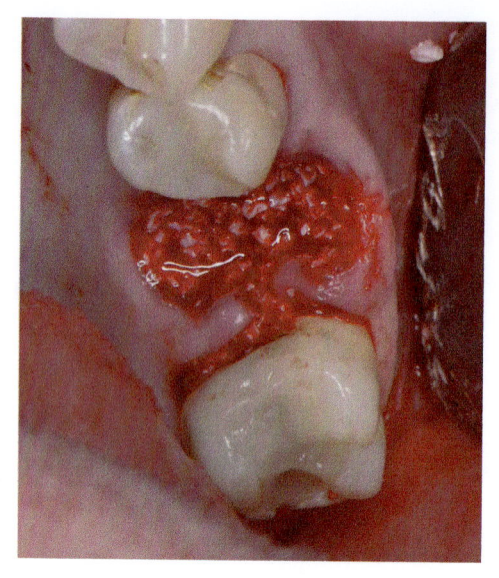

Figure 14.16 Completion of a socket bone grafting.

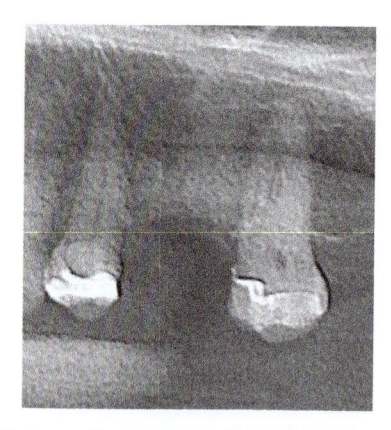

Figure 14.17 Post-operative imaging confirming sinus elevation and graft placement.

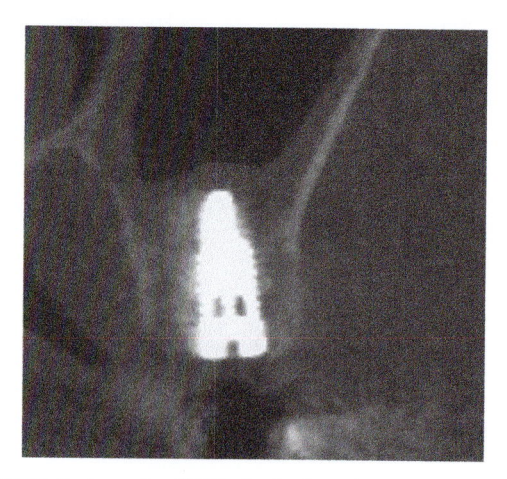

Figure 14.18 Postoperative CBCT after implant placement 3 to 6 months post sinus elevation and grafting.

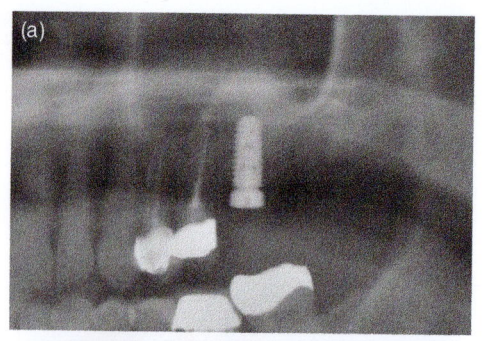

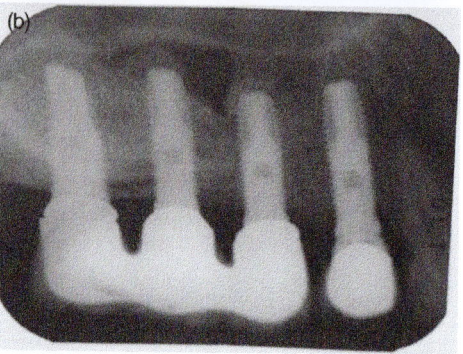

Figure 14.19 (a) Radiographic image of a "snow capped peak" on a follow-up radiograph 6+ months later indicates a well-healed (ossified) "elevated" bone after the transalveolar (crestal or trans-socket) sinus lift. The implant is placed and restored successfully "protected" by a stable peri-implant bone for lasting osseointegration. (b) Radiographic image of "snow capped peaks" of elevated and healed crestal bone above well-osseointegrated implants on a follow-up radiograph.

extraction as trans-socket sinus floor elevation with immediate bone graft and delayed dental implant placement. In addition to vertically augmenting the posterior maxillary ridge, some degree of lateral condensation of the surrounding bone is also achieved with this technique by direct bone compression. This might contribute to increased primary implant stability [17, 18]. Crestal sinus floor elevation appears to be a safe and effective technique of vertical modification of the posterior maxillary bone for implant placement.

References

1. Fugazzotto PA: Sinus floor augmentation at the time of tooth emoval, Chapter 6. In: Jensen OT (ed.), *The Sinus Bone Graft*, 2nd edn. Quintessence Publishing, Chicago, IL, 2006, pp. 67–85.
2. Tatum H Jr.: Maxillary and sinus implant reconstructions. *Dental Clinics of North America* 1986;**30**:207–229.
3. Summers RB: A new concept in maxillary implant surgery: the osteotomes technique. *Compendium Continuing Education Dentistry* 1994;**15**:152–160.
4. Raja SV: Management of the posterior maxilla with sinus lift: review of techniques. *Journal of Oral and Maxillofacial Surgery* 2009;**67**:1730–1734.
5. Hollinshead WH: The nose and paranasal sinuses, Chapter 4. In: Hollinshead WH (ed.), *Anatomy for Surgeons, The Head and Neck*, 3rd edn. Lippincott-Raven, Philadelphia, PA, 1982, pp. 259–265.
6. Krennmair G: The incidence, location, and height of maxillary sinus septa in the edentulous and dentate maxilla. *Journal of Oral and Maxillofacial Surgery* 1999;**57**:667–671.
7. Becker W: Nose, nasal sinus, and face, Chapter 2. In: Becker W (ed.), *Ear, Nose, and Throat Diseases*. Thieme Medical Publishers, Stuttgart, 1994, pp. 174–180.
8. Clemente CD: Part VII; The head and neck. In: Clemente CD (ed.), *Anatomy: A Regional Atlas of the Human Body*, 3rd edn. Lea and Feiberger, Philadelphia, 1987, pp. 686–689.

9 Aimetti M: Correlation between gingival phenotype and Schneiderian membrane thickness. *International Journal of Oral and Maxillofacial Implants* 2008;**23**(6):1128-1132.
10 Al-Nawas B: Augmentation procedures using bone substitute or autologous bone – A systematic review and meta-analysis. *European Journal of Oral Implantology* 2014 Summer; **7**(Suppl 2):S219-234, Review.
11 Lindeboom JA: A prospective placebo-controlled double-blind trial of antibiotic prophylaxis in intraoral bone grafting procedures: a pilot study. *Oral Surgery Oral Medicine Oral Pathology Oral Radiology and Endodontics* 2003 Dec;**96**(6):669-672.
12 Lindeboom JA: A randomized prospective controlled trial of antibiotic prophylaxis in intraoral bone-grafting procedures: preoperative single-dose penicillin versus preoperative single-dose clindamycin. *International Journal of Oral and Maxillofacial Surgery* 2006 May;**35**(5):433-436.
13 Sharaf B: Does the use of prophylactic antibiotics decrease implant failure? *Oral and Maxillofacial Surgery Clinics of North America* 2011 Nov;**23**(4):547-550.
14 Penarrocha M, Perez H, Gargia A: Benign paroxysmal positional vertigo as a complication of osteotome expansion of the maxillary alveolar ridge. *J Oral Maxillofac Surg* 2001;**59**:106-107.
15 Saker M, Ogle O: Benign paroxysmal positional vertigo subsequent to sinus lift via closed technique. *J Oral Maxillofac Surg* 2005 Sep;**63**(9):1385-1387.
16 Calin C: Osteotome-mediated sinus floor elevation: a systematic review and meta-analysis. *International Journal of Oral and Maxillofacial Implants* 2014 May–June;**29**(3):558-576.
17 Nevins M, Nevins ML, Schupback P, et al: The impact of bone compression on bone-to-implant contact of an osseointegrated implant: a cohort study. *Int J Periodontics Restorative Dent* 2012;**32**(6):637-645.
18 Nishioka RS, Kojima AN: Screw spreading: technical considerations and case report. *Int J Periodontics Restorative Dent* 2011;**31**(2):141-147.

CHAPTER 15

Flapless Crestal Sinus Augmentation: Hydraulic Technique

Byung-Ho Choi

Department of Oral and Maxillofacial Surgery, Yonsei University Wonju College of Medicine, Wonju, South Korea

Introduction

The optimization of maxillary sinus floor elevation protocols to achieve high implant success rates, minimize morbidity, shorten treatment periods, and allow for simultaneous implant placement is a constant challenge for clinicians. The author describes a flapless crestal sinus floor augmentation procedure using a hydraulic sinus elevation system. The minimally invasive flapless procedure significantly decreases post-operative discomfort and complications versus conventional open-flap surgery [1, 2]. In flapless crestal sinus augmentation surgery, both transcrestal osteotomy and sinus membrane elevation are performed via the implant osteotomy site without visual or tactile control [3]. For this reason, computer-guided surgery is mandatory, not just to guide drilling for implant placement but also to control the drill depth to the bony sinus floor when entering the bony sinus floor [4, 5]. To achieve high success rates in the flapless crestal sinus augmentation procedure, membrane integrity is a primary condition for success. In order to safely maintain membrane integrity, it is necessary to improve the techniques and instruments. This chapter addresses the techniques and instruments for successful flapless crestal sinus floor augmentation, using a hydraulic sinus elevation system combined with computer-guided implant surgery.

Surgical instruments

1 Osteotomy drill
2 Dome-shaped crestal approach bur
3 Hydraulic membrane lifter
4 Bone plugger, sinus curette
5 Stopper
6 Digital surgical guide

1. Osteotomy drill

This drill is used to drill to 1 mm short of the sinus floor. It comes with various lengths and diameters with a stop feature. The surgical guide guides the drill's depth, direction, and position.

2. Dome-shaped crestal approach bur

This bur is used to eliminate the remaining bone below the sinus floor (Figure 15.1). The bur has a round tip and vertical stop. The tip of the drill is characterized by a smooth cutting blade. This shape helps to avoid direct damage even if it comes in direct contact with the sinus membrane. The dome shape also makes it safe to use in either flat or steep bone walls. The bur also has a stop feature to control the drill depth through the surgical guide. To help control the drill depth precisely, a number of different stopper lengths are available. Using the stop feature and the stoppers, the drill depth can be controlled within a 1 mm range. The dome-shaped crestal approach bur has a 3.2 mm diameter, which is smaller than the diameter of implants placed in the maxillary premolar (Ø4.0 mm) and molar (Ø5.0 mm).

3. Hydraulic membrane lifter

This is for injecting liquid into the maxillary sinus. It is comprised of a syringe, tube, and a nozzle (Figure 15.2). The tip of the nozzle has a feature that can completely close the opening to the drill hole. Thus, it has a conical-shaped sealing part and an extension part that is inserted into the drill hole. The other end of the nozzle is connected with the tube, which is then connected to a saline-filled syringe. The nozzle also has a handle feature (Figure 15.3). The handle not only helps the nozzle to be positioned into the hole and secured in place but it also helps the nozzle to pressurize the opening area. The syringe should be a 5 ml disposable syringe. A 1 ml syringe is too small to apply sufficient pressure. In addition, if the extension part of the syringe that connects the tube to the syringe is too short, the tube can be easily separated when applying pressure. Therefore, if possible, use a syringe with an elongated connection part.

4. Bone plugger, sinus curette

A bone plugger is used to insert the bone-grafting material into the sinus cavity through the drill hole. A sinus curette is then used to disperse this bone-grating material in the sinus cavity (Figure 15.4). They have a stop feature to control the depth of insertion into the sinus cavity. Their diameters are Ø2.6 mm, which will allow entry into the Ø3.2 mm hole created by the 3.2 mm diameter, dome-shaped crestal approach bur. The head of the sinus curette has a dome shape.

5. Stopper

The stopper is designed to be able to connect to the crestal approach bur, bone plugger, or sinus curette. It also comes in varying lengths,

---

Vertical Alveolar Ridge Augmentation in Implant Dentistry: A Surgical Manual, First Edition. Edited by Len Tolstunov.
© 2016 John Wiley & Sons, Inc. Published 2016 by John Wiley & Sons, Inc.

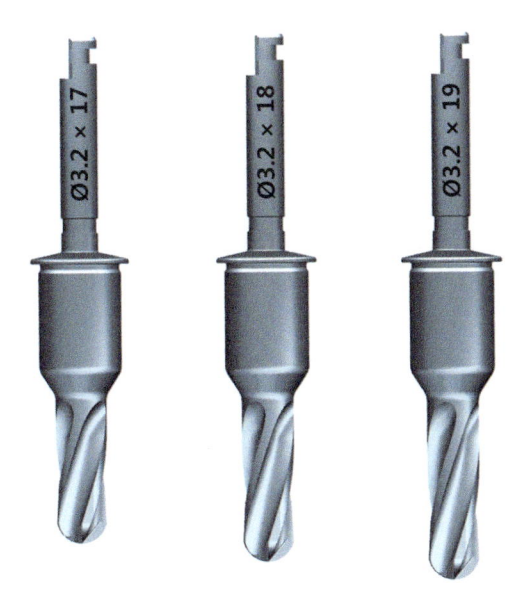

Figure 15.1 Dome-shaped crestal approach burs.

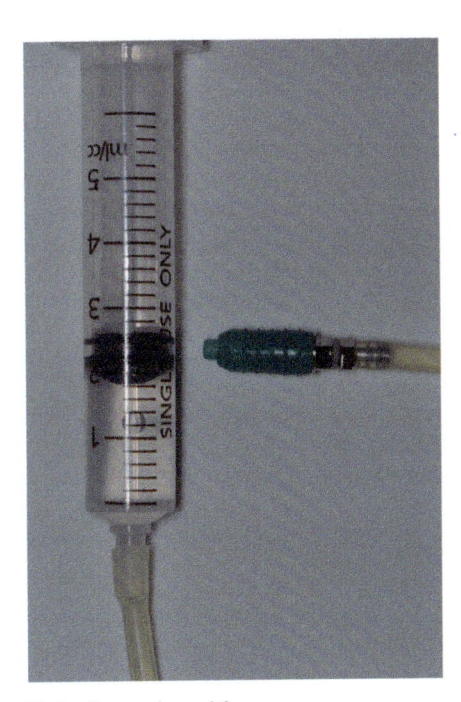

Figure 15.2 Hydraulic membrane lifter.

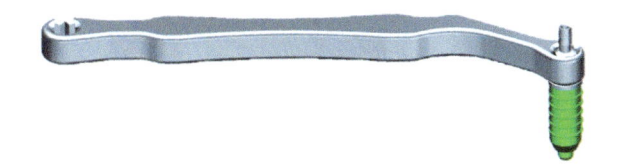

Figure 15.3 Nozzle with handle.

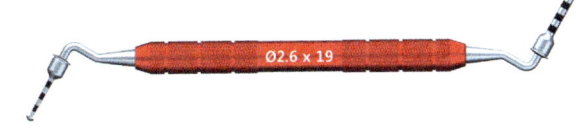

Figure 15.4 Bone plugger and sinus curette.

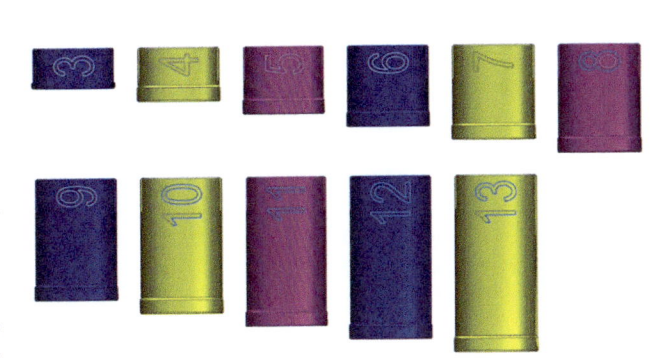

Figure 15.5 Stoppers.

which can help control the depth of insertion into the sinus cavity within a 1 mm range (Figure 15.5).

6. Digital surgical guide

The surgical guide guides the depth and direction of the osteotomy drill, crestal approach bur, and the implant. Therefore, a highly accurate and precise surgical guide must be used – the recommended vertical error value should be less than 0.5 mm. From the author's experiments, an average vertical error value of 0.44 mm was achieved if the surgical guide was digitally designed using both the cone beam computed tomography (CBCT) image and the oral scan image taken by TRIOS (3Shape, Copenhagen, Denmark) and produced using a 3D printer. The error from the digital surgical guide might have resulted from each step of the surgical guide production, including the digital impression step, the fusion of the surface scan image with the CBCT scan image, and the 3D printing process. The error value increases if the surgical guide is made with the use of stone models from alginate impressions instead of digital impressions. If the vertical error value of the surgical guide is greater than 1 mm, the risk of membrane perforation increases.

Technique

Pre-operative protocol

The best location to penetrate the bony sinus floor is determined with the help of CBCT images of the maxillary sinus while taking into consideration both the position of the final prosthesis and the anatomy of the maxillary sinus, such as the shapes of the sinus walls as well as the presence of the septum. This location will be where the implant is placed. Once the location has been determined, the drilling depth is calculated. This is important so as to avoid causing membrane perforation while drilling. Cross-sectional CBCT images can help define the length of the osteotomy up to the sinus floor. A panoramic 2D image or dental X-rays are not appropriate for this purpose as they are not precise enough. In contrast, a CBCT image can show the anatomy of the maxillary sinus with great precision in three dimensions. CBCT scans and oral digital impressions are used to perform three-dimensional implant planning and to create a

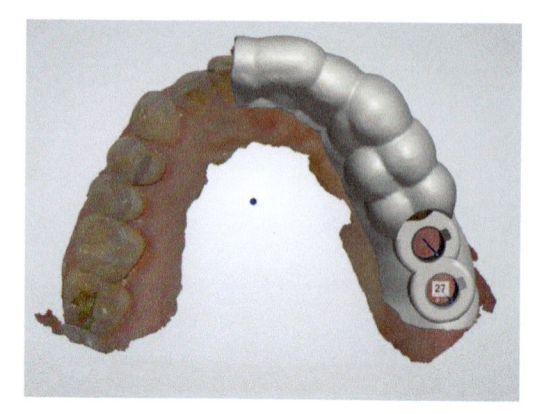

Figure 15.6 Digital surgical guide designed.

customized surgical guide (Figure 15.6). If immediate restoration is being performed, the customized abutment and provisional restoration is designed and then made using the computer-aided design/computer-aided manufacturing (CAD/CAM) milling machine. When designing the customized abutment and crown, one must consider factors such as the soft tissue profile around the proposed location of the implant and the relationship between the implant with its adjacent and opposite teeth using dental design software (Dental System, 3Shape, Copenhagen, Denmark). The surgical guide, prefabricated customized abutment and crown are prepared before implant surgery.

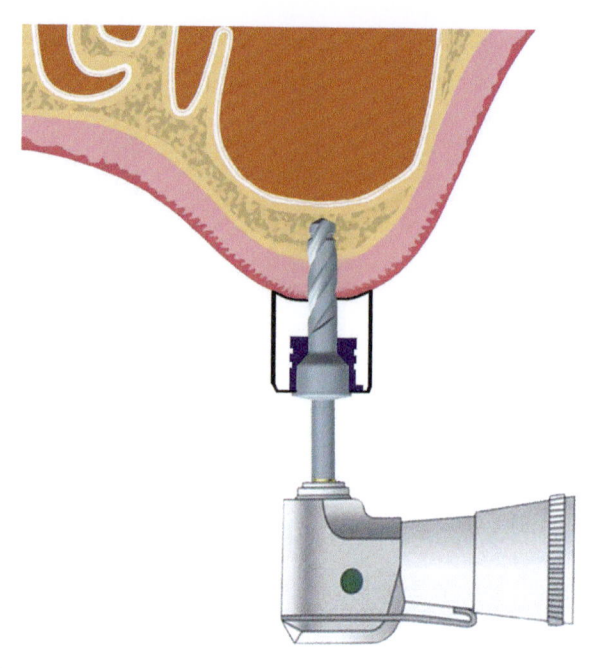

Figure 15.7 Drilling to 1 mm short of the sinus floor.

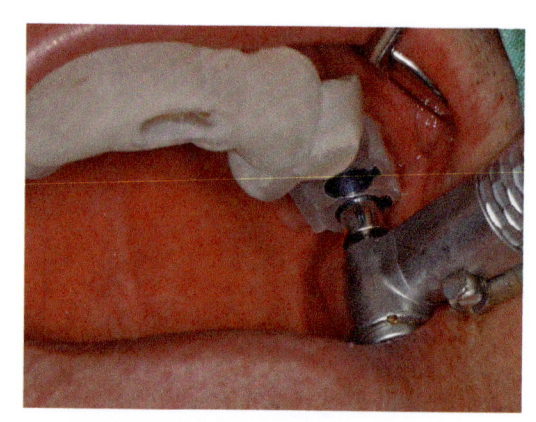

Figure 15.8 Drilling through the surgical guide.

Surgical protocol

1 Drill osteotomy. Under local anesthesia with 2% lidocaine, the stereolithographic surgical guide is placed in the mouth and checked for proper seating. The guide should be positioned accurately and securely. Accurate positioning of the guide is extremely important for precise implant placement because minor deviations can lead to errors in drilling and implant placement. The tissue punch is the first drill in sequence. The soft tissue of the proposed implant site is punched through the guide with a 3 mm soft tissue punch. After punching the soft tissue, the crestal bone is flattened with a bone-flattening drill. After flattening the bone surface, implant osteotomy is prepared up to 1 mm short of the sinus floor (Figure 15.7). The drilling is performed using sequential drills with increasing diameters through the guide. The implant osteotomy is prepared to the appropriate final diameter according to the drill sequence. The drilling depth is controlled by the drill stop in the shank that corresponds to the sum of the implant length, the gap between the guiding sleeve and the implant, and the guiding sleeve height (Figure 15.8). The drill stop precludes the drill from going deeper than intended. The final drill diameter should be approximately 0.7–1.0 mm smaller than that of the implant. For example, if a 5.0 mm implant is to be placed, use up to a 4.3 mm drill.

2 Penetrating the bony sinus floor. After drilling to 1 mm short of the sinus floor, a 3.2 mm diameter, dome-shaped crestal approach bur is used to eliminate the remaining bone below the sinus floor (Figure 15.9). After removing the remaining 1 mm, the bur is advanced into the sinus cavity using a bur with a stop, which allows it to drill down another 1 mm and expand the opening on the sinus floor. The bur is used at a speed of <10 rpm. During drilling, an upward force is applied to drill into the bony sinus floor, thus pushing the drill 1 mm beyond the sinus floor, which is controlled with drill stops and surgical guides. The bony sinus floor is perforated rather than fractured. Low-speed drilling leads to decreased friction between the bur and the membrane, when the bur comes into contact with the membrane. As a result, this technique reduces the risk of impinging on the sinus membrane, which is attributable to the risk of subsequent membrane perforation. If the bur has no stop, stopping the drill manually at the moment the last bone layer is penetrated will occur too late and the drill will still push forward and get abruptly drawn into the sinus cavity. This explains why this maneuver risks perforating the sinus membrane. The dome shape of the crestal burs, the low-speed drilling with upward force, and the perfect drilling depth control might be crucial to remove the cortical bone of the sinus floor.

3 Membrane elevation. After puncturing the sinus floor, the most reliable method should be used to elevate the Schneiderian membrane without injuring it. The most reliable method is to elevate the sinus membrane using *hydrostatic pressure* because the pressure exerted is uniformly distributed across the sinus

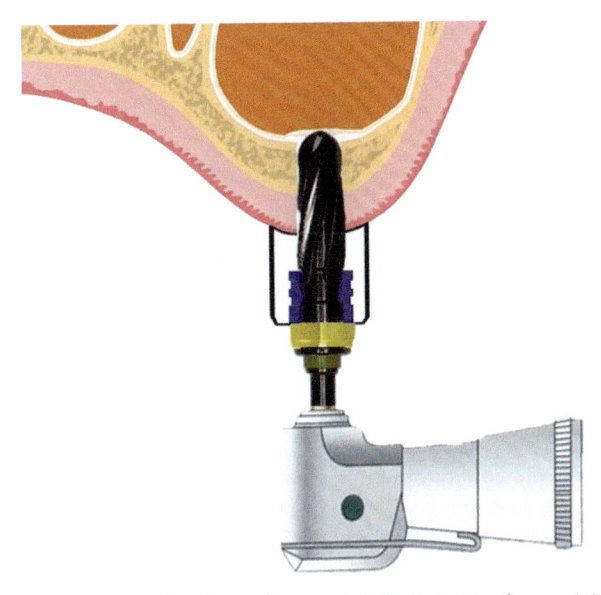

Figure 15.9 Dome-shaped crestal approach drill eliminating the remaining bone below the sinus floor.

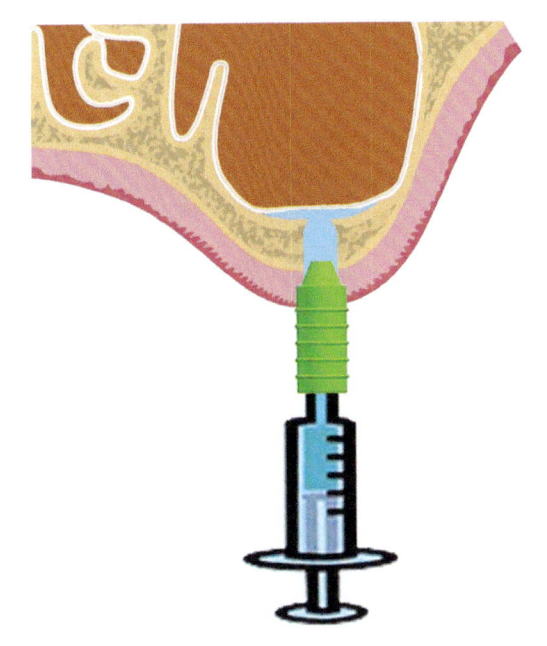

Figure 15.11 Saline injected to separate the sinus membrane from the bony sinus floor.

membrane to minimize membrane tearing during membrane elevation [6, 7]. Compared to other techniques, the hydraulic pressure generated by injecting saline into the drill hole offers the most uniform distribution of forces, resulting in uniform elevation of the sinus membrane [8]. This is supported by finite element analyses conducted by Pommer et al., which confirmed that the pressure was uniformly distributed across the elevated membrane [9].

Membrane elevation is completed without the surgical guide. First, the hydraulic membrane lifter's nozzle is connected with the handle, and then the nozzle is positioned in the opening of the drill hole and secured in place. Next, 0.8 ml of saline is slowly injected to separate the sinus membrane from the bony sinus floor and to push the membrane upward (Figure 15.10). Approximately the first 0.3–0.4 ml will go into the drill hole without feeling pressure. As the saline enters the hole and touches the sinus membrane, the membrane is elevated with feeling pressure; however, as soon as the membrane is elevated, the pressure is decreased. It is important not to inject too much saline as the pressure decreases as this can elevate the sinus membrane too much. Therefore, saline should be slowly injected 0.1 ml at a time (Figure 15.11). If the sinus floor has not been fully penetrated, the pressure can be felt after injecting 0.3–0.4 ml of saline but no more saline can be injected, in which case another attempt should be made to reinject saline after drilling an additional 1 mm into the sinus cavity using the 3.2 mm diameter, dome-shaped crestal approach bur.

4 Membrane integrity test. The most reliable way to test membrane integrity is the aspiration technique. The membrane integrity is evaluated by drawing the saline back through the drill hole. The volume of saline that was injected is fully retrieved, suggesting that the membrane remains intact. Directly viewing the sinus membrane, the Valsalva maneuver (light forceful attempted exhalation against a close nasal airway, for example), probing, or irrigation does not guarantee preservation of the sinus membrane. In the author's view, retrieving and measuring the injected saline back through the drill hole is the best test to guarantee membrane integrity.

Sinus membrane perforation is tested immediately after elevating the sinus membrane. Once 0.8 ml of saline is injected to elevate the sinus membrane, the same syringe is used to withdraw the saline. If all the saline that was just injected is withdrawn back up and the syringe shows negative pressure, then the membrane has not been perforated. There will be some blood and bubbles that get aspirated with the saline because the air that was in the hole can be pushed in with the saline and some bleeding can occur as the membrane is separated from the bone. The sinus membrane is perforated if only part of the saline is sucked back up and the syringe is unable to achieve negative air pressure. If this is the case, do not place bone-grafting material into the sinus cavity. It is possible that mucus can penetrate the graft through the perforation site and negatively affect bone formation after surgery. In addition, bone graft material can escape into the sinus cavity through the perforated area causing sinus inflammation.

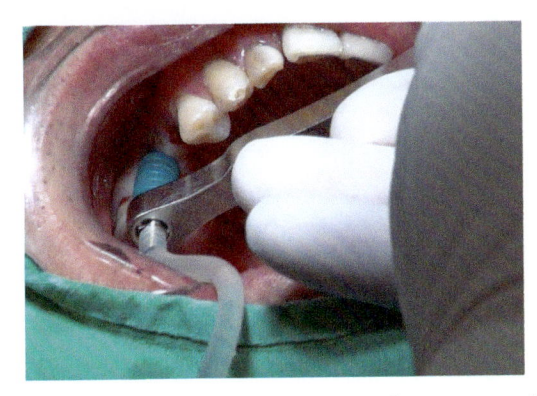

Figure 15.10 Nozzle positioned into the transcrestal osteotomy canal and secured in place.

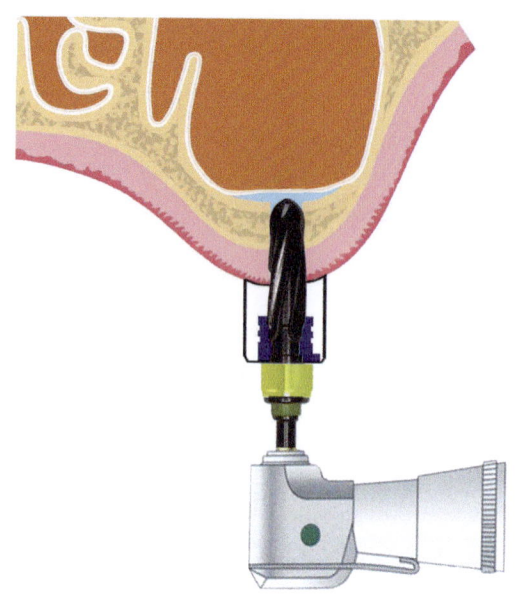

Figure 15.12 Dome-shaped crestal approach drill pushed 1 mm beyond the sinus floor.

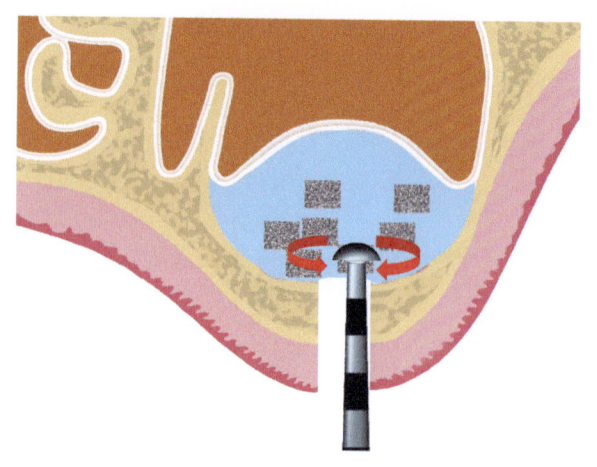

Figure 15.13 Sinus curette used to spread the graft material.

If the membrane is perforated during the membrane elevation procedure, the surgery should be reattempted after about two months. During the reattempt, the surgery is tried from a different area, away from the sinus membrane that was damaged in order to improve the success rate.

5 Expanding the opening hole of the sinus floor. Prior to inserting the grafting material into the maxillary sinus, the opening hole of the sinus floor into the sinus cavity is expanded. The surgical guide is replaced in the mouth and using the 3.2 mm diameter, dome-shaped crestal approach bur, the hole is expanded by advancing it an additional 1 mm into the sinus cavity (Figure 15.12). The bur should be advanced precisely 1 mm into the sinus cavity using the surgical guide and stop on the bur. After that, the surgical guide is removed and the bone plugger is inserted to check for the presence of any other bony barriers inside the hole – ensuring that the opening is completely clear. The bone plugger should be restricted to not insert into the sinus cavity further than the additional 1 mm using a stopper.

6 Grafting procedure. The bone grafting procedure is performed without the aid of a surgical guide. If a Bio-Oss collagen sponge (Geistlich Pharma AG, Wolhusen, Switzerland) is used as the graft material, a 1 cm^3 portion of the sponge is cut into nine pieces and then inserted into the sinus cavity through the drill hole using the bone plugger. When inserted into the sinus cavity, the grafting material has a tendency to remain pushed upwards. Therefore, it is necessary to spread the material in the sinus cavity. Whenever approximately 0.2–0.3 ml of grafting material is inserted, it is dispersed using a sinus curette by rotating the sinus curette in the sinus cavity, both clockwise and counterclockwise, drawing the largest circle possible (Figure 15.13). The amount of grafting material inserted is determined by the height of membrane elevation. When attempting to elevate the membrane by 3 mm, insert 0.3 ml; to elevate by 5 mm, insert 0.5 ml; to elevate by 7 mm, insert 0.7 ml. If only the grafting material is inserted into the sinus cavity without placing implants, an additional 0.3 ml is inserted. For example, when attempting to elevate by 7 mm, 1 ml of graft material is inserted.

7 Implant placement. Simultaneous implant placement is conducted. Before implant placement, final drilling is performed 1 mm beyond the sinus floor through the surgical guide to enlarge the sinus floor. Implants are then placed in the formed socket through the guide. It is recommended that implants be placed simultaneously with the grafting procedure because the implant will help disperse the grafting material as well as help keep the membrane elevated. However, if the vertical height of the residual bone is less than 2 mm and the implant has no primary stability, only the bone-grafting material is inserted into the sinus cavity without placing implants. Implant stability is evaluated by resistance of the implant during insertion and via measurement of the implant's insertion torque.

8 Immediate restoration or installing a healing abutment. Immediate restoration is performed using the customized abutment and preliminary restoration that was prefabricated pre-surgery if the following conditions have been met: for a single implant, immediate restoration is performed if the primary stability is greater than 30 N cm. For the implant that is splinted with neighboring implants, immediate restoration is performed if the primary stability is greater than 20 N cm. The restoration process must follow the immediate non-functional loading concept by adjusting the crown to avoid contact with the opposing teeth (Figure 15.14). Patients are asked to refrain from using the

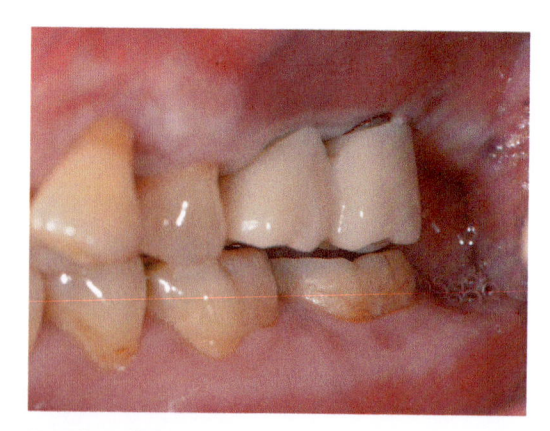

Figure 15.14 Immediate restoration with prefabricated resin temporary crowns. The occlusion and articulation of the crowns were adjusted out of contact with the opposing teeth.

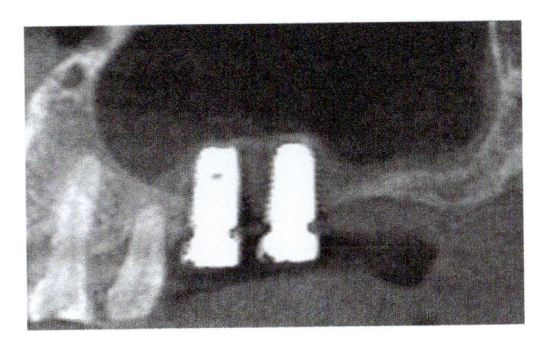

Figure 15.15 CBCT scan taken immediately after surgery.

restored teeth for 3–4 months. A cover screw or healing abutment is installed if the implant is unable to secure the primary stabilization.
9 Radiographic evaluation. Patients are scanned post-operatively with the CBCT unit to inspect and identify any sinus membrane perforations (Figure 15.15).

Advantages
Compared to a lateral approach, the flapless crestal approach offers many advantages. Pain, discomfort, and healing time are greatly reduced because of the absence of trauma resulting from the large sinus floor incisions that are used in lateral sinus elevation surgeries [10–13]. The flapless crestal approach preserves the integrity of the bony sinus structure, except at the implant site. In addition, this is a flapless procedure, which is the result of using punch incisions and simultaneous implant placement with the transmucosal components. The flapless crestal approach eliminates the need for a second surgical procedure to connect the transmucosal components, thereby reducing chair time [6, 14]. The esthetic results are also improved compared to the lateral approach [10]. Based on the author's experience, the average operative time for the flapless crestal approach was 17 ± 15 minutes. The surgical procedure substantially decreased the length of surgery compared to the previous crestal approaches. Some possible reasons for this shortened operative time might be due to using drills with stops, using surgical guides, the effective membrane elevation system, eliminating the need for sutures, and avoiding soft tissue elevation. In addition to a shorter operative time, the approach is successful in anatomically difficult sinus structures. During sinus lift surgery, problems are not encountered in the presence of antral septa or when drilling along a steep bone wall. Therefore, this procedure can be highly successful in patients with septated maxillary sinuses.

In patients with antral septum
The presence of an antral septum in the sinus cavity poses additional difficulties for a lateral approach. As a result, the lateral approach requires greater skill of the surgeon and longer operative time. Even surgeons with a lot of experience often cause sinus membrane perforation; however, with the aid of a surgical guide and hydraulic pressure, the flapless crestal approach makes the procedure simpler and faster (Figure 15.16a to c). The septum can actually be utilized to aid in shaping the grafting material in the maxillary sinus (Figure 15.17a and b). One of the reasons for the high success rate in patients with septated maxillary sinuses is that the dome-shaped crestal approach bur, which is used to drill through the sinus floor, can be safely used in steep bone walls as well (Figure 15.18). Due to its round shape, the drill works whether the surface is flat or not. Bone in the septum area tends to be hard, which can help implants achieve primary stability. If the pre-surgery CBCT scan reveals the presence of a septum, the surgeon must take this into consideration in determining the appropriate position and depth of initial drilling. When drilling through a steep sinus wall, depending on the angle, the surgeon may need to drill an additional 1 mm compared to when drilling through a flat wall.

In patients with severely atrophic maxillae
Even in patients with severely atrophic maxillae (1 to 2 mm of residual bone), the implants can be successfully inserted at the same time as maxillary sinus elevation (Figure 15.19a and b) [15]. Typically in these situations, the maxillary sinus floor wall has hardened the cortical bone remaining. To successfully place implants in 1 to 2 mm of bone in the posterior maxilla, the residual bone quality should be effectively used to achieve primary implant stability. The drilling and implant placement is performed without shaking the axis with the aid of a surgical guide. Tapered implants are used. The osteotomy for implant placement is enlarged to 0.7–1.0 mm narrower than the anticipated implant diameter.

Grafting material
It is difficult to create a desirable shape of the grafting material in the sinus cavity through the flapless crestal approach because the material is inserted without the ability to see inside the sinus cavity. The goal of the grafting procedure using the flapless crestal approach is to simply maintain the space created by the sinus

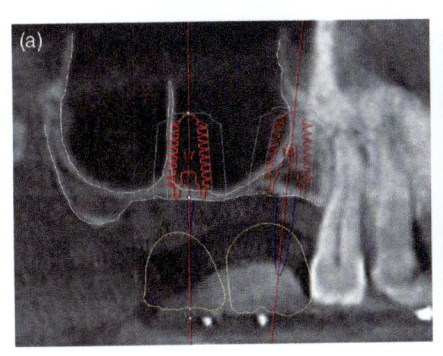

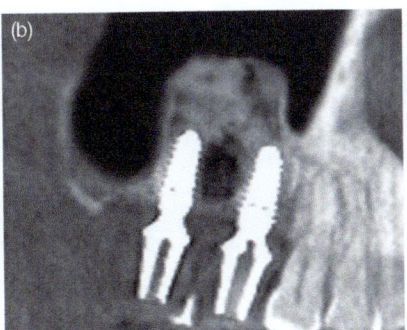

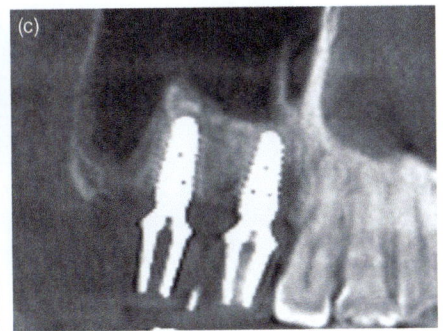

Figure 15.16 A case with antral septa: (a) before, (b) immediately, and (c) 6 months after surgery.

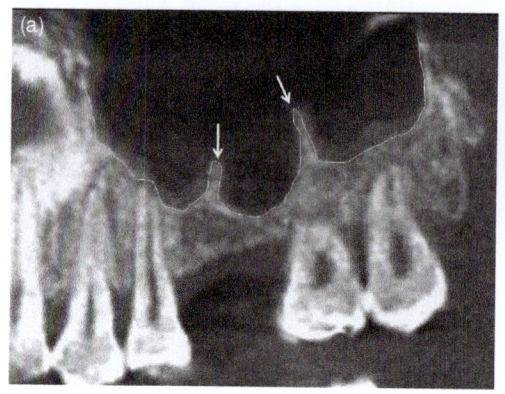

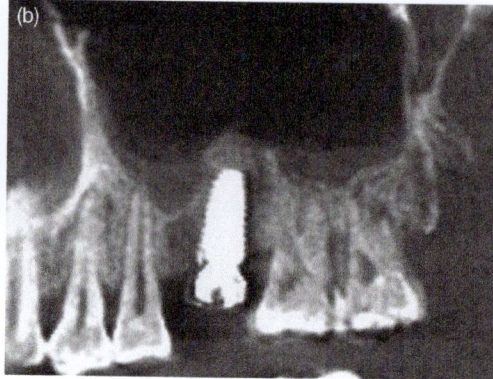

Figure 15.17 A case with antral septa: (a) before and (b) 6 months after surgery.

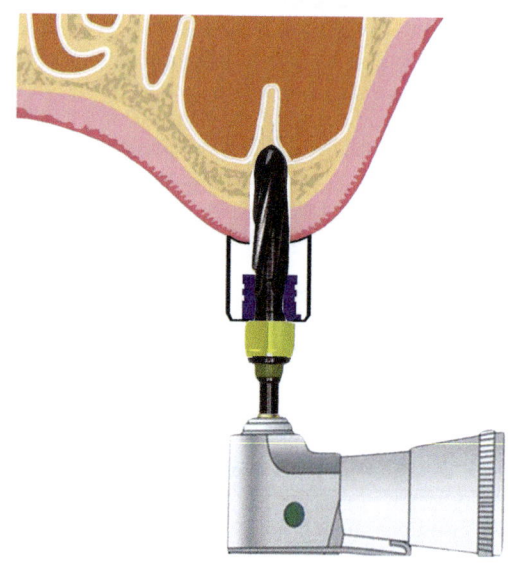

Figure 15.18 Dome-shaped crestal approach bur under the septum.

membrane elevation. In other words, the goal is to keep the sinus membrane elevated to encourage new bone formation underneath the membrane. The elevated sinus membrane can act like a tent while enabling blood flow and taking advantage of the bone's regeneration ability. The environment of the sinus cavity below the lifted sinus membrane after sinus membrane elevation is quite beneficial for bone formation [16, 17]. This is in part because the cavity is surrounded by bone and the primary source of revascularization of the graft originates from the adjacent bony walls. In addition, the sinus membrane has an intensely vascular network and contains mesenchymal progenitor cells committed to the osteogenic lineage [18]. The periosteum of the lifted sinus membrane is another source of bone-forming cells. Accordingly, new bone formation in the newly created space can be induced by only elevating the sinus membrane, provided that the space is well maintained. When the implant is placed along with grating material, both the implant and the graft material can help maintain the elevated sinus membrane. The graft material for the flapless crestal approach must be selected on the basis of its ability to maintain space, its ability to be inserted through a small opening, and its ease of dispersion inside the sinus cavity.

The graft material can be in particle, gel, or sponge form. *The particle type* can be pushed into the sinus cavity through the drill hole using a bone carrier; however, this type can be ineffective and more time-consuming as the small opening makes it difficult for the particles to be pushed in. The advantage of the *gel type* is that it can be injected into the sinus cavity through the drill hole using a syringe; however, its disadvantage is that if there is space inside the sinus cavity, the gel can shift around. In particular, in a laid-down position, the gel moves towards the back. If a thermosensitive gel is used instead, the gel may be able to solidify inside the sinus cavity and hold its shape. If the gel and particle types are mixed together,

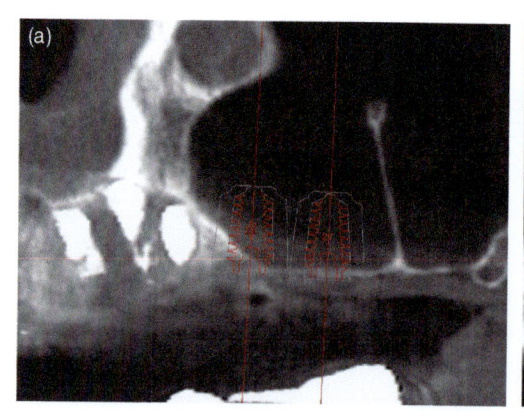

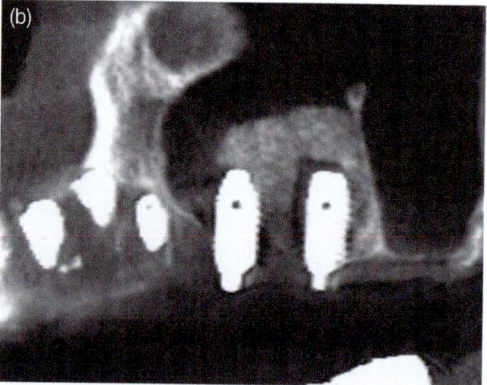

Figure 15.19 Cone beam computed tomography (CBCT) scans of the severely atrophic ridge with 1 mm of residual bone (a) before and (b) after surgery.

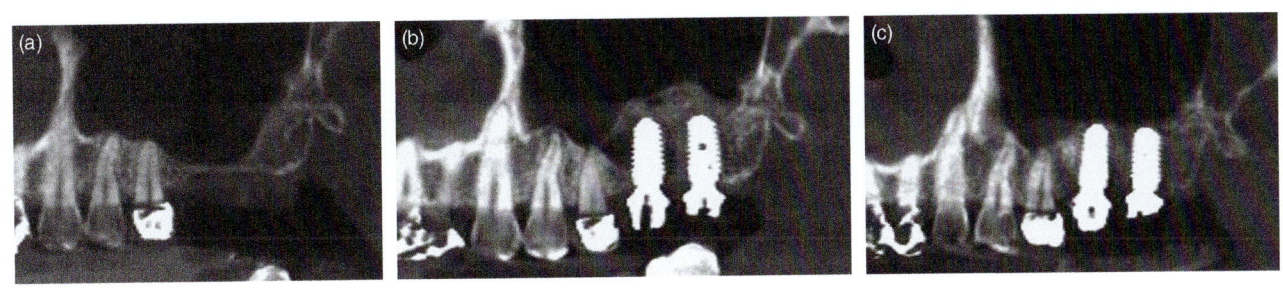

Figure 15.20 CBCT scans taken (a) before, (b) immediately, and (c) six months after surgery.

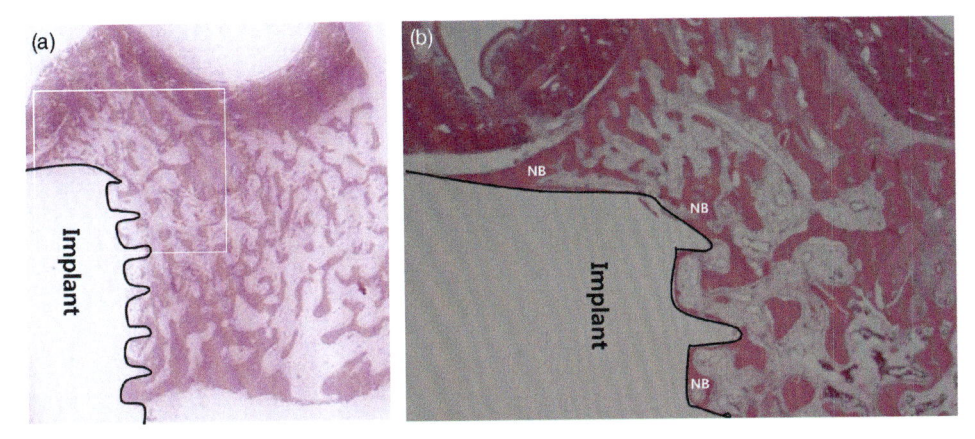

Figure 15.21 View of the specimen of Bio-Oss collagen sponge: (a) low ratio and (b) high ratio.

two things can happen. First, if the ratio of the particle type is greater than the gel type, the mixture might not be able to be injected using a syringe. Second, if the ratio of the particle type is less than the gel type, the mixture may be absorbed too easily. In contrast, if the *sponge type* material is inserted into the sinus cavity as a grafting material, the sponge can protect the membrane from the roughness of the graft material and may minimize membrane tearing during the grafting procedure. The sponge type material is soft and more elastic, which makes it easier to handle. It can be cut into a size that can easily be pushed through the hole and, when positioned, the sponge is able to maintain its space under the elevated sinus membrane. The Bio-Oss collagen sponge (Geistlich Pharma AG, Wolhusen, Switzerland) is a commonly used sponge-type grafting material. The Bio-Oss collagen sponge is made up of 90% calf cancellous bone and 10% pig collagen. Collagen sponge may not be suitable for maintaining the space because it can be absorbed quickly; however, the Bio-Oss collagen sponge is suitable because Bio-Oss bone particles are able to maintain their shape without being absorbed too quickly when inside the sinus cavity (Figure 15.20a to c). The author's animal experiment showed that when the Bio-Oss collagen sponge was used as the graft material for bone augmentation in the maxillary sinus, bone formation in the graft site was excellent and the mean osseointegration rate was more than 40% (Figure 15.21a and b).

Conclusion

The first key factor for the success of flapless crestal sinus augmentation is penetrating the bony sinus floor using the dome-shaped crestal approach bur, a low-speed drilling with upward force and a perfect drilling depth control. The second factor is that hydraulic pressure is used to safely elevate the sinus membrane and check for membrane integrity. The third factor is that a CBCT scan with high resolution, advanced surgical equipment, and a highly precise surgical guide are used for the surgery.

References

1 Bassi MA, Lopez MA: Hydraulica sinus lift: a new method proposal. *J Osteol Biomat* 2010;**1**:93–101.
2 Engelke W, Capobianco M: Flapless sinus floor augmentation using endoscopy combined with CT scan-designed surgical templates: method and report of 6 consecutive cases. *Int J Oral Maxillofac Implants* 2005;**20**:891–897.
3 Toffler M: Minimally invasive sinus floor elevation procedures for simultaneous and staged implant placement. *N Y State Dent J* 2004;**70**:38–44.
4 Cassetta M, Stefanelli LV, Giansanti M, Calasso S: Accuracy of implant placement with a stereolithographic surgical template. *Int J Oral Maxillofac Implants* 2012;**27**:655–663.
5 D'haese J, Van De Velde T, Komiyama A, Hultin M, De Bruyn H: Accuracy and complications using computer-designed stereolithographic surgical guides for oral rehabilitation by means of dental implants: a review of the literature. *Clin Implant Dent Relat Res* 2012;**14**:321–335.
6 Chen I, Cha J: An 8-year retrospective study: 1,100 patients receiving 1,557 implants using the minimally invasive hydraulic sinus condensing technique. *J Periodontol* 2005;**76**:482–491.
7 Kao DW, DeHaven HA: Controlled hydrostatic sinus elevation: a novel method of elevating the sinus membrane. *Implant Dent* 2011;**20**:425–429.
8 Watzek G. *The Percrestal Sinus Lift – From Illusion to Reality*. Quintessence Publishing, London, 2012, pp. 67–86.
9 Pommer B, Unger E, Sütö D, Hack N, Watzek G: Mechanical properties of the Schneiderian membrane *in vitro*. *Clin Oral Implants Res* 2009;**20**:633–637.
10 Fortin T, Bosson JL, Isidori M, Blanchet E: Effect of flapless surgery on pain experienced in implant placement using an image-guided system. *Int J Oral Maxillofac Implants* 2006;**21**:298–304.

11. Nkenke E, Eitner S, Radespiel-Troeger M, Vairaktaris E, Neukam FW, Fenner M: Patient-centred outcomes comparing transmucosal implant placement with an open approach in the maxilla: a prospective, non-randomized pilot study. *Clin Oral Implants Res* 2007;**18**:197–203.
12. Bensaha T: Outcomes of flapless crestal maxillary sinus elevation under hydraulic pressure. *Int J Oral Maxillofac Implants* 2012;**27**:1223–1229.
13. Brodala N: Flapless surgery and its effect on dental implant outcomes. *Int J Oral Maxillofac Implants* 2009;**24**:118–125.
14. Kfir E, Goldstein M, Yerushalmi I: Minimally invasive antral membrane balloon elevation: results of a multicenter registry. *Clin Implant Dent Relat Res* 2009;**11**: e83–91.
15. Peleg M, Mazor Z, Chaushu G, Garg AK: Sinus floor augmentation with simultaneous implant placement in the severely atrophic maxilla. *Periodontol* 1998;**69**:1397–1403.
16. Lundgren S, Andersson S, Gualini F, Sennerby L: Bone reformation with sinus membrane elevation: a new surgical technique for maxillary sinus floor augmentation. *Clin Implant Dent Relat Res* 2004;**6**:165–173.
17. Palma VC, Magro-Filho O, Oliveira JA, Lundgren S, Salata LA, Sennerby L. Bone reformation and implant integration following maxillary sinus membrane elevation: an experimental study in primates. *Clin Implant Dent Relat Res* 2006;**8**:11–24.
18. Gruber R, Kandler B, Fürst G, Fischer MB, Watzek G: Porcine sinus mucosa holds cells that respond to bone morphogenetic protein BMP-6 and BMP-7 with increased osteogenic differentiation *in vitro*. *Clin Oral Implants Res* 2004;**15**:575–580.

CHAPTER 16

Piezoelectric Surgery for Atrophic Maxilla: Minimally Invasive Sinus Lift and Ridge Augmentation, Role of Growth Factors

Dong-Seok Sohn

Department of Oral and Maxillofacial Surgery, Daegu Catholic University, School of Medicine, Daegu, Korea

Introduction

The atrophic posterior maxilla is a challenging site for oral rehabilitation with dental implants due to often insufficient vertical bone volume. Crestal or lateral window approaches for sinus augmentation are the most common surgical techniques to overcome vertical deficiency of atrophic posterior maxilla [1, 2].

Rotary bur has been generally used to cut a lateral bony window, exposing the sinus (Schneiderian) membrane and creating access for the sinus bone graft. However, surgeons with limited experience may cause sinus membrane perforation while creating the bony window using a rotary bur. The rotary bur can easily injure soft tissues such as sinus membrane, causing its perforation. Membrane perforation occurs in 10 to 44% of sinus floor elevation procedures using conventional rotary instruments [3–6].

When a perforation of the sinus membrane takes place, additional surgeries and materials are required to close the perforation. In the case of a small perforation of the sinus membrane, it is possible to continue with the sinus bone graft procedure after repairing the perforated membrane with resorbable membrane or fibrin glue. However, in the case of a large perforation, the sinus graft procedure may have to be delayed due to a bone graft material's direct contact with the sinus cavity, which often leads to a sinus infection. When sinus mucosa is perforated, higher rates of post-operative sinusitis and implant failure have been reported [8, 9].

To avoid the complications associated with sinus mucosal perforation, an ultrasonic piezoelectric surgical technique, using microvibrations generated by ultrasonic waves, is highly recommended [10–12].

A piezoelectric surgical device enables bone cutting with precision in preparation of a lateral bony window and has a low risk of sinus mucosal perforation. In addition, the ultrasonic surgical instruments produce less noise and vibration compared to conventional rotary bur instruments. Furthermore, the ultrasonic piezoelectric surgical device minimizes damage of soft tissues and other structures such as nerves and blood vessels while cutting bone during sinus augmentation, even in case of accidental contact (Figures 16.1 and 16.2).

Piezoelectric inserts for sinus augmentation

To prepare a sinus window, a round insert (tip) has been widely utilized. Studies demonstrate that the use of a piezoelectric round insert makes it possible to make bone osteotomies without injury to the sinus membrane [13–16]. However, sinus window preparation using round diamond-coated piezoelectric inserts is not effective in creating bony windows in sites with thick lateral walls of the maxillary sinus. In fact, it is time-consuming in thick lateral bone windows because of its low cutting efficacy compared to that of the sharp cutting edge of the piezoelectric saw [17]. According to the author's study on a comparison of two piezoelectric cutting inserts for lateral bony window osteotomy, the piezoelectric saw insert has some advantages over the round inserts, such as faster and more precise osteotomy, minimal bone loss, and facilitation of precise replacement of the bony window than the round insert [13]. The membrane perforation rate was not affected by the type of piezoelectric insert. That is why the author recommends using a saw insert for the preparation of a bony window to save surgical time and utilize the benefits of osteoinductive qualities of the replaceable bony window.

1. **Round diamond-coated tip.** This tip is commonly used to cut a bony window during sinus lift. However, it is slow to cut and is not recommended for the preparation of a sinus window (Figures 16.3 and 16.4).
2. **Round carbide tip,** This tip is a round tip of the carbide bur type. It cuts bone faster than the diamond round tip (S016®, S-Dental Co., Daegu, Korea). There are measuring marks from 4 mm in increments of 2 mm to estimate the cutting length. It can be used in cutting a bony window or cutting access for retrofilling during apicoectomy. It can also be used as a pilot drill in implant placement and in piezoelectric internal sinus floor elevation (PISE) (Figure 16.5).
3. **Saw insert.** This tip is the most versatile tip for various applications such as sinus graft, harvesting autogenous bone graft, oral surgery, orthognathic surgery, and ridge splitting. Thick and thin bladed saw insert are available, but the thin blade saw tip is highly recommended to prepare an osteoinductive replaceable bony window, allowing the detached bony window to be repositioned with good stability (Figures 16.6 and 16.7).

Vertical Alveolar Ridge Augmentation in Implant Dentistry: A Surgical Manual, First Edition. Edited by Len Tolstunov.
© 2016 John Wiley & Sons, Inc. Published 2016 by John Wiley & Sons, Inc.

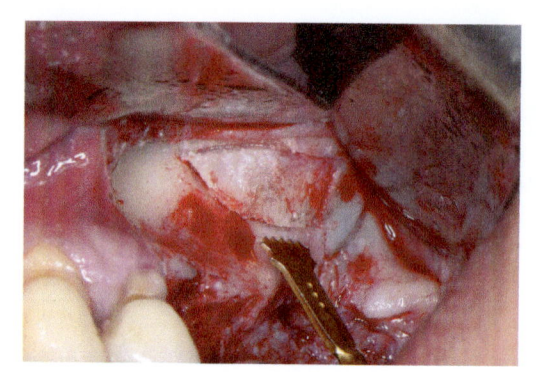

Figure 16.1 Replaceable bony window is prepared with a saw insert with a sharp blade.

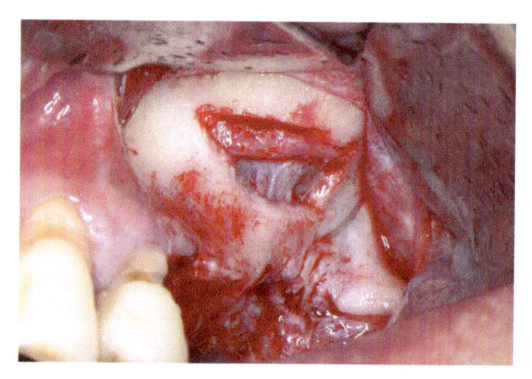

Figure 16.2 Selective and micrometric cut effect of a piezoelectric device prevents trauma of blood vessels after detachment of the bony window.

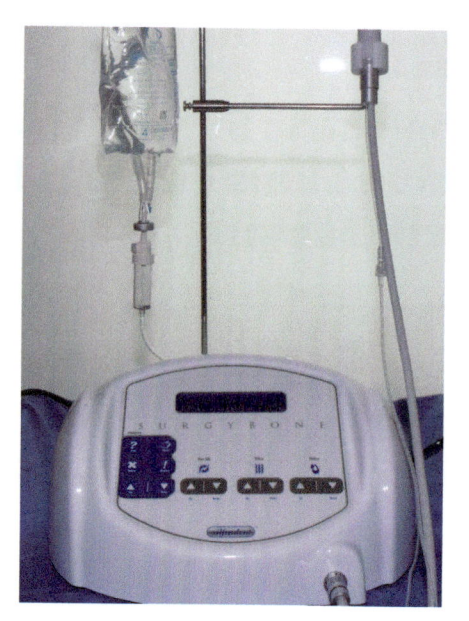

Figure 16.3 Piezoelectric surgical device.

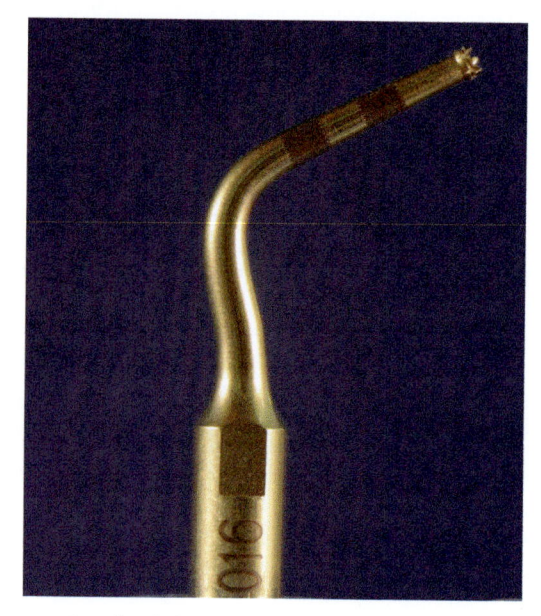

Figure 16.5 Round carbide tip. It cuts bone faster than a diamond round tip.

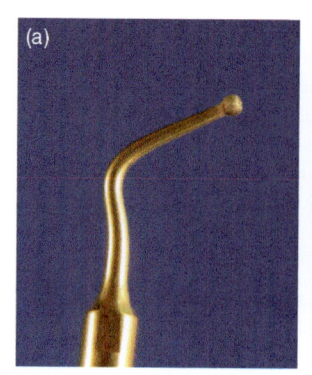

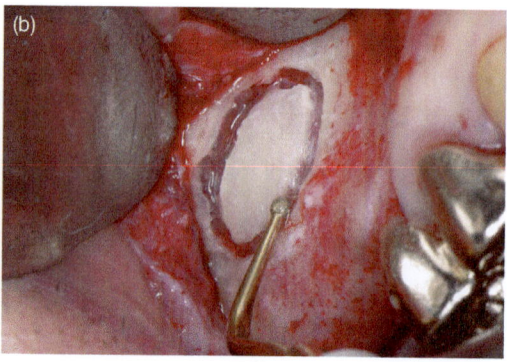

Figure 16.4 Round diamond coated tip and window preparation using the tip.

A. Lateral sinus augmentation using autologous concentrated growth factors alone

Although a bone graft is considered a prerequisite for sinus augmentation, various studies have reported the new bone formation in the maxillary sinus without a bone graft in humans and animals [18–24]. Palma et al. reported no difference in the amount of augmented bone in the maxillary sinus between grafted and nongrafted sites after 6 months of healing in primates [19]. Sohn et al. for the first time showed histologic evidence of a favorable new bone formation in the maxillary sinus without bone graft and clinical implant success *in vivo* [20]. Compared to bone-added sinus augmentation, sinus augmentation without bone substitutes has several advantages: (1) the bone harvesting procedure is not needed,

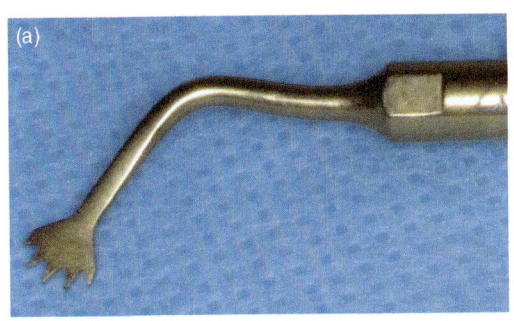

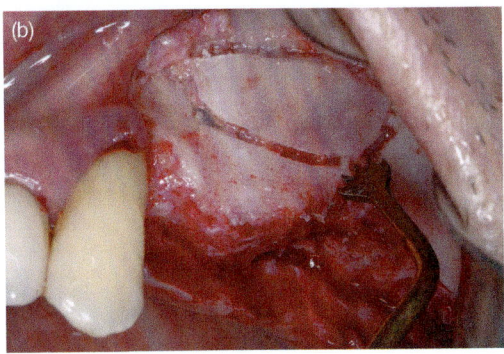

Figure 16.6 Thick bladed saw tip and its utilization for the preparation of sinus window. Note a wide osteotomy line.

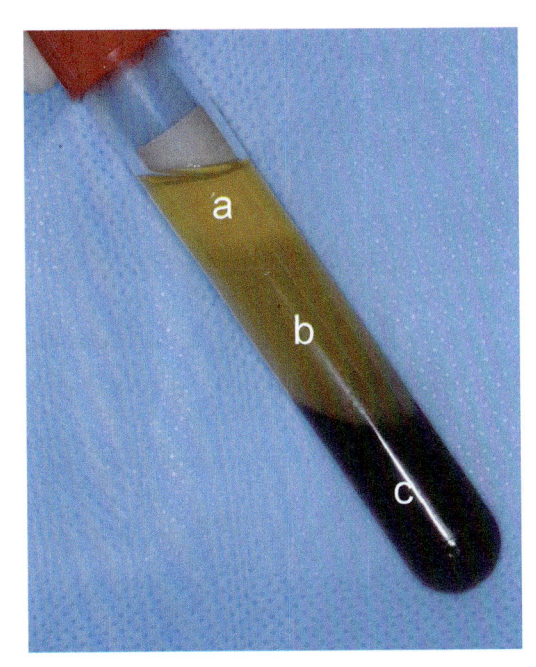

Figure 16.8 The prepared concentrated growth factors (CGFs): (a) serum layer, (b) CGF layer, which is utilized for the sinus augmentation and barrier membrane, and (c) layer of the red and white blood cells.

(2) cross-contamination between bovine and human bone is eliminated, (3) post-operative infection is very low, and (4) surgical cost and time are reduced.

Platelet aggregates, such as platelet-rich plasma (PRP) and platelet rich in growth factors (PRGF), have been used to accelerate new bone formation associated with guided bone regeneration and sinus graft for many years [24–27]. Platelet-rich fibrin (PRF) is known to slowly release growth factors such as transforming growth factor (TGF-b1), platelet-derived growth factor (PDGF), and vascular endothelial growth factor (VEGF), and accelerates new bone formation when it is mixed with bone graft in the maxillary sinus [28, 29].

In addition, fibrin-rich block with concentrated growth factors (CGFs) as the sole material showed fast new bone formation in the sinus [24]. According to the author's study on 61 sinus augmentations using fibrin-rich gel with concentrated growth factors alone, fast new bone formation in the sinus was apparent in all of the sinuses, radiographically and histologically [24]. No significant post-operative complications developed. The success rate of implants was 98.2% after an average of 10 months of loading. The study showed that the use of CGFs acts as an alternative to a bone graft and can be a predictable procedure for sinus augmentation.

Preparation of fibrin-rich block with concentrated growth factors (CGF)

CGF was prepared using Dr. Sacco's protocol [30]. Before the sinus graft or bone graft procedure was performed, 20–60 ml of the patient's venous blood was taken from the patient's vein, and the blood was divided between glass-coated test tubes without anticoagulants. The blood in the test tubes was centrifuged at 2400 to 2700 rpm using a specific centrifuge with a rotor turning at alternating and controlled speed levels for 12 minutes (Medifuge, Silfradent srl, Sofia, Italy). After centrifugation, the tubes showed three distinct layers. The uppermost layer is represented by the serum (blood plasma without fibrinogen and coagulation factors); the second (middle) layer is a fibrin buffy coat representing a very

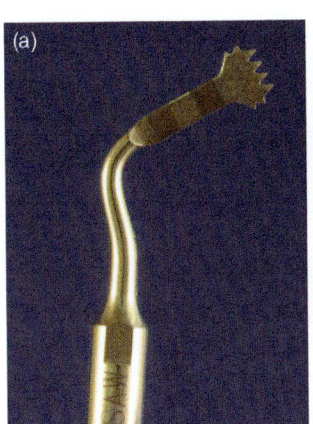

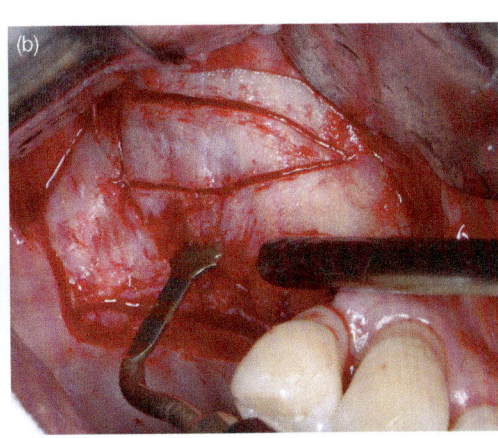

Figure 16.7 Thin bladed saw tip that is the author's preferred insert for the sinus surgery. Note, a narrow osteotomy line.

large and dense polymerized fibrin block containing the concentrated growth factors (CGFs); the third (lower) red layer consists of concentrated red and white blood cells, platelets, and clotting factors (Figure 16.8). The second layer (fibrin buffy coat) was used as alternative to bone substitutes for sinus augmentation.

Compared to platelet-rich plasma [25] or platelet-rich growth factors [26], the CGF is simple to make and does not require any synthetic or biomaterials, such as bovine thrombin and calcium chloride, to form a gel. Therefore, it is free from the risk of cross-contamination.

Case Report

A 45-year-old woman with complaints of masticatory difficulty was referred from a private dental clinic for the extraction of a hopeless right upper posterior molar and replacement with implant-supported restoration (Figures 16.9 and 16.10). Clinical examination revealed severe mobility of the present bridge restoration. A plain panoramic radiograph and cone beam computed tomography (CBCT, Combi, Pointnix Co., Seoul, Korea) showed a large mucous retention cyst (MRC) in the right maxillary sinus and severe bone resorption at the second molar area. The residual bone height at the second molar site was less than 1 mm.

The removal of a bridge restoration and sinus augmentation was performed under local anesthesia through maxillary block anesthesia by using 2% lidocaine that included 1:100 000 epinephrine. Flomoxef sodium (Flumarin®; Ildong Pharmaceutical Co., Korea, 500 mg i.v.) was administered one hour before the surgery. The bridge was extracted and the full-thickness mucoperiosteal flap was elevated to expose the lateral wall of the right maxillary sinus. The piezoelectric saw insert with a thin blade (S-Saw, S-Dental Co., Daegu, Korea) connected to a piezoelectric device (Surgybone®, Silfradent srl, Sofia, Italy) was used with copious saline irrigation to create the osteoinductive replaceable rectangular-shaped bony window at the lateral wall of the maxillary sinus (Figure 16.11). The anterior vertical osteotomy was made 3 mm distal to the anterior vertical wall of the maxillary sinus and the distal osteotomy was made approximately 20 mm away from the anterior vertical osteotomy. The height of the vertical osteotomy was approximately 10 mm. The anterior and inferior osteotomy line was created parallel to the mesial wall of the maxillary sinus and the superior and posterior osteotomies were made perpendicular to each other and the sinus walls. This design of osteotomy facilitated precise replacement of the bony window as a barrier over inserted CGF into the maxillary sinus. The bony window was detached carefully to expose the sinus membrane. Before dissecting the sinus membrane from the sinus floor, a small incision was made to aspirate the mucous retention cyst from the sinus cavity by using a suction apparatus (Figures 16.12 and 16.13).

Careful dissection of the sinus membrane was continued to reach the anterial and medial walls of the sinus cavity after removal of the mucous retention cyst. The height of the exposed sinus medial wall was at the level of the superior osteotomy line of the lateral bone window. After completion of membrane elevation, the large mucosal perforation resulting from aspiration of the cyst was repaired with resorbable collagen membrane (BioMend, Zimmer Dental, CA). Six pieces of CGF, as an alternative to a bone graft, was inserted in the new compartment under the elevated sinus mucosa in order to accelerate new bone formation. The detached bony window was repositioned with good stability (Figures 16.14 to 16.17).

Bony communication to the sinus cavity was also detected after curettage of granulation tissue in the molar extraction socket. Therefore, the implant placement was delayed in this case. For augmentation of an extraction defect, putty conditioned demineralized allograft (AllBone®, CG Bio Co., Sungnam, Korea) was used as a graft and a pedicled connective tissue graft was utilized to cover the bone graft. Flaps were sutured using interrupted mattress polytetrafluoroethylene (PTFE) sutures (Cytoplast®, Osteogenic Biomedical, Texas, USA) to achieve passive primary closure (Figures 16.18 and 16.19). The patient was instructed to follow sinus precautions (not to blow her nose, swim, or fly, to cough or sneeze with an open mouth, etc.) for two weeks after surgery. Pre-operative prophylactic antibiotic therapy was continued post-operatively for 7 days and the sutures were removed 10 days post-operatively. Post-operative CBCT was taken immediately after the surgery (Figure 16.20). A six month healing period was allowed for new bone consolidation in the sinus. CBCT of the sinus was obtained again to assess the new bone formation. An approximately 12 mm high new bone level was gained in the sinus with no graft used for the sinus. However, poor bone regeneration was observed at the augmented extraction socket due to likely fast resorption of the demineralized allograft (Figures 16.21 and 16.22). A full-thickness flap was raised to expose the implant site and a one-step undersized osteotomy was utilized to get initial stability of implants at two implant sites. Two

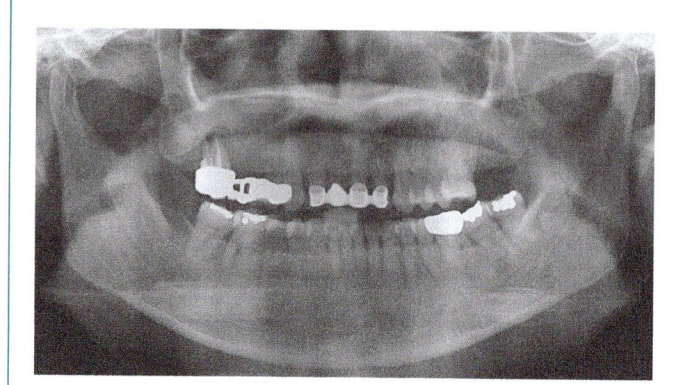

Figure 16.9 Plain radiograph and CBCT scan reveal a large mucous retention cyst in the right maxillary sinus.

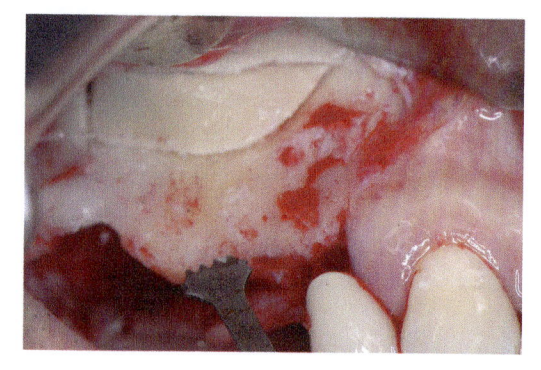

Figure 16.11 The preparation of an osteoinductive replaceable bony window. Note the beveled osteotomy at the anterior and inferior osteotomy line.

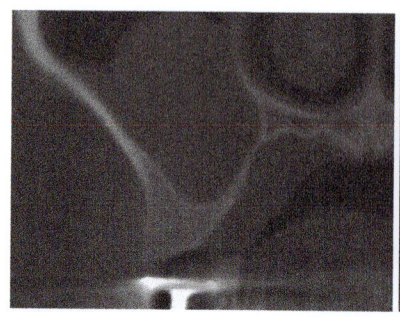

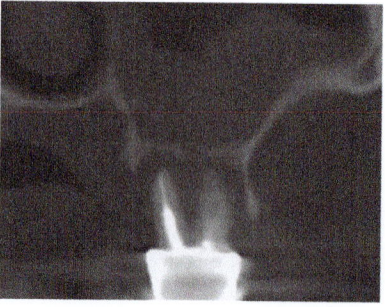

Figure 16.10 The cross-section view of CBCT at the second premolar (left) and second molar (right) reveals a large mucous retention cyst in the right maxillary sinus and severe bone resorption at the second molar site.

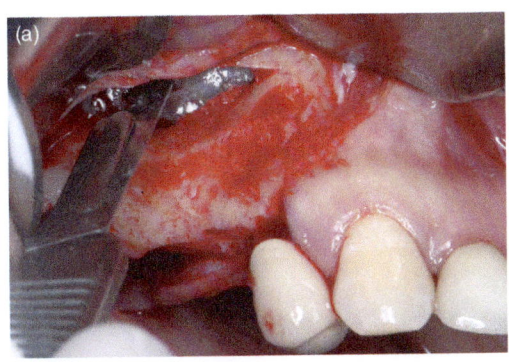

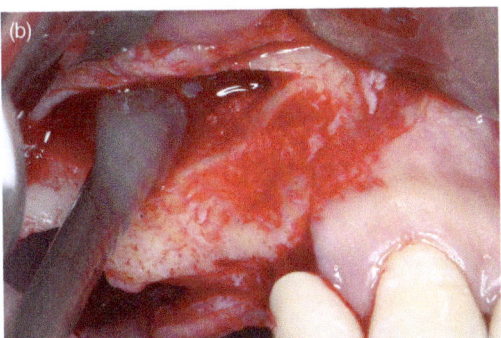

Figure 16.12 A stab incision in the sinus mucosa made to aspirate the mucous retention cyst by suction apparatus.

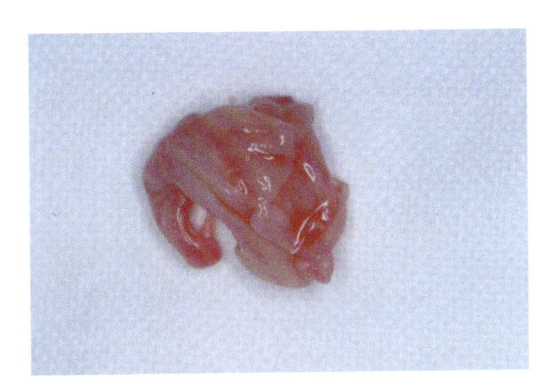

Figure 16.13 The removed cyst from the maxillary sinus.

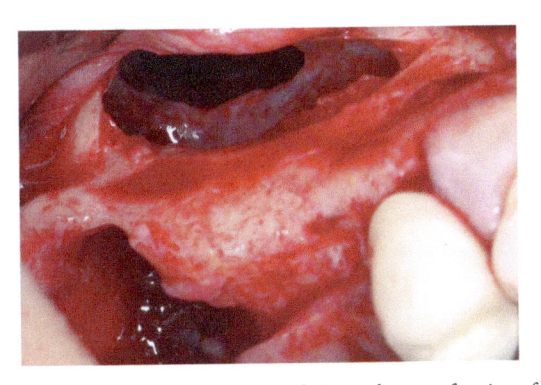

Figure 16.14 Sinus mucosa was elevated. Note a large perforation of the sinus mucosa.

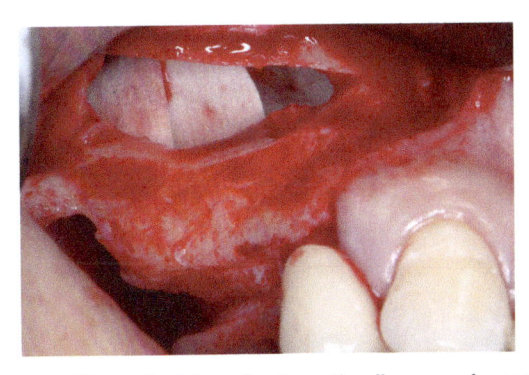

Figure 16.15 The repair of the perforation with collagen membrane to prevent dislodgement of the CGF placed into the sinus.

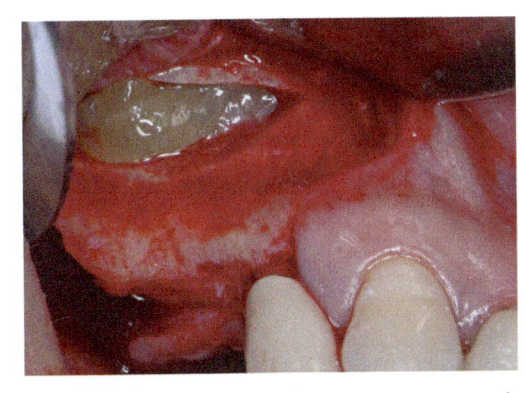

Figure 16.16 Insertion of the CGF into the new compartment under the elevated sinus mucosa.

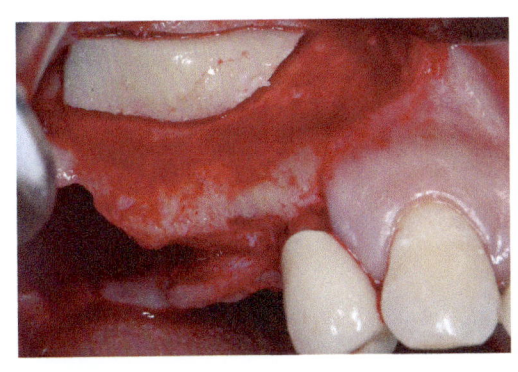

Figure 16.17 Reposition of the bony window.

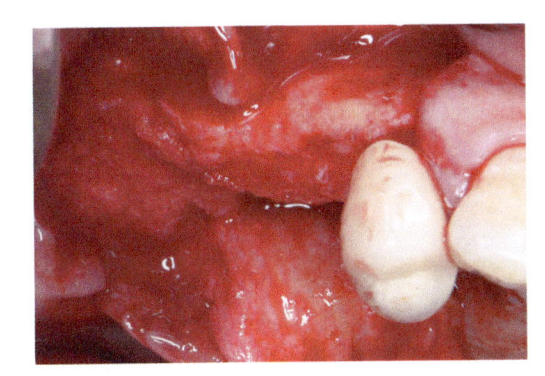

Figure 16.18 Bone graft in the extraction defect.

(continued)

(Continued)

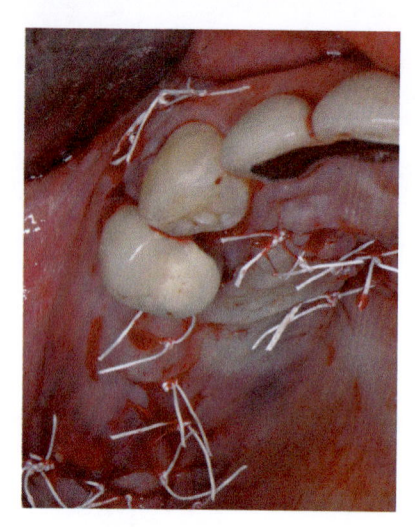

Figure 16.19 Tension free primary suture with a pedicled connective tissue graft.

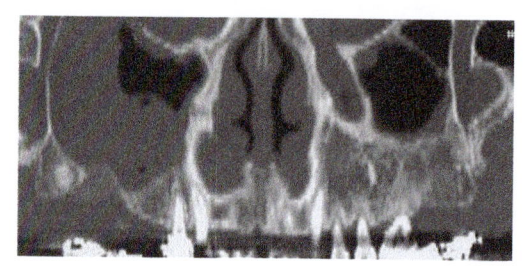

Figure 16.20 Post-operative CBCT scan.

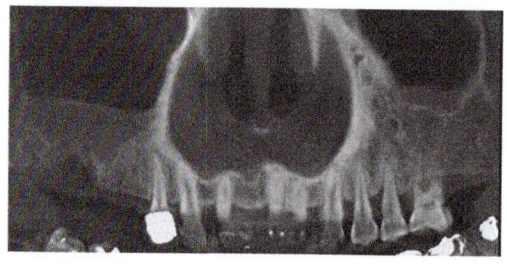

Figure 16.21 CBCT scan after 6 months of healing. Note the 12 mm high bone regeneration inside the sinus.

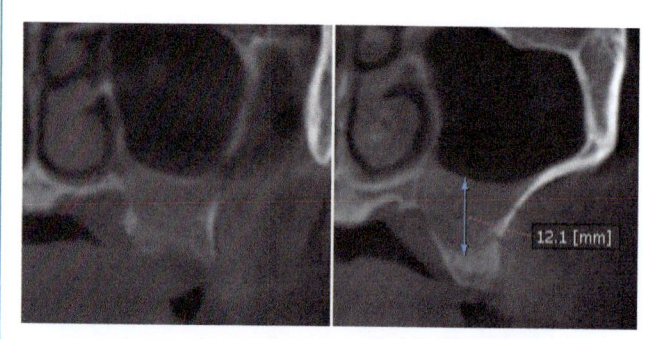

Figure 16.22 The cross-sectional view of the CBCT scan after 6 months of healing at the second molar (left) and second premolar (right) sites.

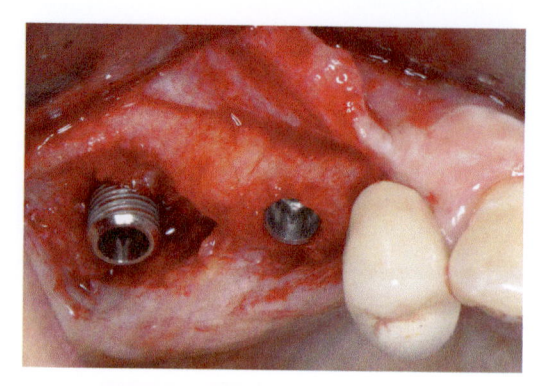

Figure 16.23 Note the bone defect after the implant placement at the second molar site.

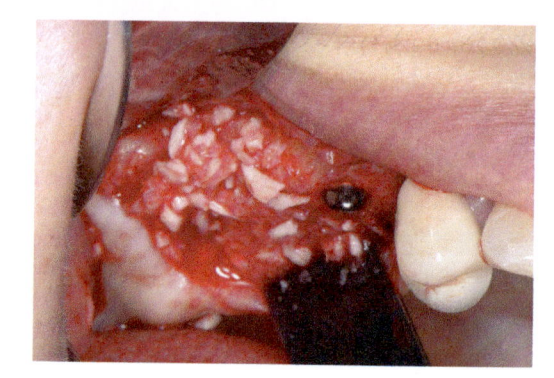

Figure 16.24 Bone graft in the defect.

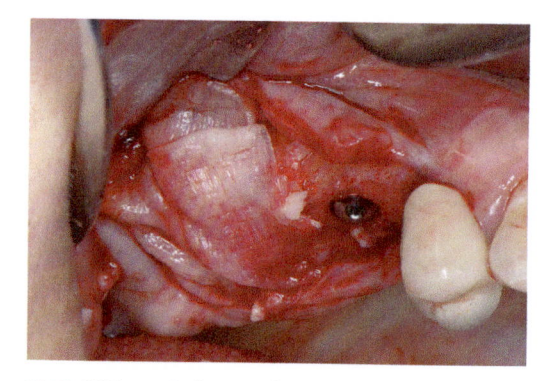

Figure 16.25 CGF over the bone graft as the barrier membrane.

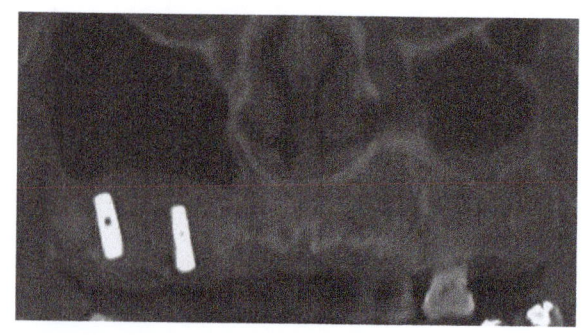

Figure 16.26 Post-operative CBCT scan taken after the implant placement.

12 mm length implants (Dentis implant, Dentis Inc, Daegu, Korea) were placed (Figure 16.23). A bone defect around the implant corresponding to the second molar was augmented with a mineral allograft (Boi Tis Co., Seoul, Korea) mixed with CGF and covered with CGF barrier membrane, not only to accelerate bone regeneration but also to prevent soft tissue ingrowth into the bone graft (Figures 16.24 to 16.27). Progressive temporary restoration was delivered after 4 months of healing. A 4-year follow-up radiograph revealed good stability of implant-supported restoration and sinus augmentation (Figures 16.28 to 16.30).

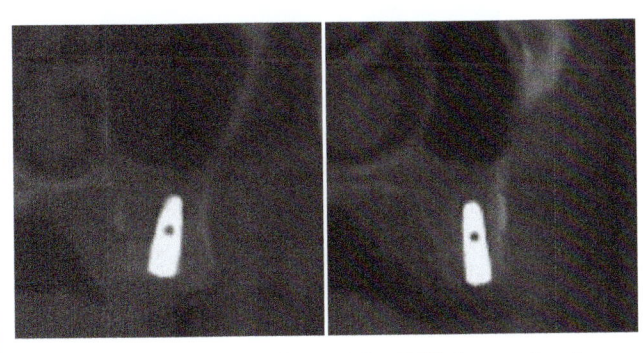

Figure 16.27 The cross-sectional view of the CBCT: the second molar site (left) and second premolar site (right).

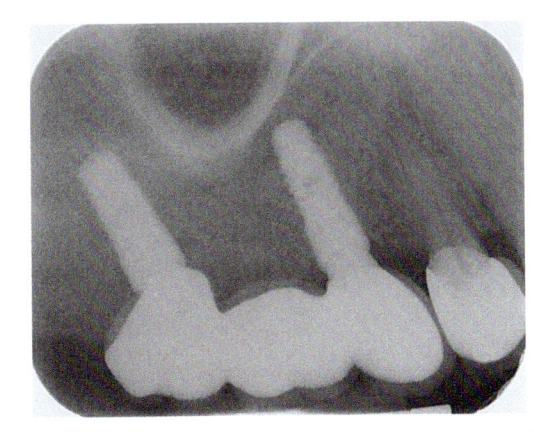

Figure 16.29 A radiograph immediately after the cementation of the final restoration.

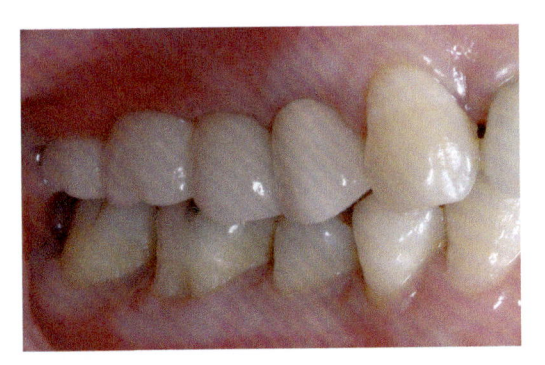

Figure 16.28 Final restoration.

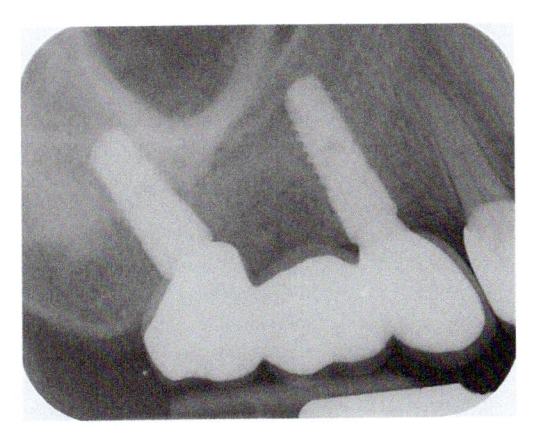

Figure 16.30 A 4-year follow-up radiograph.

B. Crestal sinus augmentation using hydrodynamic piezoelectric sinus augmentation (HPISE) and autologous concentrated growth factors

Sinus augmentation using the lateral window procedure has been predictable for several decades. However, this procedure may result in patient morbidity such as post-operative swelling, pain, and a long healing period. Some patients may prefer other options. Furthermore, surgeons with limited surgical experience tend to avoid this method due to the high risk of membrane perforations. To overcome the disadvantages of the lateral window approach in maxillary sinus augmentation, several crestal approaches, such as the osteotome technique [31], piezoelectric internal sinus elevation (PISE) [32, 33], hydraulic sinus condensing (HSC) technique [34], and hydrodynamic piezoelectric internal sinus elevation (HPISE) [35–37], have been introduced.

The crestal approach using a surgical mallet and osteotome is less invasive than the lateral approach, but it has some limitations, such as post-operative vertigo, membrane perforation from bone packing, and limited vertical augmentation due to difficult accessibility [38, 39]. In addition, the ostetome technique has lower success rates when residual bone height is 4 mm or less compared to cases with 5 mm or more [40].

Most crestal (indirect or transalveolar) techniques of sinus augmentation depend on bone compaction to elevate the sinus membrane. Too much pressure during bone compaction may lead to membrane perforation and sinusitis after the surgery. Also with these techniques, numerous pieces of equipment are needed to elevate the sinus membrane.

Unlike other crestal sinus augmentation methods, the HPISE technique does not require osteotomes or the sinus membrane elevation equipment. The HPISE technique utilizes ultrasonic

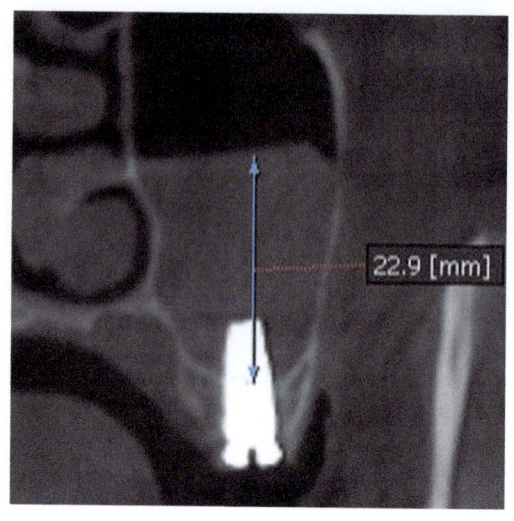

Figure 16.31 Approximately 20 mm high sinus elevation using water pressure alone. HPISE usually does not rely on bone compaction for sinus elevation.

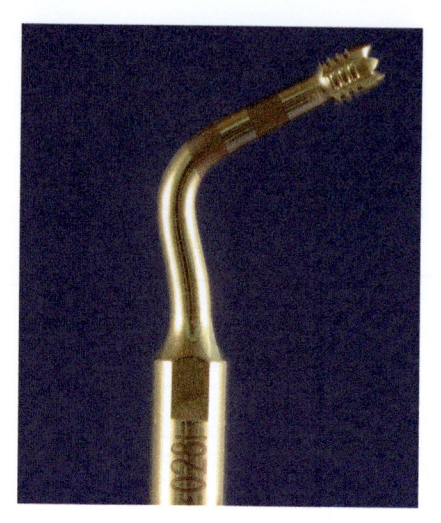

Figure 16.33 A 2.8 mm HPISE tip with internal irrigation.

microvibrations to break the sinus floor and hydraulic pressure to elevate the sinus membrane more than 20 mm (Figure 16.31). Furthermore, it does not rely on bone compaction to elevate the sinus membrane.

Surgical procedure of HPISE

After local anesthesia using lidocaine (1:100 000 epinephrine) in the surgical site, a full-thickness flap is reflected to expose the alveolar ridge. Flapless surgery is also performed when the width of the alveolar ridge is adequate, as confirmed by the CBCT. As a first step, a 1.6 mm wide carbide round insert with external irrigation (Figure 16.5), attached to a piezoelectric ultrasonic unit (Surgybone®, Silfradent srl, Sofia, Italy) or any compatible device, is used to break the sinus floor. The vibrating round insert provides a tactile sensation of the cortex of the sinus floor and the sinus membrane when the sinus floor is broken up directly (Figure 16.32). The round insert has depth-indicating lines marked at 2 mm intervals. Thus, it measures the exact residual bone height from the alveolar crest to the sinus floor. After

breaking the sinus floor with the round tip, a 2.8 mm wide cylindrical carbide insert (HPISE insert®, S-Dental Co., Daegu, Korea) is utilized to enlarge the osteotomy site and elevate the sinus membrane using hydraulic pressure (Figures 16.33 and 16.34). The HPISE insert has a 4 mm working tip height, and depth-indicating lines are marked by 2 mm intervals. Hydraulic pressure from a sterile saline solution to the sinus membrane through the internally irrigated HPISE insert causes membrane detachment from the sinus floor. Membrane perforation from the water pressure is rare. After breaking the sinus floor cortex using ultrasonic vibration, hydraulic pressure is applied for 10–20 seconds to detach the sinus membrane further from the sinus floor. After this point, the surgeon can observe up and down movement of the sinus membrane whenever a patient takes a breath.

A bone graft is dependent on the surgeon's personal preference. If sufficient sinus elevation is not achieved with the water pressure, a bone graft can be used. Bone compaction can be attained by using the ultrasonic vibration of the HPISE insert. The author prefers to

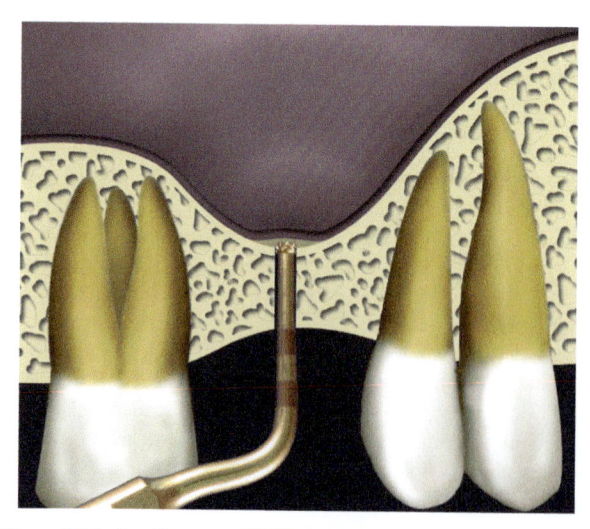

Figure 16.32 As a first step of HPISE, a 1.6 mm wide carbide round insert attached to a piezoelectric device is utilized to break the sinus floor directly.

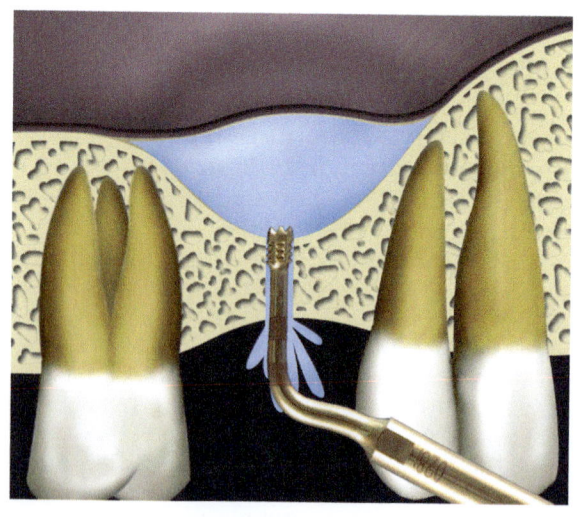

Figure 16.34 As the second step, a 2.8 mm HPISE tip is utilized to widen the implant site and elevate the sinus mucosa at the same time. This tip is a final osteotomy tip to accommodate a 3.7–4.2 mm wide tapered implant.

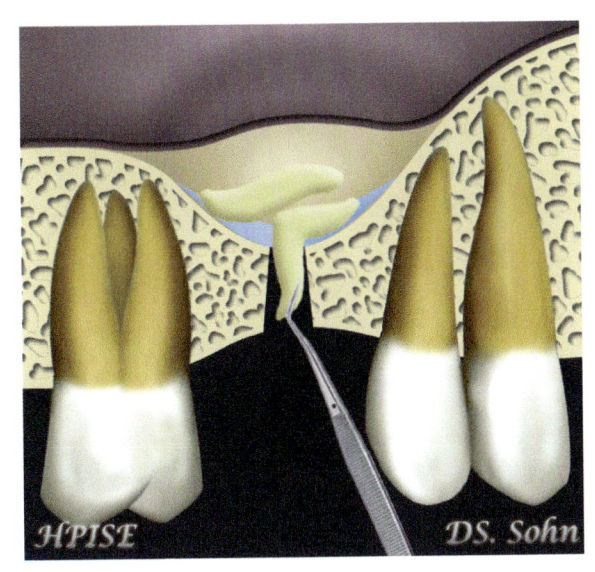

Figure 16.35 A bone graft is optional after elevation of the sinus mucosa. The author prefers to place a CGF or PRF into the sinus.

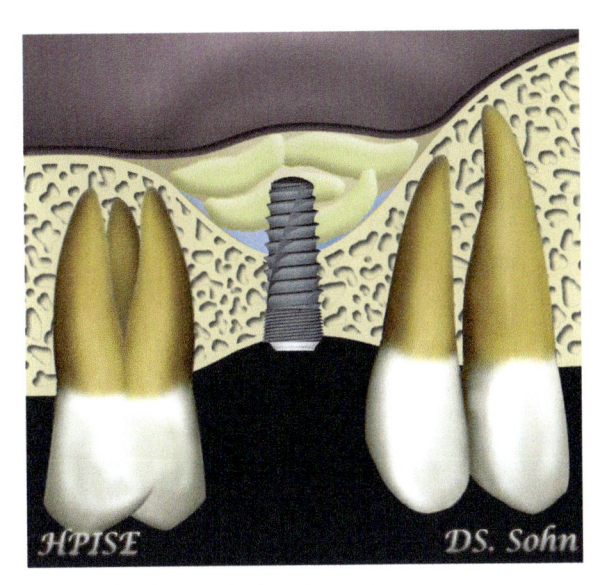

Figure 16.36 Simultaneous implant placement.

place CGF in the new compartment under the elevated sinus mucosa as an alternative to a bone graft (Figure 16.35). Implant osteotomy (undersized to get good primary stability) is done and the implant is placed simultaneously. A 2.8 mm wide HPISE tip is a final osteotomy tip to accommodate a 3.7–4.2 mm wide tapered implant (Figure 16.36). When a wider implant is placed, an additional drilling procedure is required to accommodate the wider body implant. It is always recommended that the osteotomy be undersized by one drill size to ensure adequate primary stability of the implant.

Case Report

A 44-year-old female patient presented with the missing upper right first molar (Figure 16.37a). She visited the department of periodontology at another university hospital before coming to our department and the lateral sinus augmentation was recommended to her there. However, she was afraid of post-operative discomfort from the lateral sinus augmentation and came to our department for a second opinion and possible immediate implant placement at the site of the missing tooth. Pre-operative CBCT and plain radiographs revealed approximately 3 mm of residual bone height and no sinus pathosis was seen (Figure 16.37).

HPISE with simultaneous implant placement was planned in order to minimize post-operative discomfort and shorten the healing period. The surgery was performed under local anesthesia through maxillary block anesthesia by using 2% lidocaine that included 1:100 000 epinephrine. Flomoxef sodium (Flumarin®; Ildong Pharmaceutical Co., Korea, 500 mg i.v.) was administered one hour before surgery. A full-thickness mucoperiosteal flap was elevated to expose the implant site. A 1.6 mm wide piezoelectric carbide round insert connected to the piezoelectric device was inserted through the edentulous alveolar bone to break through the sinus floor directly using the effect of a micrometric cut (Figure 16.38). An HPISE insert was used to enlarge the osteotomy site and elevate the sinus membrane using hydraulic pressure by internal irrigation at the same time (Figure 16.39). Water pressure was applied for about 10 seconds after breaking the sinus floor with this tip. Approximately 10 mm of the sinus elevation height was observed through the dental fluoroscopy (i-Scope, Seoul, Korea) by using water pressure alone (Figure 16.40). Four pieces of CGFs were inserted into the new compartment under the elevated sinus mucosa to accelerate new bone formation (Figure 16.41).

A 4.8 mm wide × 12 mm high RBM (resorbable blast media) surfaced implant (Dentis Implant Co., Daegu, Korea) was placed simultaneously with a good primary stability after underpreparation of the implant site, and the healing abutment was connected to the implant platform as a one-stage procedure (Figures 16.42 and 16.43). A post-operative CBCT scan revealed successful sinus elevation (Figure 16.44). The patient had minor post-operative discomfort and no swelling on the next day. Temporary restoration was delivered after 4 months of healing for gingival contouring (Figures 16.45). Final ceramic restoration was delivered after 2 months of use of the temporary restoration (Figures 16.46 and 16.47).

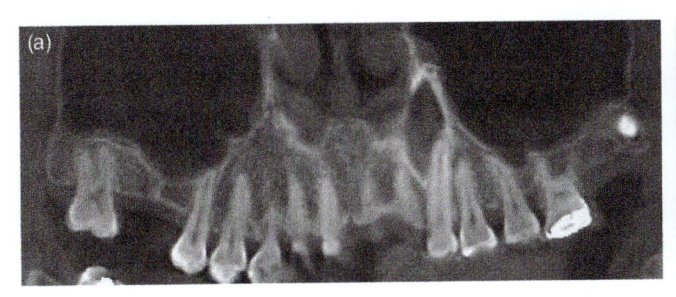

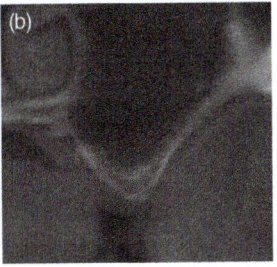

Figure 16.37 Pre-operative CBCT scan reveals approximately 3 mm of residual bone height and no sinus pathology.

(continued)

(Continued)

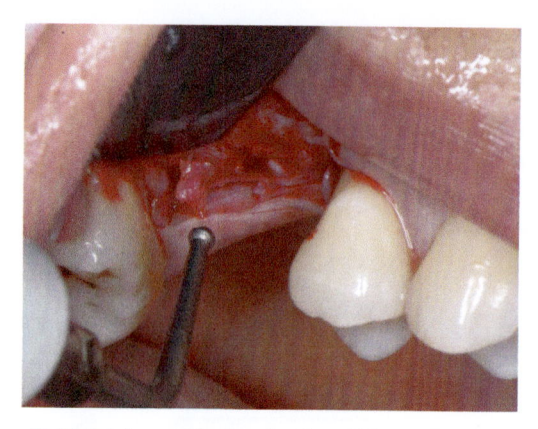

Figure 16.38 A 1.6 mm wide piezoelectric carbide round insert was inserted through the edentulous alveolar bone to break the sinus floor directly using a scratching action.

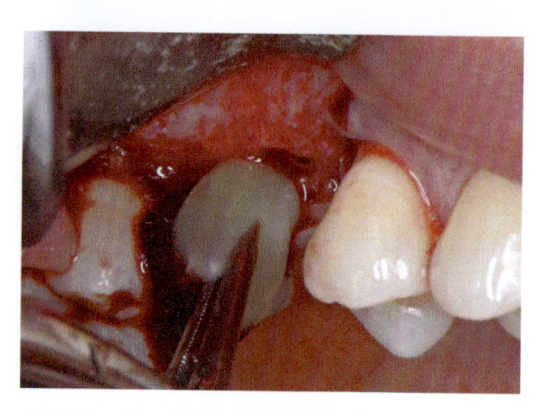

Figure 16.41 Insertion of four pieces of CGF alone into the sinus pocket.

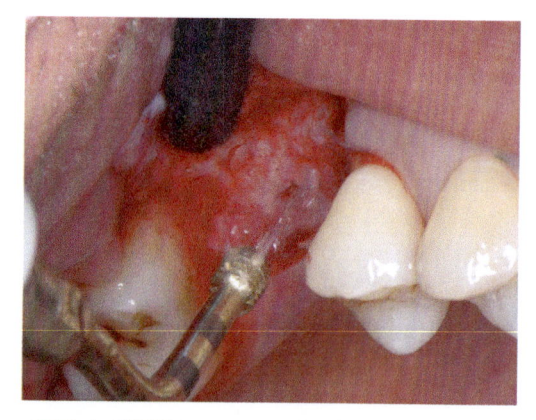

Figure 16.39 An HPISE insert was used to elevate the sinus membrane using hydraulic pressure by internal irrigation. Water pressure was applied for about 10–20 seconds after breaking the sinus floor with this tip.

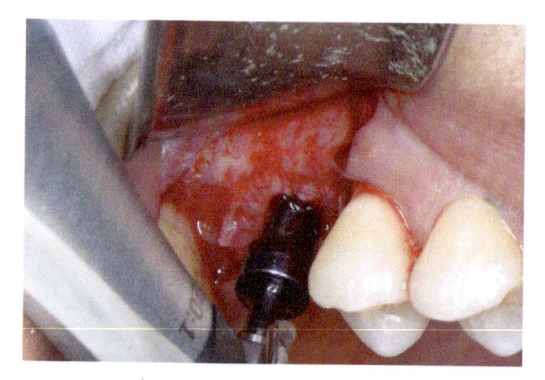

Figure 16.42 An intermediate implant drill was used to accommodate placement of a wide implant.

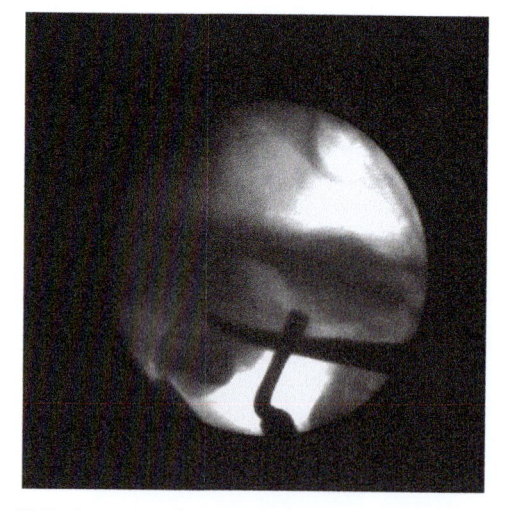

Figure 16.40 Approximately 10 mm high sinus elevation by using water pressure alone was observed in dental fluoroscopy.

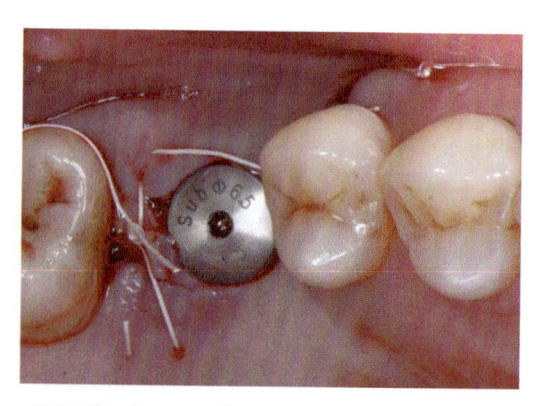

Figure 16.43 The placement of a 4.8 mm wide × 12 mm high implant.

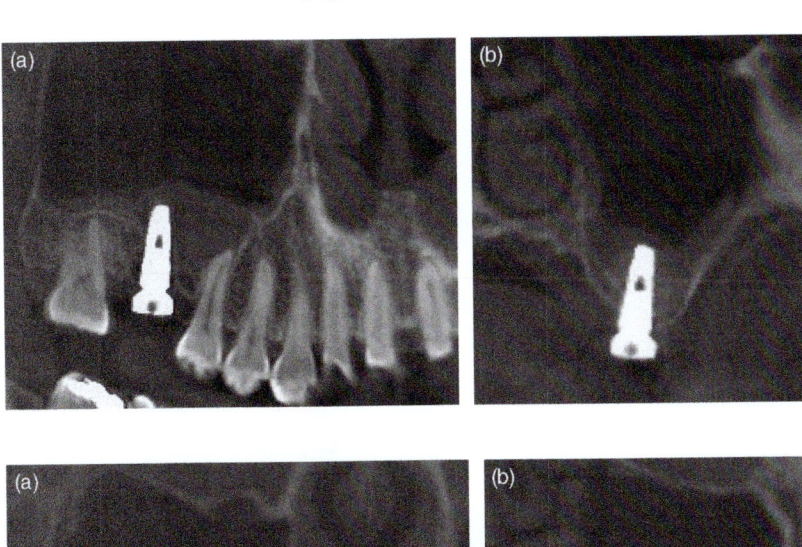

Figure 16.44 Panoramic and cross-sectional view of the post-operative CBCT scan showing successful sinus elevation.

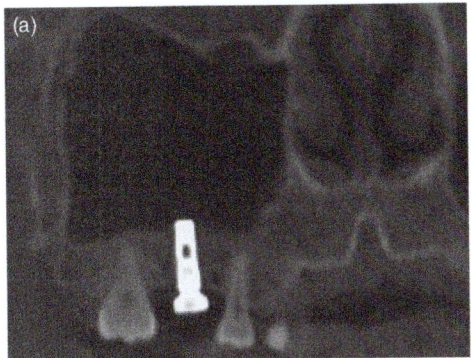

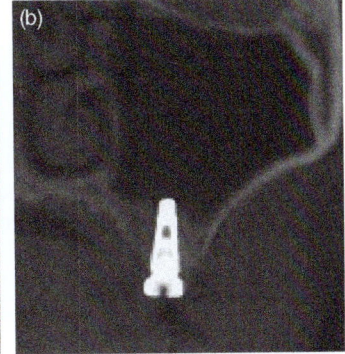

Figure 16.45 CBCT images after 4 months of healing.

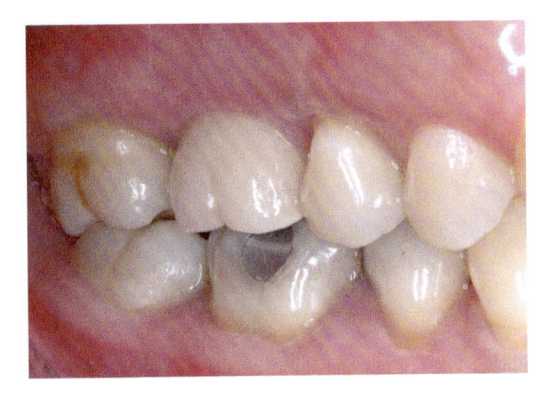

Figure 16.46 Final restoration.

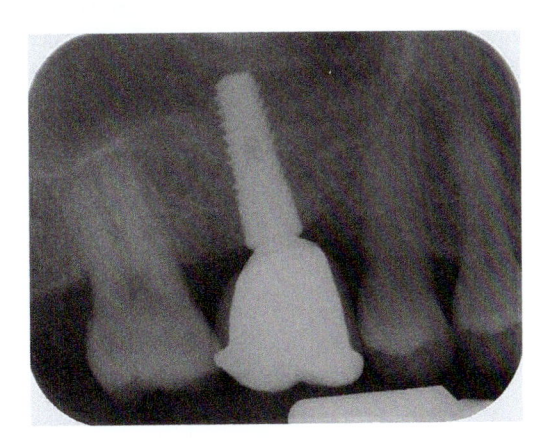

Figure 16.47 A radiograph after 4 years in function. Note a newly formed bone in the sinus.

C. Minimally invasive ridge augmentation using CGF membrane and growth factor-enriched putty conditioned bone (sticky bone™)

The alveolar ridge with severe horizontal and vertical bone resorption is a challenging site for oral rehabilitation with a dental implant due to insufficient bone volume to accommodate dental implants.

For the successful augmentation of a severe atrophic ridge, guided bone regeneration (GBR) or a block bone graft is required [41, 42]. GBR is indicated for the reconstruction of small-sized two- or three-wall bony defects. To reconstruct a large one- or two-wall bony defect, bone tacks on the collagen membrane or titanium mesh are required to contain the particulate bone graft during the healing period [43]. The block bone procedure has several disadvantages: (1) increased post-operative patient discomfort, (2) increased surgical time and cost, and (3) additional surgery from the donor site. As an alternative to the block bone procedure, titanium mesh-assisted GBR is widely accepted. However, this technique has some disadvantages, such as bone loss due to early exposure of mesh and technical difficulties.

For a successful GBR, stability of the bone graft, space maintenance, angiogenesis, and a tension-free primary suture are essential [44]. Space maintenance with a bone graft should be provided during the healing period. However, it is difficult to contain particulate bone in a one- or two-wall bony defect or vertical defect without additional use of bone tacks on the membrane or titanium mesh. For stability of a particulate bone graft inside the bone defect, a sticky bone graft has recently been introduced for the reconstruction of large bone defects. Sticky bone is biologically solidified bone graft using mixing of autologous fibrin in the liquid phase with a particulate bone powder [45]. A sticky bone graft does not disperse, even while being shaken with a cotton plier. That is why it is called a *sticky* bone. This sticky bone graft has numerous advantages: (1) easy adaptation of the bone graft to the bone defect, (2) prevention of macro- and micromigration of the bone graft during the healing period, (3) minimal bone loss and stable space maintenance during the healing period, (4) prevention of soft tissue ingrowth into the sticky bone graft, and (5) faster bone regeneration from contained autologous growth factors from fibrin in the liquid phase gained after centrifugation [27,30,45].

Preparation of sticky bone

The procedure to prepare sticky bone is the same of CGF preparation except for using an uncoated test tube. Approximately 8–9 ml of venous blood is drawn from the patient and the blood is centrifuged by a special centrifuge (Medifuge, Silfradent srl, Sofia, Italy, or any compatible centrifuge) for 3–12 minutes. At the end of the centrifugation process, there are two blood fractions: (1) the upper autologous fibrin layer and (2) the red blood cell layer (Figures 16.48 and 16.49). The upper fibrin layer is aspirated with a syringe and mixed with a particulate bone substitute. The

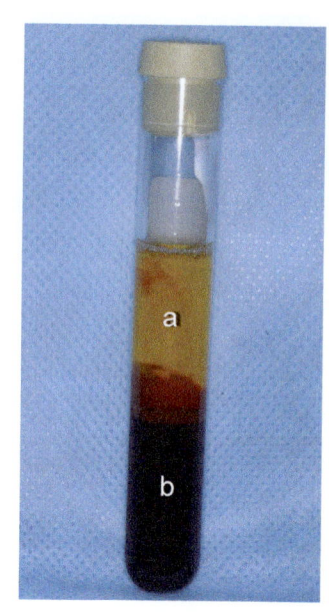

Figure 16.49 Two blood fractions after centrifugation: (**a**) the upper autologous fibrin layer, which makes sticky bone and (**b**) the red blood cell layer.

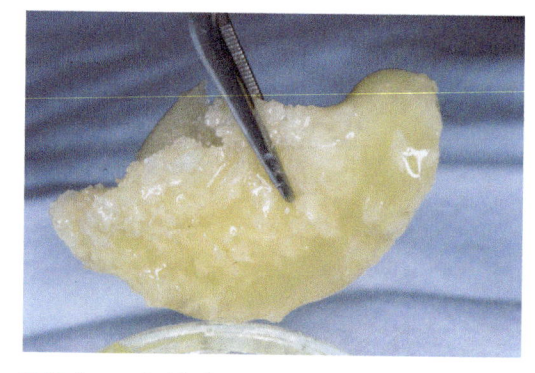

Figure 16.50 Prepared sticky bone.

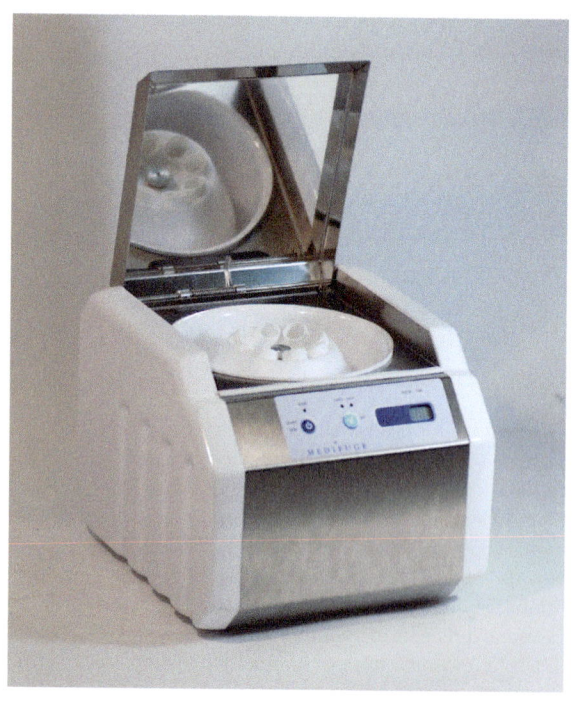

Figure 16.48 Special centrifuge to prepare CGF and sticky bone.

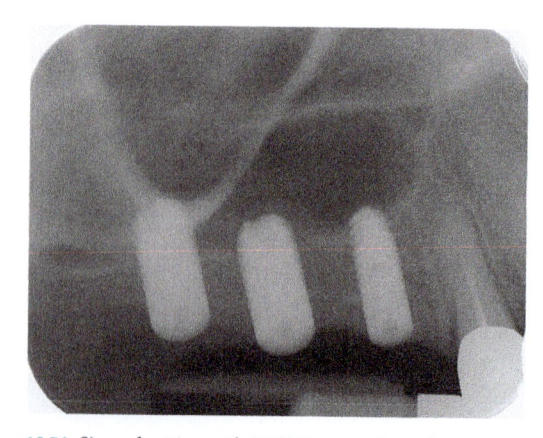

Figure 16.51 Sinus elevation with HPISE was performed.

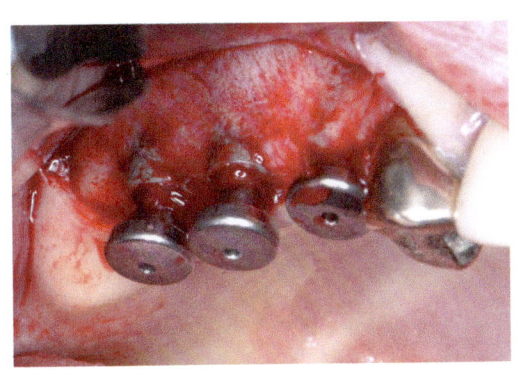

Figure 16.52 Note the horizontal bone resorption during the uncovering.

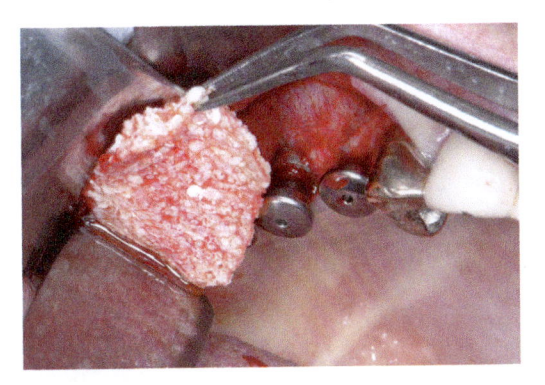

Figure 16.53 Prepared sticky bone.

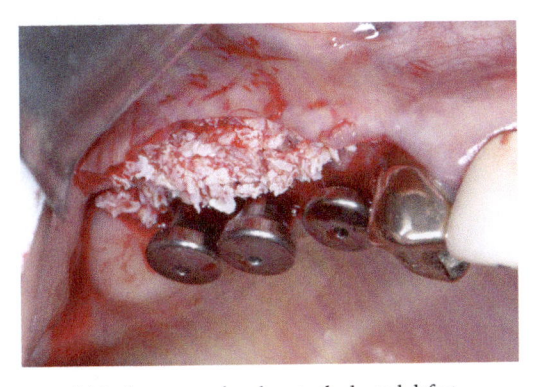

Figure 16.54 Sticky bone was placed on to the buccal defect.

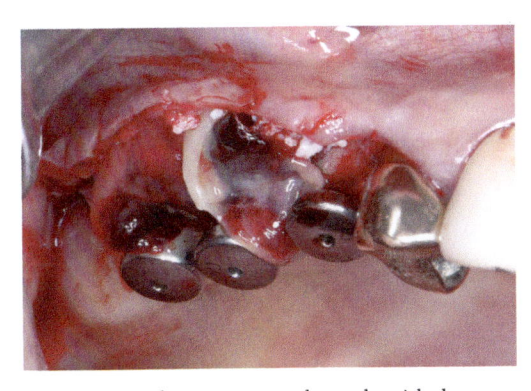

Figure 16.55 CGF membrane was covered over the sticky bone.

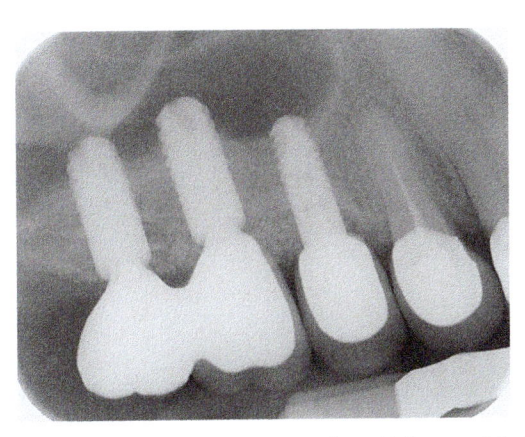

Figure 16.56 After 2 years in function. Note the stable bone graft in the interproximal area.

mixed particulate bone graft with the fibrin layer in the liquid phase is consolidated within 3 to 5 minutes into the sticky phase and well fitted into the bone defect (Figure 16.50). This sticky bone does not migrate during the healing period as compared to the particulate graft. Ti mesh, block bone, or bone tack are not needed in most cases (Figures 16.51 to 16.56). To obtain a much higher concentration of platelets in the upper fibrin layer and prevent spontaneous coagulation of the liquid-phase fibrin layer during the centrifugation, the time of centrifugation can be shortened to 3 minutes.

Case Report

A 56-year-old woman with complaints of masticatory difficulty visited our department. She had used a mini implant-supported overdenture in the maxilla but complained of poor stability of the overdenture. The patient preferred an implant-supported prosthesis. Her maxillary edentulous ridge was severely resorbed clinically. Ridge augmentation with a ridge-split procedure and simultaneous implant placement were planned.

The surgery was performed under a local anesthesia by using 2% lidocaine that included 1:100 000 epinephrine. Flomoxef sodium (Flumarin®; Ildong Pharmaceutical Co., Korea, 500 mg i.v.) was administered one hour before the surgery. A full-thickness mucoperiosteal flap was elevated to expose the atrophic maxillary ridge. The bone width was 1 to 2 mm wide (Figures 16.57 and 16.58). Before performing the ridge split, all implant sites were prepared with a 1.6 mm wide piezoelectric round tip to accommodate the rotary ridge expander. Piezoelectric crestal osteotomy was made along the alveolar crest. The depth of the crestal osteotomy was made one-half to two-thirds of the planned implant length to achieve primary stability. Anterior and posterior vertical osteotomies, connecting with the crestal osteotomy, were made in order to facilitate the ridge expansion and prevent accidental fracture of the expanded buccal plate (Figures 16.59 and 16.60). Expansion of the alveolar ridge was performed using the rotary ridge expander (Bone compressor®, MIS Implant Co., Israel) at 50 rpm. A ridge expander reduces patients' discomfort and surgical trauma (a surgical mallet is not needed) (Figure 16.61). Four implants (Dentis Implant Co., Daegu, Korea) were placed at the same time with good stability (Figure 16.62). Sticky bone using bovine bone (Biocera, Oscotec Co., Chunan) and a mineral allograft (Puros allograft, Zimmer Dental, CA) was grafted over the expanded ridge and resorbable collagen membrane (Pericardium, Zimmer Dental, CA) was placed over the bone graft (Figure 16.63). Four CGF membrane pieces were placed over the collagen membrane to accelerate soft tissue healing (Figures 16.64 to 16.66). The patient's old denture was relined and delivered immediately.

Implants were exposed after 6 months of healing by using apically repositioned flap to create the attached keratinized gingiva and vestibular space around implants. Bone regeneration over cover screws was observed because the sticky bone had not migrated during the healing period (Figure 16.67). A locator attachment-supported overdenture with a good retention was delivered successfully (Figures 16.68 and 16.79a). A 2-year follow-up radiograph showed a good preservation of bone level (Figure 16.69b).

(continued)

(Continued)

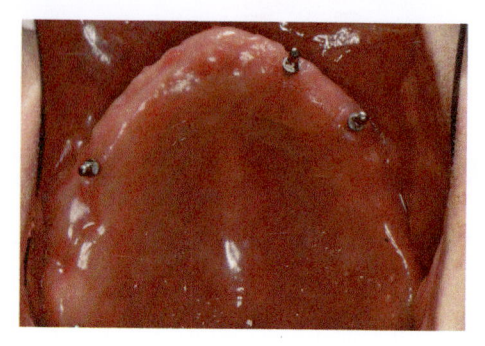

Figure 16.57 Clinical view reveals mini-implants and severe horizontal bone resorption in the maxilla.

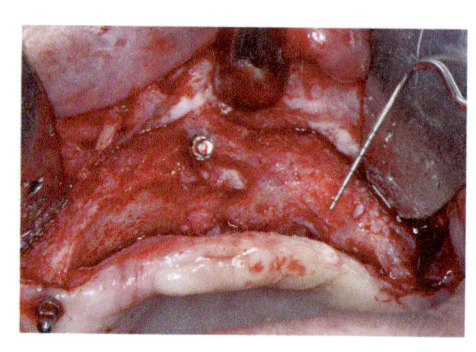

Figure 16.58 Note the 1–2 mm wide alveolar ridge. Block bone or mesh-assisted ridge augmentation were avoided to reduced post-operative patient discomfort.

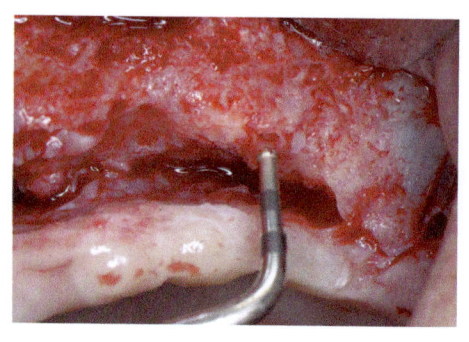

Figure 16.59 Preparation of implant sites were performed with utilization of a 1.6 mm wide piezoelectric round carbide tip before performing the ridge split. A round carbide tip does not slip down during osteotomy, even in the very narrow ridge.

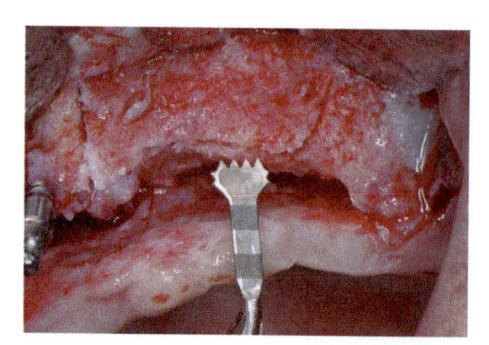

Figure 16.60 Piezoelectric crestal osteotomy and vertical osteotomy with a thin-bladed saw tip. The depth of the crestal osteotomy should be limited to one-half to two-thirds of the planned implants length.

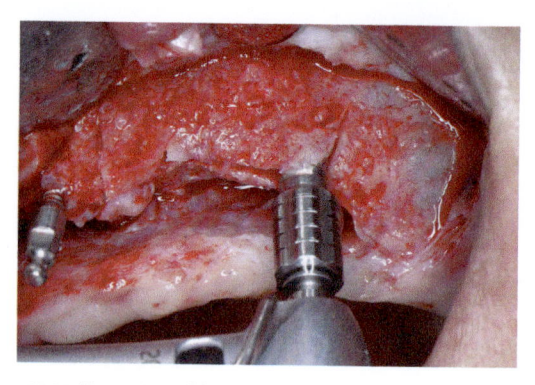

Figure 16.61 Expansion of the alveolar ridge with a rotary ridge expander at 50 rpm.

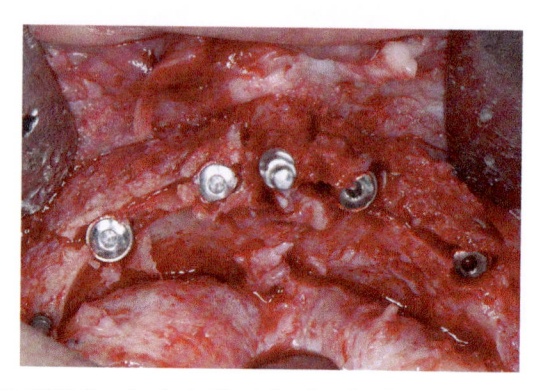

Figure 16.62 Four implants (Dentis Implant Co., Daegu, Korea) were placed with initial good stability.

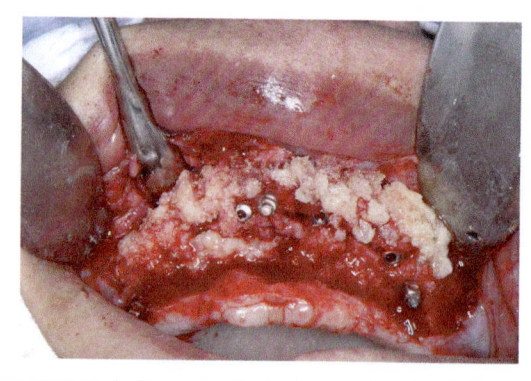

Figure 16.63 Sticky bone using bovine bone and a mineral allograft was grafted over the expanded ridge.

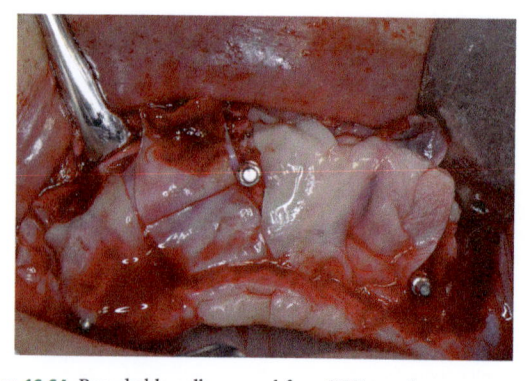

Figure 16.64 Resorbable collagen and four CGF membranes were used to cover the bone graft.

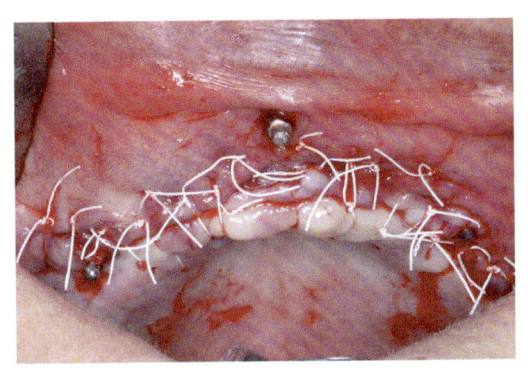

Figure 16.65 A tension-free primary closure was gained and the temporary denture was delivered immediately.

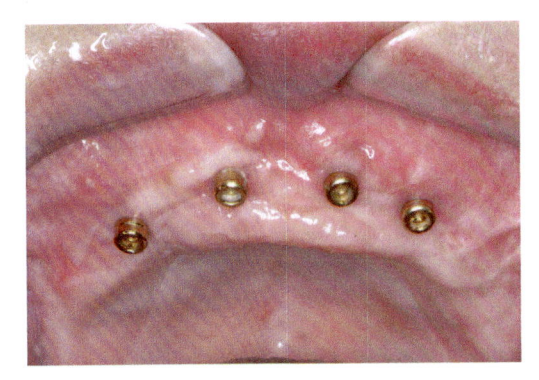

Figure 16.68 A locator attachment-supported denture is delivered.

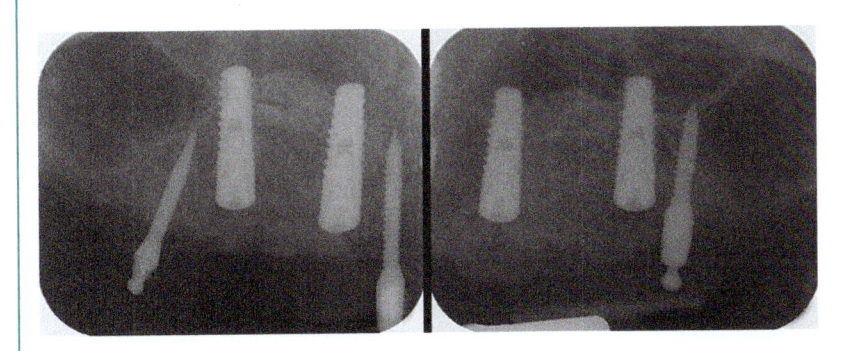

Figure 16.66 Post-operative radiograph.

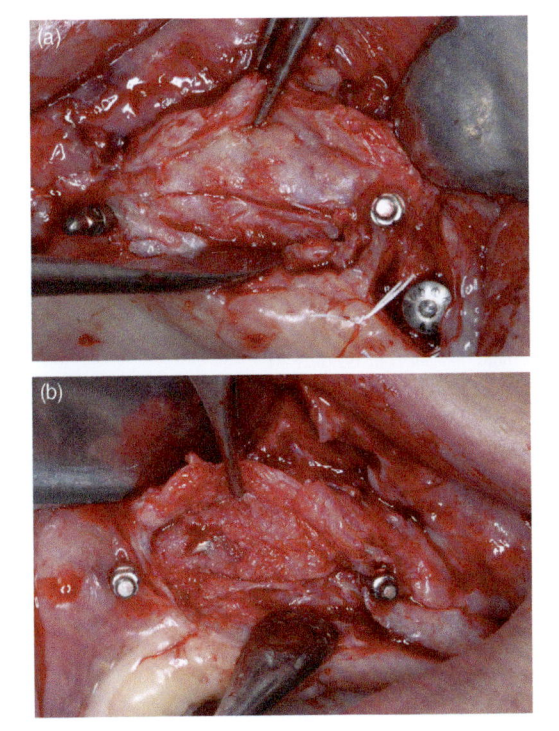

Figure 16.67 The uncovering of implants after 6 months of healing in the right and left maxilla. Note a successful bone regeneration due to sticky bone use.

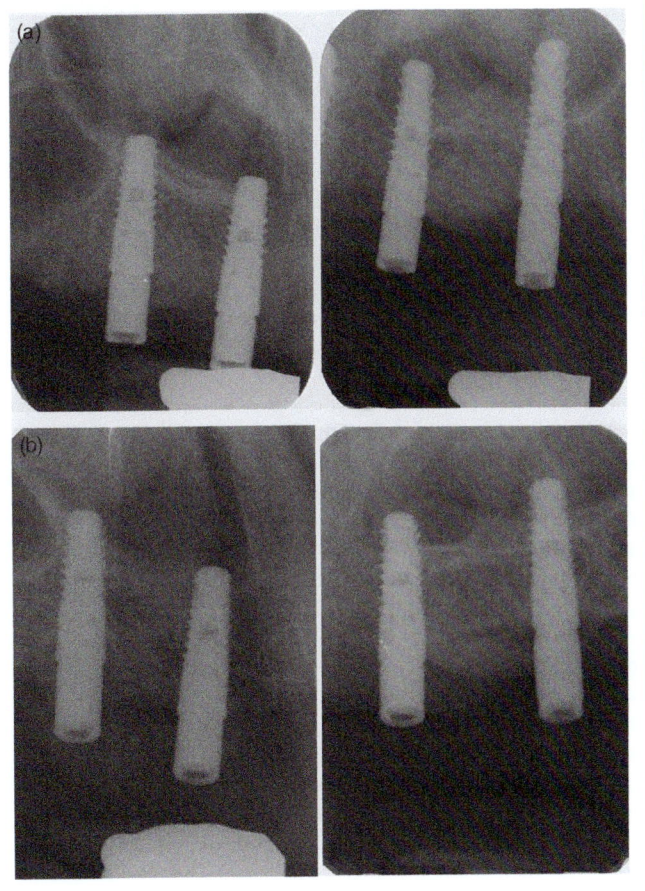

Figure 16.69 Radiographs after the delivery of implant overdenture and 2 years in function.

Discussion

Maxillary sinus membrane perforations are the most common complication of sinus augmentation [4] and have been shown to cause post-operative complications and endanger the survival rate of the endosseous implants [8, 9]. When preparing bony windows, careful management of sinus mucosa is required. Several studies reported higher membrane perforation that occurs when using rotary devices [46–48]. However, numerous studies on sinus augmentation using piezoelectric round tips showed a very low rate of mucosal perforations [11,13,15,16]. Sohn et al. compared round and thin-bladed saw tips for preparation of the lateral bony window [13]. According to the study, compared to the piezoelectric round tip, the piezoelectric thin-bladed saw tip had numerous advantages: (1) faster osteotomy when preparing the bony window, (2) precision of osteotomy, (3) minimal bone loss, and (4) facilitation of precise replacement of the bony window. The repositioned bony window acts as a homologous osteoinductive/osteoconductive barrier over the bone graft. As a barrier, the homologous bony window is free from the cross-contamination of animal or human origin, and precise adaptation of the lateral bony window prevents soft tissue ingrowth. Clinically and histologically, repositioned bony window showed complete bone healing between the replaceable bony window and the lateral sinus wall. Favorable new bone formation was observed in all specimens without any fibrous connective tissue invagination. More mature bone was observed along the floor of the replaceable bony window than at the center of the graft site [49]. According to this animal study on comparison of collagen membrane and a replaced bony window over the lateral sinus wall [50], a significantly higher and faster new bone formation was observed in the group receiving a replaced bony window.

As space makers in the new sinus compartment under the elevated sinus membrane, various bone graft materials have been used for many years. However, successful bone augmentation in the maxillary sinus *without* bone graft and osseointegration of implants have been reported in human and animal studies [12,19,23,51,52]. According to this immunochemical study on a comparison of sinus augmentation with/without bone graft in animals, a faster and greater new bone formation was observed in non-bone grafted sinus [21]. The repositioned bony window may accelerate new bone formation earlier during healing versus the placement of a collagen membrane over grafting material in the sinus. Platelet aggregates, such as platelet-rich plasma and platelet rich in growth factors, have been used to accelerate new bone formation associated with guided bone regeneration and sinus graft [24–26,36,37]. Fibrin-rich gel is known to slowly release growth factors such as transforming growth factor (TGF-b1), platelet-derived growth factor (PDGF), and vascular endothelial growth factor (VEGF). It accelerates new bone formation when it is mixed with bone graft in the maxillary sinus [28, 29]. In addition, the concentrated growth factors (CGF), as a sole "grafting" material, showed success as an alternative to bone grafts and induced fast new bone formation in the sinus [24]. Compared to the platelet-rich plasma or platelet rich in growth factors, CGF is simple to make and does not require any synthetic or biomaterials, such as bovine thrombin and calcium chloride, to form a gel condition. It is free from the risk of cross-contamination.

Compared to the lateral window approach, the crestal approach has the advantage of being minimally invasive, which contributes to less post-operative discomfort. Unlike the ostetome technique, the HPISE technique is an innovative crestal method where a surgical mallet is not required to break the sinus floor [3,35,36]. This technique is free from the risk of post-operative vertigo. The HPISE technique uses ultrasonic piezoelectric microvibrations to break the sinus floor directly and hydraulic pressure from the internal irrigation for mucosal elevation. Therefore, bone compaction is not a prerequisite for the sinus elevation in the HPISE technique unlike conventional crestal approaches.

To reconstruct severely atrophic alveolar bone, space maintenance and stability of the bone graft are essential for ridge augmentation. Although the block bone graft provides strong space maintenance in the large defect, post-operative patient discomfort associated with this procedure is increased. Titanium mesh provides strong space maintenance as well. However, the high exposure rate of the titanium mesh can cause poor bone regeneration [53]. Sticky bone using autologous fibrin interlocks particulate bone powder and micro- or macromovement of the grafted bone is prevented [45]. Therefore, the volume of sticky bone is maintained during the healing period. In addition, sticky bone contains autologous growth factors released from platelets, encouraging accelerated bone and soft tissue regeneration [30].

Conclusion

Bone graft material may not be a prerequisite for sinus augmentation. Insertion of CGF, as an alternative to a bone graft, can be a predictable procedure for sinus augmentation that can accelerate bone regeneration in the sinus. The HPISE technique is an alternative surgical method to the lateral sinus augmentation technique and can be used with or without bone graft material. The utilization of sticky bone is effective for space maintenance in the bone grafted ridge and accelerates bone regeneration and wound healing.

References

1. Boyne P, James R: Grafting of the maxillary floor with autogenous marrow and bone. *J Oral Surg* 1980;**38**:613–616.
2. Aghaloo TL, Moy PK: Which hard tissue augmentation techniques are the most successful in furnishing bony support for implant placement? *Int J Oral Maxillofac Implants* 2007;**22**:49–70.
3. Barone A, Santini S, Sbordone L, Crespi R, Covani U: A clinical study of the outcomes and complications associated with maxillary sinus augmentation. *Int J Oral Maxillofac Implants* 2006;**21**:81–85.
4. Schwartz-Arad D, Herzberg R, Dolev E: The prevalence of surgical complications of the sinus graft procedure and their impact on implant survival. *J Periodontol* 2004;**75**:511–516.
5. Shlomi B, Horowitz I, Kahn A, Dobriyan A, Chaushu G: The effect of sinus membrane perforation and repair with Lambone on the outcome of maxillary sinus floor augmentation: a radiographic assessment. *Int J Oral Maxillofac Implants* 2004;**19**:559–562.
6. Pikos MA: Maxillary sinus membrane repair: report of a technique for large perforations. *Implant Dent* 1999;**8**:29–34.
7. Levin L, Herzberg R, Dolev E, Schwartz-Arad D: Smoking and complications of onlay bone grafts and sinus lift operations. *Int J Oral Maxillofac Implants* 2004;**19**:369–373.
8. Proussaefs P, Lozada J, Kim J, Rohrer MD: Repair of the perforated sinus membrane with a resorbable collagen membrane: a human study. *Int J Oral Maxillofac Implants* 2004;**19**:413–420.
9. Kim YK, Hwang JY, Yun PY: Relationship between prognosis of dental implants and maxillary sinusitis associated with the sinus elevation procedure. *Int J Oral Maxillofac Implants* 2013;**28**(1):178–183.
10. Torrella F, Pitarch J, Cabanes G, Anitua E. Ultrasonic ostectomy for the surgical approach of the maxillary sinus: a technical note. *Int J Oral Maxillofac Implants* 1998;**13**(5):697–700.
11. Vercellotti T, De Paoli S, Nevins M: The piezoelectric bony window osteotomy and sinus membrane elevation: introduction of a new technique for simplification of the sinus augmentation procedure. *Int J Periodontics Restorative Dent* 2001;**21**(6):561–567.
12. Sohn DS, Lee JS, Ahn MR et al: New bone formation in the maxillary sinus without bone grafts. *Implant Dentistry* 2008;**17**;321–331.

13. Sohn DS, Moon JW, Lee HW, Choi BJ, Shin IH: Comparison of two piezoelectric cutting inserts for lateral bony window osteotomy: a retrospective study of 127 consecutive sites. *Int J Oral Maxillofac Implants* 2010;**25**(3):571–576.
14. Sohn DS, Ahn MR, Jang BY: Sinus bone augmentation using piezoelectric surgery. *Implantolgy* 2003;**7**:48–55.
15. Wallace SS, Mazor Z, Froum SJ, Cho SC, Tarnow DP: Schneiderian membrane perforation rate during sinus elevation using piezosurgery: clinical results of 100 consecutive cases. *Int J Periodontics Restorative Dent* 2007;**27**:413–419.
16. Blus C, Szmukler-Moncler S, Salama M, Salama H, Garber D: Sinus bone grafting procedures using ultrasonic bone surgery: 5-year experience. *Int J Periodontics Restorative Dent* 2008;**28**:221–229.
17. Sohn DS: *Color Atlas, Clinical Applications of Piezoelectric Bone Surgery*. Kunja Publishing, Seoul, South Korea, 2008, pp. 47–160.
18. Lundgren S, Andersson S, Gualini F, et al: Bone reformation with sinus membrane elevation: a new surgical technique for maxillary sinus floor augmentation. *Clin Implant Dent Relat Res* 2004;**6**:165–173.
19. Palma VC, Magro-Filho O, de Oliveira JA, et al: Bone reformation and implant integration following maxillary sinus membrane elevation: an experimental study in primates. *Clin Implant Dent Relat Res* 2006;**8**:11–24.
20. Sohn DS, Kim WS, An KM, et al: Comparative histomorphometric analysis of maxillary sinus augmentation with and without bone grafting in rabbit. *Implant Dent* 2010;**19**(3):259–270.
21. Sohn DS, Moon JW, Lee WH, Kim SS, Kim CW, Kim KT, Moon YS: Comparison of new bone formation in the maxillary sinus with and without bone grafts: immunochemical rabbit study. *Int J Oral Maxillofac Implants* 2011;**26**(5):1033–1042.
22. Hatano N, Sennerby L, Lundgren S: Maxillary sinus augmentation using sinus membrane elevation and peripheral venous blood for implant-supported rehabilitation of the atrophic posterior maxilla: case series. *Clin Implant Dent Relat Res* 2007;**9**:150–155.
23. Sohn DS, Moon JW, Moon KN, et al: New bone formation in the maxillary sinus using only absorbable gelatin sponge. *J Oral Maxillofac Surg* 2010;**68**(6):1327–1333.
24. Sohn DS, Heo JU, Kwak DH, Kim DE, et al: Bone regeneration in the maxillary sinus using an autologous fibrin-rich block with concentrated growth factors alone. *Implant Dent* 2011;**20**(5):389–395.
25. Marx RE: Platelet-rich plasma: evidence to support its use. *J Oral Maxillofac Surg* 2004;**62**(4):489–496.
26. Anitua E, Orive G, Pla R, Roman P, Serrano V, Andía I: The effects of PRGF on bone regeneration and on titanium implant osseointegration in goats: a histologic and histomorphometric study. *J Biomed Mater Res A* 2009;**91**(1):158–165.
27. You TM, Choi BH, Zhu SJ, Jung JH, Lee SH, Huh JY, Lee HJ, Li J. Platelet-enriched fibrin glue and platelet-rich plasma in the repair of bone defects adjacent to titanium dental implants. *Int J Oral Maxillofac Implants* 2007;**22**(3):417–422.
28. Dohan DM, Choukroun J, Diss A, Dohan SL, Dohan AJ, Mouhyi J, Gogly B: Platelet-rich fibrin (PRF): a second-generation platelet concentrate. Part I: technological concepts and evolution. *Oral Surg Oral Med Oral Pathol Oral Radiol Endod* 2006;**101**(3):e37–44.
29. Choukroun J, Diss A, Simonpieri A, Girard MO, Schoeffler C, Dohan SL, Dohan AJ, Mouhyi J, Dohan DM: Platelet-rich fibrin (PRF): a second-generation platelet concentrate. Part V: histologic evaluations of PRF effects on bone allograft maturation in sinus lift. *Oral Surg Oral Med Oral Pathol Oral Radiol Endod* 2006;**101**(3):299–303.
30. Corigliano M., Sacco L., Baldoni E: CGF – una proposta terapeutica per la medicina rigenerativa. *Odontoiatria* no. 1 – anno XXIX– Maggio, 2010, pp. 69–81.
31. Summers RB: The osteotome technique: Part 3 – Less invasive methods of elevating the sinus floor. *Compendium* 1994;**15**:698–708.
32. Sohn DS: Lecture titled with clinical applications of piezoelectric bone surgery. In: 8th Internationa Congress of Oral Implantologists, Singapore, August 28 2004.
33. Sohn DS, Lee JS, An KM, Choi BJ: Piezoelectric internal sinus elevation (PISE) technique: a new method for internal sinus elevation. *Implant Dent* 2009;**18**:458–463.
34. Chen L, Cha J: An 8-year retrospective study: 1100 patients receiving 1557 implants using the minimally invasive hydraulic sinus condensing technique. *J Periodontol* 2005;**76**:482–491.
35. Sohn DS, Maupin P, Fayos RP, et al: Minimally invasive sinus augmentation using ultrasonic piezoelectric vibration and hydraulic pressure. *J Implant Adv Clin Dent*: 2010;**2**:27–40.
36. Kim JM, Sohn DS, Heo JU, Park JS, Jung HS, Moon JW, Lee JH, Park IS: Minimally invasive sinus augmentation using ultrasonic piezoelectric vibration and hydraulic pressure: a multicenter retrospective study. *Implant Dent* 2012;**21**(6):536–542.
37. Kim JM, Sohn DS, Bae MS, Moon JW, Lee JH, Park IS: Flapless transcrestal sinus augmentation using hydrodynamic piezoelectric internal sinus elevation with autologous concentrated growth factors alone. *Implant Dent* 2014;**23**(2):168–174.
38. Peñarrocha M, Pérez H, García A, et al: Benign paroxysmal positional vertigo as a complication of osteotome expansion of the maxillary alveolar ridge. *J Oral Maxillofac Surg* 2001;**59**:106–107.
39. Saker M, Oqle O: Benign paroxysmal positional vertigo subsequent to sinus lift via closed technique. *J Oral Maxillofac Surg* 2005;**63**:1385–1387.
40. Rosen PS, Summers R, Mellado JR, Salkin LM, Shanaman RH, Marks MH, Fugazzotto PA: The bone-added osteotome sinus floor elevation technique: multicenter retrospective report of consecutively treated patients. *Int J Oral Maxillofac Implants* 1999;**14**(6):853–858.
41. Pikos MA. Block autografts for localized ridge augmentation: Part II. The posterior mandible. *Implant Dent* 2000;**9**:67–75.
42. Dahlin C, Linde A, Gottlow J, Nyman S: Healing of bone defects by guided tissue regeneration. *Plast Reconstr Surg* 1988;**81**(5):672–676.
43. Rasia-dal Polo M, Poli PP, Rancitelli D, Beretta M, Maiorana C: Alveolar ridge reconstruction with titanium meshes: a systematic review of the literature. *Med Oral Patol Oral Cir Bucal* 2014, 1;**19**(6):e639–4635.
44. Wang HL, Boyapati L: "PASS" principles for predictable bone regeneration. *Implant Dent* 2006;**15**(1):8–17.
45. Sohn DS: Lecture titled With sinus and ridge augmentation with CGF and AFG. In: Symposium on CGF and AFG, Tokyo, June 6, 2010.
46. Hernández-Alfaro F, Torradeflot MM, Marti C: Prevalence and management of Schneiderian membrane perforations during sinus-lift procedures. *Clin Oral Implants Res* 2008;**19**(1):91–98.
47. Viña-Almunia J, Peñarrocha-Diago M, Peñarrocha-Diago M: Influence of perforation of the sinus membrane on the survival rate of implants placed after direct sinus lift. Literature update. *Med Oral Pathol Oral Cir Bucal* 2009: 1;**14**(3): E133–136.
48. Wen SC1 Lin YH, Yang YC, Wang HL: The influence of sinus membrane thickness upon membrane perforation during transcrestal sinus lift procedure. *Clin Oral Implants Res* 2015;**26**(10):1158–1164.
49. Kim JM, Sohn DS, Heo JU, Moon JW, Lee JH, Park IS: Benefit of the replaceable bony window in lateral maxillary sinus augmentation: clinical and histologic study. *Implant Dent* 2014;**23**(3):277–282.
50. Moon YS, Sohn DS, Moon JW, Lee JH, Park IS, Lee JK: Comparative histomorphometric analysis of maxillary sinus augmentation with absorbable collagen membrane and osteoinductive replaceable bony window in rabbits. *Implant Dent* 2014;**23**(1):29–36.
51. Cricchio G, Sennerby L, Lundgren S: Sinus bone formation and implant survival after sinus membrane elevation and implant placement: a 1- to 6-year follow-up study. *Clin Oral Implants Res* 2011;**22**(10):1200–1212.
52. Lin IC, Gonzalez AM, Chang HJ, et al: A 5-year follow-up of 80 implants in 44 patients placed immediately after the lateral trap-door window procedure to accomplish maxillary sinus elevation without bone grafting. *Int J Oral Maxillofac Implants* 2011;**26**(5):1079–1086.
53. Lizio G, Corinaldesi G, Marchetti C: Alveolar ridge reconstruction with titanium mesh: a three-dimensional evaluation of factors affecting bone augmentation. *Int J Oral Maxillofac Implants* 2014;**29**(6):1354–1363.

CHAPTER 17

Sinus Floor Elevation and Grafting: The Lateral Approach

Michael Beckley[1] and Len Tolstunov[2]

[1]Department of Oral and Maxillofacial Surgery, University of the Pacific, Arthur A. Dugoni School of Dentistry Private Practice, Oral and Maxillofacial Surgery, Livermore, California, USA
[2]Private Practice, Oral and Maxillofacial Surgery, San Francisco, California, USA
Department of Oral and Maxillofacial Surgery, University of California San Francisco, School of Dentistry, University of the Pacific, Arthur A. Dugoni School of Dentistry Private Practice, Oral and Maxillofacial Surgery, San Francisco, California, USA

Prior to implant placement in the posterior maxilla, bone volume and sinus anatomy must be evaluated. Lack of internal loading after tooth removal, pressure resorption from removable prostheses, and pneumatization of the maxillary sinus may result in multidimensional bone deficiency. Bone may be deficient at the alveolar crest, lateral alveolus, and sinus floor. Predictable, functional, and esthetic outcomes are rooted in comprehensive clinical and radiographic diagnosis prior to surgery. Sinus elevation and grafting through a lateral window approach is a predictable technique to vertically augment the posterior maxilla prior to and often simultaneously with implant placement. Successful dental implant placement and osseointegration after sinus augmentation and grafting with a lateral approach has been reported to be between 78.1 and 100% [1–8].

Tatum modified the Caldwell–Luc operation for dental implant treatment in the posterior maxilla with a limited amount of vertical bone stock in 1975, which he described in detail in 1986 [9]. Tatum used the lateral maxillary bone window that was rotated medially into the sinus elevating the sinus membrane. In 1980, Boyne reported maxillary sinus grafting in 48 patients using autologous bone and non-resorbable hydroxylapatite (HA) particles. After three months of healing, HA-coated titanium implants were placed. A 6.4% implant failure rate was reported with implants placed in the grafted sinus floor [10]. Subsequent to this paper the literature has become replete with different techniques, grafts materials, and protocols for augmenting the posterior maxilla and sinus prior to and with implant placement.

Indications and contraindications

Prior to surgery the patient's medical history should be reviewed. There are very few absolute contraindications to lateral sinus floor elevation and grafting. Common systemic contraindications include the following conditions when presented in an uncontrolled state: hypertension, diabetes mellitus, thyroid disease, and adrenal disease. Other conditions can include coagulopathies, immunocompromised diseases, neoplastic disease, medication-related osteonecrosis of the jaws (MRONJ), early or late pregnancy, substance abuse, and untreated mental illness. In general, patients with well-controlled chronic diseases are candidates for sinus elevation and grafting.

Local contraindications include: acute sinusitis, non-patent osteomeatal complex (OMC), prior radiation therapy, and incomplete craniofacial growth. Acute and chronic sinusitis should be resolved prior to surgery. This may not be possible in all situations. However, if there is any doubt about the patency of the OMC, treatment should be postponed until patency has been confirmed or established, if possible (Figure 17.1). Otolaryngology referral should be considered for patients with suspected sinus disease.

Patients with minimal residual alveolar bone below the sinus floor in the posterior maxilla may benefit from sinus elevation and grafting first, and implant placement after graft healing (Figure 17.2). In patients with residual alveolar bone height sufficient for primary implant stabilization, combining lateral sinus lifting with grafting and simultaneous implant placement should be considered (Figure 17.3).

Applied surgical anatomy

Sinus means "pocket" in Latin. The maxillary sinus is usually the largest of the paranasal sinuses (Figure 17.4). The average height of the adult maxillary sinus is 33 mm, width 23 mm, and 34 mm from anterior to posterior. The second premolar and first and second molars are the teeth most often in proximity to the sinus and often the cause of odontogenic sinusitis. The relationship of the floor of the sinus to teeth is variable. The tooth roots may be covered in bone or project into the sinus with little or no bone covering them. Ridges and septa are common and may partition the sinus into two compartments. These may pose challenges when elevating and grafting the sinus floor. Pre-operative three-dimensional imaging can be helpful in identifying septa and ridges [11]. The innervation and blood supply is from the posterior superior alveolar, infraorbital, and anterior superior alveolar arteries and nerves. During the development of the facial skeleton, the maxillary sinus is very small until the primary and then the secondary dentition appears and develops to its final form with the eruption of permanent dentition [12]. After tooth loss in the posterior maxilla and with the aging process, the sinus often enlarges or become pneumatized, "taking

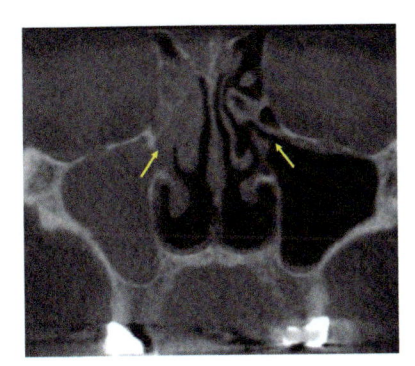

Figure 17.1 Cone beam computed tomography (CBCT) scan (coronal section) indicating diseased right maxillary sinus with obstruction of the ostium and healthy left maxillary sinus with patent osteomeatal complex (OMC).

over" the alveolar bone below the sinus floor, which slowly resorbs [13] (Figure 17.5).

The ostium of the maxillary sinus deserves particular attention because a patent ostium is necessary for a healthy sinus. The ostium is located in the superior part of the medial wall of the sinus and opens into the middle meatus and drains into the nasal cavity through the ethmoid infundibulum (Figure 17.1). The ostium is located high enough on the medial wall of the sinus that inadvertent obstruction with graft material is unlikely. The location of the osteomeatal complex (OMC) does not provide for gravity-dependent sinus drainage. Drainage of the sinus is primarily through the mucociliary action. The sinus is lined with pseudostratified ciliated columnar epithelium with many goblet cells and an underlying connective tissue layer with many mucous glands. The lining of the sinus is commonly referred to as the Schneiderian membrane. A correlation between Schneiderian membrane thickness and gingival phenotype has been reported [14].

Sinus grafting may not be required in all cases of lateral sinus floor elevation. It has been reported that superior positioning of the lateral window or isolated elevation of the Schneiderian membrane may result in bone formation sufficient for implant placement [4, 15]. Many biologic and synthetic materials have used for sinus grafting. Graft sources can be divided into the following categories:
- Autologous bone (intraoral, extraoral sites)
- Allografts (MFDB, DFDB)
- Xenografts (bovine, equine, porcine)
- Biomimetics (BMP, PRP, PRF)

Success has been reported with many biologic and synthetic materials used for sinus augmentation. However, no one material has demonstrated clinical superiority [5, 6, 16–21].

Surgical technique: lateral sinus floor elevation and grafting

Lateral sinus floor elevation and grafting can be performed with local anesthesia or local anesthesia combined with intravenous sedation. Currently, there is no standard of care for preoperative imaging prior to sinus elevation, grafting, and implant placement. Decisions regarding pre-operative imaging should be patient specific and based on the clinician's experience. However, cone beam computed tomography offers excellent visualization of the regional anatomy and allows the

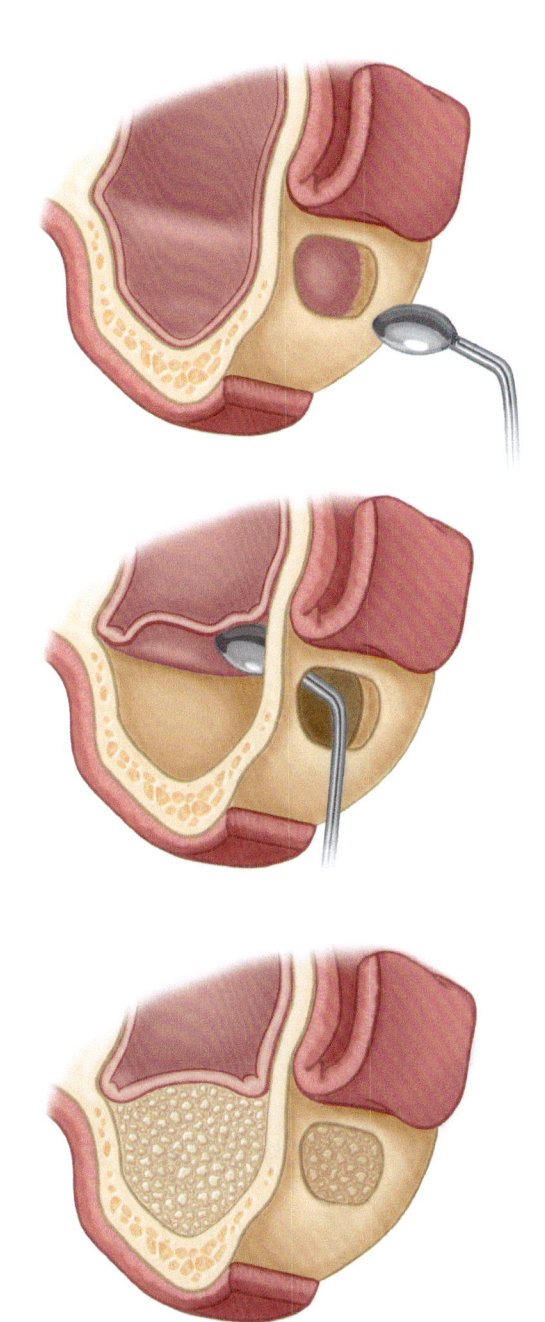

Figure 17.2 Illustration of lateral sinus floor elevation and grafting for delayed implant placement: limited amount of bone present in the posterior maxilla.

clinician to identify septa, pathology, and confirm patency of the osteomeatal complex [11, 13] (Figure 17.6).

These authors were unable to find any randomized controlled clinical trials comparing lateral sinus elevation and grafting with and without antibiotic administration. However, the available scientific evidence does support antibiotic administration prior to dental implant placement [22]. What antibiotic is most appropriate and whether a post-operative course improves outcomes is unknown. It has been reported that post-operative infection and antibiotic use is increased in patients who have experienced Schneiderian membrane perforation during sinus elevation and grafting surgeries [23].

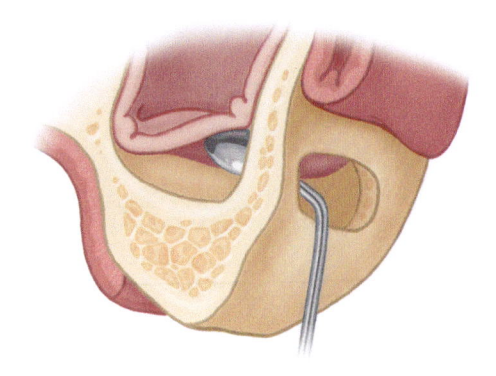

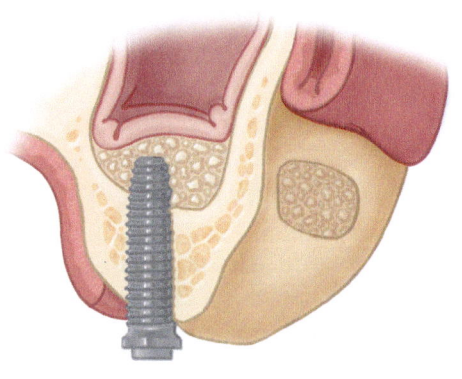

Figure 17.3 Illustration of lateral sinus floor elevation, grafting, and immediate implant placement: sufficient amount of bone present in the posterior maxilla for an immediate implant insertion.

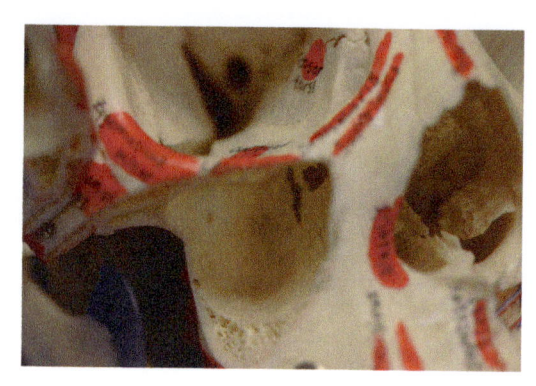

Figure 17.4 Skull, maxillary sinus.

Membrane placement over the osteotomy of the lateral maxillary wall has been advocated after sinus elevation and grafting. The rationale for this is based on guided tissue regeneration of osseous defects. Membrane placement may also be helpful to manage perforations of the Schneiderian membrane. There is evidence to support the routine use of resorbable and nonresorbable membrane placement to cover the lateral wall osteotomy. In a systematic review conducted by Wallace in 2003, he reported an increase in implant survival rate when barrier membranes were used to cover the lateral window after sinus augmentation [24]. However, others have reported no difference in implant survival with the placement of resorbable or non-resorbable membranes over the lateral window in cases of sinus grafting without membrane perforation [25].

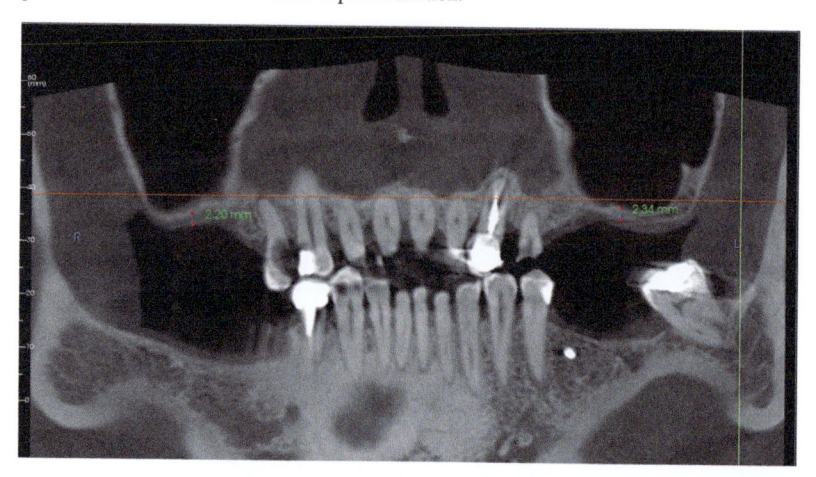

Figure 17.5 CBCT image demonstrating extensive bilateral maxillary sinus pneumatization and deficiency of alveolar bone for immediate implant placement.

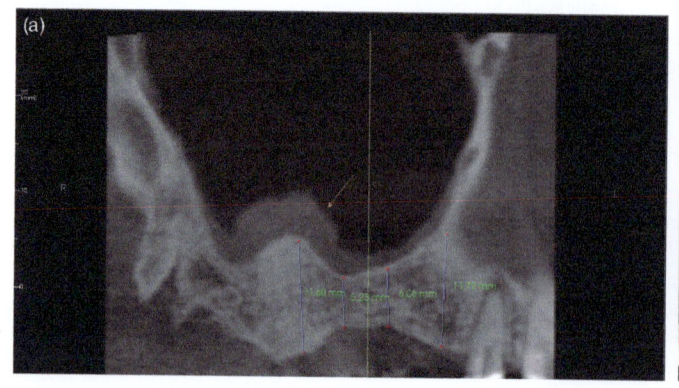

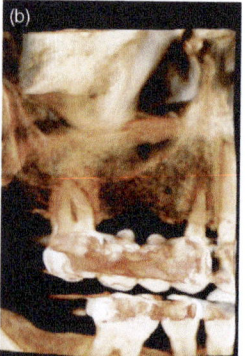

Figure 17.6 (a) CBCT image sand (b) CBCT 3D image of the maxillary sinus and adjacent alveolar bone. Precise evaluation and measurements can be done at the implant planning stage.

Sinus Floor Elevation and Grafting: The Lateral Approach   181

Case Report: Lateral approach to sinus floor elevation for delayed implant placement

The following case illustrates a lateral approach to sinus floor elevation for delayed implant placement after graft healing in the first molar region of the right maxilla (Figure 17.7). The patient underwent surgical procedure under IV sedation, 900 mg IV clindamycin phosphate was administered, and local anesthesia was given. A full-thickness mucoperiosteal flap was elevated (Figure 17.8a). The next step is careful removal of the lateral maxillary wall, taking care not to perforate the Schneiderian membrane.

There are two main surgical approaches to expose the sinus membrane. One is complete obliteration of the bone window and the other is bone window formation and elevation into the maxillary sinus like a trapdoor (Figure 17.8b). The choice of technique is based on the surgeon's preference and experience. In this case report, the first approach was utilized and was accomplished with a round burr. A diamond burr is often preferred to the stainless steel one due to its more "gentle" properties towards the thin Schneiderian membrane. Piezoelectric instruments are often also used at this stage of surgery to prevent membrane perforation.

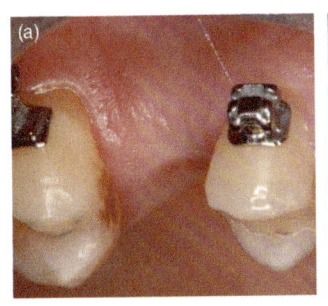

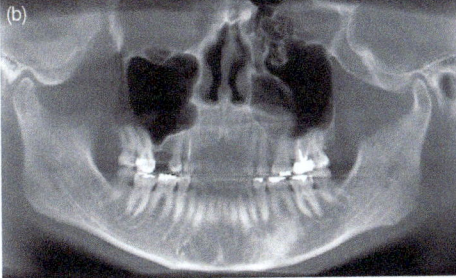

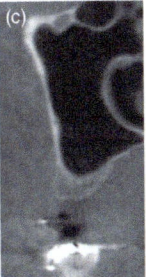

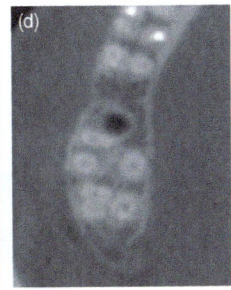

Figure 17.7 (a) Intraoral photograph of the missing right first maxillary molar; clinically, bone width appears to be present. It is important to check bone height using radiographic images. (b) Panoramic CBCT image indicating missing right first maxillary molar and advanced sinus pneumatization. (c) CBCT cross-sectional (coronal) image indicating extensive sinus pneumatization involving the alveolar ridge if an implant is contemplated. (d) Axial CBCT slice indicating involvement of the alveolar bone in the sinus pneumatization process necessitating the sinus lift procedure if an implant is contemplated.

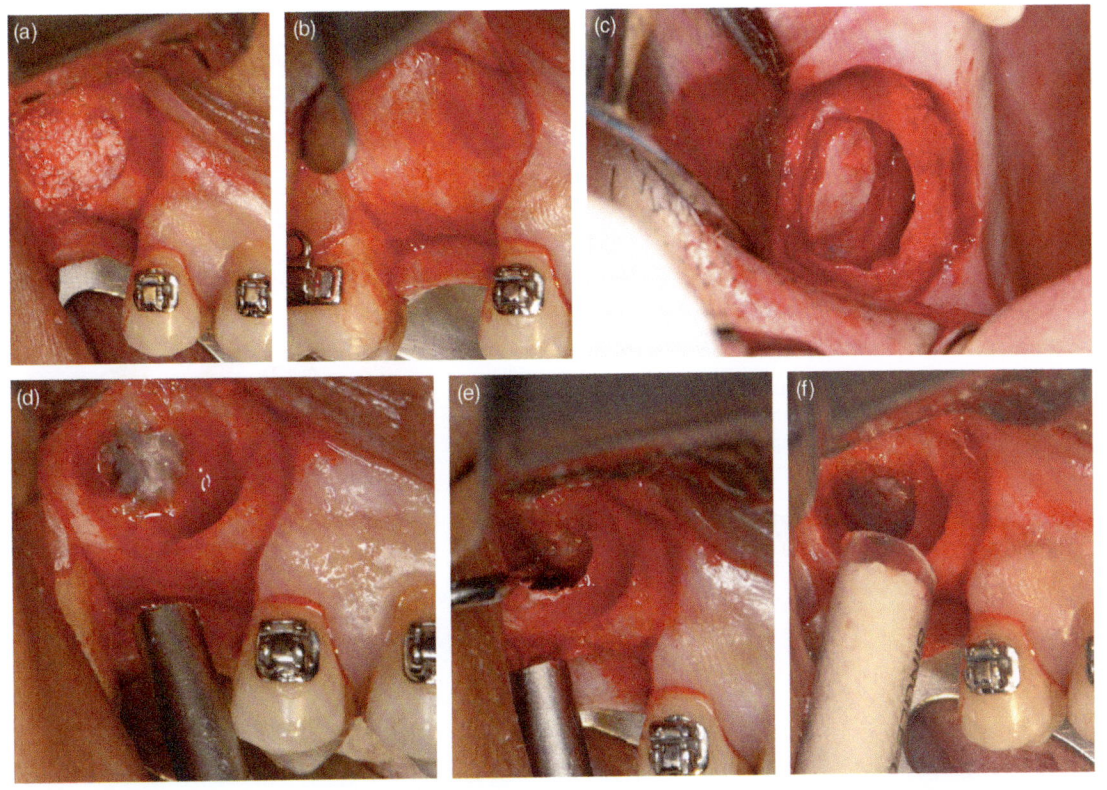

Figure 17.8 Intraoperative photographs demonstrating a lateral approach to the subantral augmentation (sinus lift) and bone grafting in surgical steps: (a) the buccal full thickness mucoperiosteal flap is elevated, exposing the anterior wall of the maxillary bone; (b) the "trapdoor" approach to sinus elevation preserving the osteotomized bone and elevating it inwards with the intact sinus membrane creating a subantral space (pocket); (c) intact Schneiderian membrane; (d) continuation of elevation of the intact Schneiderian membrane; (e) bone grafting of the subantral pocket is initiated; (f) bone grafting of the subantral space is completed.

(continued)

(continued)

After the bone of the lateral maxillary wall was removed, the Schneiderian membrane was exposed (Figure 17.8c). The next step was to gently elevate the membrane with specialized sinus curettes (Figure 17.8d). This may be facilitated by asking the patient to breathe in forcefully through the nose, thus creating negative pressure within the sinus cavity, which can result in the membrane moving superiorly. There are many techniques that can be used for a careful detachment of the thin sinus membrane around the bony window. Some prefer to start displacement of the membrane at the bottom of the bony window and some at the top. A slow and careful approach is the key here. A surgeon who takes his or her time at this stage of the surgery could be more successful in preventing the membrane perforation.

After the *intact* sinus membrane was successfully elevated, the graft could be placed. It is important to place the graft slowly and with minimal force to avoid membrane perforation. In this case, cancellous bovine bone was used (Figure 17.8e and f). Some grafting material can contain sharp bone particles in the graft mixture. If the cancellous (or corticocancellous) graft is dry, particles can cause pinpoint perforations in the membrane. Sterile saline solution can be generously added to the graft to moisture it and avoid the presence of sharp dry particles. No membrane was placed in this case.

Figure 17.9 demonstrate another case of a direct (lateral) subantral bone augmentation with an atraumatic bone window preparation, careful Schneiderian membrane elevation with a series of sinus curettes, and cautious layered bone grafting. Subantral augmentation (sinus lift) with a bone graft can triple the vertical dimension of the alveolar ridge, allowing placement of a longer implant at a later stage (Figure 17.10).

In some cases, placement of a protective Collagen membrane over the bone window can help to protect the graft and prevent its displacement (Figure 17.11). The wound closure is usually done with 4.0 chromic gut sutures (Figure 17.12). Primary watertight suture closure is advised. The site is usually allowed to heal for four to six months before implant placement (Figures 17.13 and 17.14). After the osseointegration is achieved, the implant can be restored with an implant crown (Figure 17.15).

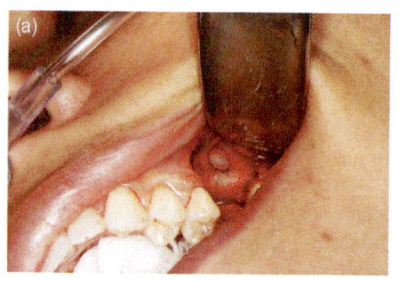

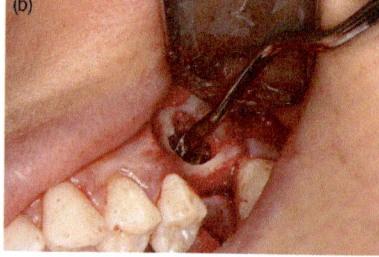

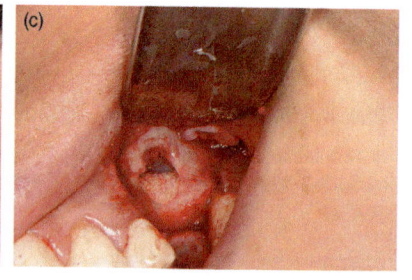

Figure 17.9 (**a**) Case showing an intraoperative photo of the lateral sinus lift procedure where the lateral bony wall is outlined and fully removed. (**b**) Sinus curettes are used for membrane elevation. (**c**) Formed subantral pocket is filled with bone grafting material.

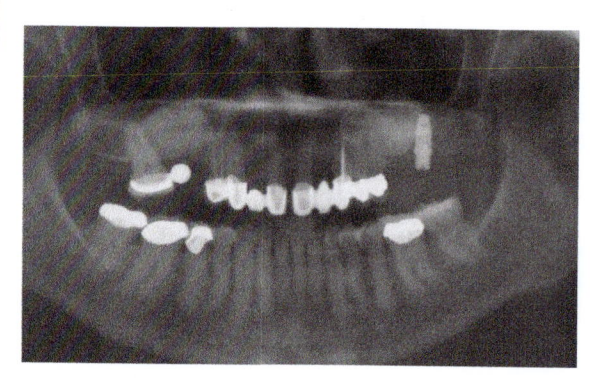

Figure 17.10 Panoramic radiograph showing the bilateral sinus lift and bone graft that can significantly enhance the vertical dimension of the alveolar ridge allowing for successful implant reconstruction.

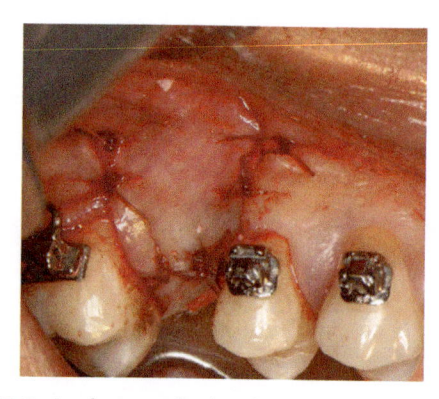

Figure 17.12 Another example when the surgical site was closed primarily without membrane use.

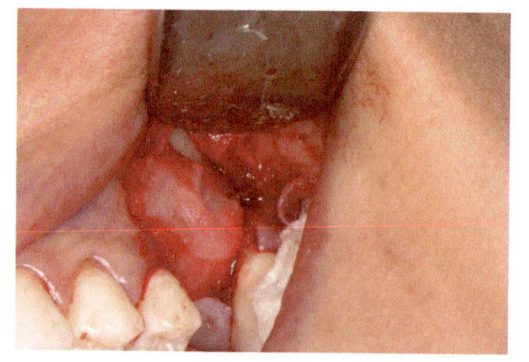

Figure 17.11 The surgical site was closed with Collagen membrane placement on top of the bone window.

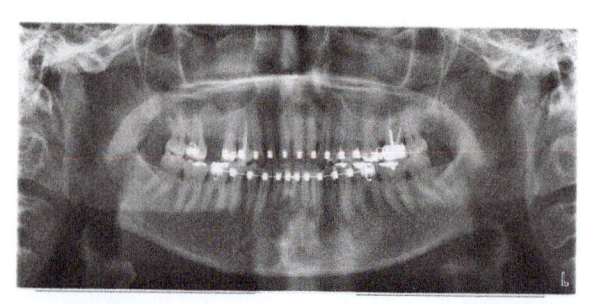

Figure 17.13 Post-operative imaging showing sinus elevation and graft placement.

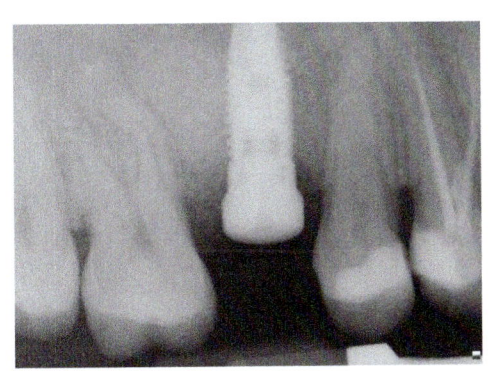

Figure 17.14 Implant placement four months after sinus elevation and grafting.

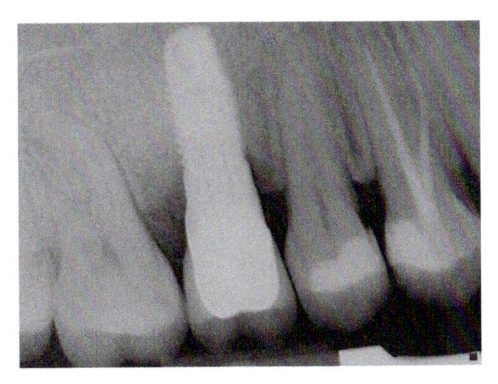

Figure 17.15 Periapical radiograph three years after lateral sinus lift and bone graft and delayed implant reconstruction.

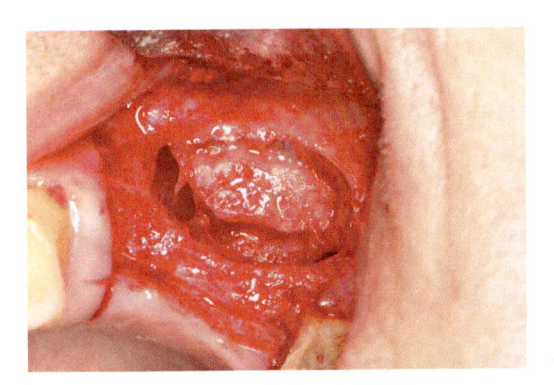

Figure 17.16 Intraoperative photograph of a sinus perforation as a complication of the sinus lift procedure.

There are a variety of techniques that are designed to decrease perforation of the sinus membrane. One of them (Dr. Arthur T. Forrest) is called 4ST ("simplifies-safer-sinus-surgery") technique. This intra-operative method utilizes slow expanding capabilities of compressed sinuscube sponges (dense reticulated polyurethane foam). Utilizing soft "wiggling" motion, 2-to-4 compressed guided sponges are sequentially inserted under the delicate Schneiderian membrane ensuring its safer lift from the sinus floor and walls. "Soft and slow" handling of the sinus membrane during the direct (lateral) sinus lift is tremendously important in prevention of membrane perforations and success of the procedure.

Complications

Like any surgical technique, lateral sinus elevation has its own complications. Complications include sinus perforation, postoperative sinusitis, graft displacement within the sinus, graft failure due to resorption, and implant failure. The most common intraoperative complication is sinus membrane perforation, which can occur in 10 to 60% of cases [26] (Figure 17.16). Though rare, the most significant complication is the development of an oral–antral fistula that can lead to a chronic sinus infection. More extensive discussion on complications of sinus lift procedures will be presented in the last chapter of this section of the book.

Conclusion

The lateral approach to sinus elevation is a predictable oral surgical technique to increase a vertical bone stock for implant placement in the posterior maxilla. In patients with minimal (less than 4 mm) residual alveolar bone, grafting and delayed implant placement is advised. For patients with residual alveolar bone sufficient for initial primary implant stabilization (more than 4–5 mm), atraumatic sinus membrane elevation, particulate bone grafting, and implant placement can be carried out in one surgery. The lateral sinus lift procedure can double, triple, and, in some cases, quadruple the amount of available subantral bone in the posterior maxilla for successful implant reconstruction (Figure 17.17). The surgeon's experience and expertise should help to avoid sinus membrane perforation and other complications of this surgical technique, as well as select an immediate versus delayed implant placement protocol.

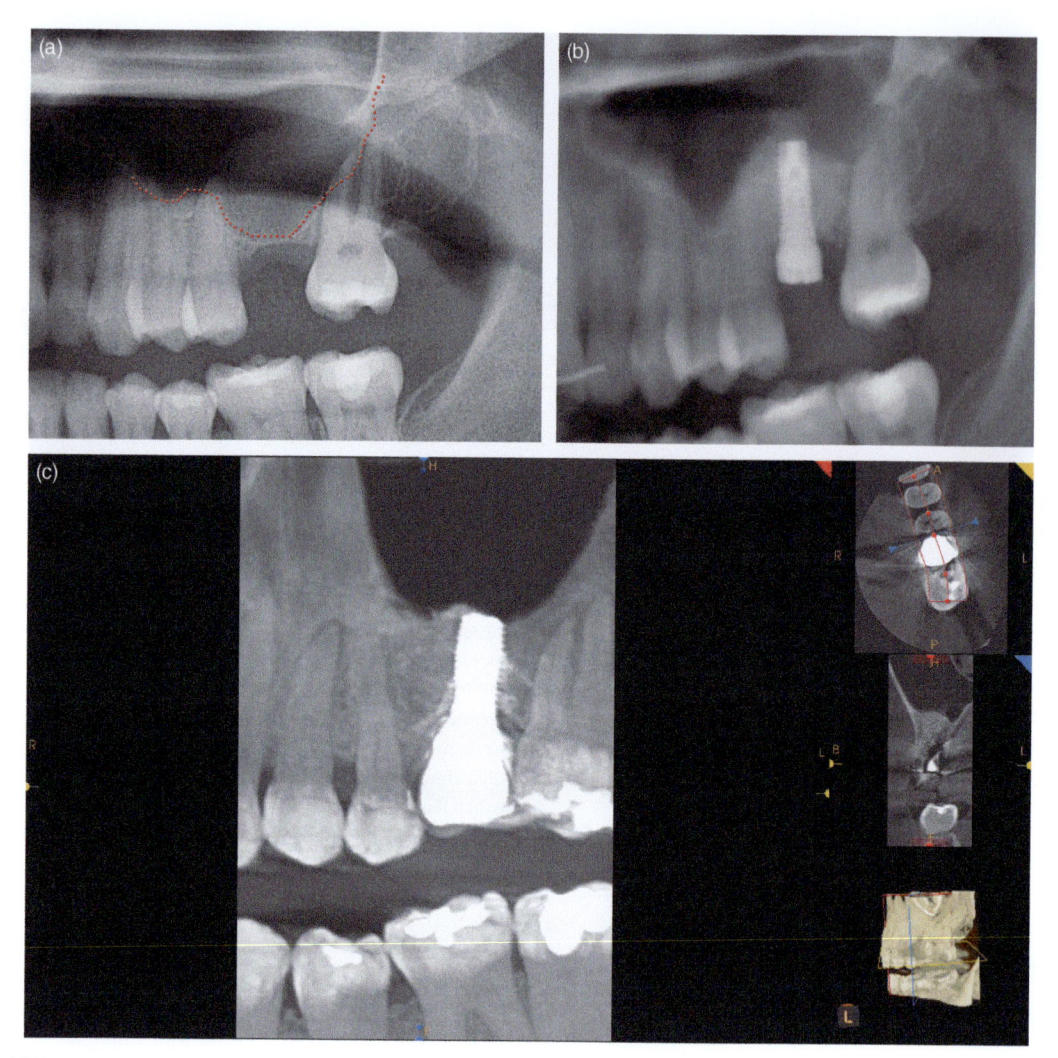

Figure 17.17 (a) Pre-operative panoramic radiographs of the edentulous first molar space indicating extensive pneumatization of the maxillary sinus. (b) Post-operative radiographs of the same case indicating that the amount of vertical alveolar bone can be significantly enhanced using the lateral sinus lift procedure to accommodate placement of a 10+ mm implant. (c) CBCT image of the same case after completion of the restorative procedure; the well-osseointegrated implant is completely surrounded by the grafted bone.

References

1. Chen TW, Chang HS, Leung KW, Lai YL, Kao SY: Implant placement immediately after the lateral approach of the trap door window procedure to create a maxillary sinus lift without bone grafting: a 2-year retrospective evaluation of 47 implants in 33 patients. *Journal of Oral and Maxillofacial Surgery: Official Journal of the American Association of Oral and Maxillofacial Surgeons* 2007 Nov; **65**(11):2324–2328. PubMed PMID: 17954333. Epub 2007/10/24. eng.
2. Fugazzotto PA, Vlassis J: Long-term success of sinus augmentation using various surgical approaches and grafting materials. *The International Journal of Oral and Maxillofacial Implants* 1998 Jan–Feb; **13**(1):52–58. PubMed PMID: 9509780. Epub 1998/03/24. eng.
3. Geminiani A, Papadimitriou DE, Ercoli C: Maxillary sinus augmentation with a sonic handpiece for the osteotomy of the lateral window: a clinical report. *The Journal of Prosthetic Dentistry* 2011 Nov;**106**(5):279–283. PubMed PMID: 22024176. Epub 2011/10/26. eng.
4. Lin IC, Gonzalez AM, Chang HJ, Kao SY, Chen TW: A 5-year follow-up of 80 implants in 44 patients placed immediately after the lateral trap-door window procedure to accomplish maxillary sinus elevation without bone grafting. *The International Journal of Oral and Maxillofacial Implants* 2011 Sep–Oct;**26**(5):1079–1086. PubMed PMID: 22010092. Epub 2011/10/20. eng.
5. Sohn DS, Heo JU, Kwak DH, Kim DE, Kim JM, Moon JW, et al: Bone regeneration in the maxillary sinus using an autologous fibrin-rich block with concentrated growth factors alone. *Implant Dentistry* 2011 Oct;**20**(5):389–395. PubMed PMID: 21881519. Epub 2011/09/02. eng.
6. Tawil G, Mawla M: Sinus floor elevation using a bovine bone mineral (Bio-Oss) with or without the concomitant use of a bilayered collagen barrier (Bio-Gide): a clinical report of immediate and delayed implant placement. *The International Journal of Oral and Maxillofacial Implants* 2001 Sep–Oct;**16**(5):713–721. PubMed PMID: 11669254. Epub 2001/10/24. eng.
7. Tetsch J, Tetsch P, Lysek DA: Long-term results after lateral and osteotome technique sinus floor elevation: a retrospective analysis of 2190 implants over a time period of 15 years. *Clinical Oral Implants Research* 2010 May;**21**(5):497–503. PubMed PMID: 20443802. Epub 2010/05/07.eng.
8. Uckan S, Tamer Y, Deniz K: Survival rates of implants inserted in the maxillary sinus area by internal or external approach. *Implant Dentistry* 2011 Dec;**20**(6):476–479. PubMed PMID: 22051745. Epub 2011/11/05. eng.
9. Tatum H, Jr: Maxillary and sinus implant reconstructions. *Dental Clinics of North America* 1986 Apr;**30**(2):207–229. PubMed PMID: 3516738.
10. Boyne PJ, James RA: Grafting of the maxillary sinus floor with autogenous marrow and bone. *Journal of Oral Surgery (American Dental Association, 1965)* 1980 Aug;**38**(8):613–616. PubMed PMID: 6993637. Epub 1980/08/01. eng.
11. Vogiatzi T, Kloukos D, Scarfe WC, Bornstein MM: Incidence of anatomical variations and disease of the maxillary sinuses as identified by cone beam computed tomography: a systematic review. *The International Journal of Oral and Maxillofacial Implants*. 2014 Nov–Dec;**29**(6):1301–1314. PubMed PMID: 25397794. Epub 2014/11/15. eng.
12. Hollinshead WH: The nose and paranasal sinuses, Chapter 4. In: Hollinshead WH (ed.), *Anatomy for Surgeons: The Head and Neck*, 3rd edn. Lippincott-Raven, Philadelphia, PA, 1982, pp. 259–265.

13. Krennmair G, Ulm CW, Lugmayr H, Solar P. The incidence, location, and height of maxillary sinus septa in the edentulous and dentate maxilla. *Journal of Oral and Maxillofacial Surgery: Official Journal of the American Association of Oral and Maxillofacial Surgeons* 1999 Jun;57(6):667–671; discussion 71–72. PubMed PMID: 10368090. Epub 1999/06/15. eng.
14. Aimetti M, Massei G, Morra M, Cardesi E, Romano F: Correlation between gingival phenotype and Schneiderian membrane thickness. *The International Journal of Oral and Maxillofacial Implants* 2008 Nov–Dec;23(6):1128–1132. PubMed PMID: 19216284. Epub 2009/02/17. eng.
15. Lundgren S, Andersson S, Sennerby L: Spontaneous bone formation in the maxillary sinus after removal of a cyst: coincidence or consequence? *Clinical Implant Dentistry and Related Research* 2003;5(2):78–81. PubMed PMID: 14536041. Epub 2003/10/11. eng.
16. Al-Nawas B, Schiegnitz E: Augmentation procedures using bone substitute materials or autogenous bone – a systematic review and meta-analysis. *European Journal of Oral Implantology* 2014 Summer;7(Suppl 2):S219–234. PubMed PMID: 24977257. Epub 2014/07/01. eng.
17. Badr M, Coulthard P, Alissa R, Oliver R: The efficacy of platelet-rich plasma in grafted maxillae. A randomised clinical trial. *European Journal of Oral Implantology* 2010 Autumn;3(3):233–244. PubMed PMID: 20847993. Epub 2010/09/18. eng.
18. Esposito M, Piattelli M, Pistilli R, Pellegrino G, Felice P: Sinus lift with guided bone regeneration or anorganic bovine bone: 1-year post-loading results of a pilot randomised clinical trial. *European Journal of Oral Implantology* 2010 Winter;3(4):297–305. PubMed PMID: 21180682. Epub 2010/12/25. eng.
19. Fugazzotto PA: Maxillary sinus grafting with and without simultaneous implant placement: technical considerations and case reports. *The International Journal of Periodontics and Restorative Dentistry* 1994 Dec;14(6):544–551. PubMed PMID: 7751119. Epub 1994/12/01. eng.
20. Montesani L, Schulze-Spate U, Dibart S: Sinus augmentation in two patients with severe posterior maxillary height atrophy using tissue-engineered bone derived from autologous bone cells: a case report. *The International Journal of Periodontics and Restorative Dentistry* 2011 Jul–Aug;31(4):391–399. PubMed PMID: 21837305. Epub 2011/08/13. eng.
21. Nkenke E, Stelzle F: Clinical outcomes of sinus floor augmentation for implant placement using autogenous bone or bone substitutes: a systematic review. *Clinical Oral Implants Research*. 2009 Sep;20(Suppl 4):124–133. PubMed PMID: 19663959. Epub 2009/08/12. eng.
22. Sharaf B, Dodson TB: Does the use of prophylactic antibiotics decrease implant failure? *Oral and Maxillofacial Surgery Clinics of North America* 2011 Nov;23(4):547–550, vi. PubMed PMID: 21982607. Epub 2011/10/11. eng.
23. Nolan PJ, Freeman K, Kraut RA: Correlation between Schneiderian membrane perforation and sinus lift graft outcome: a retrospective evaluation of 359 augmented sinus. *Journal of Oral and Maxillofacial Surgery: Official Journal of the American Association of Oral and Maxillofacial Surgeons* 2014 Jan;72(1):47–52. PubMed PMID: 24071378. Epub 2013/09/28. eng.
24. Wallace SS, Froum SJ: Effect of maxillary sinus augmentation on the survival of endosseous dental implants. A systematic review. *Annals of Periodontology/The American Academy of Periodontology* 2003 Dec;8(1):328–343. PubMed PMID: 14971260. Epub 2004/02/20. eng.
25. Cho YS, Park HK, Park CJ: Bony window repositioning without using a barrier membrane in the lateral approach for maxillary sinus bone grafts: clinical and radiologic results at 6 months. *The International Journal of Oral and Maxillofacial Implants* 2012 Jan–Feb;27(1):211–217. PubMed PMID: 22299099. Epub 2012/02/03. eng.
26. Moreno Vazquez JC, Gonzalez de Rivera AS, Gil HS, Mifsut RS: Complication rate in 200 consecutive sinus lift procedures: guidelines for prevention and treatment. *Journal of Oral and Maxillofacial Surgery: Official Journal of the American Association of Oral and Maxillofacial Surgeons* 2014 May;72(5):892–901. PubMed PMID: 24583086. Epub 2014/03/04. eng.

CHAPTER 18

Posterior Maxillary Sandwich Osteotomy Combined with Sinus Floor Grafting for Severe Alveolar Atrophy

Ole T. Jensen

School of Dentistry, University of Utah, Salt Lake City, Utah, USA

Introduction

The posterior maxilla in a state of atrophy with a prominent sinus cavity can be treated with combined alveolar and sinus floor augmentation to gain enough bone stock for dental implant restoration [1,2]. One way to augment the alveolus to avoid a vertical onlay graft, which is often challenging for the posterior maxilla, is to perform a sandwich osteotomy with an interpositional bone graft, essentially a vertically extended sinus floor graft [3,4].

The biological rationale of the posterior segmental osteotomy, as described by S. Wunderer, was confirmed in the laboratory by W. Bell [5–7]. When this procedure is done with a sinus membrane elevation for sinus floor grafting (that is, also has a well-founded biological basis), the combined procedure for the posterior segment appears to be an optimal strategy for implant reconstruction [8,9]. The problem, however, is a technical one. The procedure has almost never been attempted. For this reason the technical aspect of this procedure will be presented here with clinical correlations.

Technique

Models are made and a mock surgery is planned and completed on the models as it is done in an orthognathic surgery work-up. The technique for the posterior sandwich osteotomy is shown in Figure 18.1a and b [2]. One of the most important aspects to plan is the anterior–posterior extent of the segment as well as the location of the vertical cuts to the crest of the alveolus away from dental roots. Vertical cuts should be 2 mm away from dental elements [10]. Following administration of intravenous anesthesia and local anesthesia, a lateral approach is made to the sinus cavity for a lateral antrostomy [11]. This is done through a vestibular incision carried down to bone, reflecting mostly superiorly to maintain mucosal drape on the residual alveolar process. Once the lateral wall of the maxilla is identified, a lateral window osteotomy is made, about 10 mm vertical × 15 mm horizontal that does not extend to the vertical segmental osteotomy cuts that have been planned. The sinus membrane is then elevated and reflected anterior and posterior to clear room for the segmental osteotomies, which will pass through the sinus cavity. Next, a frown-shaped cut extends from the sinus osteotomy window forward, curving to the alveolar crest to about 2 mm posteriorly from the most distal tooth. The posterior cut extends posterior to the tuberosity region in front of the pterygoid plate. The cut then curves down to the alveolar crest. These cuts are made without reflecting mucosa – easily done with a piezo-knife submucosally [12]. Once the lateral cuts are complete a similar cut is made trans-sinus of the palatal bone. This usually requires a combination of piezosurgery and hand osteotomies to free the segment. A curved oscillating sagittal saw can also aid in making this cut. The palatal cut needs not to be complete in most cases (create a greenstick fracture is enough) as the palatal wall is usually quite thin. The segment is then down-fractured, rotating the segment medially. The palatal mucosa is not released. The segment can be brought down about 10 mm maximally but usually 6–8 mm is sufficient to greatly improve the alveolar dimension vertically. The alveolar crest will end up slightly palatal, which can be corrected at the time of implant placements about 5 months later. This is usually done by soft tissue transfer and additional alveolar facial bone grafting using GBR [1].

Clinical application

A 30-year-old female presents with an impacted decayed bicuspid tooth that requires removal of almost all the remaining alveolus in the presence of a prominent sinus cavity (Figure 18.2). Socket bone grafting is done at the time of tooth removal using allograft and autograft particles. Following three months healing from tooth removal the patient returns for reconstruction of the left posterior maxilla (Figure 18.3a and b). A vestibular incision is made and curved osteotomies are performed laterally followed by sinus membrane elevation and trans-sinus palatal osteotomy (Figure 18.4a). The segment is down-fractured (Figure 18.4b). A fixation plate is placed (Figure 18.5a). Interpositional grafting combined with sinus floor grafting are done using BMP-2/allograft in a 50:50 ratio using bovine collagen sponge as a carrier for the BMP-2 (Figure 18.5b) [13]. The wound is closed and the observable improved alveolar height is demonstrated (Figure 18.6). Five

---

Vertical Alveolar Ridge Augmentation in Implant Dentistry: A Surgical Manual, First Edition. Edited by Len Tolstunov.
© 2016 John Wiley & Sons, Inc. Published 2016 by John Wiley & Sons, Inc.

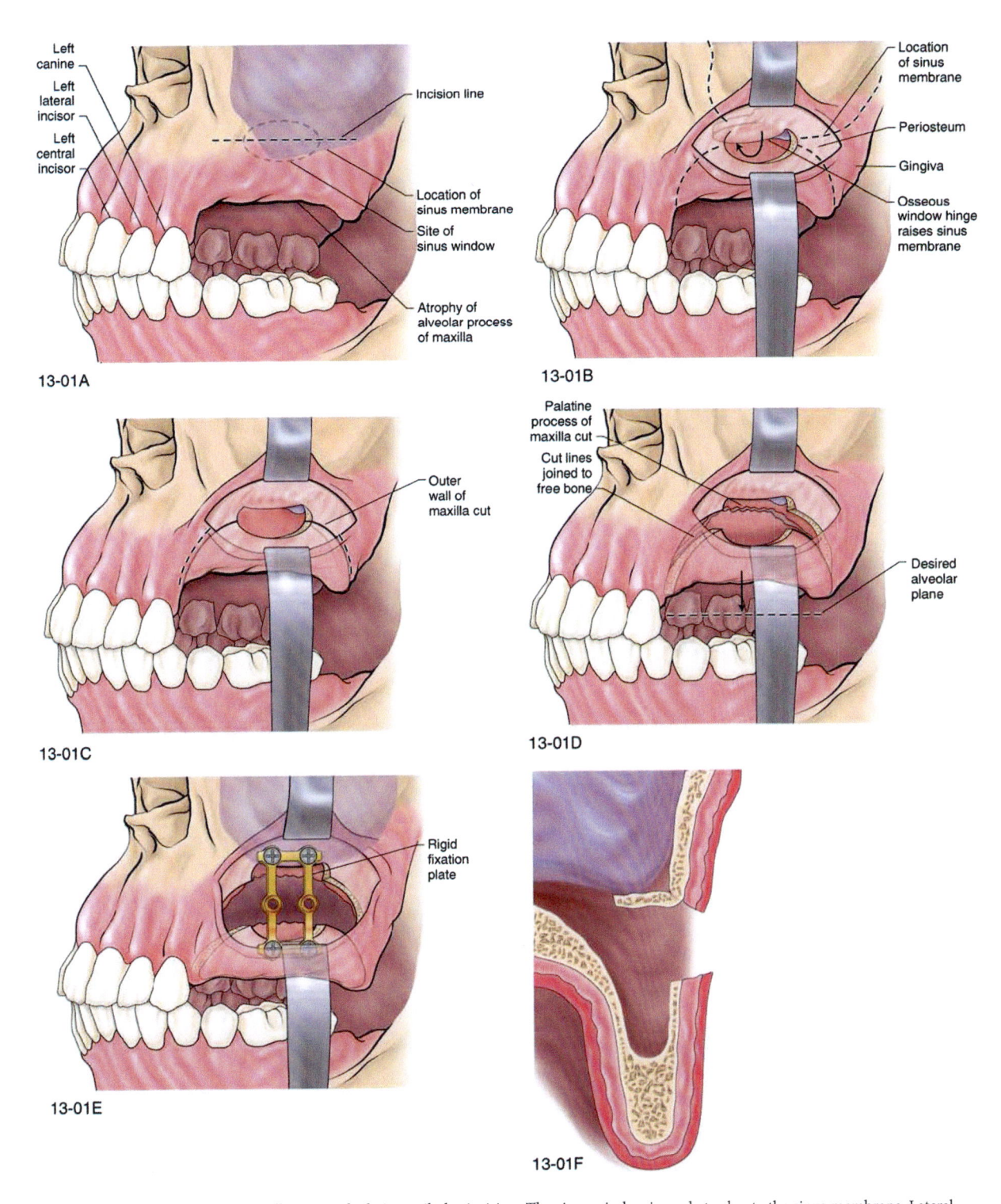

Figure 18.1 (a) Vertically deficient maxilla approached via vestibular incision. The sinus window is made to elevate the sinus membrane. Lateral osteotomy is made using piezosurgery from the window anterior and posterior curving down to the alveolar crest. (b) Palatal osteotomy is done trans-sinus, curving down towards the alveolar crest using piezo surgery. Segment is freed with osteotomes and down-fractured. Segment is fixed with bone plate and interpositionally grafted. Vestibular wound is closed primarily. Source: Jensen 2010. Reproduced with permission from Quintessence Publishing Inc.

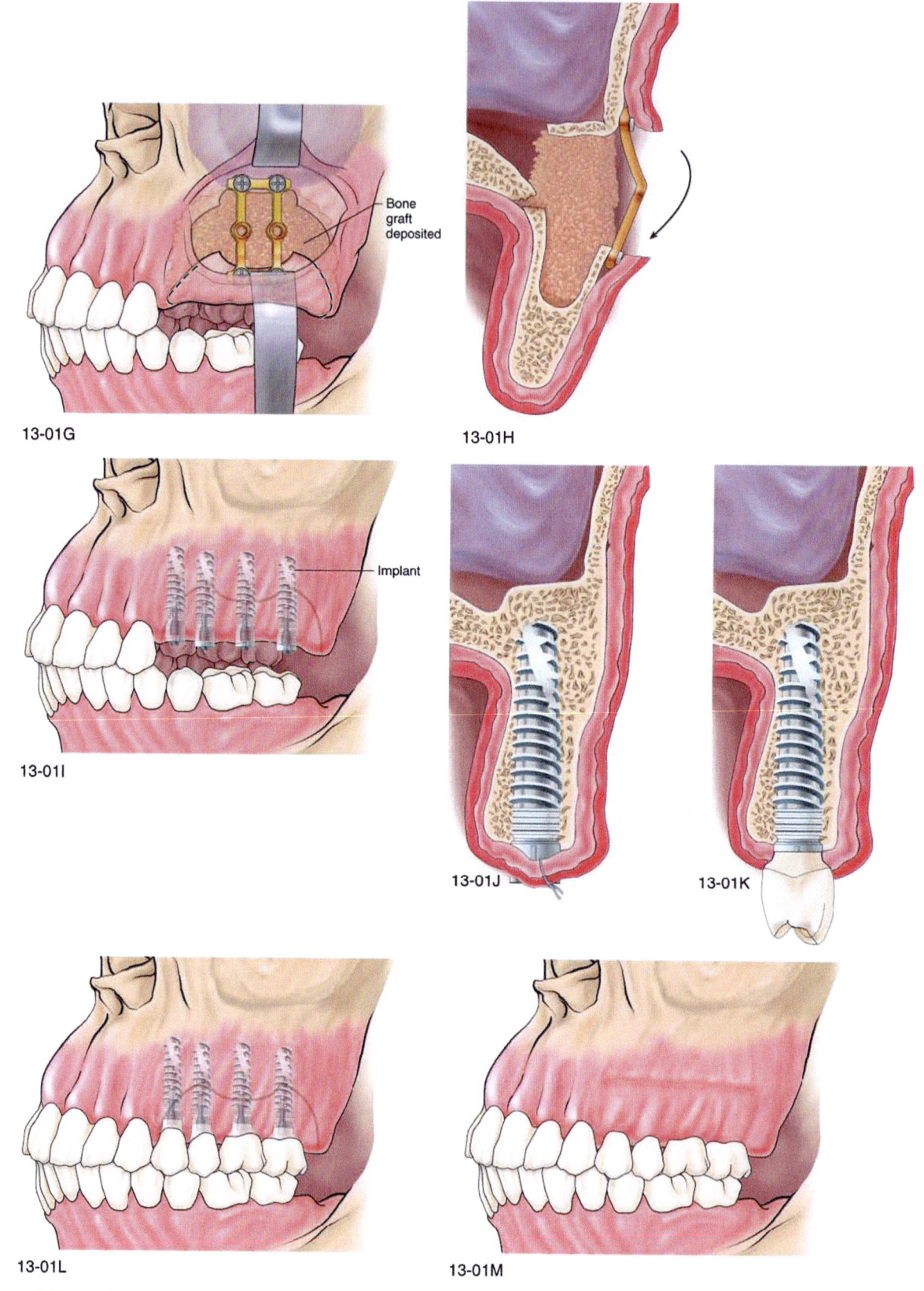

188 Subantral Grafting (Sinus Lift) for Vertical Ridge Augmentation

13-01G

Bone graft deposited

13-01H

13-01I

Implant

13-01J

13-01K

13-01L

13-01M

Figure 18.1 *Continued*

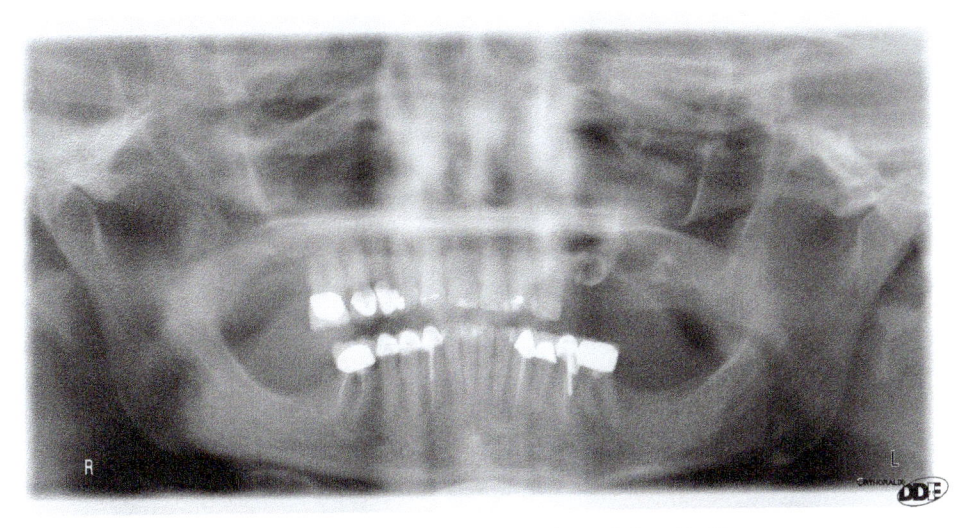

Figure 18.2 Pre-operative panoramic image showing impacted tooth in left sinus with very little residual bone.

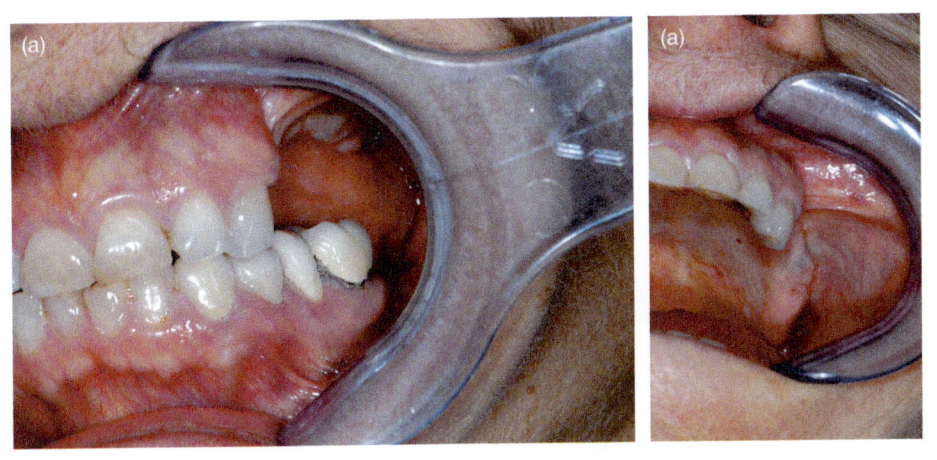

Figure 18.3 (a) Pre-operative lateral view (intraoral photograph). (b) Pre-operative occlusal view (intraoral photograph).

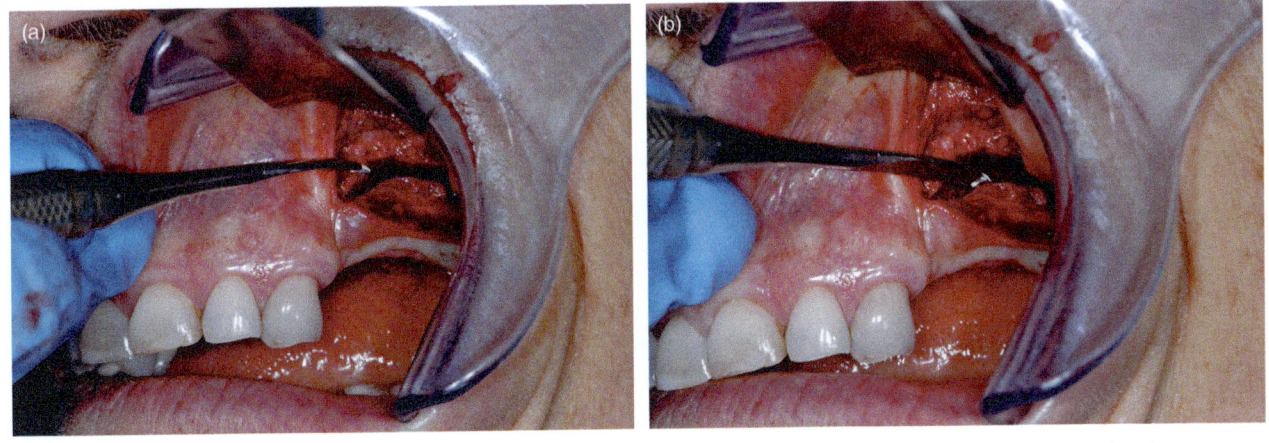

Figure 18.4 (a) Intraoperative photograph showing curved lateral osteotomy of the buccal wall that is followed by a trans-sinus palatal vault osteotomy. (b) Intraoperative photograph demonstrating a bone segment down-fracture to increase vertical height of the vertically deficient posterior maxilla.

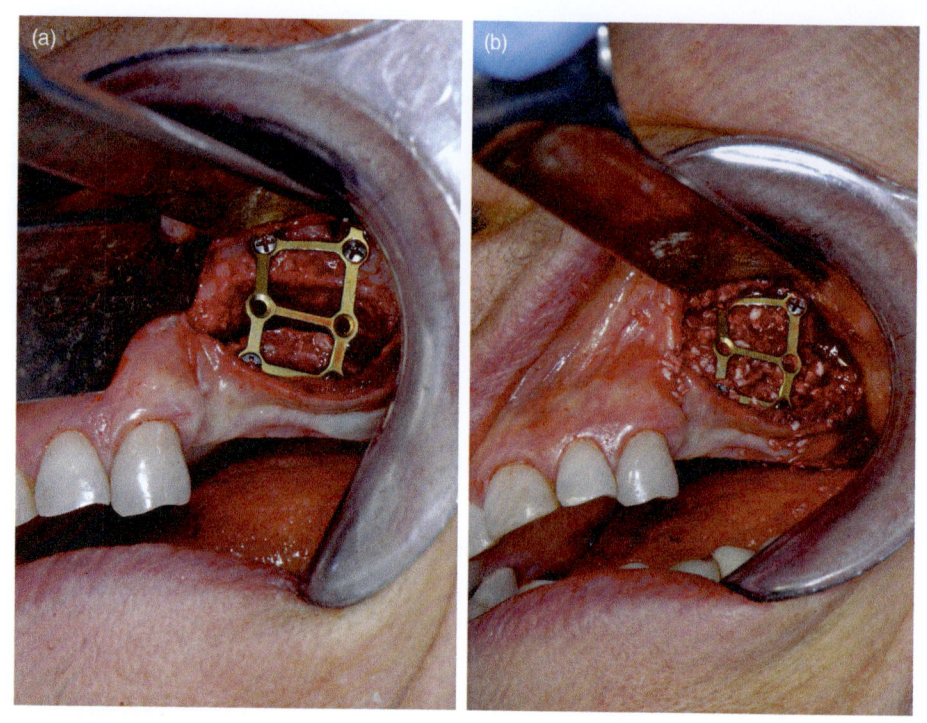

Figure 18.5 (a) Intraoperative photograph depicting a segment of bone that was fixated with a bone plate at an appropriate vertical height. (b) Intraoperative photograph showing an interpositional grafting.

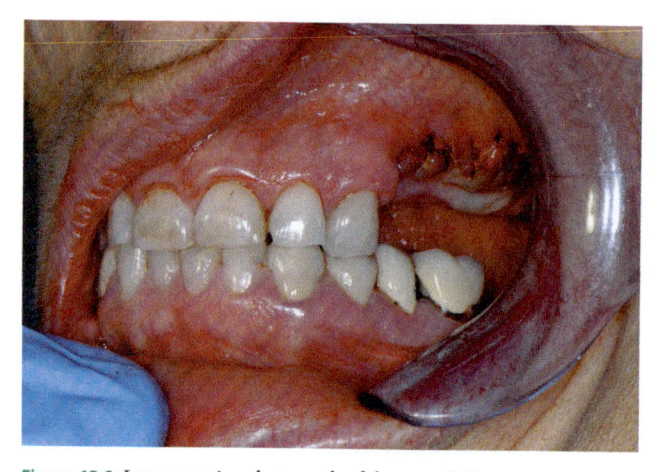

Figure 18.6 Intraoperative photograph of the wound closure.

months later CAT scan images reveal bone graft consolidation (Figure 18.7). At this stage, through a slightly palatally positioned crestal incision, the fixation plate is removed revealing a well-ossified bone (Figure 18.8). Three implants are placed (Figure 18.9) and an additional bone xenograft is added laterally to improve the buccal projection of the alveolar ridge (Figure 18.10). Postoperative radiographs shows two implants in the grafted bone (Figure 18.11). Final restoration as a splinted three-unit bridge was done 4 months later and depicted in the photograph after 1 year in function (Figure 18.12).

Discussion

What makes the posterior maxilla so difficult in the face of a vertical defect is the combined nature of limited alveolar bone stock and pneumatization of maxillary sinuses. This procedure, better than any other approach, can address both bone deficiencies. Other procedures may not provide the same success. For example, the use of iliac block grafts has been shown to have a high incidence for bone resorption whereas the osteotomy interpositional graft is much more stable [14]. The use of sinus grafting alone can be done but this does not correct alveolar height and leads to an increase in the crown–implant ratio [15]. Other approaches, like titanium mesh or guided bone regeneration with barrier membranes, are helpful for a modest amount of vertical correction and should probably be limited to smaller defect cases [16,17]. In addition, with GBR or mesh, there is a higher incidence of infection or mesh exposure, possibly not observed as much in the sandwich osteotomy technique [18,19].

One reason BMP-2 is recommended in these cases is that the graft tends to be quite large and the use of xenograft alone, for example, may not be sufficient. BMP-2 grafts are well suited for consolidation and healing of the segments, as is iliac particulate graft material, whereas alloplasts, allograft, and xenografts alone do not do as well.

One advantage of this approach as well is the secondary grafting that can be done at the time of implant placements. This will shape the alveolus in what is volumetrically a much less extensive graft than what would be required otherwise. Therefore, the definitive peri-implant grafting is more likely to avoid complications [1].

The main disadvantage of the interpositional graft is lack of expertise by surgeons unfamiliar with orthognathic surgery. Any

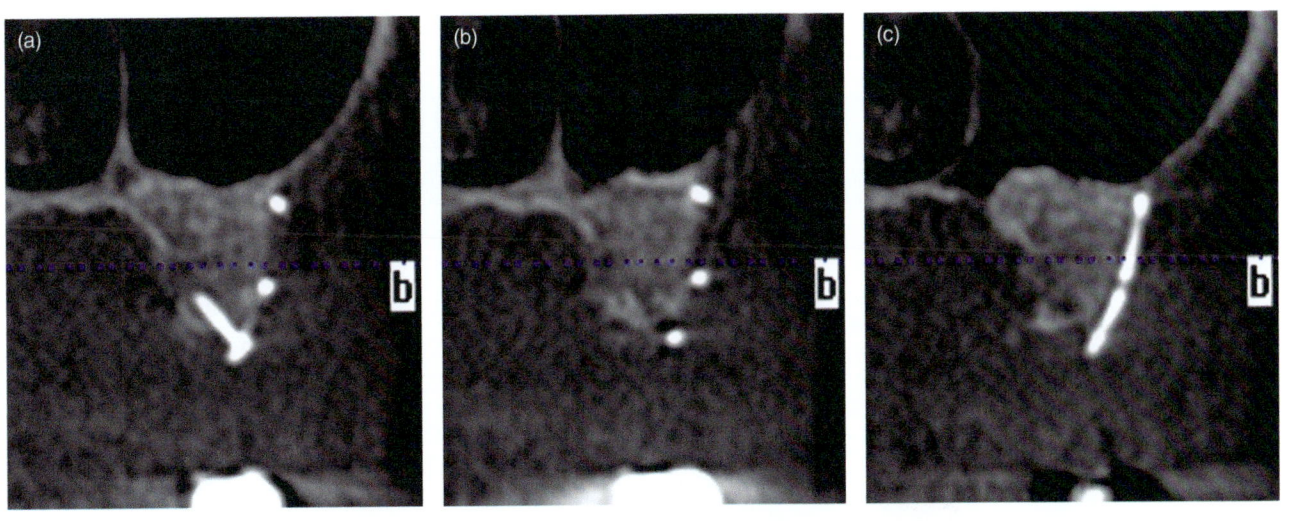

Figure 18.7 Cross-sectional (coronal) cone beam computed tomography (CBCT) slices of bone consolidation four months after surgery.

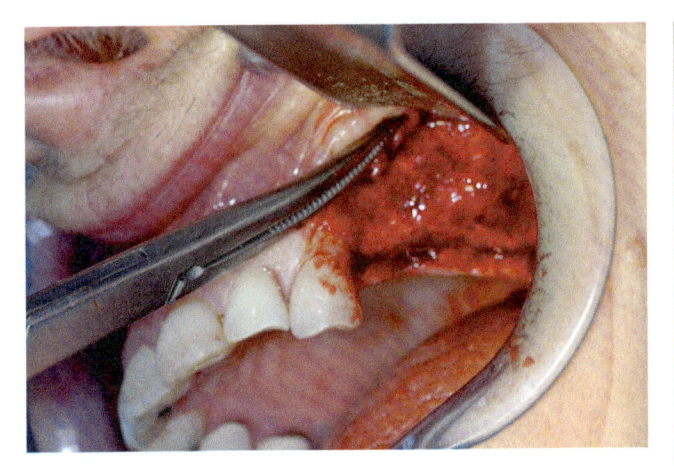

Figure 18.8 Intraoperative photograph of removal of hardware and exposure of the healed alveolar process.

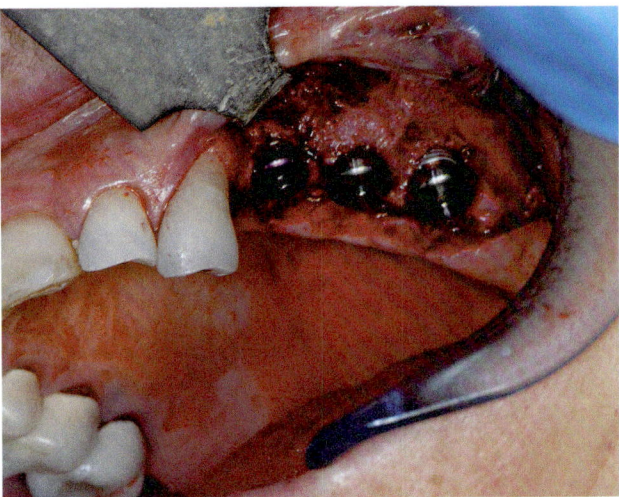

Figure 18.9 Intraoperative photograph demonstrating placement of three endosseous implants.

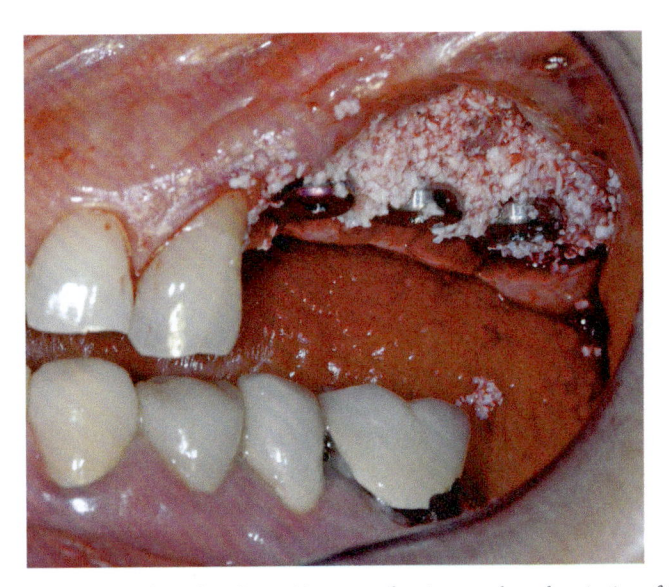

Figure 18.10 Intraoperative photograph of secondary buccal grafting with xenograft to improve buccal projection of the alveolar ridge.

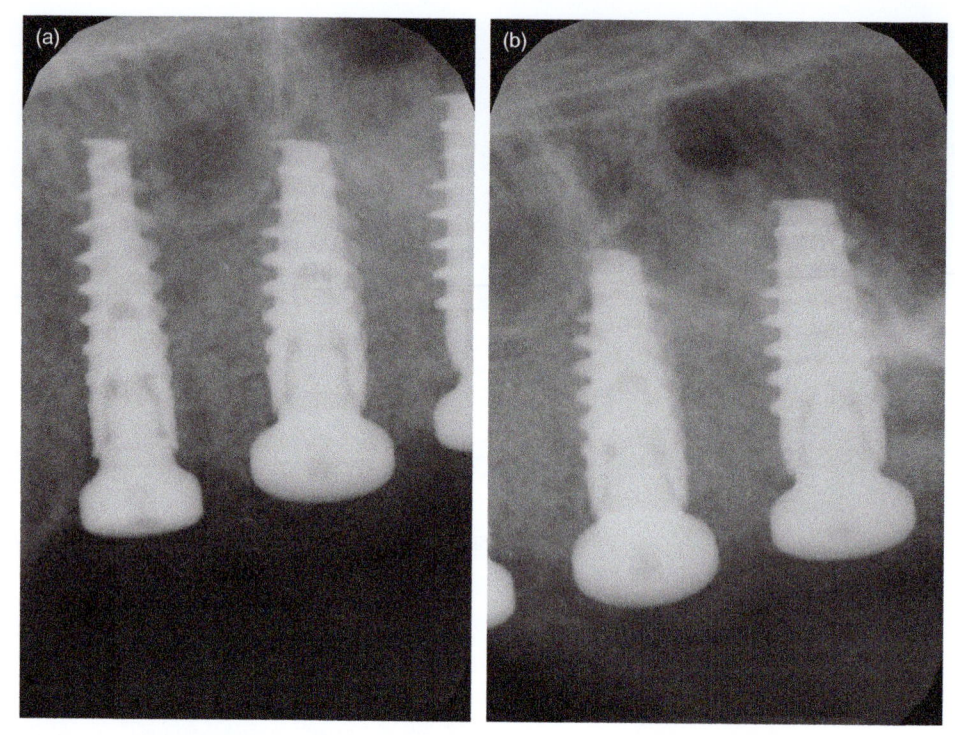

Figure 18.11 Post-operative periapical radiographs of placed dental implants.

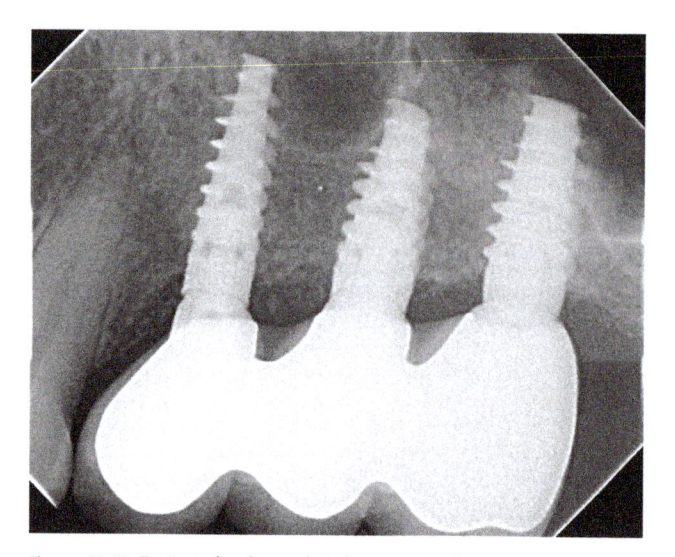

Figure 18.12 Periapical radiograph indicating a final restoration (three-unit bridge) after one year in function.

surgeon facile with Le Fort procedures and alveolar segmental surgery can easily learn this procedure, which need not be done in a hospital setting.

In summary, the posterior alveolar osteotomy, the so-called sandwich osteotomy, can be done with sinus membrane elevation and combined interpositional and sinus floor grafting to a favorable effect. Bone stock can be increased up to 10 mm vertically to satisfy successful implant placement for dental restorative reconstruction.

References

1. Jensen OT, Cottam J: Posterior maxillary sandwich osteotomy combined with sinus grafting with bone morphogenetic protein-2 for alveolar reconstruction for dental implants: report of four cases. *Int J Oral Maxillofac Implants* 2013 Nov–Dec;**28**(6):e14–23.
2. Jensen OT, Cottam JR: Sinus graft combined with osteoperiosteal flaps. In: Jensen OT (ed.), *The Osteo Periosteal Flap*. Quintessence Publishing, Chicago, IL, 2011, pp. 189–202.
3. Cordaro L, Torsello F, Accorsi Ribeiro C, Libertore M, Mirisola di Torresanto V: Inlay–onlay grafting for three dimensional reconstruction of the posterior atrophic maxilla with mandibular bone. *Int J Oral Maxillofac Surg* 2010 Apr;**39**(4):350–357.
4. Dasmah A, Thor A, Ekestubbe A, Sennerby L, Rasmusson L: Particulate vs. block bone grafts: three-dimensional changes in graft volume after reconstruction of the atrophic maxilla, a 2-year radiographic follow-up. *J Craniomaxillofac Surg* 2012 Dec;**40**(8):654–659.
5. Wunderer S: Die Prognathieopertion mittels frontal gestltem maxillafragment. *Osterr A Stomatol* 1962;**59**:98–102.
6. Quejada JG, Kawamura H, Finn RA, Bell WH: Wound healing associated with segmental total maxillary osteotomy. *J Oral Maxillofac Surg* 1986 May;**44**(5):366–377.
7. Bell WH, Levy BM: Revascularization and bone healing after posterior maxillary osteotomy. *J Oral Surg* 1971;**29**:313–320.
8. Nevins M, Kirker-Head C, Nevins M, Wozney JA, Palmer R, Graham D: Bone formation in the goat maxillary sinus induced by absorbable collagen sponge implants impregnated with recombinant human bone morphogenetic protein-2. *Int J Periodontics Restorative Dent* 1996 Feb;**16**(1):8–19.
9. Boyne PJ, Lilly LC, Marx RE, Moy PK, Nevins M, Spagnoli DB, Triplett RG: De novo bone formation by recombinant human bone morphogenetic protein-2 (rhBMP-2) in maxillary sinus floor augmentation. *J Oral Maxillofac Surg* 2005 Dec;**63**(12):1693–1707.
10. Ho MW, Boyle MA, Cooper JC, Dodd MD, Richardson D: Surgical complications of segmental Lefort I osteotomy. *Br J Oral Maxillofac Surg* 2011 Oct;**49**(7):562–566.
11. Kim JM, Sohn DS, Heo JU, Moon JW, Lee JH, Park IS: Benefit of the replaceable bony window in lateral maxillary sinus augmentation: clinical and histological study. *Implant Dent* 2014 Jun;**23**(3):277–282.
12. Pavlikova G, Foltan R, Horka M, Hanzelka T, Borunska H, Sedy J: Piezosurgery in oral and maxillofacial surgery. *Int J Oral Maxillofac Surg* 2011 May;**40**(5):451–457.

13 Jensen OT, Lehman H, Ringeman JL, Casap N: Fabrication of printed titanium shells for containment of BMP-2 composite graft materials for alveolar bone reconstruction. *Int J Oral Maxillofac Implants* 2014 Jan-Feb;**29**(1):e103–105.

14 Felice P, Marchetti C, Piattelli A, Pellegrino G, Checchi V, Worthington H, Esposito M: Vertical ridge augmentation of the atrophic posterior mandible with interpositional block grafts: bone from the iliac crest versus bovine and organic bone. *Eur J Oral Implantol* 2008 Autumn;**1**(3):183–198.

15 Antua E., Alkhraust MH, Pinas L, Begona L, Orive G: Implant survival and crestal bone loss around extra short implants supporting a fixed denture: the effect of crown height space, crown-to-implant ratio, and offset placement of the prosthesis. *Int J Oral Maxillofac Implants* 2014 May–Jun;**23**(3):682–689.

16 Her S, Kang T, Fien MJ: Titanium mesh as an alternative to membrane for ridge augmentation. *J Oral Maxillofac Surg* 2012 Apr;**70**(4):803–810.

17 Roccuzzo M, Ramieri G, Bunino M, Berrone S: Autogenous bone graft alone or associated with titanium mesh for vertical alveolar ridge augmentation: a controlled clinical trial. *Clin Oral Implants Res* 2007 Jun;**18**(3):286–294.

18 Khojasteh A, Scheilifar S, Mohajerani H, Nowzari H: The effectiveness of barrier membranes on bone regeneration in localized bony defects: a systematic review. *Int J Oral Maxillofac Implants* 2013 Jul–Aug **28**(4):1076–1089.

19 Nazirkar G, Singh S, Dole V, Nikam A: Effortless effort in bone regeneration: a review. *J Int Oral Health* 2014 Jun;**6**(3):120–124.

CHAPTER 19

Management of Complications of Sinus Lift Procedures

Douglas E. Kendrick

Department of Oral and Maxillofacial Surgery, The University of Iowa Hospitals and Clinics, Iowa City, Iowa, USA

Introduction

Dental implant surgery is considered to be safe with a high success rate and minimal complications. However, complications can arise both in implant surgery and during adjunctive procedures such as sinus augmentation. These complications are usually minimal, but more severe complications can also occur. The sinus lift procedure of the maxillary sinus is a delicate procedure. Careful pre-operative planning and intraoperative surgical technique can help decrease or prevent complications.

Risks and complications include perforation of the sinus membrane, intraoperative or post-operative hemorrhage, infection, graft resorption, and loss of the graft or implants. Reports have shown that approximately 50% of complications associated with sinus lift procedures are due to perioperative complications; approximately 50% of those complications are sinus membrane perforations [1]. Although there are many complications that can occur during sinus lift procedures, implants have a 90 to 97% success rate after 3 years of function in a site that had a sinus graft procedure [1].

Perforation

The sinus (Schneiderian) membrane consists of periosteum with a thin layer of ciliated pseudostratified epithelium overlying the periosteum. The sinus membrane is important in maintaining proper function of the maxillary sinus [2]. The membrane ranges in thickness from 0.3 to 0.8 mm and can easily be torn during elevation [3]. Perforation of the sinus membrane is the most common complication in sinus grafting procedures and occurs in 10 to 60% of procedures [2, 4–7] (Figures 19.1 to 19.3). Perforations most commonly happen during development of the bony window but can also happen during elevation of the sinus membrane or placement of the bone graft [8]. There is an increased risk of perforation when there is a septum, spine, or sharp edge present in the sinus [9, 10]. Absence of a residual alveolar ridge or a small residual ridge of 3 mm or less has an increased risk for perforation than ridges that have greater height [8, 10]. Perforations can allow for bacterial infection, mucosal inflammation, and graft migration. Extremely thin or thick walls also increase the risk of sinus perforation [11]. Perforations can allow for bacterial contamination of the graft site and subsequent surgical infection. The graft material may also migrate into the maxillary sinus, leading to graft loss and sinusitis.

The surgeon should evaluate pre-operative radiographs and CT images to evaluate the thickness of the sinus wall, location of septa, and membrane thickness (Figures 19.4 and 19.5). CT imaging in a form of cone beam computed tomography (CBCT) is recommended to identify bony irregularities such as septa as panoramic radiographs have been shown to be inaccurate in identifying them [12]. Reduction of the thick lateral sinus wall prior to osteotomy may aid in prevention of sinus perforations [13].

The use of a round diamond bur is often the instrument of choice in creating the lateral window. Piezoelectric surgery may decrease the risk of perforation [13, 14]. If a perforation does occur, the osteotomy can be enlarged in size to reestablish contact with the membrane [15]. Small perforations (less than 4–5 mm) of the sinus membrane can be managed by placing a fast absorbing collagen membrane to act as a barrier (Figures 19.1 and 19.6 to 19.8). Larger tears require a more rigid, longer lasting collagen membrane [16]. This can be followed with placement of the bone graft material as planned. If a larger perforation occurs that cannot be managed with an occlusive membrane, the procedure must be aborted, the site closed, and the sinus allowed to heal so another attempt can be made at a later date. A healing period of 6 to 9 months is recommended for large sinus membrane perforations [16]. Re-entry into the maxillary sinus may be technically more difficult.

If membrane perforation occurs, the surgeon should consider placing implants after the graft site has healed due to the increased risk of infection [16]. The site should be allowed to heal for 4–6 months prior to implant placement if there is concern for infection [1, 16].

Sinusitis and infection

Post-operative sinusitis is the most common post-operative complication and is most likely to occur in patients who are already prone to sinusitis due to anatomical reasons such as septal deviation, oversized turbinates, or allergies [14, 17]. Acute sinusitis can occur after sinus grafting and may be due to obstruction of the maxillary ostium from mucosal inflammation, hematoma, seroma, or overfilling with graft material. Perforation of the sinus membrane increases the risk of sinusitis [10]. Infection can either be localized to the surgical site or become more fulminant if left untreated. Infection usually presents 3 to 7 days post-operatively [16]. Contamination with bone grafting material or inoculation with bacteria

---

Vertical Alveolar Ridge Augmentation in Implant Dentistry: A Surgical Manual, First Edition. Edited by Len Tolstunov.
© 2016 John Wiley & Sons, Inc. Published 2016 by John Wiley & Sons, Inc.

Management of Complications of Sinus Lift Procedures   195

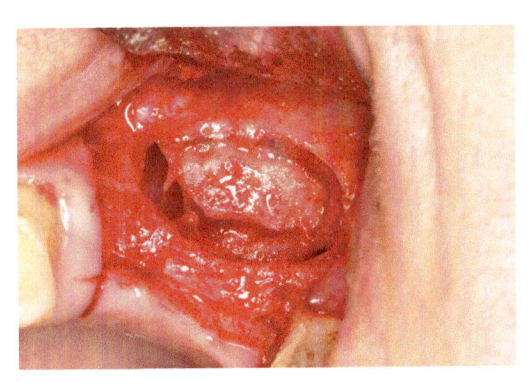

Figure 19.1 Intraoperative photograph of a sinus membrane perforation during the osteotomy.

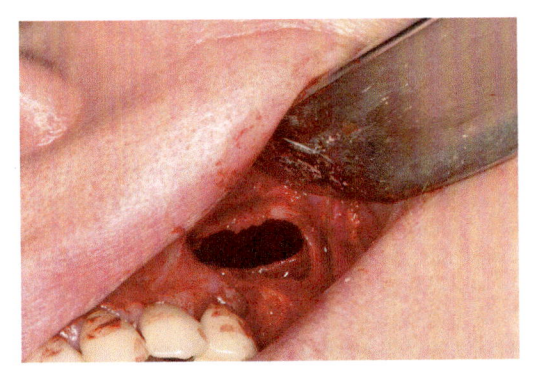

Figure 19.2 Intraoperative photograph of a large sinus membrane perforation during membrane elevation.

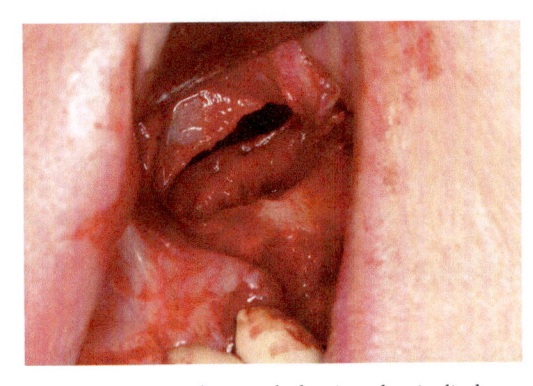

Figure 19.3 Intraoperative photograph showing a longitudinal tear of the sinus membrane.

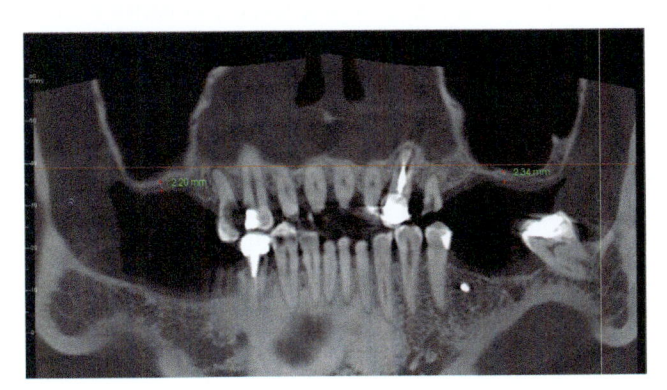

Figure 19.4 Pre-operative evaluation of the sinus morphology with a panoramic reconstruction from a cone beam computed tomography (CBCT) image.

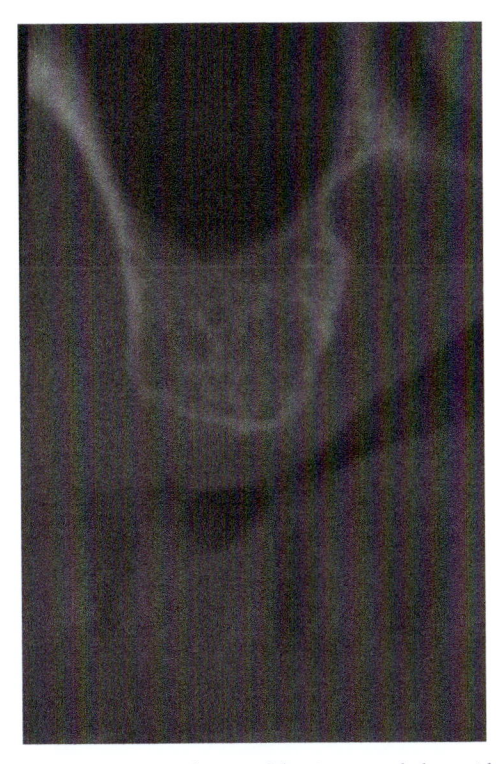

Figure 19.5 Pre-operative evaluation of the sinus morphology with a cone beam computed tomography (CBCT) image in the coronal plane.

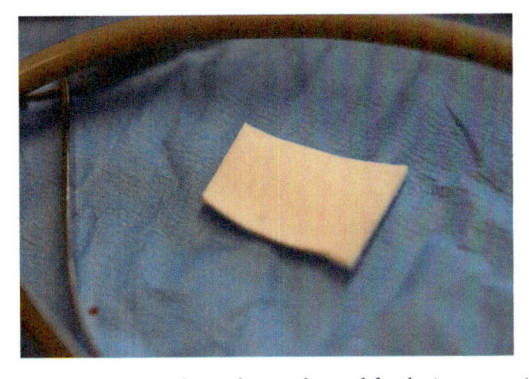

Figure 19.6 Collagen membrane that can be used for the intraoperative occlusion (closure) of small sinus membrane perforations.

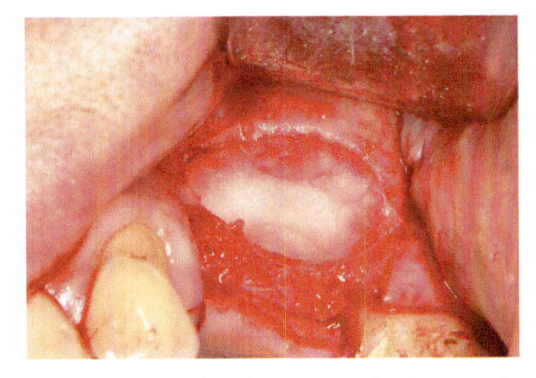

Figure 19.7 Intraoperative photo demonstrating the placement of a collagen membrane for occlusion of a small sinus membrane perforation.

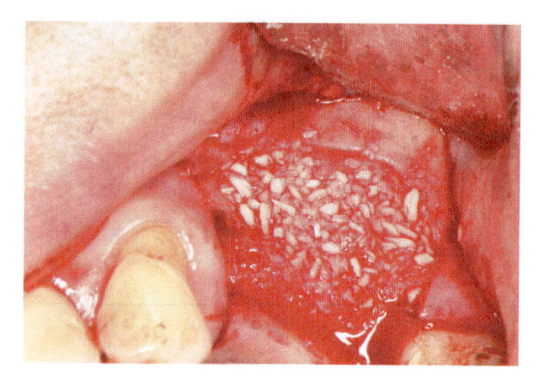

Figure 19.8 Intraoperative photo demonstrating the placement of the bone graft material after placement of a collagen membrane.

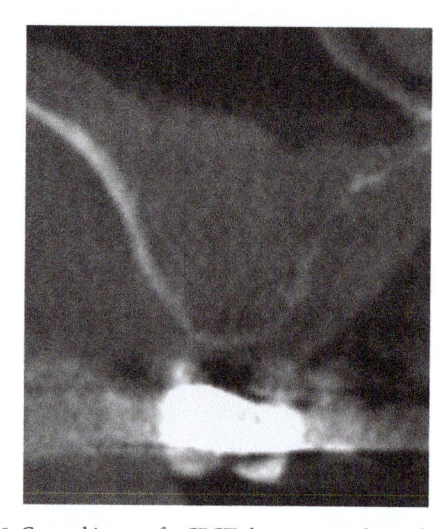

Figure 19.9 Coronal image of a CBCT showing partial opacification of the right maxillary sinus.

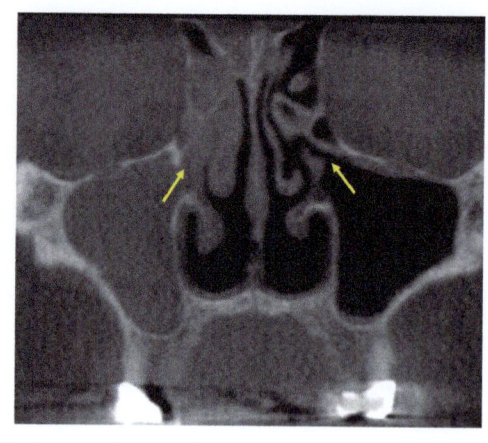

Figure 19.10 Coronal image of a CBCT showing pathology with complete opacification of the right maxillary sinus. There is obstruction of the right ostium and patency of the left ostium (yellow arrows).

can also lead to infection and sinusitis; therefore, strict aseptic techniques should be followed.

Pre-operative discussion with the patient regarding the history of sinus disease is required prior to surgery. Radiographic examination to evaluate the sinus for pathology and patency of osteomeatal complex (OMC) is required and best evaluated by CBCT scans (Figures 19.9 and 19.10). The adjacent teeth should also be tested for vitality and examined clinically and radiographically for any periodontal or periapical pathology. A healthy sinus will usually clear when presented with inflammation or bacterial insult. Failure to diagnose chronic sinus disease may lead to post-operative infection and graft failure.

Pre-operative antibiotics and chlorhexidine gluconate 0.12% mouth rinse should be used. The use of pre-operative chlorhexidine has been shown to decrease complications of infections from 8.7 to 4.1% [18]. Post-operative antibiotics should be used and amoxicillin is the drug of choice. Clindamycin should be used in patients who have allergies to penicillin. Systemic decongestants such as pseudoephedrine and nasal sprays such as phenylephrine can be used post-operatively to reduce the amount of maxillary sinus edema.

If infections do occur, the most common initial finding seen during an infected graft site is intraoral swelling, erythema, and pain [16]. Amoxicillin with clavulanic acid (875 mg/125 mg twice daily) or clindamycin (300 mg three times daily) may be used for empiric therapy. Metronidazole (500 mg three times daily) may also be added and has excellent coverage for anaerobic bacteria. Small, localized infection may resolve with antibiotics.

Infections that do not resolve or continue to progress with antibiotics should be surgically drained. The surgical site is entered through the original incision. Entering the sinus directly over the sinus window must be avoided and may induce an oroantral fistula. Gram stain, cultures for anaerobic and aerobic bacteria, and sensitivities should be obtained from the infected site. Any infected bone graft and membrane should be removed. Implants that were placed at the time of the graft should also be removed. The site is copiously irrigated and closed. A slow resorbing collagen membrane may be placed over the sinus window. A second sinus graft can be attempted 3–4 months later once the sinus has healed and inflammation has subsided.

Chronic infection and sinusitis can occur that may be unresponsive to antibiotics. These infections require surgical treatment and intravenous antibiotics. Functional endoscopic sinus surgery (FESS) may be required for refractory sinusitis. Referral to the ENT surgeon may be needed in these cases.

Bleeding

Significant bleeding during the sinus lift procedure is rare (less than 2%) and unlikely to be life threatening. Bleeding can affect visualization during surgery and may lead to post-operative hematoma if not controlled prior to soft tissue closure. Soft tissue bleeding is usually minimal and may be caused by supraperiosteal dissection, a buccal flap tear, or severing small vessels during flap elevation. The sinus membrane can also bleed, especially if a laceration occurs. Bone bleeding can be from cancellous bone or from intraosseous vessels. The maxillary alveolar bone is primarily supplied by branches and anastomoses from the infraorbital and posterior superior alveolar arteries [19]. Bleeding from these anastomoses can occur during the lateral sinus lift. The average distance from the alveolus to this anastomosis is 16.4 to 18.9 mm [19, 20]. These vessels become closer to the crest of the alveolus as the alveolus undergoes resorption. The vessels are located greater than 15 mm from the alveolar crest in mildly resorbed alveolar ridges. In more resorbed alveolar ridges, the vessels can be located as close as 7 mm from the alveolar crest [20].

The superior portion of the lateral maxillary osteotomy should, therefore, be placed no higher than 15 mm on mildly resorbed ridges and even lower for severely resorbed ridges. Bleeding may also occur from the nose if there is a sinus membrane perforation.

Bleeding can be managed using pressure with a moist gauze, cauterization, bone wax, local anesthetic with epinephrine and topical hemostatic agents. If bleeding occurs during osteotomy for indirect sinus lift with an implant placement, the osteotome or implant can be placed into the site to tamponade the bleeding. Careful planning should be taken for any patient with bleeding disorders and there should be appropriate consultation with the patient's primary care physician or hematologist. The surgeon should also consider modification of any antiplatelet or anticoagulant medications that the patient is taking after consulting the patient's physician.

Hematoma

A hematoma may present if hemostasis is not achieved prior to soft tissue closure. Hematomas are usually self-limiting, but may increase the risk of infection as they are a good culture medium for bacteria. The bleeding from the posterior superior alveolar artery and the infraorbital artery and their anastomoses are usually the main source for hematoma formation. Amoxicillin and clavulanic acid (875 mg/125 mg twice daily) for 7–10 days can be prescribed to prevent post-operative infection [17].

Neurosensory changes

The primary nerves that can be traumatized while performing sinus lift surgery are the infraorbital nerve and the superior alveolar nerve branches. Neurosensory changes in the distribution of the infraorbital nerve include the skin of the anterior portion of the cheek and infraorbital area, lower eyelid, lateral nose, upper lip, teeth, and oral mucosa on the affected side. Trauma to the superior alveolar nerves can result in sensory changes to the teeth and oral mucosa in the posterior alveolar region. The neurosensory changes can range from mild paresthesia, to dysesthesia, to complete anesthesia depending on the level insult on the nerve. The neurosensory changes are usually transient and resolve within 6 months [21].

Neurosensory defects can be due to either direct or indirect trauma. The direct sinus lift requires reflection of the periosteum and soft tissue overlying the maxillary sinus wall. Direct trauma may occur during reflection due to traumatic soft tissue retraction, intraneural injection, or damage during osteotomy. Care should be taken to avoid soft tissue retraction in the direction of the infraorbital nerve. The surgeon must also understand that the infraorbital nerve becomes closer in proximity to the crest of the alveolus in a severely resorbed maxilla. Indirect trauma can be secondary to hematoma or post-surgical edema and is almost always temporary.

Oroantral fistula

Oroantral fistulas can arise any time the maxillary sinus is accessed during grafting procedures. These can be caused by poor soft tissue closure, wound dehiscence, or infection.

Small oroantral fistulas may resolve spontaneously over the course of several weeks with the use of antibiotics and chlorhexidine gluconate rinses. Large fistulas may require additional surgery such as buccal advancement flaps, palatal pedicle flaps, and buccal fat pad advancement flaps.

Flap dehiscence and graft exposure

Flap dehiscence may occur in the first week following surgery, resulting in exposure of the alveolar bone or even the graft site. Factors that can contribute to flap dehiscence and graft exposure include flap and suture tension, mechanical trauma from mastication or dentures, poor tissue handling by the surgeon, or infection.

Dehiscence of the flap can be avoided by obtaining tension-free closure with releasing incisions anteriorly or posteriorly as well as periosteal releases as necessary. Mattress sutures can aid in obtaining tight primary closure. Any complete dentures and partial dentures should be relieved in the area of the graft to avoid pressure on the graft site. The flange of the denture should also be removed in the area to prevent any trauma to the graft site and flap. A tissue conditioner material may be considered in the area. Avoiding wearing the denture may be a viable option, especially in the posterior maxilla, where esthetics are less concerning.

A small dehiscence can be closed primarily within 24 to 48 hours. If the wound is larger than 2–3 cm or the wound has been open for more than 2 days, then the wound margins should be excised and the margins sutured again [22]. The use of chlorhexidine rinse and antibiotics should be considered, especially if the wound cannot be closed primarily. This can allow for an uneventful healing by secondary intention.

Injury to adjacent teeth

Sinus lift procedures have an inherent risk to adjacent teeth due to the close proximity of the osteotomies to roots adjacent to the surgical site. Roots can be damaged during the implant osteotomy or during lateral sinus osteotomy. Long roots, dilacerated roots, and convergence of adjacent roots can increase the likelihood of tooth damage. Careful evaluation of pre-operative imaging and intra-operative evaluation of root prominences can aid in placement of osteotomies in the correct location.

Implant loss

Implant loss can occur at any time after a sinus lift procedure with immediate placement of implants. There can also be implant loss with a two-stage procedure in which the implants were placed several months following the sinus lift procedure. Lack of osseointegration can be due to insufficient volume of bone graft, insufficient density of the native posterior maxillary bone, poor surgical technique, infection, trauma from mastication, pressure from a dental prosthesis, or implant migration due to lack of initial implant stability.

Mucocele formation

True sinus mucoceles can form after surgery involving the maxillary sinus. Sinus mucoceles are true cysts that form within the maxillary sinus. They are lined by respiratory epithelium and filled with mucin. True mucoceles slowly grow in size. Bony expansion of the maxillary sinus walls and resorption of bone may occur once the cyst becomes large. They may mimic malignancies of the maxillary sinus [23]. Radiographically, the maxillary sinus will appear cloudy.

The surgical ciliated cyst (post-operative maxillary cyst) is a type of mucocele and consists of a cystic lining comprised of respiratory epithelium identical to the maxillary sinus. These lesions may present years after trauma or surgery to the maxillary sinus. A portion of the maxillary sinus epithelium is separated from the main body of the sinus and develops into a cystic cavity in which mucin is secreted [23]. The patient may complain of swelling, pain, or tenderness in the area. The lesion is most commonly associated with a Caldwell–Luc operation, but may occur after any procedure in which the sinus membrane is violated, such as a tooth extraction [23]. This lesion presents as a spherical radiolucency on radiographic imaging.

Both the mucoceles and surgical ciliated cysts require surgical treatment because they are destructive in nature. Treatment is simple curettage and the site can be bone grafted at the time of removal.

Conclusion

The sinus lift procedure of the maxillary sinus is a delicate procedure. The most common complication of the sinus lift procedure (about 50% of cases) is a perforation of the sinus membrane. Careful preoperative planning with CBCT images and a vigilant intraoperative surgical technique can help decrease or prevent complications.

References

1. Jensen OT, Shulman LB, Block MS, et al: Report of the Sinus Consensus Conference of 1996. *Int J Oral Maxillofac Implants* 1998;13(Suppl):11–45.
2. Ardekian L, Oved-Peleg E, Mactei E, et al: The clinical significance of sinus membrane perforation during augmentation of the maxillary sinus. *J Oral Maxillofac Surg* 2006;64:277–282.
3. Morgensen E, Tos M: Quantitative histology of the maxillary sinus. *Rhinology* 1977;15:129.
4. Pikos M: Maxillary sinus membrane repair: report of a technique for large perforations. *Implant Dent* 1999;8:29–34.
5. Proussaefs P, Lozada J, Kim J, et al: Repair of the perforated sinus membrane with resorbable collagen membrane: a human study. *Int J Oral Maxillofac Implants* 2004;19:413–420.
6. Block MS, Ken JN: Sinus augmentation for dental implants: the use of autogenous bone. *J Oral Maxillofac Surg* 1998;55:1281–1286.
7. Timmenga NM, Raghoebar GM, Boering G, et al: Maxillary sinus function after sinus lifts for the insertion of dental implants. *J Oral Maxillofac Surg* 1997;55:936–939.
8. Ardekian, L, Efrat OP, Mactei EE, et al: The clinical significance of sinus membrane perforation during augmentation of the maxillary sinus. *J Oral Maxillofac Surg* 2006;64:277–282.
9. Chanavaz M: Maxillary sinus: anatomy, physiology, surgery, and bone grafting related to implantology – eleven years of surgical experience. *J Oral Implantol* 1990;16:199–209.
10. Van den Bergh JP, ten Bruggenkate CM, Disch FJ, et al: Anatomical aspects of sinus floor elevations. *Clin Oral Implants Res* 2000;11: 256–265.
11. Kim SG: Clinical complications of dental implants. In: Turkyilmaz I (ed.), *Implant Dentistry – A Rapidly Evolving Practice*. Intech, Rijeka, Croatia, 2011, pp. 467–490.
12. Ulm CW, Olar P, Gsellman B, et al: The edentulous maxillary alveolar process in the region of the maxillary sinus – a study of physical dimension. *Int J Oral Maxillofac Surg* 1995;24:270–282.
13. Zijderveld SA, van den Bergh JP, Schulten EA, et al: Anatomical and surgical findings and complications in 100 consecutive maxillary sinus floor elevation procedures. *J Oral Maxillofac Surg* 2008;66:1426–1438.
14. Fugazzotto P, Melnick PR, Al-Sabbagh M.: Complications when augmenting the posterior maxilla. *Dent Clin N Am* 2015;59:97–130.
15. Greenstein G, Cavallar J, Ramanos G, et al: Clinical recommendations for avoiding and managing surgical complications associated with implant dentistry: a review. *J Periodont* 2008;79:1317–1329.
16. Pikos MA. Complications of maxillary sinus augmentation, Chapter 9. In: Jensen OT (ed.), *The Sinus Bone Graft*, 2nd edn. Quintessence Publishing Co., Chicago, IL, 2006, pp. 103–114.
17. Timmenga NM, Raghoebar GM, van Weissenbruch R, et al: Maxillary sinusitis after augmentation of the maxillary sinus floor: a report of 2 cases. *J Oral Maxillofac Surg* 2001;59:200–204.
18. Lambert PM, Morris HF, Ochi S: The influence of 0.12% chlorhexidine digluconate rinses on the incidence of infectious complications and implant success. *J Oral Maxillofac Surg* 1997;55:25–30.
19. Solar P, Geyerhofer U, Traxler H, et al: Blood supply to the maxillary sinus relevant to sinus floor elevation procedures. *Clin Oral Implants Res* 1999;10:34–44.
20. Mardinger O, Abba M, Hirschberg A, et al: Prevalence, diameter, and course of the maxillary intraosseous vascular canal with relation to sinus augmentation procedure: a radiographic study. *Int J Oral Maxillofac Surg* 2007;36:735–738.
21. Stern A, Green J: Sinus lift procedures: an overview of current techniques. *Dent Clin N Am* 2012;56:219–233.
22. Sadig W, Almas K: Risk factors and management of dehiscent wounds in implant dentistry. *Implant Dent* 2004;13:140–147.
23. Neville BW, Damm DD, Allen CM, et al: Physical and chemical injuries, Chapter 8. In: Neville B (ed.), *Oral and Maxillofacial Pathology*, 2nd edn. Saunders, Philadelphia, PA, 2001, pp. 320–323.

SECTION IV

Alveolar Distraction Osteogenesis for Vertical Alveolar Ridge Augmentation

CHAPTER 20

Distraction Osteogenesis for Implant Site Development: Diagnosis and Treatment Planning

Stephanie J. Drew

Private Practice, The New York Center for Orthognathic and Maxillofacial Surgery, West Islip, New York
Stony Brook University Hospital and Hofstra Medical School, New York, USA

Introduction

Post-traumatic or post-extraction alveolar bone loss is a significant problem in implant dentistry. Horizontal bone deficiency can be easer to circumvent with different bone grafting techniques. Vertical alveolar bone defects are especially challenging to reconstruct. Implant dentistry is a prosthetically driven discipline and bone stock is needed where implants are to be placed in a functional position.

When implants are placed into non-reconstructed bone defects, they become a prosthetic and hygienic failure. The prosthetic components have to be very long to make up for the loss of tissues; the implants and prostheses become food traps. Often functional deficits can interfere with speech. Many of these cases become mechanical failures by losing tissues or having components fracture due to the forces placed upon them during normal function.

While traditional onlay bone grafting is an option in some cases, when there is a significant deficit of soft and hard tissue these techniques may not be as predictable. Even with the advent of titanium tacks, meshes, various membranes, and both allogeneic bone grafting materials and rhBMP2 as a supplement, the soft tissue coverage remains the largest barrier to achieving predictable success for these large defects.

The discovery of the technique of distraction osteogenesis (DO) surgery by Dr. G. Ilizarov paved the way to enable surgeons to solve very difficult challenges patients faced when there was a lack of soft tissue and bone to reconstruct [1]. Specifically, choices were limited and unpredictable when a large volume of tissue and bone were missing. Originally this technique was used to lengthen the limbs of patients [1]. In the late 1970s, this technique was used in the facial cadaveric bones first and was then translated to clinical cases [2]. In the 1980s, distraction surgery was then further perfected and applied to various types of craniofacial anomalies including hemifacial microsomia, as well as cleft and craniosynostosis problems and in tumor resection surgery for the reconstruction of segmental defects via transport distraction [3]. During this time, it was also discovered that transport distraction could be used on a smaller scale in the area of the alveolus [4–6]. Thus, alveolar distraction in oral applications was born, and today continues to be used for implant site development with predictable results [7–13].

Basic principles of distraction osteogenesis

The distraction osteogenesis surgery relies on the following four basic principles:

1 **An injury (osteotomy) to the bone via a precisely placed osteotomy.** A distraction device is placed on the two bone segments that can separate the two pieces along a planned vector at a specific rate and rhythm. A delicate and precise osteotomy should be done with care not to burn the bone. The use of the piezo knife has been shown to be a great alternative to standard instrumentation for these types of procedures [14–16].
2 **Latency period.** This allows the initial inflammatory reaction to the osteotomy trauma to occur between the bone segments. At this time, healing begins by recruiting the needed osteoprogenitor cells into action. The original work on long bones called for a 7 day latency period. This was based on the scientific knowledge of the biology of the phases of bone healing. The 7th day is when fibroblasts and angiogenesis are in full force and the body is ready to start laying down new bone. This is the beginning of the next phase.
3 **The distraction period.** This is the time when the bones are separated very slowly from one another at a specific rate and rhythm. It was found during this time period that when a traction forced is applied at the specific rate and rhythm, the fibroblasts align and the soft tissue responds by expanding and growing simultaneously with new bone formation [17–22]. If too slow the bone calcifies too fast and if too quickly the body only forms fibrous tissue. In traditional distraction, the rate in adult patients that has been found to work predictably is 1 mm per day. It can be broken down into several increments over a 24-hour period of time. The distractor screw pitch is designed to allow a full rotation to meet this requirement.

In alveolar distraction the timing is slightly different. The screw pitch design only allows for 0.3 mm per rotation of the distraction screw. This allows for 0.9 mm per day. Any faster distraction and the tight alveolar or palatal soft tissues will typically not respond well to too much pressure.
4 **Period of consolidation.** The timing of consolidation is important so that the newly formed immature bone can calcify and allow the result to remain stable over time [23–25]. Often the distractor itself serves as the stabilizing device. The device is no longer advanced and holds the segment in place while the bone matures in the center

---

Vertical Alveolar Ridge Augmentation in Implant Dentistry: A Surgical Manual, First Edition. Edited by Len Tolstunov.
© 2016 John Wiley & Sons, Inc. Published 2016 by John Wiley & Sons, Inc.

chamber. It is at the end of consolidation that the distractor can be finally removed. The timing of this last period is dependent on age, the type of bone moved, whether the tissues were radiated, and the distance it has moved. The bone calcifies from the center of the cut edges toward the middle. Radiographic confirmation of calcification is the best way to confirm when to remove the distractor when relying on a free segment being advanced.

However, under some circumstances the edges of the bone may be in contact with other areas of bone, as in alveolar distraction or Le Fort distraction, and these areas of contact will calcify faster than the distraction chamber, creating stability earlier. As a rule at least 12 weeks of consolidation are needed in these cases.

It is at the end of consolidation that the distractor hardware is removed. Typically, one should allow the soft tissues to heal before placing implant fixtures. The soft tissues may also need some connective tissue grafting since many patients not only lose bone but also soft tissue.

Indications for alveolar distraction surgery for implant site development

1 Lack of bone height
2 Lack of bone width
3 Lack of both height and width
4 Lack of soft tissue coverage for traditional onlay bone grafting
5 Previously failed onlay grafting
6 Moving a segment of ankylosed teeth
7 Moving malpositioned integrated implants
8 Patient's compliance

Contraindications for alveolar distraction surgery

1 Problem can be solved easily with traditional grafting
2 No compliance
3 No bone stock available to distract
4 Radiated area (relative contraindication)
5 Sandwich osteotomy can solve the problem of alveolar height

There have been many cases of alveolar bone distraction osteogenesis surgery reported in the literature. The reader is provided here with key published case reports. Reading these papers will enhance understanding of the technique [26–43].

Alveolar distraction depends upon the development of a transport disk that will remain viable and stable during the distraction process. The disk should not be so small that it becomes devascularized during the surgery. The transport disk should be no smaller than 7 mm high by 10 mm wide to maintain vascularity. Although there have been smaller segments distracted, it is not advised. Single tooth segments are very difficult to distract.

The width of the distracted bone should be wide enough to surround at least a narrow platform fixture once elevated into the correct vertical position. The goal is to bring the soft tissues up with the section of bone (transport disk) that is thickest at the base to gain both height and width to surround the fixtures (Figure 20.1).

Soft tissue grafting of attached (keratinized) tissue should be delayed until the bone is brought into position and it is completely healed and revascularized. If the transport segment is too small the distractor arm may not be able to be anchored to it to move it. Available bone stock is key in making decisions as to whether to use distraction as a technique.

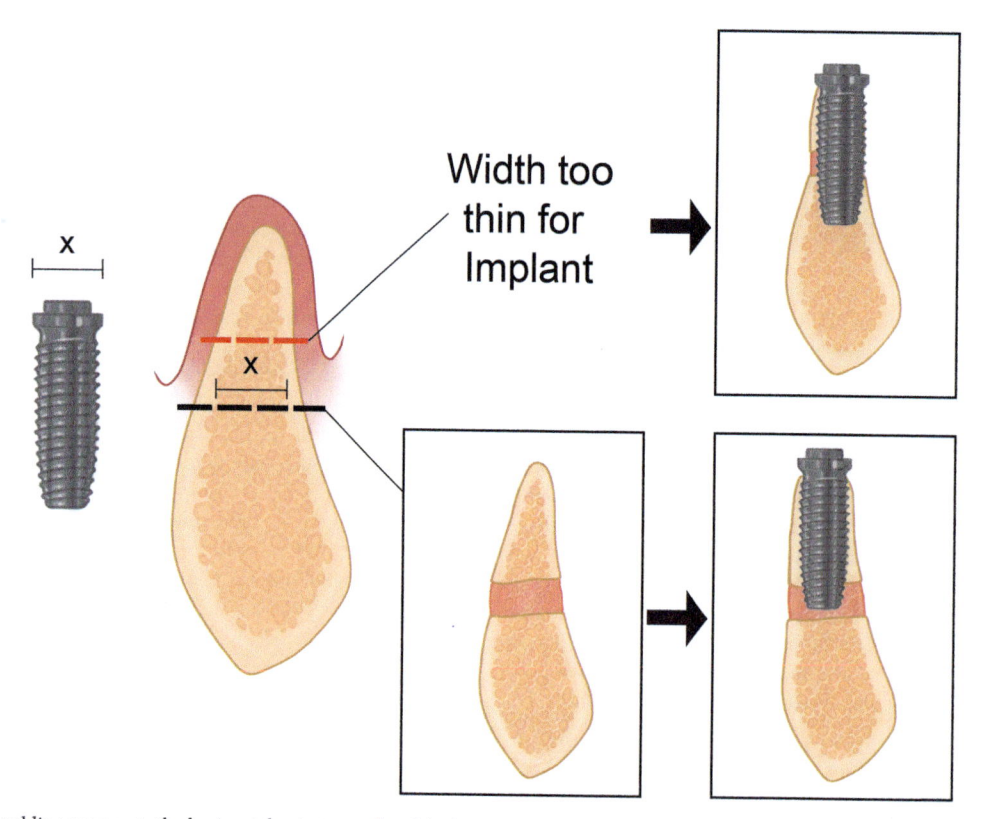

Figure 20.1 The red line represents the horizontal osteotomy placed in the wrong position to bring up the bone. It will be too thin to surround the threads of the future implant. The black dotted line shows a better choice for the horizontal cut that would support the width of the planned fixture.

Diagnosis and treatment planning for alveolar distraction

Work-up dogma: *"Let the prosthetic plan guide you in all bone and soft tissue reconstruction plans in implant dentistry."*

To plan the DO procedure, you must answer the following four questions:
1. How large is the deficiency?
2. Is there enough bone to distract?
3. What is the direction or vector of distraction?
4. What device will be best to use for this purpose?

Clinical examination

Evaluation of soft tissue
Look for tissue deficiencies and scarring. Scars may interfere with soft tissue viability. Lack of attached tissues should be dealt with after the distraction is complete for a healthy implant–soft tissue interface. Look for damage from radiation treatment. Consider hyperbaric oxygen (HBO) therapy. Document the case with intraoral photographs to record initial defects and progress.

Evaluation of hard tissue
Determine bone deficiency, both vertical and horizontal. Visual inspection and manual palpation are used to start making a diagnosis. Planning implant surgery requires looking at not only the intraoral soft and hard tissue but also the relationship to the lips and cheeks. Look at jaw interarch relationships to guide device placement. Patients with skeletal discrepancies may post challenges for activation arm placement.

Prosthetic requirements for final prosthesis
Let the final prosthetic plan guide the vector planning and site development. Use the restorative dentist's expertise in facebow mounting the case to come up with the ideal final restoration. Then work backward from this plan. There are times when the plan will need to be modified accordingly, depending upon anatomic restrictions as well as tissue limitations. The restorative dentist can also make guides for implant placement by either working in the lab or with virtual "surgery" utilizing planning software translated to make stereolithographic guides.

Radiographs
A computed tomography (cone beam or medical) scan is mandatory to determine bone stock. These scans allow us to identify the amount of bone stock available. It helps also to see the quality of the bone. The DICOM data can be used in various software programs to plan surgery or have stereolithographic models fabricated. The ability to see the three-dimensional nature of the problems we are trying to solve are of great value in creating a predictable and accurate outcome for implant placement prior to distraction surgery.

Regional anatomic considerations specific to alveolar distraction

The anterior maxilla
The floor of the nose may interfere with placement of the base plate. For the incisive canal and foramen, distracting this area lengthens the canal not the bone.

The posterior maxilla
For the maxillary sinus, if a surgeon decides to include the sinus in the superior part of the osteotomy, then the sinus floor will be distracted (instead of bone) and it will make the sinus cavity larger.

The anterior mandible
For genial tubercles and floor of the mouth, the tubercles will move up with the distracted segment when included in the disk. This may come to interfer with the final prosthesis and further surgery may need to be done. It is best to avoid it.

The posterior mandible
For the inferior alveolar nerve, working around this nerve and dealing with small segments of transport disk necessitates not only CT scans and three-dimensional imaging but also a cutting and drilling guide for placing the screws. This helps to stabilize the base plate to the inferior border in the correct position. Right angled screw drivers are quite helpful in these cases [44, 45]. The lingual nerve may be positioned directly on the medial surface of the posterior vertical cut. It is important to be careful completing these cuts.

Stereolithic models
Three-dimensional anatomically correct models are very helpful in planning vectors and device placement, as well as in device bending, especially for the novice surgeon [46, 47].

Planning surgery
Virtual reality using the DICOM data from the CT scan is available to use to plan osteotomy placement, vector alignment, and distractor choice. There are also times when both virtual planning as well as stereolithic modeling are needed in more complicated cases. The surgeon must determine from the clinical, radiographic, and possibly 3D model data the vector of distraction and the type of distractor to use. Once these are known, then the distractors can be bent and prepared for surgery.

Vector in alveolar distraction
The direction of movement of the transport disk must be planned and then controlled by placing the distractor in the correct orientation [48–51]. There are some distractors on the market that can be adjusted in a second plane; however, these tend to be bulky. In the maxilla or mandible, as the distraction disk is moving vertically, the tissues of the hard palate or the lingual tissue expand also but are often very tight, and at times may cause the disk and rod to rotate palatally or lingually. The distractor arm should be supported by the footplate or an appliance superiorly, such as an orthodontic wire or an occlusal splint, to avoid this complication. Orthodontic appliances and wires can be used to hold the distraction arm in the correct vector alignment. An occlusal splint with a distractor arm holding area can also be used to help keep the device properly oriented.

Choosing a distractor
Which distractor to use depends upon how you need to move the bone and how much bone stock is available [52–55]. The distractor needs to be stable during movement and consolidation. The distraction arms come in different lengths to achieve the needed height of distraction. The footplates may come in different sizes. Some

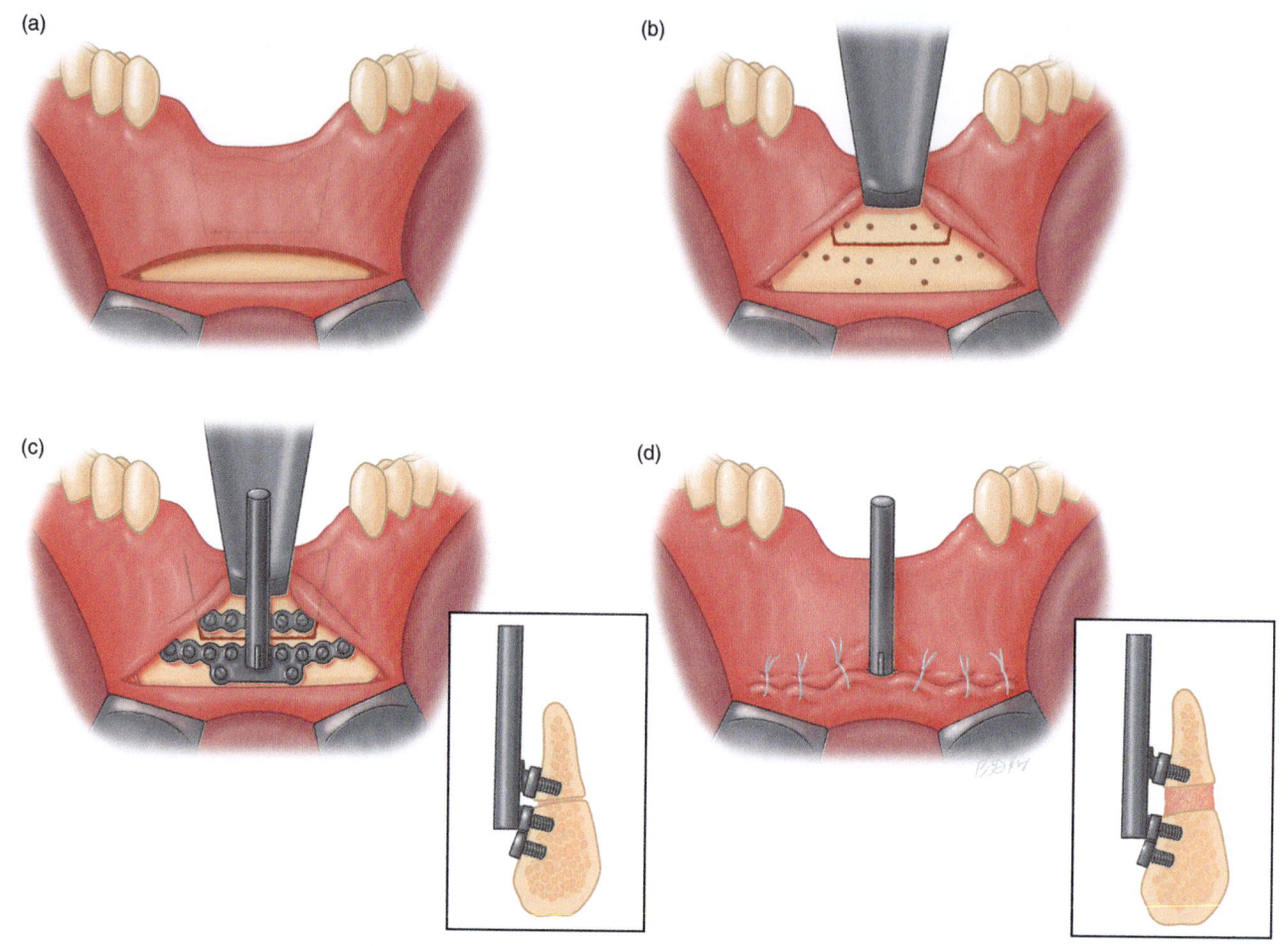

Figure 20.2 Step-by-step surgical technique of distraction osteogenesis. (**a**) Incision placement: keep the tissues attached superiorly. (**b**) Align the distractor and mark out holes for screws and osteotomy. Remove the distractor and complete the osteotomies. (**c**) Place the distractor and activate to make sure the transport disk will move in the right vector and not bind. (**d**) Close the incision around the distraction activation arm.

distractor rods may be placed into the transport disk but most are placed on the lateral aspect. Some distractors are adjustable. The point here is that one size does not fit all. Pick the distractor that best fits the situation. You will need to become familiar with what is out in the marketplace and some companies may even be willing to customize a distractor if there is enough lead time. There also may be times when the base footplate goes on the bone and the moving plate is anchored to the teeth that are in the moving segment.

Alveolar distractors today come in three types:
1 Extraosseous. The device attaches completely extraosseously to the lateral surface of the bone. This is the most common type.
2 Endosseous. The device attaches through the middle of the transport disk to the moving plate via the distraction screw. The stable base plate is secured on the lateral aspect and have been used to move smaller pieces of bone.
3 Implant distractor. These are implants that serve as the distraction devices.

Preparing the distractor for surgery
The alveolar distractors have the following parts:
1 A base plate that does not move.
2 The distractor arm that houses the activation screw and the moving plate that is soldered on to an internally threaded ring that is threaded onto the activation screw. As the screw is turned the plate moves along the screw to separate the plates from one another (Figure 20.2). The three-dimensional anatomy of the jaws does not allow for just a straight placement of these devices on to the surface to maintain the required vectors for success.

The base plate and moving plate of the DO devices need to be bent to obtain the correct occlusal vector orientation. This is where the stereolithic model may help the device to become oriented more precisely. One can bend these "chair side" during surgery, but in novice hands it may lead to poor vector orientation and thus a need to reposition the devices after activation if not noted at the time of surgery.

Osteotomy design
Second to vector orientation, the osteotomy design is the key to a smoothly moving disk and even most important a viable disk. When planning the vertical cuts of the osteotomy, a converging osteotomy towards the lingual or palatal is best in order to keep the bone from moving that way when it is rising on the distraction rod. Parallel walls come in second. The lower horizontal cut is planned to give the largest disk possible so that it is viable and the widest part of the bone can be lifted into position to grow the new bone to support dental implants. If a thin area is cut then a thin piece of bone will be grown. "You get what you cut" (Figure 20.3).

OSTEOTOMY DESIGN

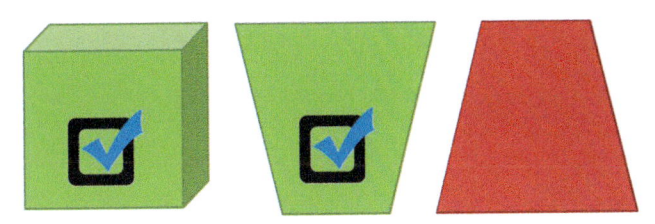

Figure 20.3 Osteotomy designs: parallel (acceptable), divergent (preferable), convergent (incorrect).

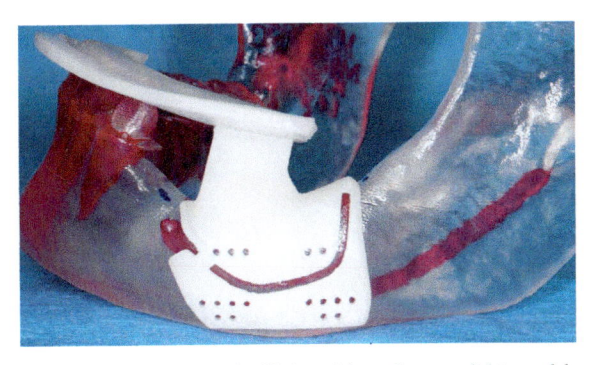

Figure 20.4 Cutting jigs may be fabricated from the stereolithic models when planning the DO procedure to help orient the drill bits or saw blades when cutting the osteotomies.

The remaining bone must be large enough to support the base plate of the distractor. If the mandible is too thin, it is at risk of fracture. In the maxilla, the challenge is placing the base plate so that the support screws do not engage the floor of the nose or the sinus, leading to an unstable distractor.

Cutting jigs may be fabricated from the stereolithic models when planning the DO procedure to help orient the drill bits or saw blades when cutting the osteotomies (Figure 20.4).

Device positioning jigs can also be made to allow for correct vector orientation. It is more difficult to confirm placement in the actual surgery due to visual impedance of the soft tissue flaps.

Occlusal clearance is a very important concept that may be overlooked and create some truly functional issues during the distraction process. This may necessitate additional surgery to reposition the device. The device activation arm needs clearance from mastication so that it is not bitten during function.

The "over distraction" concept is also an important concept [56]. The leading edge of the distraction disk is typically thin as the tissue rises and the overlying pressure from the soft tissue starts to remodel this sharp edge by compressing against it. The height of this piece consequently changes and shrinks a little. Sometimes, it even rotates toward the lingual or palatal so that the buccal plate becomes the superior surface. This is a function of the tight soft tissue on the opposite side of the cut. These facts are very helpful in implant site development, but if an operator chooses a distraction activation arm that is too short then the bone height will not be adequate. It is important to plan for over distraction by at least a few millimeters. It is easy to remove an excess bone but much harder to add it.

Screw size

Choosing the right length of screws to put into the moving transport disk is also an important concept. If you use very short screws that only engage the buccal cortex, they can loosen and perhaps cause failure of the distraction. Consider using screws that are longer to maintain the position of the segment on the moving bone plate. Lastly, it is important that these screws are not close to osteotomy edges, as the edges will remodel as the bone moves and the stability of the appliance can be lost.

Steps of distraction osteogenesis surgery (also see Figure 20.2)

1. An incision is made in the unattached mucosa to expose inferiorly for the non-moving base plate. Tunnel underneath soft tissue to the superior edge for vertical cuts.
2. Take a pre-bend distractor and lay against the bone in the correct vector orientation.
3. Mark the screw holes and horizontal osteotomy using a very thin fissure bur. Sometimes a cutting jig (Figure 20.4) in combination with a screw hole locator can be used to mark these sites.
4. Remove the distractor and start the horizontal osteotomy outlining with copious irrigation; a piezo knife is preferred. If it is very deep then complete with an osteotome to avoid overheating bone and soft tissue.
5. Complete the vertical divergent cuts to the superior surface making sure there is a clearance so the segment will move.
6. Separate the moving segment with gentle pressure to release the bone. Make sure to keep the medial soft tissues intact so the segment does not become devascularized.
7. Place the distractor and secure the screws to the lower site first and then the disk. Make sure as the lower screws are placed that the vector is not changed. It is at this time any minor adjustments can be made to get the vector perfect.
8. Activate the distractor to make sure the segment and the distractor are moving smoothly. Then close it back down to the zero point. Close the soft tissue.

Case Report 1: DO of the anterior mandible (Figures 20.5 to 20.17)

This patient is a 26-year-old female that presented to her dentist with a complaint of loosening anterior teeth. Panoramic examination revealed significant bone loss around the lower incisor teeth (Figure 20.5a). The central and lateral incisors were removed with soft tissue for biopsy (Figure 20.5b). The diagnosis of squamous odontogenic tumor necessitated a marginal resection, leaving the patient with a vertical and horizontal bone and soft tissue defect of the mandible from the mesial of the lower left first premolar to the lower right lateral incisor (Figure 20.6a and b).

Cone beam CT was evaluated to plan out implant placement and reconstructive surgery. It was felt that distraction surgery was the best way to achieve both height and width needed for the fixtures. The prosthodontist wanted to place three fixtures in this area to create a stable prosthesis. The distraction is retro-engineered to meet the requirements of where the fixtures were to be placed. This determined how much height was needed to be achieved. Then the distractor was chosen.

The surgery was done at least 4 months after the tumor removal to allow soft tissue remodeling and revascularization. The osteotomy was planned from the cone beam CT radiographs and accomplished with a piezo knife. The distractor was then placed along the planned vector (Figure 20.7a to e). The period of latency was 7 days. The distractor was then turned 3 times per day for a total of 0.9 mm/day. This is determined by the pitch of the screw threads on the various

(continued)

(Continued)

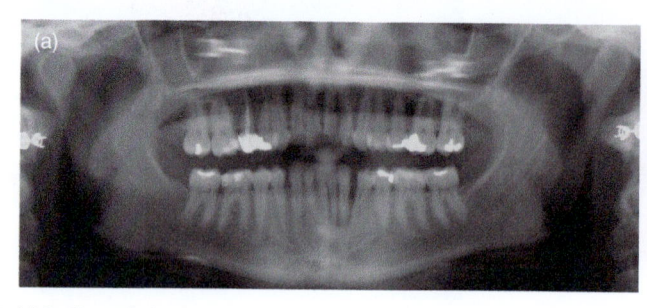

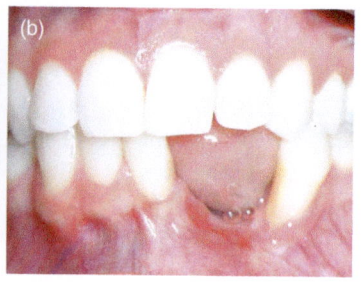

Figure 20.5 (a) Radiograph demonstrating squamous odontogenic tumor in the anterior mandible involving the left canine to the right central incisor. (b) Soft tissue defect after biopsy.

alveolar distractors (Figure 20.8). Attempt not to move the alveolar segments faster than 1 mm per day as the gingiva will tend to break down and the transport segment can be lost due to lack of vascularity (Figure 20.9).

Once the distraction is completed, consolidation occurs. In alveolar distraction, this is approximately a 12-week period that allows the bone to be mature or strong enough to maintain the movement. Cone beam CT (CBCT) can show appropriate bone calcification (Figure 20.10a to g). The advantage of the alveolar distraction is that the vertical walls maintain contact and will consolidate in about 8 weeks. If necessary, the distraction device can be removed at that time. We tend to be very conservative and wait the 12-week period to allow the most healing to occur before moving the mucosa around the distraction chamber (Figure 20.11a to f).

Once the distractor device is removed, it is advisable to wait for soft tissue healing before placing implants into the bone (Figure 20.12a to c). It usually takes about 4–6 additional weeks. It is especially important to wait for soft tissue maturation if a surgeon plans to move a flap or further graft on to the chamber if it does not fill in completely (Figure 20.13a and b).

The implants in this case were placed with a guide fabricated by the prosthodontist. Impants were restored after a period of 4 months of osseointegration (Figures 20.14 to 20.17).

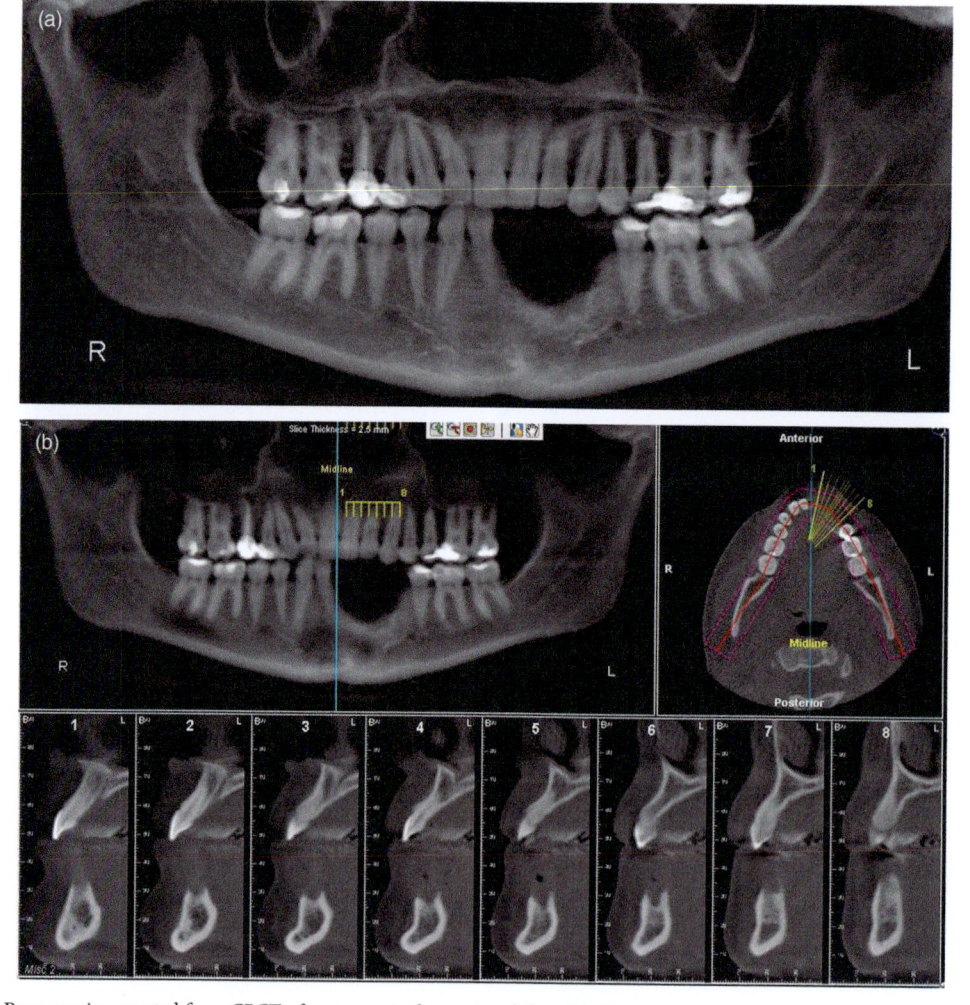

Figure 20.6 (a) Panorex view created from CBCT of post-marginal resection defect. (b) CBCT view to document and quantify vertical and horizontal deficiency and determine if distraction is possible.

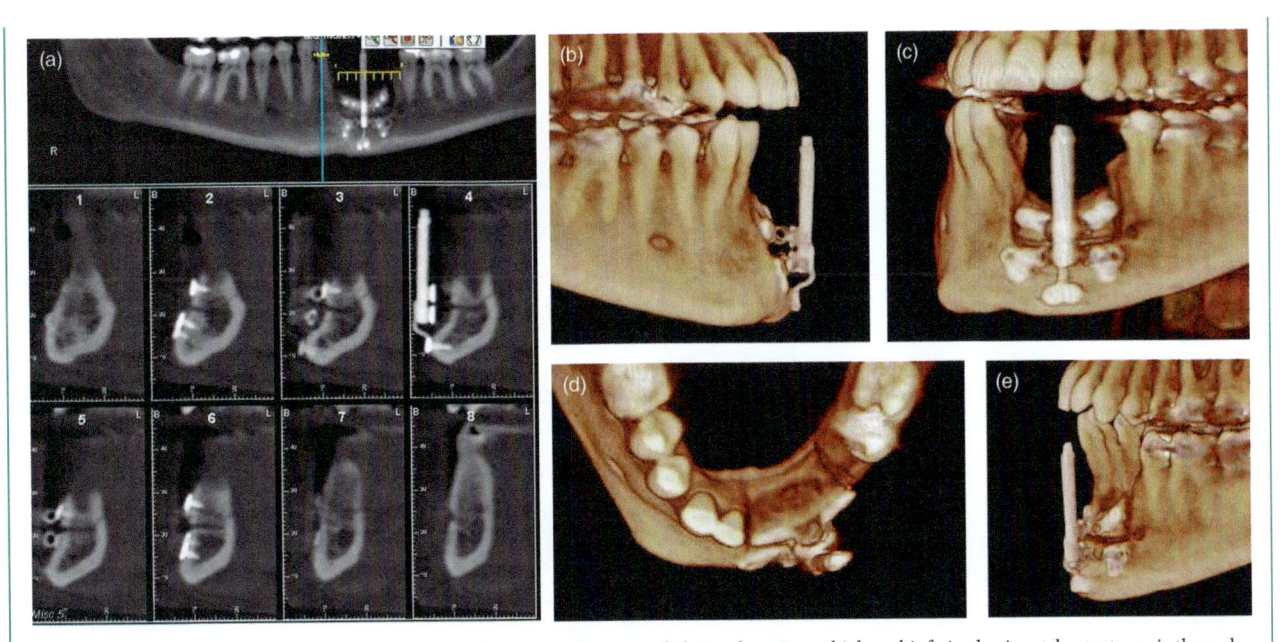

Figure 20.7 (a) Post-distractor placement. The rod is the vector. Transport disk is at least 7 mm high and inferior horizontal osteotomy is through the wide part of the bone so that a wide chamber can be created while height is achieved. (b) Distractor in 3D view. Note arms are bent so that the rod controls the vector as the segment rises. (c) Anterior 3D view. Note that vertical osteotomies are parallel or slightly divergent so the disk does not bind as it rises. If you find that the area may bind then just remove more bone to open space. (d) Superior 3D view. Note vertical osteotomies converge a bit toward the lingual. This is a way to keep the block from moving lingually as the transport disk rises and the lingual tissue pulls it that way. (e) Lateral 3D view. Note that the distractor is closed down after placing and checking on the bone.

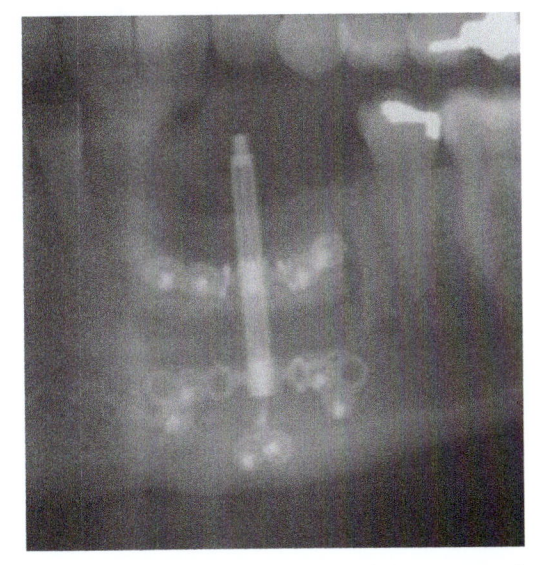

Figure 20.8 Mid-distraction radiograph. The disk is moving without binding and the chamber is expanding as the bone rises along the rod.

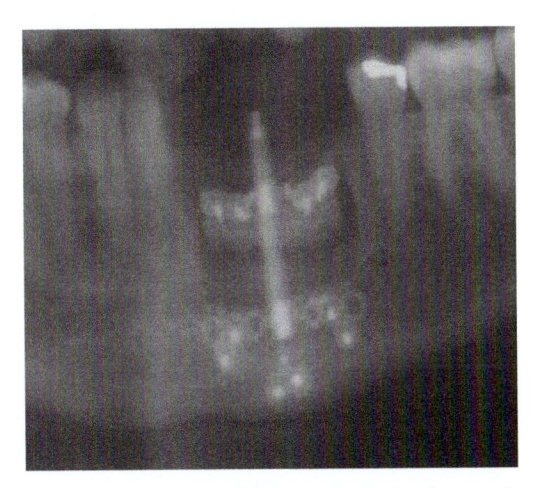

Figure 20.9 Toward the end of distraction, note that the posterior lip appears to be touching the bone ledge next to the bicuspid. If this is confirmed, simply use local anesthesia to then allow the creation of a small opening over the area and clear the bone with a fine fissure bur to release. Then continue distracting. Be very careful not to injure surrounding soft tissues.

(continued)

(Continued)

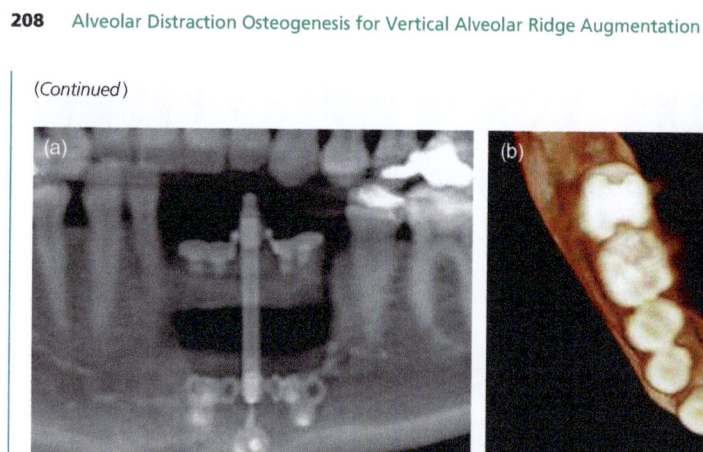

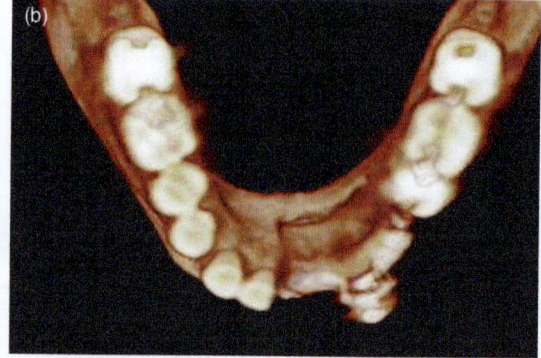

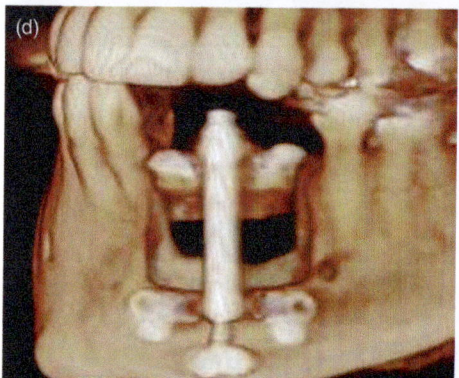

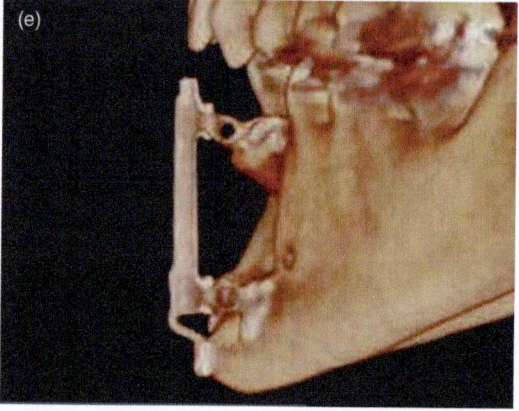

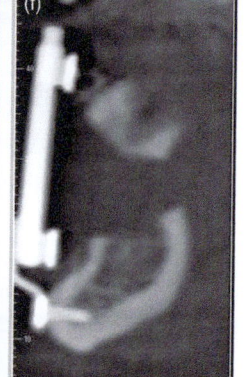

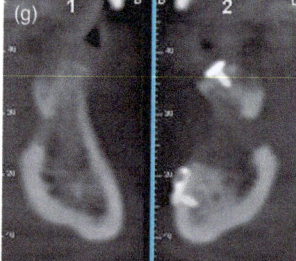

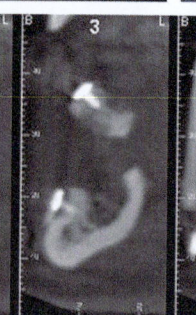

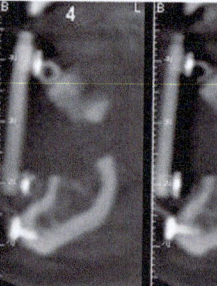

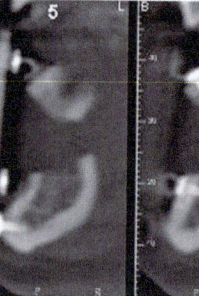

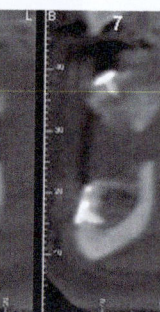

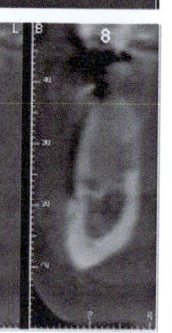

Figure 20.10 The width achieved after distraction surgery. Note that the disk appears to have torque so that the plate is on top. This happened because of the tight tissues on the lingual. Although the chamber looks empty, it is not. It is full of new bone, but the bone has not yet calcified.

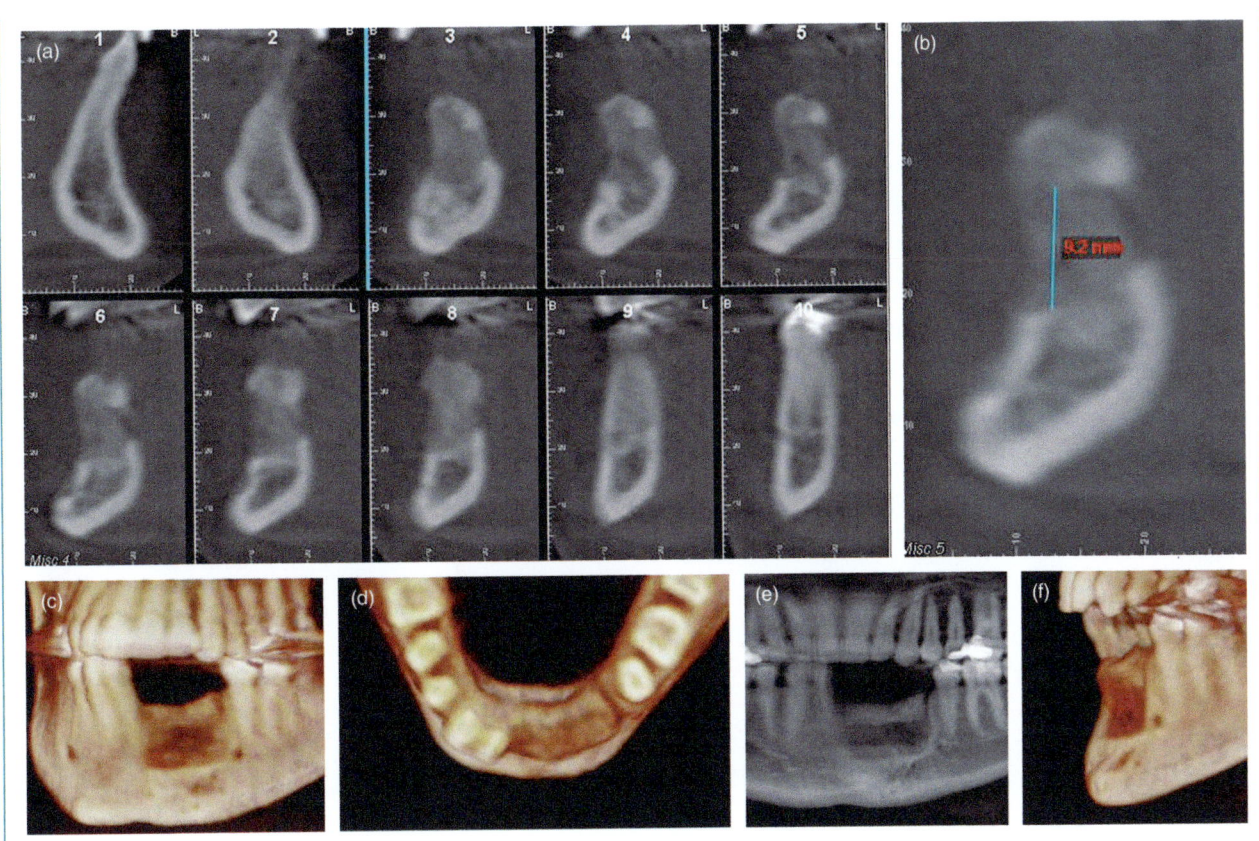

Figure 20.11 The end of consolidation showing (a) the placement of implants with direction indicators in place, (b) implants in position and (c) implants in bone on the radiograph. Note that the chamber is now filled with calcified bone. Now is the time when the distractor can be safely removed.

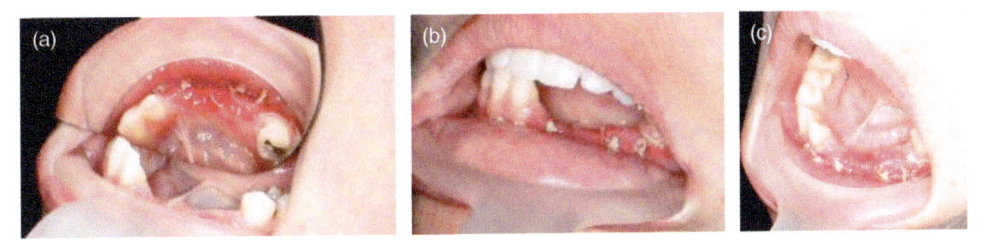

Figure 20.12 Distractor removal through original incision and closure, where (a) shows the stage of a reconstructive radiograph and (b) clinical pictures with a temporary prosthesis. Let these tissues heal to revascularize before placing the implants through a superior incision. Stripping up and over the new bone and transport disk is not recommended as it may strip the blood supply too much. A wait of about 6 weeks is recommended.

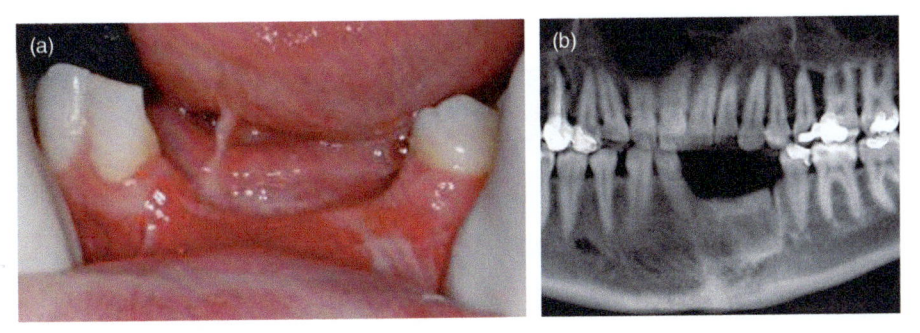

Figure 20.13 (a) The final prosthesis radiograph and (b) clinical photos of the final prosthesis at the time of implant placement. Note the further consolidation and good tissue healing.

(continued)

210 Alveolar Distraction Osteogenesis for Vertical Alveolar Ridge Augmentation

(Continued)

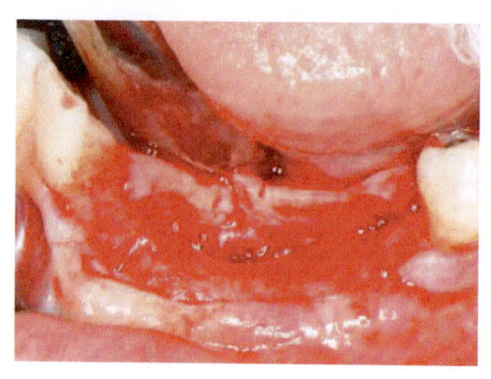

Figure 20.14 Incision for the implant is crestal. Plan soft tissue grafting if needed at this time. Note the remnant of vertical osteotomy on the distal of site next to the premolar. This can be grafted with allogeneic bone at this time as well.

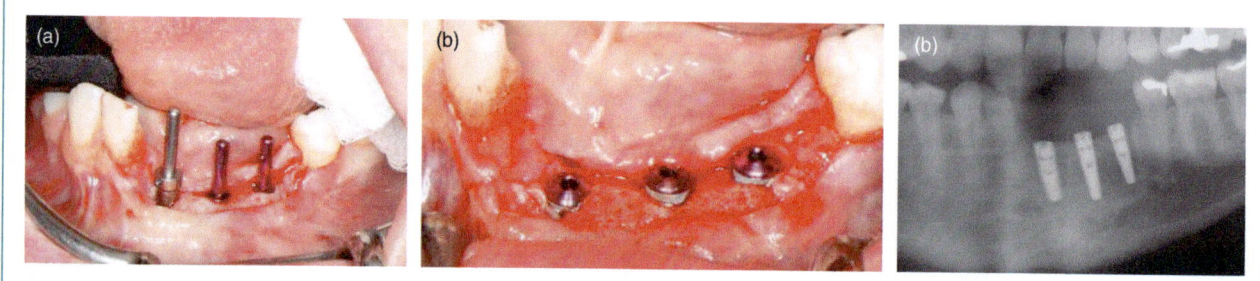

Figure 20.15 Radiograph demonstrating the amount of bone loss and deficiency needed for the reconstruction and placement of implants. A guide was created for location by the prosthodontist.

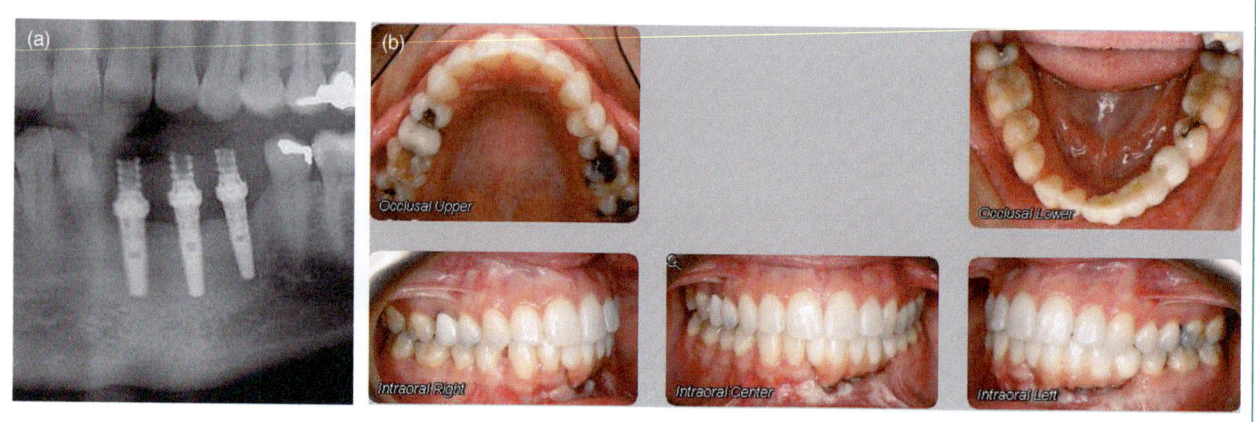

Figure 20.16 (a) Measurements on the cone beam for planning distraction. (b) Temporary restoration where the horizontal line shows where to place the osteotomy and the vertical blue line indicates the amount needed to bring it inferiorly during distraction, the goal of the surgery. (c) Clinical picture of what the alveolar defect looks like.

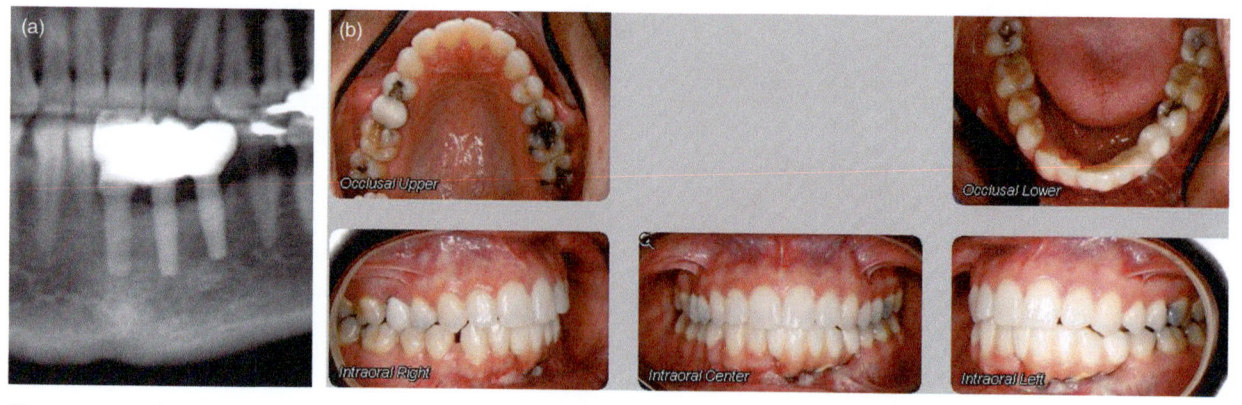

Figure 20.17 Final restoration showing the different widths at different heights measured. Choose the width that will get the most width.

Case Report 2: DO of the posterior maxilla (Figures 20.18 to 20.30)

This patient had failed implants in the left premolar–canine region of the maxilla (Figure 20.18a and b). The lateral incisor was also periodontally involved and deemed non-salvageable (Figure 20.19). As part of the preparation for the distraction surgery, the lateral incisor was removed and socket grafted with allogeneic bone. The soft tissues were allowed to heal for two months.

The distraction surgery was planned by using cone beam radiography to measure the bone defect and plan the osteotomies (Figure 20.20a to c). The scan was used to determine where to place the horizontal osteotomy and develop the transport disk (Figure 20.21). Careful planning was needed to ensure that the disk was going to be large enough to be viable. The DICOM data was sent to the medical modeling engineers to develop a vector plan for the distractor and create a guide (Figures 20.22 and 20.23).

The distractor was placed and a latency period of 7 days was used (Figure 20.24). The distractor was turned 3 times per day at a rate of 0.3 mm/turn (Figure 20.25a and b). During the distraction period, the distractor remained stable and the planned height was achieved (Figure 20.26a and b). The palatal soft tissues were very tight in the region and one could see that the soft tissue would try to pull the segment palatally (Figure 20.27a and b). The end of consolidation was confirmed with radiographs (Figure 20.28a to c). The cone beam was used to plan out the implant placement (Figure 20.29). The implants were then placed and left to integrate for 4 months before restoration were constructed (Figure 20.30a to d).

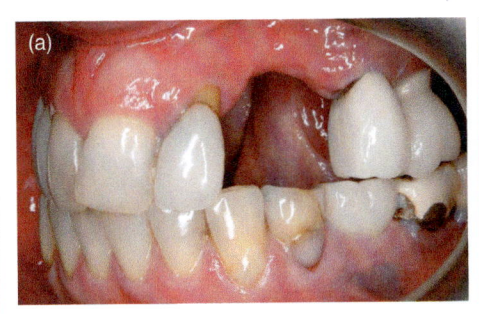

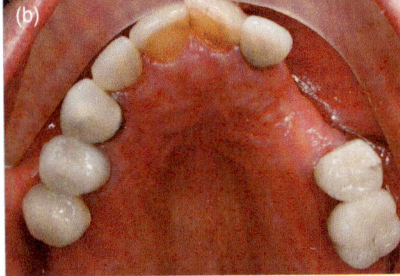

Figure 20.18 Soft tissue defect from previously failed implants showing computer planning of the distractor placement, osteotomy placement, and vector planning.

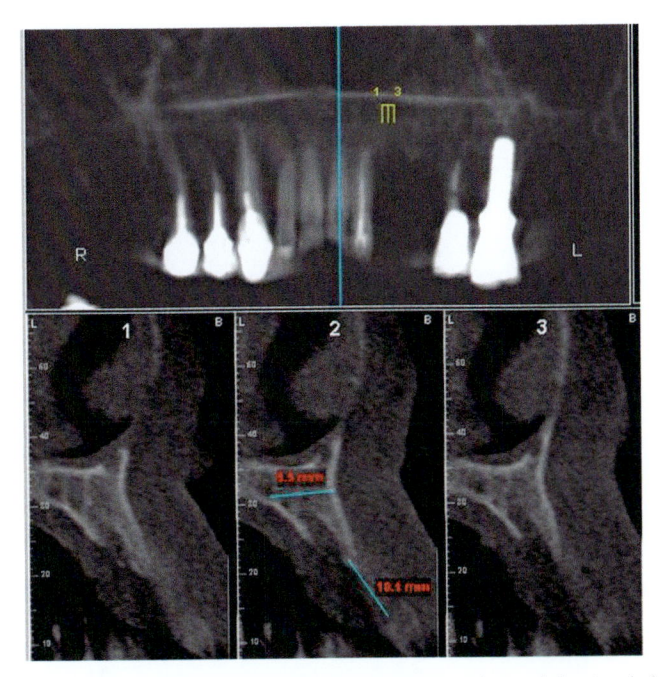

Figure 20.19 Pre-treatment CBCT with definition of the defect, showing the distractor in place and the virtual plan with the segment in the goal position. The lateral incisor was not salvageable. It was removed and socket grafted.

(continued)

(Continued)

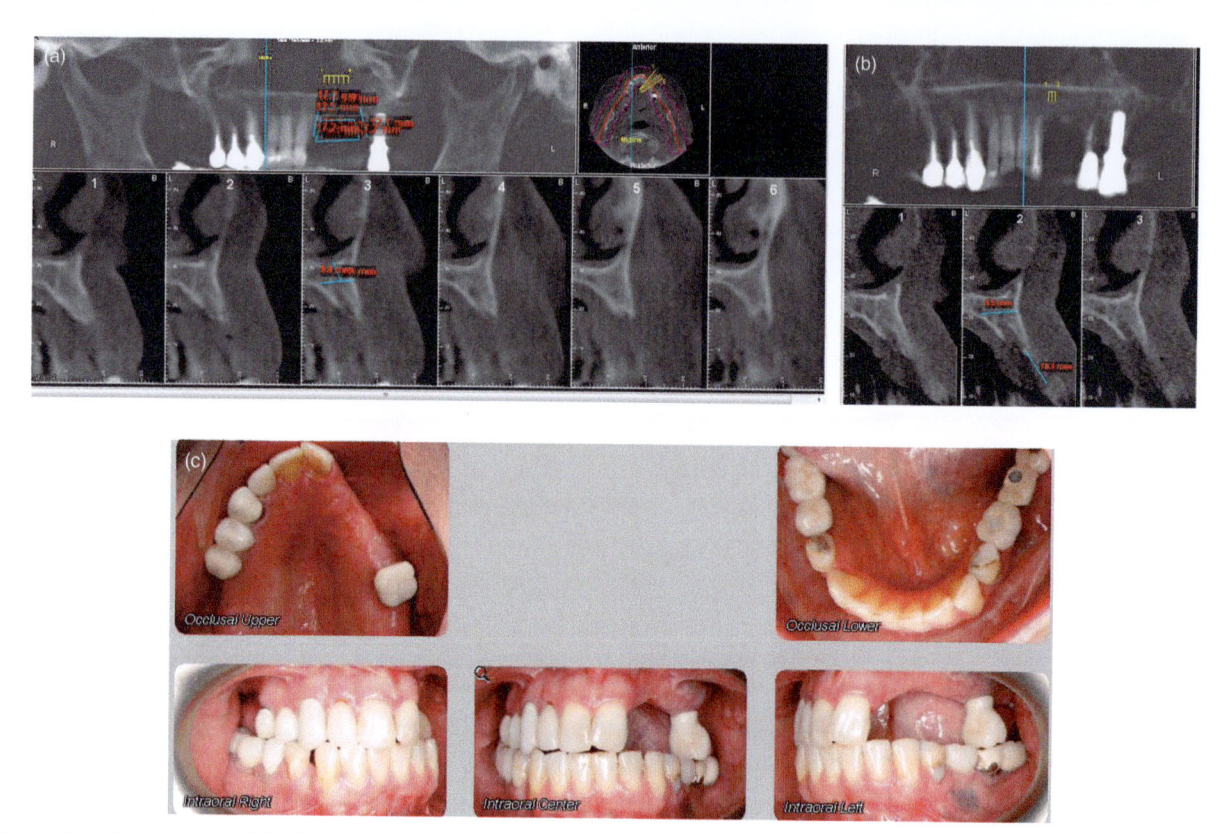

Figure 20.20 Measurements of the defect after the lateral was removed and the graft consolidated, with the distractor in position post-placement.

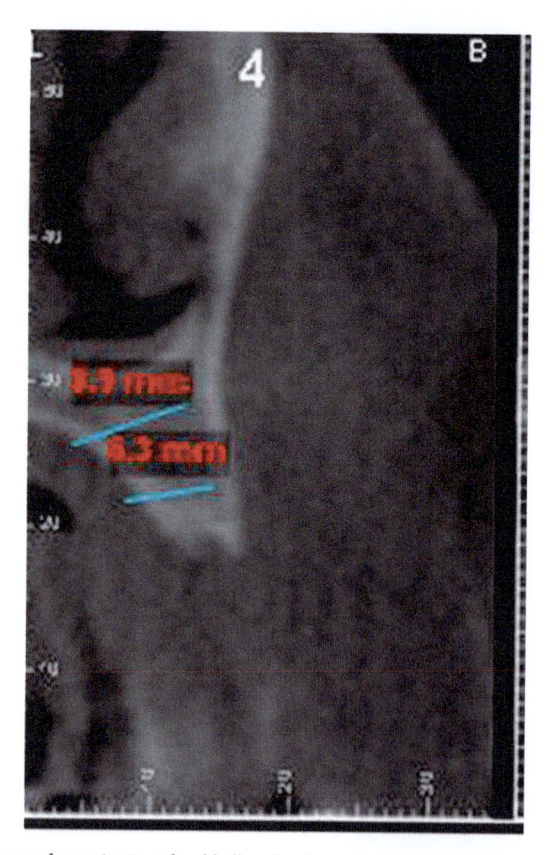

Figure 20.21 Note that horizontal osteotomy determination should allow for the wider part of the bone to move down and also for enough vertical bone height and stock to hold on to superior bone plate screws of the distractor.

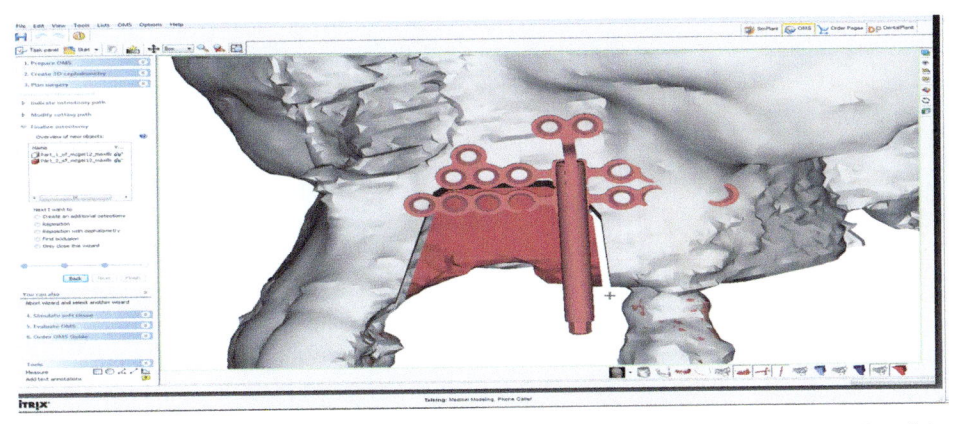

Figure 20.22 Virtual planning distraction placement and vector. The cut is determined to be close to the sinus posteriorly and the cutting jig is created to make the cut more precise.

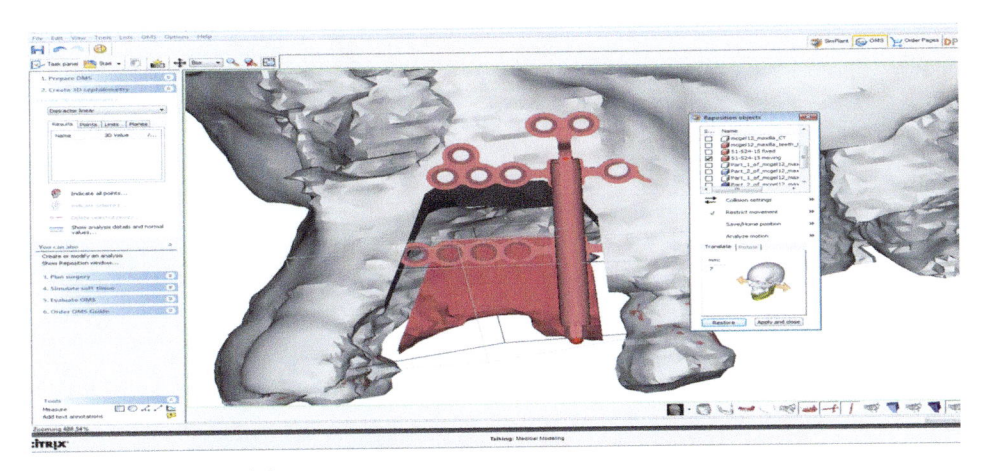

Figure 20.23 Vector and movement of the disk.

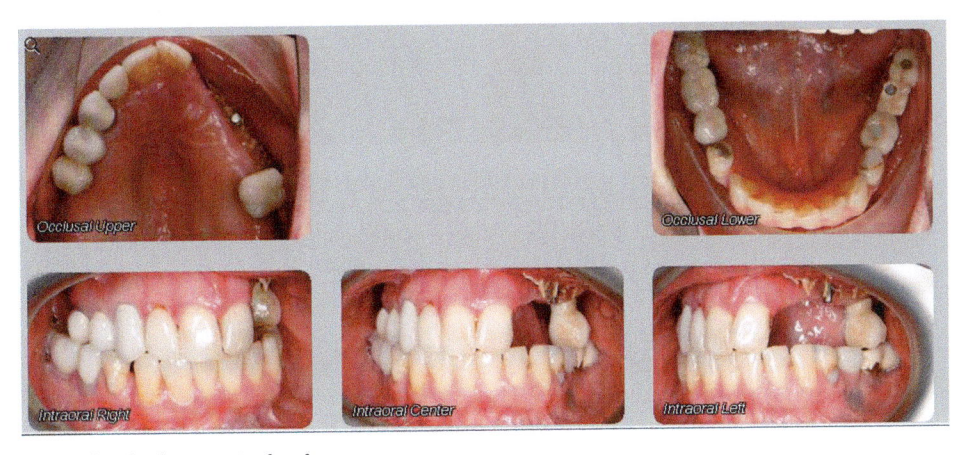

Figure 20.24 Soft tissue after the distractor is placed.

(*continued*)

(Continued)

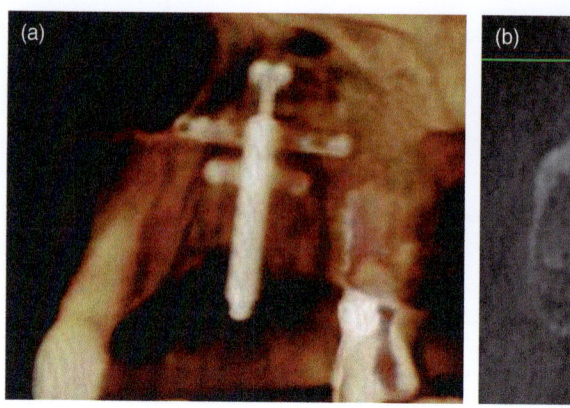

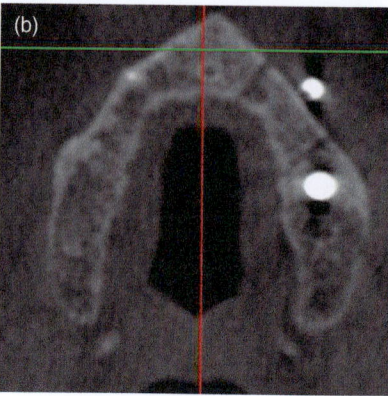

Figure 20.25 Cone beam cut of implant planning on a scan into distracted bone showing 3D of distractor placement. (a) Note that the vertical cuts on the 3D view diverge from the base to create a smooth path. (b) On the axial view note that vertical cuts are created to keep the disk from moving palatally.

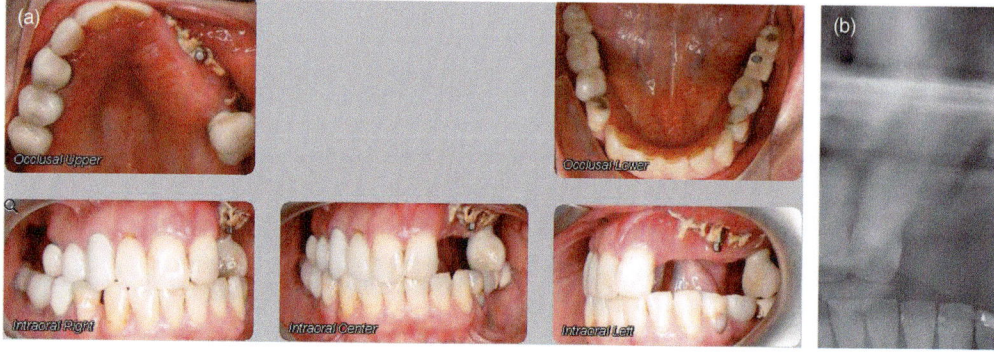

Figure 20.26 (a) Soft tissue healing one week before starting DO. (b) Radiograph of bone before DO week 1.

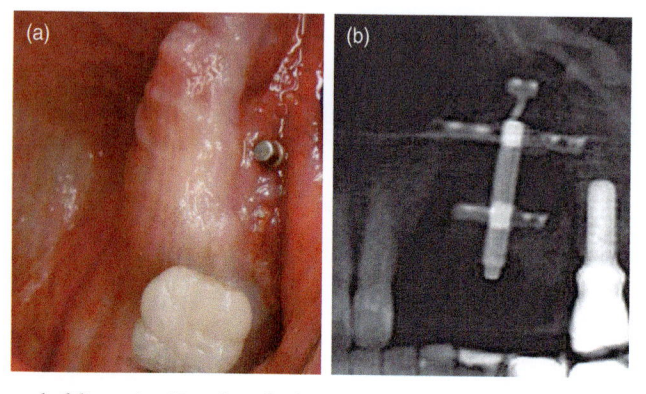

Figure 20.27 (a) Soft tissue near the end of distraction. Note the palatal position of the soft tissue and segment due to tough tissues of the hard palate. (b) Radiograph of area distracted. See over distraction in vertical of segment to account for the necessary width.

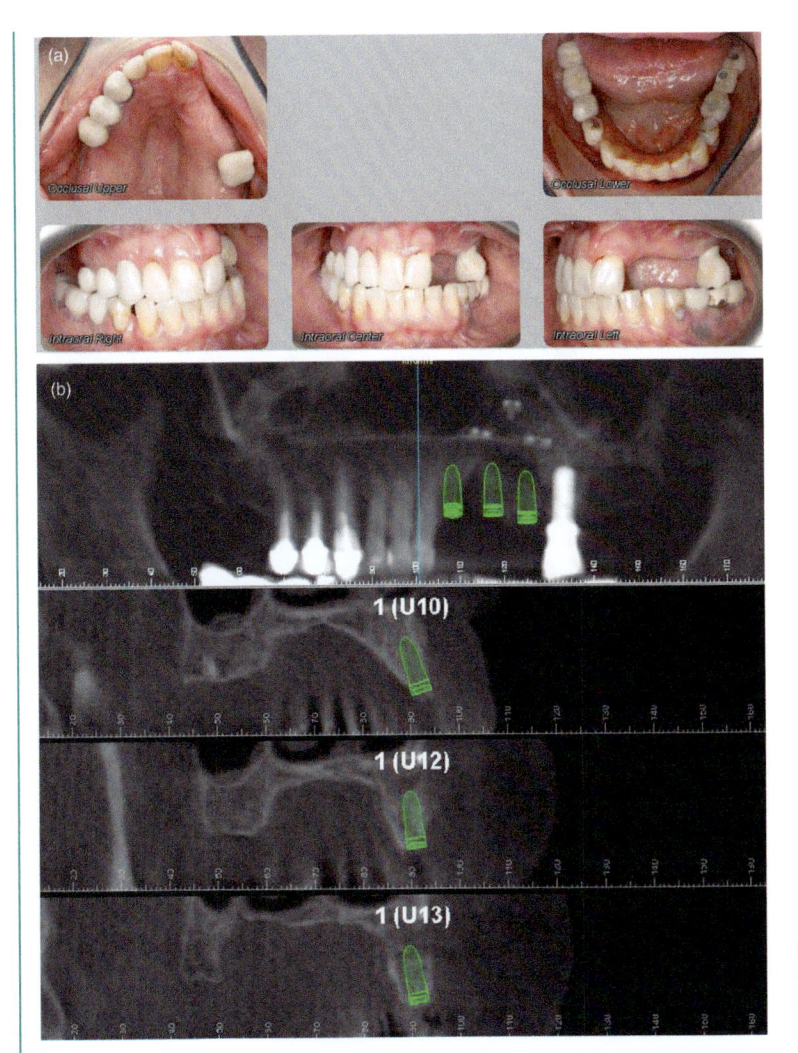

Figure 20.28 (a) Soft tissue at the end of distraction. (b) Radiograph of bone consolidating at the end of distraction. (c) Consolidation and ridge shape noted on the cone beam radiograph.

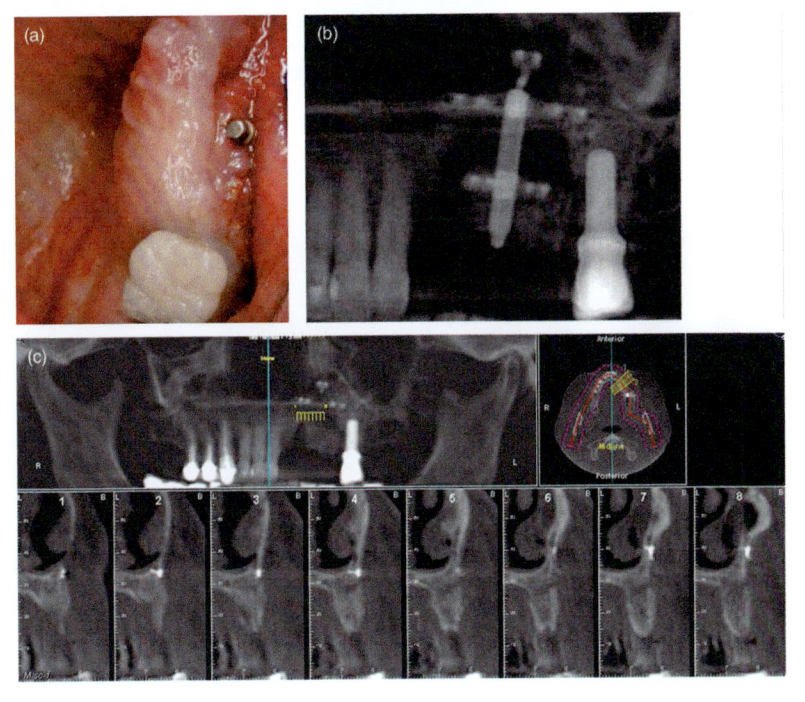

Figure 20.29 Implant treatment plan.

(continued)

Figure 20.30 (a) Implant placement. (b) Occlusal relationship. (c) Prosthesis. (d) Radiograph.

Case Report 3: DO of the ankylosed teeth (Figures 20.31 to 20.41)

A young patient had a previous injury and intruded his incisors (Figure 20.31). He had undergone previous orthognathic surgery before the distraction surgery was planned (Figure 20.32). The osteotomies were well healed. The teeth were deemed non-salvageable by the prosthodontist. It was determined that these teeth would act as a guide to bring down the bone and soft tissue into position to prepare for the implant placement.

The osteotomy was created to include both incisors (Figure 20.33) and the distractor stabilized above the roots to push down the segment into position (Figure 20.34). The incisor edges were ground down as the segment came down with turning the distractor until the correct height was achieved (Figure 20.35a and b). The distraction allowed enough soft tissue and bone to develop (Figure 20.36). The period of consolidation was 12 weeks. The distractor was then removed. A soft tissue healing prior to proceeding with the implant dentistry was allowed (Figure 20.37). The gingival architecture was enhanced enough to prepare for a predictable implant surgery (Figure 20.38).

A period of 8 weeks passed before the teeth were removed and the implants placed at the same time (Figure 20.39). The final restoration and radiographs show an esthetic result for this young patient (Figure 20.40a and b and 20.41).

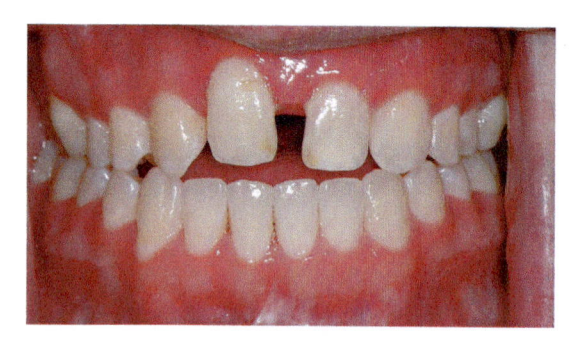

Figure 20.31 Ankylosed central incisors secondary to trauma.

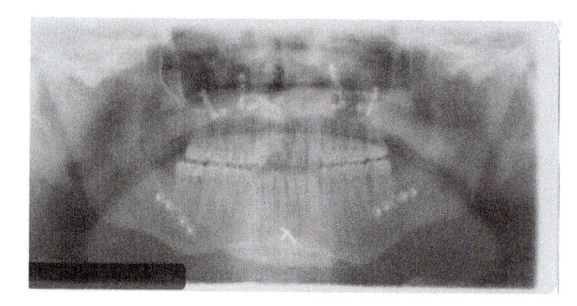

Figure 20.32 Panoramic view of dentition.

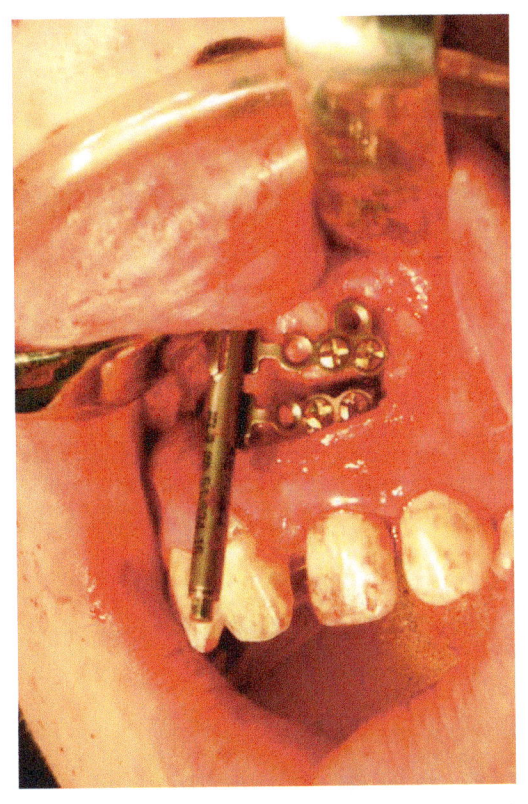

Distraction Osteogenesis for Implant Site Development **217**

Figure 20.33 Placement of device. Plan to move teeth down and reshape incisor edges until the gingiva and bone are at the correct height for implants.

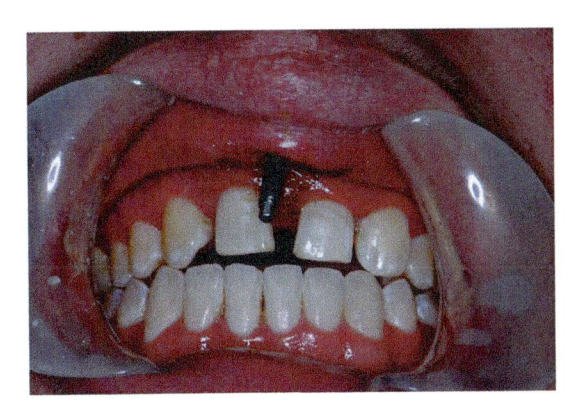

Figure 20.34 Beginning of DO.

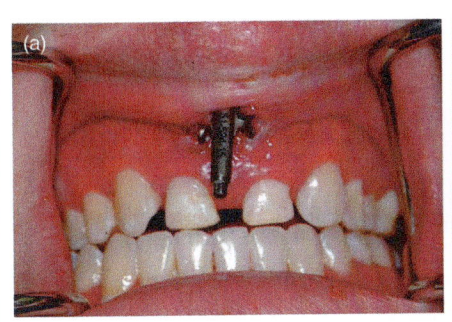

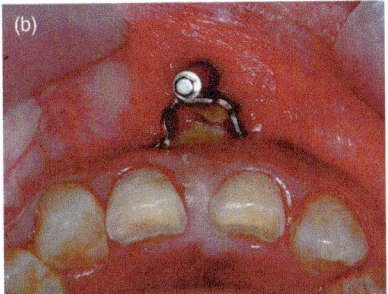

Figure 20.35 (a) End of DO. (b) Note the position of the rod to maintain the vector and incisor edges of teeth that had to be recontoured to allow downward movement.

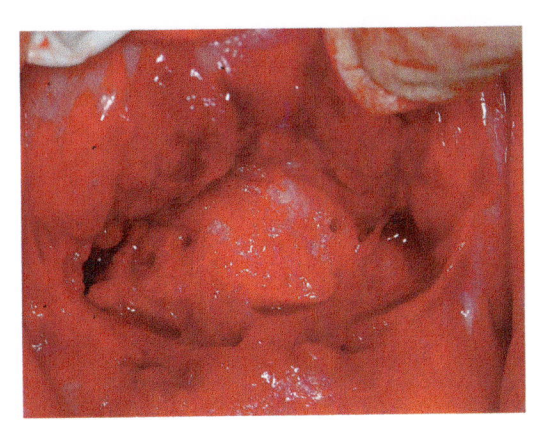

Figure 20.36 Removal of distractor. Not all of the new bone is formed.

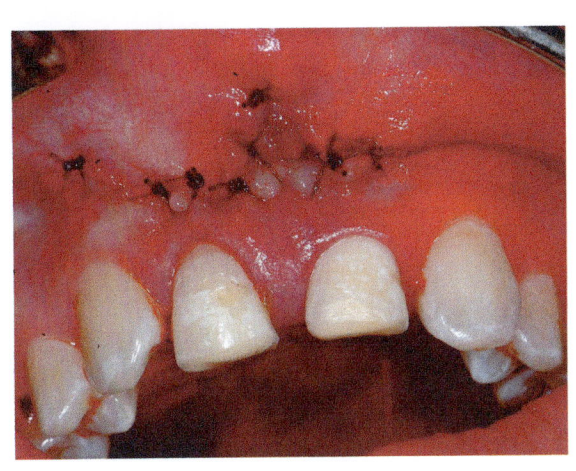

Figure 20.37 Closure after distractor removal.

(continued)

(Continued)

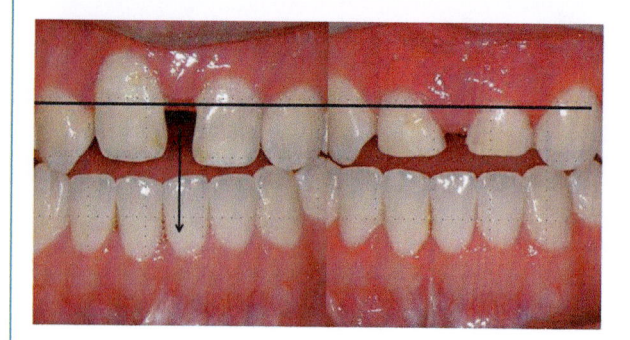

Figure 20.38 Before and after distraction.

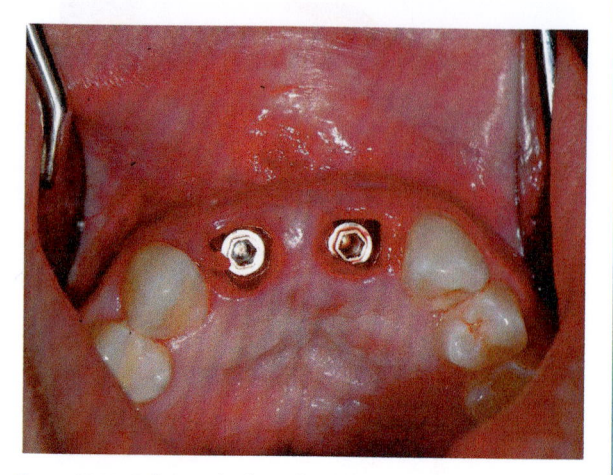

Figure 20.39 Soft tissue healing after distractor removal. Removal of teeth and immediate placement of implants.

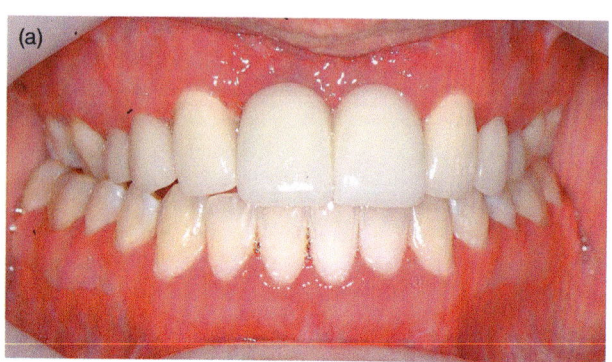

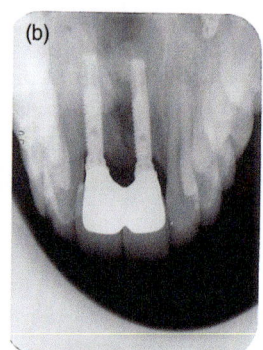

Figure 20.40 (a) Final restoration. (b) Final radiograph.

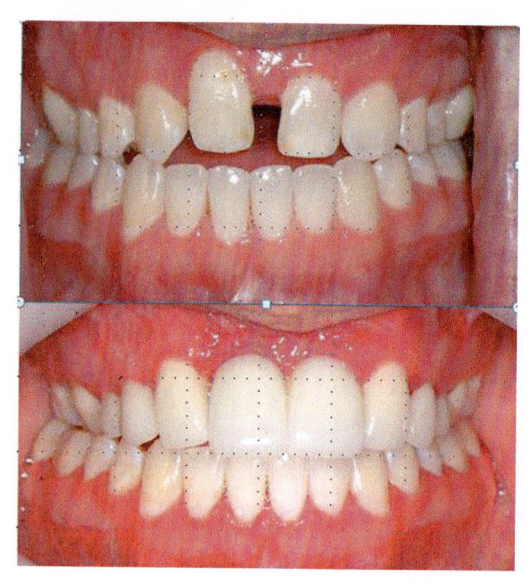

Figure 20.41 Before and after DO and the final restoration in place.

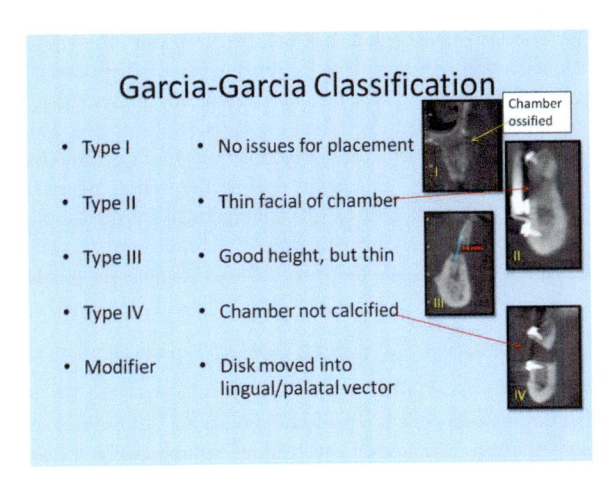

Figure 20.42 Garcia-Garcia classification of post-distraction defects.

Planning implant placement into distracted alveolar bone

Placing dental implants into the distracted bone has been proven to be predictable and just as reliable as into grafted bone [57]. However, to increase the predictability of placing implants and avoiding the potential complications of dehiscence of implants within the distracted bone Garcia-Garcia et al. [57] have suggested using a classification system of post-distraction defects (Figures 20.42 to 20.46). The system describes a classification of Type I for bone with no defect in the distraction chamber, Type II for having a good cortical rim with a small concavity on the facial, Type III for a narrow rim and lateral bone concavity, and Type IV for having a bone bridge with no bone in the distraction chamber site. A subcategory D was used as a modifier when the transport disk had become displaced lingually or palatally.

Type I shaped bone has no issues for implant placement (Figure 20.43). Type II shape has a good superior ridge but there is a thin

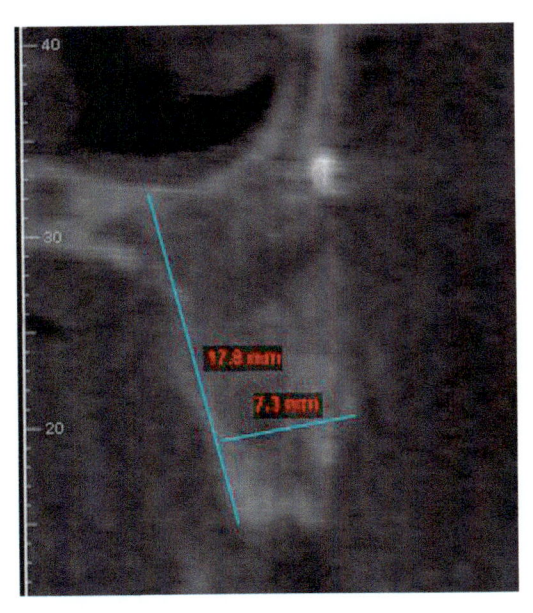

Figure 20.43 Type I distracted bone with no defect in the distraction chamber.

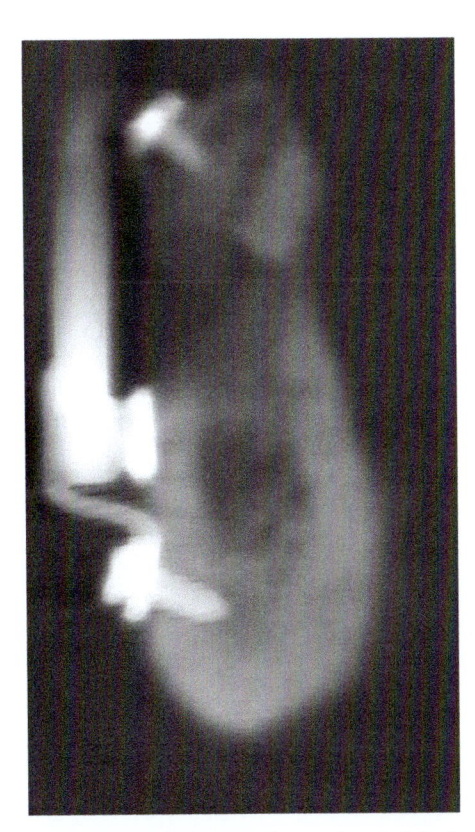

Figure 20.44 Type II distracted bone with a good cortical rim but small concavity on the facial (thin facial bone).

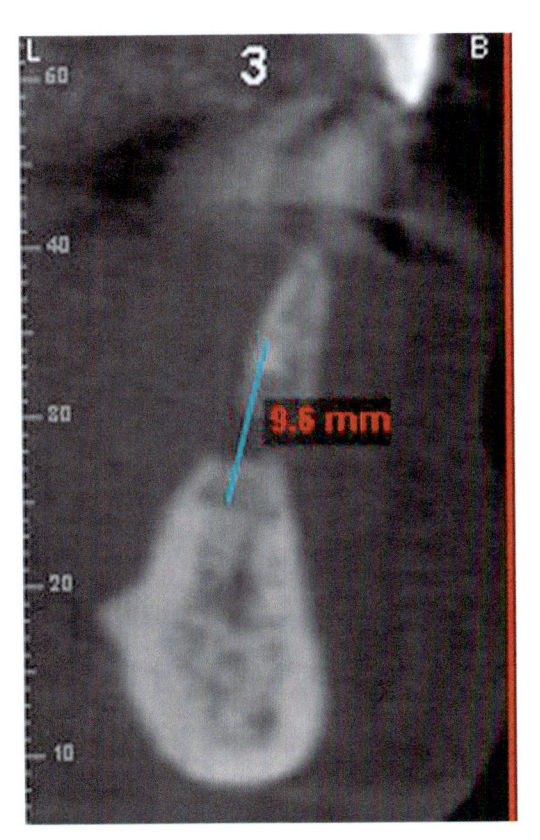

Figure 20.45 Type III distracted bone has a narrow rim and lateral bone concavity.

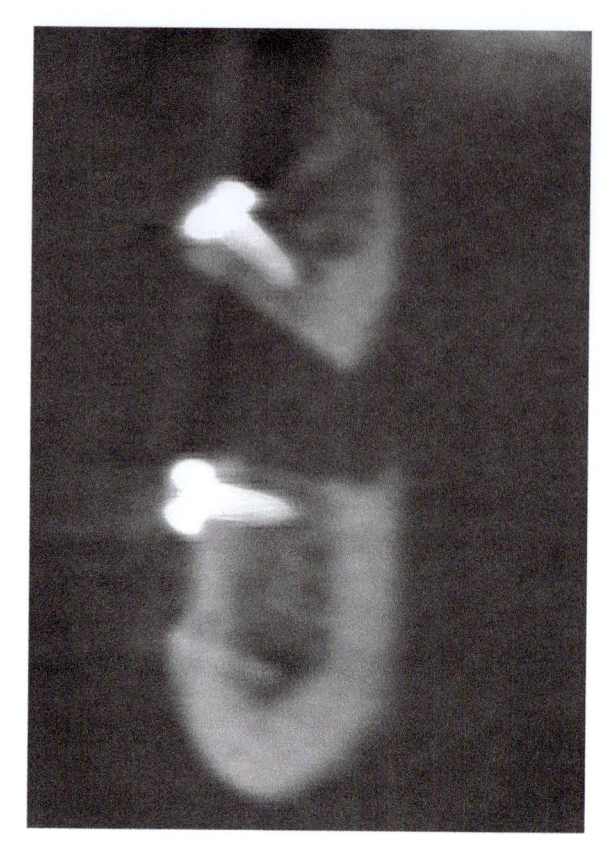

Figure 20.46 Type IV distracted bone with a bone bridge with no bone in the distraction chamber site (bone has not yet been fully ossified).

area on the facial aspect of the chamber (Figure 20.44). When implants are placed into this type of bone, the middle threads on the facial site may become exposed. This can be resolved with bone grafting and membrane placement at the time of implant placement. Good implant stability should be achieved initially. If this is not the case, then it is important to graft the chamber and come back secondarily to place implants. One will typically see these deformities on a CT scan during implant planning. This can be addressed at the time of distractor removal.

Type III shape is more difficult to place implants into (Figure 20.45). The bone has adequate vertical height, but the ridge is thin. We typically see this when a thin piece of bone is used as the transport disk. Again, it is important to remember, "You get what you distract." The horizontal cut has to be in wide enough bone to rise up to create an adequate alveolar ridge for implant stability. In these cases, onlay grafting, either particulate or block grafting, may be used to widen the site. Then implants can be placed after these grafts are integrated to the natural bone.

Type IV is a fascinating type of defect, where the bone is adequate at the crest but the chamber has not ossified (Figure 20.46). One wonders if the timing of consolidation here was the issue in the report (waiting period was only 12 weeks). The chamber could take almost 6 months to completely calcify, depending on the height of the distraction chamber created. Nonetheless, if the chamber is filled with fibrous tissue, it will need to be removed and the site grafted to enable implant placement. The decision to place implants simultaneously in these cases should be based on having a large wide amount of bone superiorly to stabilize the fixture and not run the risk of devascularization and subsequent bone loss.

The modifier of the lingual position of the transport disk has been mentioned under vector control. However, when this happens, if the ridge is in the wrong position, a new osteotomy may need to be created to align this segment. Then implants can be placed. This is only necessary if implants cannot be positioned in a prosthetically rehabilitative position. If caught during the actual distraction process, the distractor arm can be manipulated by repositioning the footplate or controlled with skeletal screws or extra skeletal means, like a splint or orthodontic appliances, to move the segment.

Conclusions on planning DO for dental implants

Distraction osteogenesis is a powerful tool to have in the surgeon's armamentarium. If indicated and planned appropriately, the technique will enable patients, who otherwise could not have implant restorations, a chance of good function, comfort, and esthetics. Though this technique is time consuming, once executed properly the patient's satisfaction is high.

References

1. Ilizarov GA, Ledyasev VI, Shitin VP: Experimental studies of bone lengthening. *Eksp Khir Aestheziol* 1969;**14**:3.
2. Snyder CC, Levine GA, Swanson HM, Browne E Jr: Mandibular lengthening by gradual distraction. Preliminary report. *Plast Reconstr Surg* 1973;**51**:506–508.
3. McCarthy JG, Schreiber J, Karp N, Thorne CH, Grayson BH: Lengthening the human mandible by gradual distraction. *Plast Reconstr Surg* 1992;**89**:1–8.
4. Block MS, Chang A, Crawford C: Mandibular alveolar ridge augmentation in the dog using distraction osteogenesis. *J Oral Maxillofac Surg* 1996 Mar;**54**(3):309–314.
5. Herford AS: Distraction osteogenesis: a surgical option for restoring missing tissue in the anterior esthetic zone. *J Calif Dent Assoc* 2005 Nov;**33**(11):889–895.
6. Walker DA: Mandibular distraction osteogenesis for endosseous dental implants. *J Can Dent Assoc* 2005 Mar;**71**(3):171–175.
7. Vega LG, Bilao A: Alveolar distraction osteogenesis for dental implant preparation: an update. *Oral Maxillofac Surg Clin North Am* 2010 Aug;**22**(3); 369–385.
8. Esposito M, Grusovin MG, Felice P, Karatzopoulos G, Worthington HV, Coulthard P: The efficacy of horizontal and vertical bone augmentation procedures for dental implants – a Cochrane systematic review. *Eur J Oral Implantol* 2009 Aug;**2**(3):167–184.
9. Elo JA, Herford AS, Boyne PJ: Implant success in distracted bone versus autogenous bone –grafted sites. *J Oral Implantol* 2009;**35**(4):181–184.
10. Saulacic N, Lizuka T, Martin MS, Garcia AG: Alveolar distraction osteogenesis: a systematic review. *Int J Oral Maxillofac Surg* 2008 Jan;**37**(1):1–7.
11. Kim JW, Cho MH, Kim SJ, Kim MR: Alveolar distraction osteogenesis versus autogenous onlay bone graft for vertical augmentation of severely atrophied alveolar ridges after 12 years of long-term follow up. *Oral Surg Oral Med Oral Pathol Oral Radiol* 2013 Nov: **116**(5):540–549.
12. Zwetyenga N, Vidal N, Ella B, Siberchiot F, Emparanza A: Results of oral implant-supported prosthesis after mandibular vertical alveolar ridge distraction: a propos of 54 sites. *Oral surg Oral Med Oral Pathol Oral Radiol* 2012 Dec;**114**(6):725–732.
13. Ergun G, Nagas IC, Pilmaxz D, Oztruk M: Prosthetic rehabilitation of edentulous ridges following alveolar distraction osteogenesis: clinical report of three cases. *J Oral Implantol* 2011 Mar4;**37**(Spec No): 183–191.
14. Gonzalez-Garcia A, Diniz-Freitas M, Somoza-Martin M, Garcia-Garcia A: Piezoelectric bone surgery applied. I. Alveolar distraction osteogenesis: a technical note. *Int J Oral Maxillofac Implants* 2007 Nov–Dec;**22**(6):1012–1016.
15. Lee HJ, Ahn MR, Sohn DS: Piezoelectric distraction osteogenesis in the atrophic maxillary anterior area: a case report. *Implant Dent* 2007 Sep;**16**(3):227–234.
16. Gonzalez-Garcia A, Diniz-Freitas M, Sooza-Martin M, Garcia-Garcia A: Piezoelectric and conventional osteotomy in alveolar distraction osteogenesis in a series of 17 patients. *Int J Oral Maxillofac Implants* 2008 Sep–Oct;**23**(5):891–896.
17. Marchetti C, Corinaldesi G, Pieri F, Degidi M, Piattelli A: Alveolar distraction osteogenesis for bone augmentation of severely atrophic ridges in 10 consecutive cases: a histologic and histomorphometric study. *J Periodontol* 2007 Feb;**78**(2):360–366.
18. Amir LR, Becking AG, Jovanovic A, Perdijk FB, Everts V, Bronckers AL: Vertical distraction osteogenesis in the human mandible: a prospective morphometric study. *Clin Oral Implants Res* 2006 Aug;**17**(4):417–425.

19 Sezer B, Koyuncu BO, Gunbay T, Sezak M: Alveolar distraction osteogenesis in the human mandible: a clinical and histomorphometric study. *Implant Dent* 2012 Aug;21(4):317–322.

20 Amir LR, Becking AG, Jovaovic A, Perdijk FB, Everts B, Bronckers AL: Formation of new bone during vertical distraction osteogenesis of the human mandible is related to the presence of blood vessels. *Clin Oral Implants Res* 2006 Aug;17(4):410–416.

21 Chiapasco M, Lang NP, Bosshardt DD: Quality and quantity of bone following alveolar distraction osteogenesis in the human mandible. *Clin Oral Implants Res* 2006 Aug;17(4):394–402.

22 Spencer AC, Campbell PM, Dechow P, Ellis ML, Buschang PH: How does the rate of dentoalveolar distraction affect the bone regenerate produced? *Am J Orthod Dentofacial Orthop* 2011 Nov;140(5):e211–221.

23 Veziroglu F, Yilmaz D: Biomechanical evaluation of the consolidation period of alveolar distraction osteogenesis with three-dimensional finite element analysis. *Int J Oral Maxillofac Surg* 2008 May;37(5):448–452.

24 Cano J, Campo J, Gonzalo JC, Bascones A: Consolidation period in alveolar distraction: a pilot histomorphometric study in the mandible of the beagle dog. *Int J Oral Maxillofac Implants* 2006 May–Jun;21(3):380–391.

25 Faysal U, Cem SB, Atilla S: Effects of different consolidation periods on bone formation and implant success in alveolar distraction osteogenesis: a clinical study. *J Craniomaxillofac Surg* 2013 Apr;41(3):194–197.

26 Iida S, Nakano T, Amano K, Kogo M: Repeated distraction osteogenesis for excessive vertical alveolar augmentation: a case report. *Int J Oral Maxillofac Implants* 2006 May–Jun;21(3):471–475.

27 Kocyigit ID, Tuz HH, Atil F, Tekin U, Coskunses FM: Correction of postsurgical alveolar ridge defect with vertical alveolar distraction of the onlay block graft *J Cranofac Surg* 2012 Sep;23(5):1550–1552.

28 Pektaas ZO, Kircellli BH, Bayram B, Kircelli C, Uckan S: Alveolar cleft closure by distraction osteogenesis with skeletal anchorage during consolidation. *Int J Oral Maxillofac Implants* 2007;22(Suppl): 49–70.

29 Rachmiel A, Emodi O, Gutmacher Z, Blumenfeld I, Aizenbut D: Oral and dental restoration of wide alveolar cleft using distraction osteogenesis and temporary anchorage devices. *J Craniomaxillofac Surg* 2013 Jul: 42(7):897–900.

30 Rachmiel A, Emodi O, Aizenbud D. Three-dimensional reconstruction of large secondary alveolar cleft by two-stage distraction. *Cleft Palate Craniofac J* 2014 Jan;51(1):36–42.

31 Fujioka M, Kanno T, Mitsugi M, Sukegawa S, Furuki Y: Oral rehabilitation of a maxillectomy defect using bone transport distraction and dental implants. *J Oral Maxillofac Surg* 2010 Sep;68(9):2278–2282.

32 Kunkel M, Wahlmann U, Teichert TE, Wegener J, Wagner W: Reconstruction of mandibular defect following tumor ablation by vertical distraction osteogenesis using intraosseous distraction devices. *Clin Oral Implants Res* 2005 Feb;16(1):89–97.

33 Natashekar M, Chowdhary R, Chandraker NK. Rehabilitation of recurrent unicystic ameloblastoma using distraction osteogenesis and dental implants. *Niger J Clin Pract* 2011 Oct–Dec;14(4):486–491.

34 Kongshei A, Banerjee S, Gupta T, Banerjee A: Implant supported prosthesis after ridge augmentation procedure by distraction osteogenesis for atrophic mandible. *J Indian Prosthodont Soc* 2013 Dec;13(4):617–620.

35 Marianetti TM, Leuzzi F, Foresta E, Gasparini G, Cervelli D, Amoroso PF, Pelo S: Vertical distraction osteoenesis combined with bilateral 2-step osteotomy for preprosthetic rehabilitation of edentulous mandible. *J Craniofac Surg* 2013 Jul;24(4):1175–1178.

36 Felice P, Lizio G, Checchi L: Alveolar distraction osteogenesis in posterior atrophic mandible: a case report on a new technical approach. *Implant Dent* 2013 Aug;22(4):332–338.

37 Perez-Sayans M, Leon-Camacho Mde L, Somoza-Martin JM, Fernendez-Gonzalez B, Bianes-Vazques-Gundin S, Gandara-Rey JM, Garcia-Garcia A: Dental implants placed on bone subjected to vertical alveolar distraction show the same performance as those placed on primitive bone. *Med Oral Patol Oral Cir Bucal* 2013 Jul 1;18(4):686–692.

38 Mampilly MO, Rao LP, Sequiera J, Rao BH, Chandra J, Rai G: Rehabilitation of edentulous atropic anterior mandible – the role of vertical alveolar distraction osteogenesis. *J Clin Diagn Res* 2014 Nov;8(11):ZR01–ZR03.

39 Seniski NE, Kocer G, Kaya BU: Ankylosed maxillary incisor with severe root resorption treated with single-tooth dento-osseous osteotomy, vertical alveolar distraction oteogenesis and mini-implant anchorage. *Am J Orthod Dentofacial Orthop* 2014 Sep: 146(3):371–384.

40 Agabiti IC, Cappare P, Gherlone EF, Mortellaro C, Bruschi GB, Crepsi R: New surgical technique and distraction osteogenesis for ankylosed dental movement. *J Craniofac Surg* 2014 May;25(3):828–830.

41 Fong JH, Lui MT, Wu JH, Chou IC, Yeung TC, Kao SY: Using distraction osteogenesis for repositioning the multiple dental implants – retained premaxilla with autogenous bone graft and keratinized palatal mucosa graft vestibuloplasty in a trauma patient: report of a case. *J Oral Maxillofac Surg* 2006 May;64(5):794–798.

42 Marcantonio E, Dela Coleta R, Spin-Neto R, Marcantonio E Jr, Dela Coleta Pizzol KE, Boeck EM: Use of a tooth-implant supported bone distractor in oral rehabilitation: a description of a personalized technique. *J Oral Maxillofac Surg* 2008 Nov;66(11); 2339–2344.

43 Oduncuoglu BF, Alaaddinoglu EE, Oguz Y, Uckan S, Erkut S: Repositioning a prosthetically unfavorable implant by vertical distraction soteodenesis. *J Oral Maxillofac Surg* 2011 Jun;69(6):1628–1632.

44 Lautner N, McCoy M, Gaggl A, Krenkel C: Intramandibular course of the mandibular nerve; clinical significance for distraction and implantology. *Rev Stomatol Chir Maxillofac* 2012 Jun;113(3):161–168.

45 Kim DH, Park MS, Won SY, Hu KS, Han DH, Kim HJ: Alveolar regions of the mandible for the installation of immediate-implant fixtures and bone screws of alveolar distractors. *J Cranioac Surg* 2011 May;22(3):1056–1060.

46 Gaggl A, Schultes G, Santler G, Karcher H: Three-dimensional planning of alveolar ridge distraction by means of distraction implants. *Comp Aided Surg* 2000;5(1):35–41.

47 Poukens J, Haex J, Tiediger D: the use of rapid prototyping in the preoperative planning of distraction osteogenesis of the craniomaxillofacial skeleton. *Comput Aided Surg* 2003;8(3):146–154.

48 Kanno T, Mitsugi M, Sukegawa S, Hosoe M, Furuki Y: Computer-simulated bi-directional alveolar distraction osteogenesis. *Clin Oral Implants Res* 2008 Dec;19(12):1211–1218.

49 Kocyigit ID, Tuz HH, Ozqul O, Coskumses FM, Kisnisci RS: A simple solution for vector control in vertical alveolar distraction osteogenesis. *J Oral Implantol* 2014 Oct;40(5):557–560.

50 Kawashima W, Takayama K, Fujii R, Matsubara Y, Kirita T: Vector-controlled alveolar distraction osteogenesis using an implant-fixed provisional prosthesis: a case report. *Implant Dent* 2013 Feb;22(1):26–30.

51 Oh HK, Park HJ, Cho JY, Park YJ, Kook MS: Vector control of malpositioned segment during alveolar distraction osteogenesis by using rubber traction. *J Oral Maxillofac Surg* 2009 Mar;67(3):60.

52 Uckan S, Oguz Y, Bayram B: Comparison of intraosseous and extraosseous alveolar distraction osteogenesis. *J Oral Maxillofac Surg* 2007 Apr;65(4):671–674.

53 Perdjik FB, Jeijer GJ, van Strijen PJ, Kooke R: Effect of extraosseous devices designed for vertical distraction of extremely resorbed mandibles on backward rotation of upper bone segments. *Br J Oral Maxillofac Surg* 2009 Jan;47(1):31–36.

54 Perez-Sayans M, Martins-Horta D, Somoza-Martin M, Fernandez-Gonzales B, Reboioras-Lopez D, Vila PG, Garcia-Garcia A: Clinical study comparing alveolar distraction using the lead system and MODUS MDO 1.5/2.0. *J Craniofac Surg* 2014 Nov;25(6):584–588.

55 Robiony M, Toro C, Stucki-McCormick SU, Zerman N, Costa F, Politi M: The"FAD"(floating alveolar device): a bidirectional distraction system for distraction osteogenesis of the alveolar process. *J Oral Maxillofac Surg* 2004 Spring;62(9 Suppl 2):136–142.

56 Kannno T, Mitsugi M, Firuki Y, Hosoe M, Akamatsu, H, Takenobu T: Over-correction in vertical alveolar distraction osteogenesis for dental implants. *Int J Oral Maxillofac Surg* 2007 May;36(5):398–402.

57 Garcia-Garcia A, Somoza Martin M, Gadara Vila P, Gandara Rey JM: A preliminary morphologic classification of the alveolar ridge after distraction osteogenesis. *J Oral Maxillofac Surg* 2004 May;62(5):563–566.

CHAPTER 21

Alveolar Distraction Osteogenesis for Vertical Ridge Augmentation: Surgical Principles and Technique

Shravan Renapurkar[1] and Maria J. Troulis[2]

[1]Department of Oral and Maxillofacial Surgery, Virginia Commonwealth University, Richmond, VA, USA
[2]Department of Oral and Maxillofacial Surgery, Massachusetts General Hospital, Walter C. Guralnick Professor and Chair of Oral and Maxillofacial Surgery, Harvard School of Dental Medicine, Boston, MA, USA

Introduction

Distraction osteogenesis (DO) was first described by Codivilla in 1905 [1] and later popularized via the extensive research performed by Ilizarov in orthopedic literature [2, 3]. Craniofacial DO was first done by Snyder [4] in 1973 in a canine model and later reported in humans by Guerrero [5] (1990), McCarthy et al. [6] (1992), Kaban et al. [7] (1993). There are diverse indications for application of DO in the craniofacial skeleton today including augmentation of alveolar bone for various pre-prosthetic indications. Alveolar distraction was initially reported via animal studies conducted by Block et al. [8] and later described via a clinical report by Chin et al. [9] in 1996. Several retrospective and prospective human studies over the years have proved the efficacy and established biological feasibility of alveolar distraction osteogenesis [10–19].

Surgical rationale of alveolar DO

Loss of bone and associated soft tissue secondary to loss of teeth from periodontal disease, caries, and trauma make prosthetic rehabilitation challenging. The most challenging dentoalveolar defects are composite defects that lack both hard and soft tissue, often due to trauma and failed previously placed bone grafts. Preservation and reconstruction of alveolar bone in the vertical and horizontal dimensions is one of the critical steps in dental implant placement for functional prosthetic restoration.

Current techniques to augment the deficient alveolar ridge include autogenous block bone grafts (ABGs), guided bone regeneration (GBR) using particulate grafts, osteotomy and immediate correction of defects, alveolar distraction osteogenesis (ADO), and vascularized free flap reconstruction. Autogenous bone grafts not only involve donor site morbidity and associated risks but are also known to show variable resorption over time [15,20–22]. Chiapasco et al. [10–12] in their prospective studies comparing the outcomes in alveolar ridge augmentation methods between ADO and ABG found that prior to implant placement the ABG group showed more resorption of bone compared to the ADO group although the final implant success rates were comparable in between the two groups. In another subsequent study comparing ADO and GBR it was found that ADO offers more predictable bone gain maintenance over the long term when compared to GBR [10]. Guided bone regeneration has been largely successful for smaller bony defects [10, 20]. In severely atrophic alveolar ridges, bone grafts and osteotomies have the limitation of not being able to enhance and in fact being limited by lack of adequate soft tissue coverage. Lack of adequate soft tissue coverage not only prevents primary wound closure at the time of augmentation but also compromises the final outcome after implant restoration. ADO has the distinct advantage of being able to improve both the availability of bone as well as the associated soft tissue.

Biological rationale of alveolar DO

As in long bones and craniofacial skeleton, DO in the alveolar bone is based on the tension–stress principle, which involves gradual traction between two vital surfaces of bone after an osteotomy. The biology of DO has been elaborately studied by several investigators in orthopedics, beginning with Ilizarov in 1988 [2, 3]. The biology of craniofacial DO has been studied using a Yucatan minipig model at the Skeletal Biology Research Center, Massachusetts General Hospital, Boston, MA [23–28].

The biology specific to ADO was described by Block et al. in animals utilizing both extraosseous and intraosseous devices [8]. Their study concluded that bone and soft tissue formed from ADO was histologically similar to normal tissue. The distracted bone level was able to be maintained around implants placed subsequently over a period of 1 year. Gaggl et al. described the correlation of clinical, radiographic, and histologic findings in sheep using distraction implants. They found that radiopacity in the DO site appeared at the end of a 1-month post-distraction and increased up to 6 months when the regenerate appeared homogenously radiopaque. Six months after distraction, good osseous integration was noted with an implant bone surface area of about 70% [29].

Human studies on alveolar bone distraction have proved it to be a reliable technique for the correction of vertically deficient edentulous ridges [10–19]. The newly formed bone withstood the functional demands of implant loading. The survival and success rates of dental implants placed in the distracted areas have been shown to be consistent with those of implants placed in native bone [10, 30]. Amir et al. found a positive correlation between blood vessel density and bone volume density in newly formed bone after vertical mandibular distraction, which supports the concept that vascularity is necessary for the formation of new bone [31]. Lindeboom and

Vertical Alveolar Ridge Augmentation in Implant Dentistry: A Surgical Manual, First Edition. Edited by Len Tolstunov.
© 2016 John Wiley & Sons, Inc. Published 2016 by John Wiley & Sons, Inc.

colleagues studied microvascular changes in capillary density in alveolar distraction sites from post-operative day 1 until the end of consolidation. This study showed that the major increase in vascularity was during the activation phase and that the vessel density during consolidation was comparable with pre-operative levels [32]. Chiapasco and colleagues in their prospective study on human ADO showed that after 12 weeks into healing the newly formed bone consisted of woven bone reinforced by parallel-fibered bone with bone marrow spaces between the trabeculae. In the same study the bone area fraction in the alveolar distraction region ranged from 21.6 to 57.8% [33].

Indications and contraindications

Alveolar augmentation for placement of dental implants is one of the most common indications. ADO has been shown to be effective in treating moderate to severe maxillary and mandibular alveolar ridge atrophy, mostly in the anterior region [10,11,18,30]. ADO has been mostly used for correcting *vertical* alveolar ridge defects but can be used for increasing the width as well [34–36]. A traditional ADO distractor can to some degree simultaneously correct an alveolar bone horizontally due to often observed pyramidally shaped (widening to its base, like an iceberg) morphology of the alveolar bone. If an alveolar transport bone segment is very narrow at the top, by quickly widening to its base (like a pinnacle) during vertical distraction and vertical bone repositioning, this transport bone segment moves occlusally, widening the alveolar ridge. This might bring enough or not bone stock for future implant placement.

Reports have been published for use of ADO in segmental defects reconstructed with a free fibula flap to further augment the fibula vertically [37]. The biggest benefit of ADO is its ability to increase soft tissue as well as bone.

ADO is contraindicated in cases where the bone loss is so severe that the device cannot be placed or if the transport segment is not at least 5 mm in size. Lack of a safe distance in bone between vital structures like the inferior alveolar nerve/maxillary sinus/nasal floor prevents successful application of the device and affects the outcome of ADO. Patients unable to follow the distractor activation protocol should not be considered.

Surgical principles and treatment planning for lveolar DO

Planning for ADO begins with an evaluation of the form of residual alveolus. The amount of bone and soft tissue available and required for obtaining the restorative and surgical goals should be determined. Mounted dental models of the patient with a wax-up of the missing teeth and alveolus will determine the goal of alveolar augmentation and help determine the type of distractor.

Jensen and Block presented an alveolar site classification system that could be applied in making treatment decisions: Class I – mild alveolar deficiency with up to 5 mm of vertical bone loss; Class II – moderate deficiency with 6–10 mm of vertical bone loss; Class III – severe deficiency with greater than 10 mm of vertical bone loss; Class IV – severe bone loss at the edentulous alveolar ridge as well as significant bone loss on adjacent teeth [19].

Class I defects are smaller and treated with traditional sandwich osteotomy or with conventional bone grafting techniques. Class II defects are the ones that are more amenable to be reconstructed with ADO. Treatment of Class III defects depends on the availability of bone stock in the defect. If there is enough bone, distraction can be performed but may have to be supplemented by bone grafts later or else will need bone grafting first with secondary ADO. Class IV defects are complicated by adjacent teeth that have a poor prognosis. These teeth can be extracted to convert the defect into a Class III type defect and continue treatment as above.

Maxillary anterior defects command the greatest attention as they fall into the esthetic zone and require adequate soft tissue. Maxillary posterior defects can be difficult to address with ADO depending on the proximity of the sinus. Posterior mandibular defects can be treated with ADO but one needs to consider the position of the inferior alveolar nerve, size and width of the transport segment, and the interocclusal clearance. A minimum of 5 mm of bone superior to IAN is needed [15, 38]. Interdental defects can be managed with intraosseous distractors but larger defects and posterior edentulous defects will require an extraosseous distractor. Combined defects may need a combination of bone grafts and ADO. Completely edentulous posterior ridge distraction involves a difference in the osteotomy design, which is in the form of an "L" that will allow differential distraction in the anterior and posterior parts of the transport segment [13]. Horizontal alveolar distraction both in the maxilla or mandible has not been as widely studied as vertical ADO. Only a few case reports exist [34–36].

Phases of alveolar DO

Surgery (phase 1)

Special consideration should be given to the incision placement as it could not only affect the blood supply to the transport segment but also will determine the type of soft tissue regenerated during distraction. The incision should be placed such that the flap has a broad base preserving the periosteum on the transport segment. Preferably, the incision is placed in the attached gingiva and away from the osteotomy. Vertical incisions should not coincide with the vertical osteotomies as this could lead to periodontal defects. The position of the osteotomy should be based on an adequately sized transport segment as well as adequate basal bone and avoiding injury to adjacent structures (Figure 21.1).

Latency (phase 2)

Varying periods of latency have been studied in ADO that ranged from immediate distraction to as far as 14 days of latency in cases where there was a question about the integrity of the soft tissue pedicle. A 7-day latency period in ADO allows gingival/mucosal healing. In a review by Saulacic et al. [14] it was shown that a 7-day latency period showed good quality of bone.

Distraction (phase 3)

The amount of alveolar distraction is determined by the amount of bone and soft tissue augmentation needed for implant placement and prosthetic rehabilitation. The ideal rate of distraction is a balance between risks of premature fusion from too slow a rate against the non-union from too fast a rate. Conventionally agreed upon, a rate of 1 mm/day is based upon animal and clinical experiments in long bones and craniofacial skeleton [2,3,8,11,29], but in ADO 0.5 mm/day is considered a standard rate. Amir et al. [31] found that in elderly patients with severely atrophic mandibles undergoing vertical distraction osteogenesis, decreasing the standard distraction rate of 1 mm/day down to 0.5 mm/day may

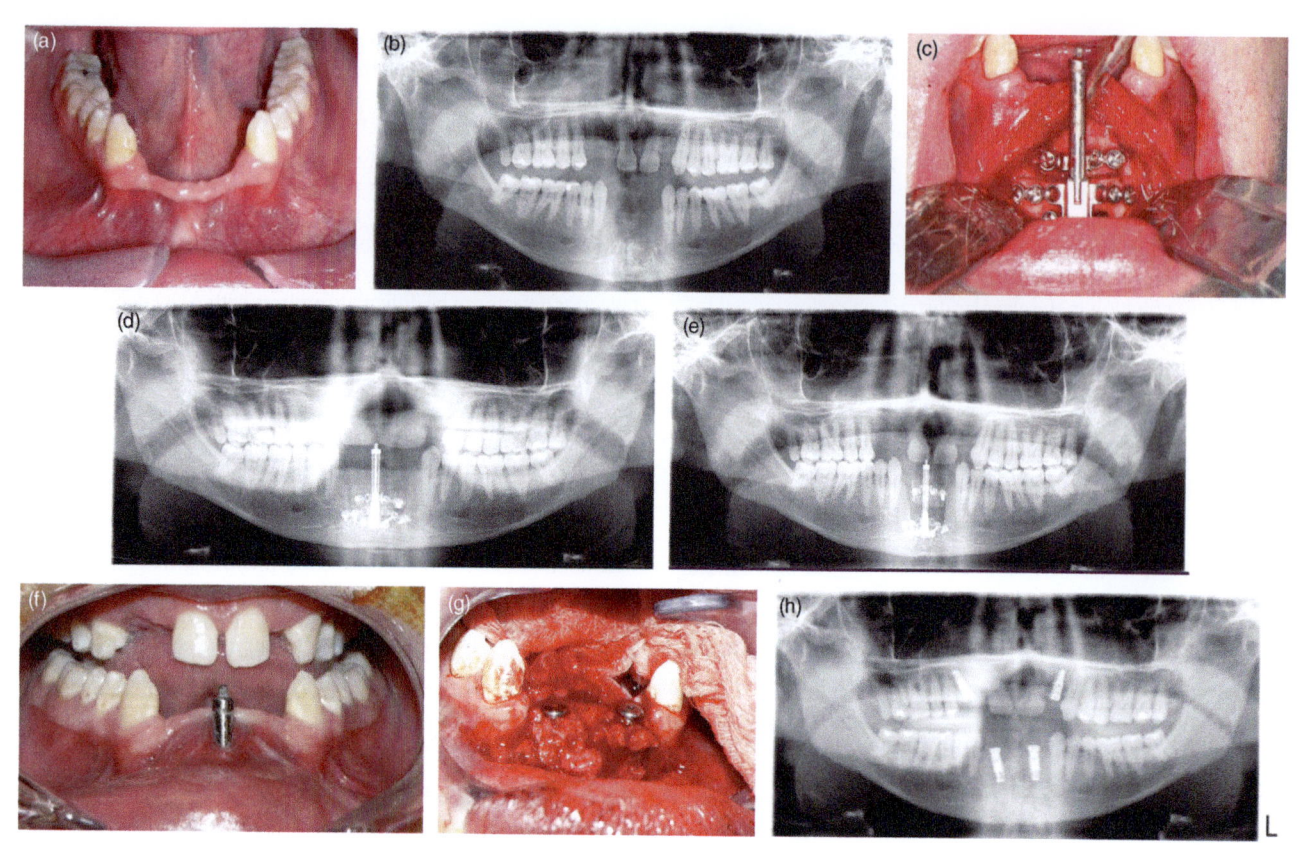

Figure 21.1 A 29-year-old man with h/o trauma resulting in teeth and bone loss in the mandibular anterior alveolus planned for implant reconstruction. F(a) Clinical evaluation reveals deficient bone both in the vertical and horizontal dimensions in the edentulous ridge between mandibular canines. The patient was planned to undergo an alveolar distraction osteogenesis (ADO) for augmentation of the bone prior to implant placement. (b) A panoramic radiograph with deficiency in the anterior mandibular alveolus. (c) Extraosseous alveolar distractor was placed via a labial vestibular incision. Distractor adapted to the osteotomy site first. Osteotomy was then completed with lingual and apical convergence. (d, e) Distraction started at a rate of 1 mm/day after a latency period of 2 days. Total distraction was calculated to be 13 mm. (f) Consolidation period was for 3 months prior to removal of the distractor and placement of endosseous dental implants. (g, h) Dental implants placed in the edentulous ridge after removal of the distractor. "Fig. 21.1a, 21.1c, 21.1f, 21.1g, Permission to publish was obtained from Haggerty CJ, Block MS: Alveolar distraction osteogenesis. In: *Minimally Invasive Maxillofacial Surgery*. PMPH-USA, 2013, pp. 177–188 [30]."

be beneficial for bone growth as histologic evaluation revealed higher blood vessel volume in the bone distracted at the rate of 0.5 mm/day, which in turn showed higher bone density.

Consolidation (phase 4)

There has been no single universal protocol for the duration of consolidation. Block et al. animal studies suggested an 8-week consolidation period [8]. Amir et al.'s experiment revealed that 10 weeks of consolidation is required for new bone to bridge a 10 mm distraction gap [31]. Chiapasco et al. [33] reported that 3 months following mandibular distraction the regenerate demonstrated woven bone reinforced by parallel-fiber bone undergoing maturation. Raghoebar and colleagues [39] showed that bone biopsies taken 2 months after distraction revealed more connective tissue in the fibrous interzone. Radiographic examination at the end of 8 weeks would be strongly recommended prior to removal of the distractor. For patient comfort, the distractor can be removed early and implants placed so as to engage the native bone stock.

Advantages and disadvantages of ADO

When compared to conventional alveolar augmentation techniques, ADO has several advantages. ADO avoids donor site morbidity and surgical risks associated with autogenous bone graft harvest. Simultaneous distraction of bone and soft tissues in ADO decreases or eliminates the need for soft tissue grafting in contrast to other bone augmentation techniques. The distraction device is maintained and activated by patients themselves at home. Disadvantages include the additional cost of the device, patient compliance, and difficulty in controlling the vector of distraction.

Alveolar DO devices

ADO devices are of two basic types:

1 Extraosseous distractors (e.g., alveolar ridge distractor; Synthes®, distractor track; KLS/Martin®, Tuttlingen, Germany) (Figure 21.2). These devices are placed subperiosteally on the lateral surface of the bone and anchored to the bone via small plates, which are connected to a rod with an internal screw. This screw when activated creates distraction by moving the plates apart. Extraosseous devices are used in severe alveolar defects and can provide both vertical and horizontal vectors depending on the placement technique, although there is not a great amount of horizontal augmentation achieved. Extraosseous devices are easier to place, as the plates are flexible to be adapted over the remaining bone. The plates can be contoured to control the vector of distraction. The distraction rod of the device extends through the mucosa into the oral cavity.

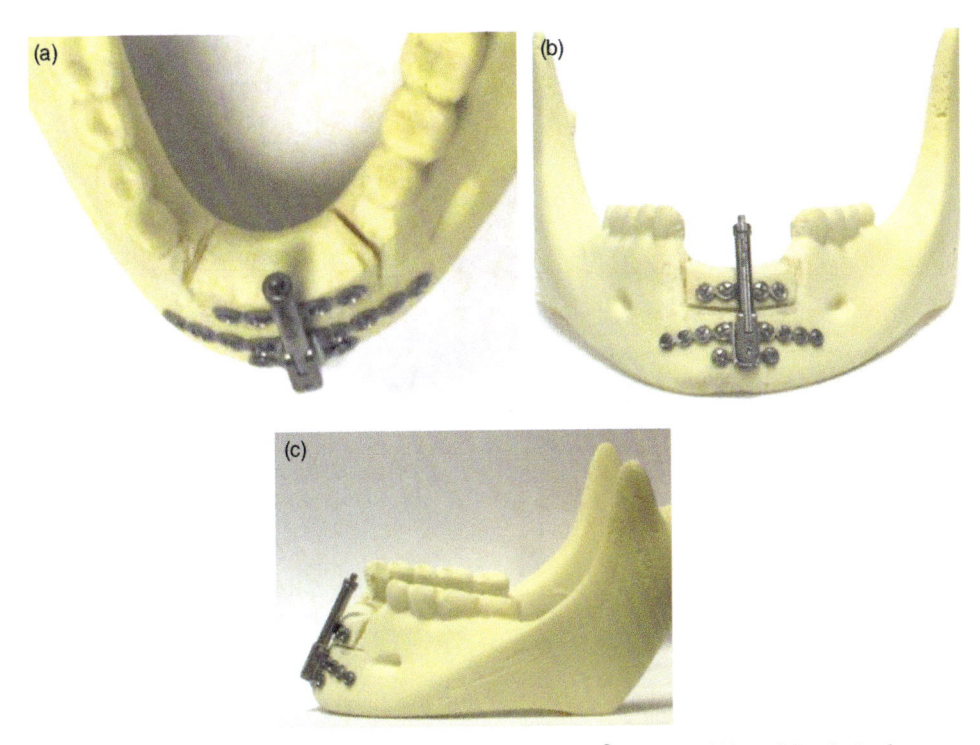

Figure 21.2 Placement of an extraosseous alveolar distractor (Synthes alveolar distractor ®) on a mandible model to depict the osteotomy and orientation of the distractor. The osteotomy is made with lingual and apical convergence to avoid interference and also helps in distractor vector maintenance (**a**) Axial view shows the convergence of osteotomy in a lingual direction while (**b**) shows the convergence in the apical direction. (**c**) The plates on the distractor are adapted to the basal bone as well as the transport segment.

2 Intraosseous devices (eg, LEAD® System, Leibinger, Kalamazoo, MI; DIS-SIS distraction implant; SIS Systems Trade GmbH, Klagenfurt, Austria) (Figure 21.3). These devices are placed through the transport segment and fixed to the basal bone with a microplate. Distraction with a modified version of the dental implant, which distracts the bone and then continues to function as an implant, has also been reported [31]. Intraosseous distractors work best in smaller segments. The LEAD distractor system® has a threaded rod, a threaded transport plate, and an unthreaded stabilizing base plate. The threaded rod goes through the transport plate and segment via a channel drilled through the segment and connects to the stabilizing base plate. The threaded rod is rotated to obtain distraction.

Control of the vector

Vector control of the transport segment in ADO is critical. Achieving an adequate amount of new tissue in an appropriate position requires pre-operative planning. A surgical guide/temporary prosthesis, proper positioning, and adaptation of fixation plates in the extraosseous distractor, and the direction of the threaded rod in intraosseous distractors can help control the vector [40, 41]. Lingual tipping of the transport segment is common and can be prevented by a lingually convergent design of the osteotomy, using a lingual guiding splint or orthodontic arch wires. In edentulous patients temporary implants can be used as anchorage to guide the distraction. In cases where the lingual tipping has developed, repositioning of the transport segment can be done manually.

Implant placement

Implants are the treatment of choice for restoring function and reconstructing edentulous areas of the maxilla and mandible. The timing of implant placement in the distracted bone has been controversial. ADO facilitates earlier placement of dental implants compared to the bone grafting techniques. Various reports have quoted the waiting times to be anywhere between immediate to 12 weeks. Chiapasco et al. reported that 3 months following distraction woven bone reinforced by parallel-fibered bone undergoing maturation was noted [33]. In a prospective multicenter study, Chiapasco et al. reported success rate of 94.2% in 138 implants placed in distracted bone after 2–3 months of consolidation with a mean follow-up of 34 months [42]. Systematic review by Salucic et al. reviewed a total of 469 implants placed in distracted bone. Failed implants were reportedly placed in the ridges following a mean consolidation period of 8.10 ± 2.51 weeks, compared to 12.43 ± 5.62 weeks of consolidation for successful implants. This difference had statistical significance ($P = 0.01$). Stable peri-implant bone was retained in 95% of implants in the review [14].

Complications

The complication rates in ADO have been reported to be anywhere between 30 and 100% but the majority of them are reported to be minor [16, 17, 38, 43–52]. Thinning of the transport segment or the basal bone and excessive force during osteotomy make the transport segment or the mandible more vulnerable to fracture. If the fractured fragment of the transport segment is small in size it could be discarded and treatment continued as planned, but if it is significantly large it needs to be reduced and stabilized along with abortion of the planned procedure. This complication can be prevented by meticulous case selection with an adequate amount of available bone and appropriate execution of the osteotomy.

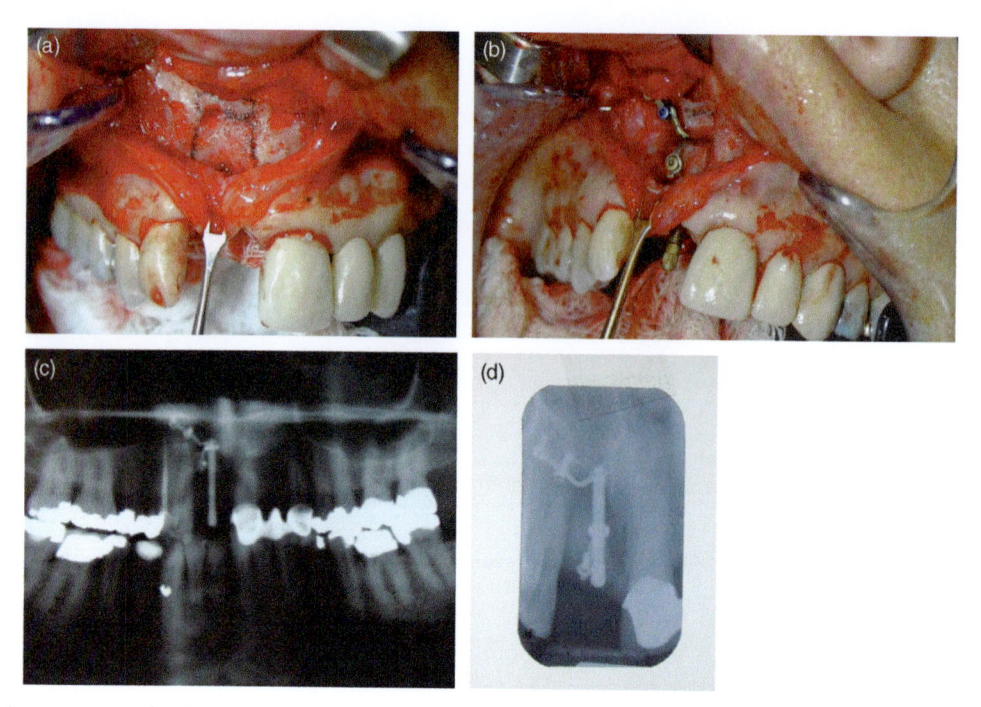

Figure 21.3 (**a,b**) An intraosseous alveolar distractor placed in the maxillary anterior alveolar ridge using a labial approach staying inferior to the nasal floor. An intraosseous distractor was used as the edentulous space was singe tooth. Notice the activation arm projecting through the crestal surface of the gingiva. (**c**) Radiographic change after placement of the distractor. (**d**) Periapical radiograph depicting the distracted transport segment with evidence of progressing bone fill in the osteotomy.

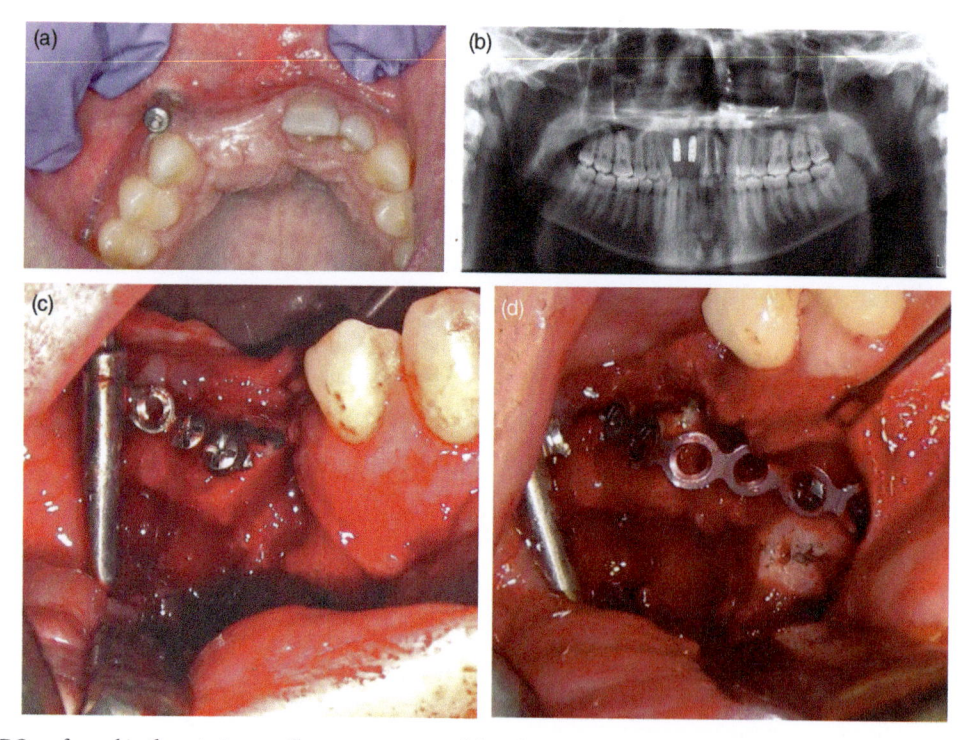

Figure 21.4 (**a**) ADO performed in the anterior maxillary post-traumatic defect shows palatal movement of the transport segment, which is a common challenge during the alveolar distraction. (**b**) In this particular case implants were able to be placed due to a minimal amount of palatal inclination in the alveolus. (**c and d**) Right posterior mandibular dentoalveolar defect treated with ADO using an extraosseous distractor. There was more distraction at the posterior osteotomy than the anterior along with mucosal dehiscence. Re-exploration of the area showed (**c**) a fractured anterior plate in the distractor. (**d**) The fractured part of the distractor was removed and the regenerate was molded along with fixation of the transport segment using plates and screws on the anterior osteotomy. Source: Haggerty CJ, Block MS: Alveolar distraction osteogenesis. In: *Minimally Invasive Maxillofacial Surgery*. PMPH-USA, 2013, pp. 177188 [30]. Reproduced with permission from PMPH-USA.

Avoiding sharp angles in the osteotomy is reported to reduce the incidence of fractures [38].

Excessive length of the threaded rod of the distractor can cause occlusal interference, discomfort to the patient, and limit distraction. This can be prevented by appropriate selection or modification of the length of the threaded rod by fitting and/or trimming with application on mounted dental models. Damage to adjacent soft and hard tissue structures occurs usually due to an improper technique or use of excessive force during osteotomy. Using an osteotome for completion of the lingual part of the osteotomy or using a piezoelectric saw blade may help reduce this complication.

Poor vector control/direction of distraction is mostly secondary to the pull from the palatal mucosa on the maxilla (Figure 21.4a and b) or the lingual musculature on the mandible. The frequency of this vector deviation towards palatal/lingual surfaces has been reported to be between 13 and 50% for extraosseous devices and between 19 and 50% of cases for intraosseous devices varying based on the study [48]. Dehiscence or perforation of the mucosa by the transport segment/distractor is secondary to poor soft tissue coverage over the osteotomy and sharp edges of bone or excessive tension at closure over the distractor. Reducing the rate of distraction and reduction of the sharp bony edges may be required. Distractor device failure can occur due to breakage and could occur secondary to incomplete osteotomy or corticotomy or metal fatigue from repeated bending (Figure 21.4c and d). A buccal bone surface defect or deficiency is one of the most common complications with ADO. This has been hypothesized to be secondary to stripping of the periosteum over the buccal surface and manipulation of bone or also due to poor vector control. Additional bone grafting may be done to manage the defect, if clinically indicated, for the prosthetically driven implant placement.

Conclusions

The ability to increase the amount of available soft tissue in addition to augmentation of bone is the distinctive benefit of ADO when compared to the conventional techniques of bone augmentation including bone grafts and osteotomies. Alveolar distraction osteogenesis is a technique-sensitive procedure involving proper case selection, meticulous treatment planning, and patient compliance. Animal and clinical research have established ADO as a very efficient tool for the surgeon in attaining alveolar augmentation. Patient compliance and attention to vector control during DO play critical roles in managing the outcomes. Although the overall complication rates in ADO patients has been reported to be higher in frequency in comparison to bone grafting, most of these were reported to be minor and easily manageable. The success rates of implants placed in distracted bone is equivalent to those placed in native bone. ADO continues to be under evolution as more human studies are needed to standardize its protocol in order to minimize the complications and improve outcomes.

References

1 Codivilla A: On the means of lengthening in the lower limbs, the muscles and tissues which are shortened through deformity. *Am J Orthop Surg* 1905;**2**:353–369.
2 Ilizarov GA: The tension stress effect on the genesis and growth of tissues. Part I. The influence of stability of fixation and soft tissue preservation. *Clin Orthop* 1989;**238**:249–281.
3 Ilizarov GA: The tension stress effect on the genesis and growth of tissues. Part II. The influence of the rate and frequency of distraction. *Clin Orthop* 1989;**239**:263–285.
4 Snyder CC, Levine GA, Swanson HM, Browne EZ Jr: Mandibular lengthening by gradual distraction. Preliminary report. *Plast Reconstr Surg* 1973;**51**:506–508.
5 Guerrero CA: Expansion rapida mandibular. *Rev Venez Ortod* 1990;**12**:48.
6 McCarthy JG, Schreiber J, Karp N, Thorne CH, Grayson BH: Lengthening the human mandible by gradual distraction. *Plast Reconstr Surg* 1992;**89**:1–8.
7 Perrott DH, Berger R, Vargervik K, Kaban LB: Use of a skeletal distraction device to widen the mandible: a case report. *J Oral Maxillofac Surg* 1993;**51**(4):e435–439.
8 Troulis MJ, Glowacki J, Perrott DH, et al: Effects of latency and rate on bone formation in a porcine mandibular distraction model. *J Oral Maxillofac Surg* 2000;**58**:507.
9 Kaban LB, Thurmüller P, Troulis MJ, et al: Correlation of biomechanical stiffness with plain radiographic and ultrasound data in an experimental mandibular distraction wound. *Int J Oral Maxillofac Surg* 2003;**32**:296.
10 Glowacki J, Shusterman EM, Troulis MJ, et al: Distraction osteogenesis of the porcine mandible: histomorphometric evaluation of bone. *Plast Reconstr Surg* 2004;**113**:566.
11 Zimmermann CE, Thurmüller P, Troulis MJ, et al: Histology of the porcine mandibular distraction wound. *Int J Oral Maxillofac Surg* 2005;**34**:411.
12 Tayebaty FT, Williams WB, Baumann A, et al: Histologic and histomorphometric analysis of the porcine mandibular distraction wound. *J Oral Maxillofac Surg* 2006;**64**:43.
13 Lawler ME, Tayebaty FT, Williams WB, et al: Histomorphometric analysis of the porcine mandibular distraction wound. *J Oral Maxillofac Surg* 2010;**68**:1543.
14 Block MS, Chang A, Crawford C: Mandibular alveolar ridge augmentation in the dog using distraction osteogenesis. *J Oral Maxillofac Surg* 1996;**54**:309–314.
15 Gaggl A, Schultes G, Regauer S, Karcher H: Healing process after alveolar ridge distraction in sheep. *Oral Surgery, Oral Medicine, Oral Pathology, Oral Radiology and Endodontology* 2000;**90**(4):420–429.
16 Chin M, Toth BA: Distraction osteogenesis in maxillofacial surgery: using internal devices. *J Oral Maxillofac Surg* 1996;**54**:45–53.
17 Haggerty CJ, Block MS: Alveolar distraction osteogenesis. In: *Minimally Invasive Maxillofacial Surgery*. PMPH-USA, 2013, pp. 177–188.
18 Chiapasco M, Zaniboni M, Boisco M: Augmentation procedures for the rehabilitation of deficient edentulous ridges with oral implants. *Clin Oral Implant Res* 2006;**17**(Suppl 2):136–59.
19 Chiapasco M, Zaniboni M, Rimondini L: Autogenous onlay bone grafts vs. alveolar distraction osteogenesis for the correction of vertically deficient edentulous ridges: a 2–4-year prospective study on humans. *Clin. Oral Impl. Res.* 2007;**18**:432–440.
20 Chiapasco M, Romeo E, Casentini P, Rimondini L: Alveolar distraction osteogenesis vs. vertical guided bone regeneration for the correction of vertically deficient edentulous ridges: a 1–3-year prospective study on humans. *Clin Oral Implants Res* 2004;**15**:82–95.
21 Schwartz-Arad R, Levin L: Multitier technique for bone augmentation using intraoral autogenous bone blocks. *Implant Dent* 2007;**14**:5–8.
22 Saulacic N, Iizuka T, Martin MS, et al: Alveolar distraction osteogenesis: a systematic review. *Int J Oral Maxillofac Surg* 2008;**37**(1):1–7.
23 Rachmiel A, Srouji S, Peled M: Alveolar ridge augmentation by distraction osteogenesis. *Int J Oral Maxillofac Surg* 2001;**30**:510–517.
24 Batal HS, Cottrell DA: Alveolar distraction osteogenesis for implant site development. *Oral Maxillofac Surg Clin North Am* 2004;**16**(1):91–109.
25 Vega LG, Bilbao A: Alveolar distraction osteogenesis for dental implant preparation: an update. *Oral Maxillofac Surg Clin North Am* 2010 Aug;**22**(3):369–385.
26 Jensen OT, Cockrell R, Kuhlke L, Reed C: Anterior maxillary alveolar distraction osteogenesis: a prospective 5-year clinical study. *International Journal of Oral and Maxillofacial Implants* 2002 Jan-Feb;**17**(1):52–68.
27 Jensen, OT, Block M: Alveolar modification by distraction osteogenesis. *Atlas of the Oral and Maxillofacial Surgery Clinics of North America* 2008;**16**(2):185–214.
28 Saulacic N, Zix J, Iizuka T: Complication rates and associated factors in alveolar distraction osteogenesis: a comprehensive review. *International Journal of Oral and Maxillofacial Surgery* 2009 Mar;**38**(3):210–217.
29 Herford AS, Audia F: Maintaining vector control during alveolar distraction osteogenesis: a technical note. *Int J Oral Maxillofac Implants* 2004;**19**:e758–762.
30 Uckan S, Veziroglu F, Dayangac, E: Alveolar distraction osteogenesis versus autogenous onlay bone grafting for alveolar ridge augmentation: technique, complications, and implant survival rates. *Oral Surgery, Oral Medicine, Oral Pathology, Oral Radiology and Endodontology* 2008;**106**(4):511–515.
31 Alkan A, Baş B, Inal S: Alveolar distraction osteogenesis of bone graft reconstructed mandible. *Oral Surgery, Oral Medicine, Oral Pathology, Oral Radiology, and Endodontics* 2005;**100**(3):e39–42.
32 Bell RB, Blakey GH, White RP, Hillebrand DG, Molina A: Staged reconstruction of the severely atrophic mandible with autogenous bone graft and endosteal implants. *Journal of Oral and Maxillofacial Surgery* 2002;**60**(10):1135–1141.

33. Amir LR, Becking AG, Jovanovic A, et al: Formation of new bone during vertical distraction osteogenesis of the human mandible is related to the presence of blood vessels. *Clin Oral Implants Res* 2006;17(4):410–416.
34. Lindeboom JA, Mathura KR, Milstein DMJ, et al: Microvascular soft tissue changes in alveolar distraction osteogenesis. *Oral Surg Oral Med Oral Pathol Oral Radiol Endod* 2008;106(3):350–355.
35. Chiapasco M, Lang NP, Bosshardt DD: Quality and quantity of bone following alveolar distraction osteogenesis in the human mandible. *Clin Oral Implants Res* 2006 Aug;17(4):394–402.
36. Mehra and Figueroa: Vector control in distraction osteogenesis. *J Oral Maxillofac Surg* 2008;66:776–779.
37. Takahashi TI, Funaki K, Shintani H, Haruoka T: Use of horizontal alveolar distraction osteogenesis for implant placement in a narrow alveolar ridge: a case report. *Int J Oral Maxillofac Implants* 2004 Mar–Apr;19(2):291–294.
38. Cheung LK, Chua HD, Hariri F, Pow EH, Zheng L: Alveolar distraction osteogenesis for dental implant rehabilitation following fibular reconstruction: a case series. *J Oral Maxillofac Surg* 2013 Feb;71(2):255–271.
39. Enislidis G, Fock N, Millesi-Schobel G, Klug C, Wittwer G, Yerit K: Analysis of complications following alveolar distraction osteogenesis and implant placement in the partially edentulous mandible. *Oral Surg Oral Med Oral Pathol Oral Radiol Endod* 2005;100:e25–30.
40. Froum SJ, Rosenberg ES, Elian N, Tarnow D, Cho SC: Distraction osteogenesis for ridge augmentation: prevention and treatment of complications. Thirty case reports. *Int J Periodont Rest Dent* 2008;2:e337–345.
41. Günbay T, Koyuncu BO, Akay MC, et al: Results and complications of alveolar distraction osteogenesis to enhance vertical bone height. *Oral Surg Oral Med Oral Pathol Oral Radiol Endod* 2008;105(5):e7–13.
42. Izuka T, Hallermann W, Seto I, Smolka W, Smolka K, Bosshardt DD: Bi-directional distraction osteogenesis of the alveolar bone using extraosseous device. *Clin Oral Implants Res* 2005;16:e700–707.
43. Mazzonetto R, Allais M, Maurette PE, Moreira RWF: A retrospective study of the potential complications during alveolar distraction osteogenesis in 55 patients. *Int J Oral Maxillofac Surg* 2007;36:6–10.
44. Wolvius EB, Scholtemeijer M, Weijland M, et al: Complications and relapse in alveolar distraction osteogenesis in partially dentulous patients. *Int J Oral Maxillofac Surg* 2007;36(8):700–705.
45. Ettl T, Gerlach T, Schüsselbauer T, et al: Bone resorption and complications in alveolar distraction osteogenesis. *Clin Oral Investig* 2010;14(5):481–489.
46. Perdijk FB, Meijer GJ, Strijen PJ, et al: Complications in alveolar distraction osteogenesis of the atrophic mandible. *Int J Oral Maxillofac Surg* 2007;36(10):916–921.
47. Garcia AG, Martin MS, Vila PG, Maceiras JL: Minor complications arising in alveolar distraction osteogenesis. *J Oral Maxillofacial Surg* 2002;60(5):496–501.
48. Saulacic N, Martin MS, Vila PG, Garcia-Garcia A: Bone defect formation during implant placement following alveolar distraction. *International Journal of Oral and Maxillofacial Implants*, 2007;22(1):47–52.
49. Jensen OT, Ellis E: The book flap: a technical note. *Journal of Oral and Maxillofacial Surgery* 2008;66(5):1010–1014.
50. Laster Z, Rachmiel A, Jensen OT: Alveolar width distraction osteogenesis for early implant placement. *Journal of Oral and Maxillofacial Surgery* 2005;63(12):1724–1730.
51. Raghoebar GM, Liem RSB, Vissink A: Vertical distraction of the severely resorbed edentulous mandible. *Clinical Oral Implants Research* 2002;13:558–565.
52. Chiapasco M, Consolo U, Bianchi A, Ronchi, P: Alveolar distraction osteogenesis for the correction of vertically deficient edentulous ridges: a multicenter prospective study on humans. *International Journal of Oral and Maxillofacial Implants* 2004;19(3):399–407.

CHAPTER 22

Management of Maxillary and Mandibular Post-Traumatic Alveolar Bone Defects with Distraction Osteogenesis Technique

Adi Rachmiel[1,2] and Dekel Shilo[1]

[1]Department of Oral and Maxillofacial Surgery, Rambam Health Care Campus, Haifa, Israel
[2]Bruce Rappaport Faculty of Medicine, Technion–Israel Institute of Technology, Haifa, Israel

Introduction

The use of endosseous implants for dental restorations has become popular in recent decades, with evident long-term stability and survival [1, 2]. Many patients lack the vertical and horizontal bone dimensions required for endosseous implant insertion. Alveolar ridge reconstruction may be indicated for the atrophic alveolar process resulting from maxillofacial trauma, periodontal disease, and post-resection of aggressive large jaw cysts or tumors. The alveolar ridge deficiency may interfere with safe and correct positioning of implants; therefore bone augmentation is essential to guarantee adequate bone volume, which provides patients with proper interarch relations and allows for satisfactory aesthetic, prosthetic, and occlusal results.

There are different modalities for reconstructing the atrophic alveolar bone. Among them are autogenous block bone grafting, guided bone regeneration (GBR) with a particulate graft, ridge splitting or expansion technique, osteotomies of the ridge or the jaws, and distraction osteogenesis [3].

Distraction osteogenesis (DO) is a technique in which bone is generated by progressive elongation of two bone fragments following an osteotomy or corticotomy [4, 5]. The first description of distraction osteogenesis was published in 1869 by Von Langenbeck [6], whose method was explored in long bones [7] and later in the craniofacial region. Significant contributions in the development of distraction osteogenesis were made by Ilizarov [4, 5], who described two biologic effects of DO known as the "Ilizarov effects": (a) the tension–stress effect on the genesis and growth of tissues and (b) the influence of blood supply and loading on the shape of bones and joints. In addition, two other principles of Ilizarov should be respected: the distraction device should be stable and not rigid, and there should be full control on the vector of lengthening.

McCarthy was the first to clinically apply distraction osteogenesis in craniofacial anomalies [8]. Since the clinical application of DO in the craniofacial complex, a number of experimental and clinical investigations have demonstrated that gradual mechanical traction of bone segments at an osteotomy site created in the craniofacial complex generated new bone, parallel to the direction of traction [9–11].

In cases of mild-to-moderate alveolar bone loss up to 6 mm, a possible method for bone reconstruction is an onlay block bone graft or a sandwich osteotomy combined with an interpositional autogenous graft [12, 13]. In these methods, the donor site morbidity is unavoidable and some resorption of the autogenous grafted bone occurs.

Alveolar distraction osteogenesis (ADO) is a method used for reconstructing alveolar bone in moderate-to-severe alveolar bone deficiency cases [14–16]. The new bone is formed between the surfaces of bone segments that are gradually separated by incremental traction. DO is a useful solution in a number of pathological conditions other than alveolar bone deficiency: maxillary cleft deficiency [17–19], a compromised airway [20–22], and craniofacial anomalies [8, 23, 24].

ADO is generally indicated in cases of vertical bone deficiency, an unfavorable implant to crown ratio and aesthetically compromised rehabilitation [16, 25–27]. It is frequently performed for vertical elongation following loss of teeth due to trauma or after tooth extraction due to periodontal causes [16, 26, 28]. Following maxillary trauma, the loss of teeth and alveolar bone together with fibrotic scar formation can result in adverse changes to the interarch space, occlusal plane, arch relationship, and arch form that complicates rehabilitation and can compromise the esthetic outcome.

In the anterior region, alveolar distraction osteogenesis is most frequently used in the anterior maxilla for major reconstruction procedures in which the bone deficiency has mainly the vertical component with some degree of the horizontal (anterior–posterior) component [27]. In the anterior mandible, distraction osteogenesis is mostly used to allow for interforaminal implant placement for an overdenture [29–33].

In the posterior region, ADO is applied more frequently in the mandible [26, 34] rather than in the maxilla [35], to permit placement of implants with increased length and reduced crown height (improved crown–implant ratio). The aim of alveolar ridge distraction is to reconstruct the alveolus and to control the vector of elongation to achieve three-dimensional alveolar rehabilitation.

Alveolar distraction can be unidirectional, bidirectional, or horizontal:

1 Unidirectional distraction device. An atrophic alveolar segment up to 3 cm transversely can be treated by one unidirectional distraction device. In a larger alveolar segment over 3 cm, the use of two distraction devices on both sides of the osteotomy may be

---

Vertical Alveolar Ridge Augmentation in Implant Dentistry: A Surgical Manual, First Edition. Edited by Len Tolstunov.
© 2016 John Wiley & Sons, Inc. Published 2016 by John Wiley & Sons, Inc.

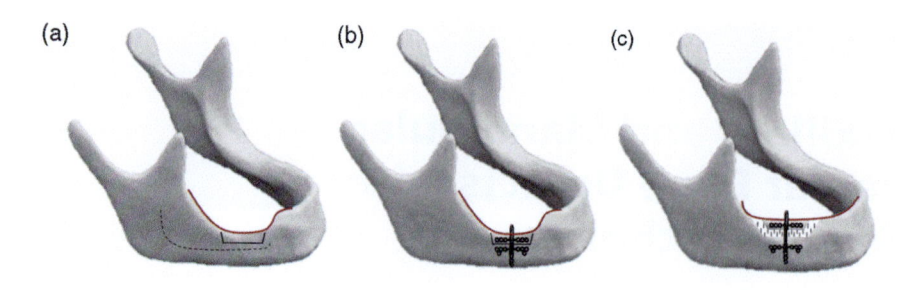

Figure 22.1 Unidirectional extraosseous distraction osteogenesis. (a) The trapezoid osteotomy is composed of two vertical and one horizontal osteotomies. In the posterior mandible the horizontal osteotomy should be at least 2 mm above the inferior alveolar nerve. (b) The extraosseous distractor is fixed to the bone. One plate is fixed with screws to the basal bone and the other to the transported segment. (c) Bone elongation is commenced at the desired rate and in the created gap new bone is generated. Grey rods represent the newly formed trabecular bone.

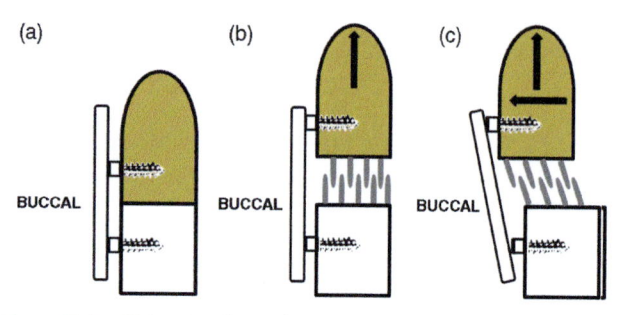

Figure 22.2 – Bidirectional crest distractor. (a) The osteotomies are created similarly to the ones described in Figure 22.1 and the distractor is placed in the same manner. (b) Vertical elongation of the alveolus is commenced. (c) The distractor allows a buccal correction of the transported segment vector of elongation. Grey rods represent the newly formed trabecular bone.

needed to control the sagittal plane on both sides of the vector of elongation (Figure 22.1).
2 Bidirectional distraction device. Used for concomitant vertical and buccal vector control of elongation [36] (Figure 22.2).
3 Horizontal alveolar distraction is conducted by a crest distractor to enlarge the buccolingual alveolar ridge horizontally [37, 38] (Figure 22.3).

Different distraction devices

There are different devices used for distraction osteogenesis, they can be divided into:
- Intraosseous: central application of the device, for example, the LEAD System (Stryker CMF, Portage, MI, USA) [14, 16] (Figure 22.4).
- Intraosseous distraction by using implants: for example, Ace (Ace Surgical Supply Co., Brockton, MA, USA), Dis-Sys Distraction Implant (Sis Inc., Klagenfort, Austria) and the 3i Implant Distractor

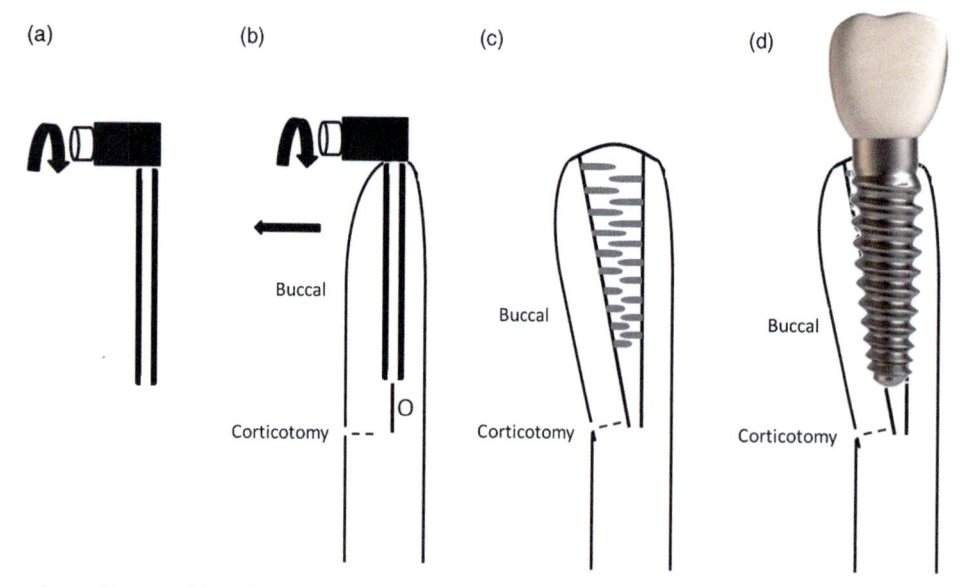

Figure 22.3 Horizontal crest distractor. (a) A schematic representation of the horizontal crest distractor. The distractor is composed of two parallel arms that are inserted inside the sagittal osteotomy. (b) Placement of the distractor in the alveolar crest after the sagittal osteotomy and the corticotomy at the buccal side. The two arms of the distraction device should be inserted at least two-thirds of the depth of the osteotomy in order to enlarge the width of the upper alveolar ridge. (c) The enlarged crest with the newly created bone between the two bone fragments. (d) Placement of an implant in the enlarged alveolar crest. The upper circular arrow represents the direction of turning of the lengthening screw. The lower arrow near the buccal cortex represents the direction of horizontal elongation of the buccal alveolar plate. Buccal shows the buccal aspect of the ridge; corticotomy represents the horizontal corticotomy; O represents the lower part of the osteotomy; grey rods represent the newly formed trabecular bone.

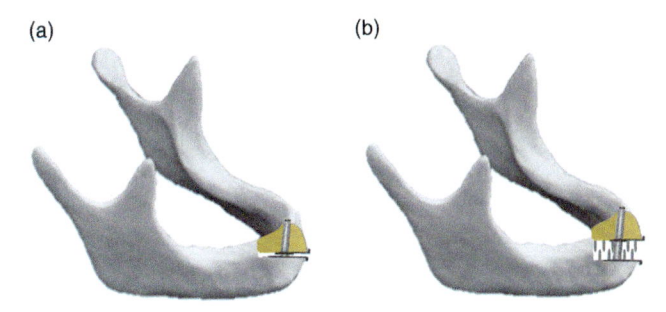

Figure 22.4 Intraosseous distraction with a distraction device. (a) The osteotomies are created similarly to the ones described in Figure 22.1 and the distraction rod is placed transmucosal at the alveolar crest between two plates, which are fixed by screws, one to the basal bone and the other to the transported segment. (b) Bone elongation is commenced by turning the distraction rod. Grey rods represent the newly formed trabecular bone.

Table 22.1 Protocol for alveolar distraction osteogenesis procedure.

Surgery	Latency period	Rate of bone elongation	Consolidation period	Device removal	Implant placement
	4 days	0.5 mm/day as necessary	3–4 months		

(Implant Innovations, West Palm Beach, FL, USA) [27,39–41] (Figure 22.5).

- Extraosseous: eccentric application of the device, for example, the Track distractors by KLS Martin (Tuttlingen, Germany) [15] and Medicon distracters (Tuttlingen, Germany) (Figure 22.1).

When comparing the three described devices, intraosseous and implant activated devices depend on substantial basal bone support and are vulnerable to lateral forces that may lead to a wrong vector of distraction and may increase bone resorption around the device. Implant-dependent distractors are known to cause crestal bone resorption and it is hard to control their final position after distraction is completed for prosthetic purposes. Implant distraction devices can also be left for later prosthetic rehabilitation or are removed and later replaced by osseointegrated implants [41]. Extraosseous distraction devices are the most common and popular devices. Their drawbacks are need for a substantial subperiosteal space, propensity to interfere with a blood supply, and possible exposure of the device [42].

Description of the method of alveolar distraction osteogenesis (ADO)

A paracrestal mucoperiosteal incision on the buccal side is performed leaving the crestal attached mucosa intact, followed by two vertical release incisions, 4 mm lateral to the planned osteotomy. Mucoperiosteal reflection is performed up to the base of the mandible or in the maxilla up to the base of the pyriform aperture. Using a fine cylindrical bur or a reciprocating saw two vertical and one horizontal osteotomies are performed, creating a trapezoidal osteotomy that forms the transported segment (Figure 22.1a). The transported segment should have at least 6 mm in height to achieve adequate space for placement of the plate and screws. The transported segment should stay attached to the crestal and lingual mucosa and periosteum. Failure to preserve the lingual or palatal periosteum attached to the bony segment results in a free bone graft and a risk of necrosis of the transported bone. Great care is also taken to avoid fracture of the basal bone at the mandible and maxilla. In the mandible, the horizontal osteotomy needs to be a minimum of 2 mm above the mandibular canal to avoid damage to the inferior alveolar nerve (Figure 22.1a). Next, the distraction device is adapted in size and desired vector and fixated by insertion of screws (Figure 22.1b). In the case of intraosseous devices, a transmucosal rod or distraction implant is inserted through the crestal mucosa and the fixation is done using screws next to the horizontal osteotomy site [41].

In patients with an extensive alveolar defect, two distraction devices can be placed for better control of the vector of elongation on both sides of the defect. In patients with severe atrophy or after bone resection or bone loss due to trauma, two stages of jaw reconstruction can be performed: bone graft as the first stage followed by distraction osteogenesis as a second stage.

Bone elongation is initiated after a four-day latency period at a rate of 0.5 mm/day and continues as necessary and according to the length of the distraction device (Figure 22.1c). Following the bone elongation, a consolidation period of 3 to 4 months is required. Subsequently, the devices are removed and endosseous implants can be placed followed by prosthetic restoration (Table 22.1). It is important to be aware of the vector of distraction, the stability of the bone, the final alveolar height, and the timing of placement of dental implants.

Latency period, rate of bone elongation, and consolidation period

Many works dealt with the latency period, rate of bone elongation and the consolidation period. Yang [43] reviewed 59 articles on horizontal distraction, vertical distraction, and interdental distraction. In his article, he showed that the mean latency period was 6.26

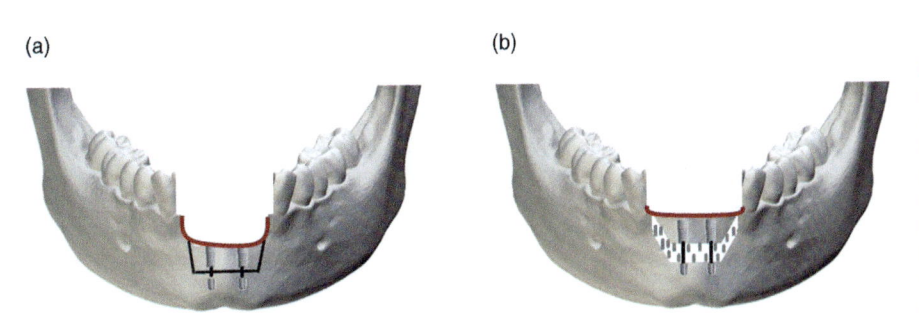

Figure 22.5 Intraosseous distraction with implants. (a) The osteotomies are created similarly to the ones described in Figure 22.1 and the implant distractors are placed transmucosal at the alveolar crest. (b) Bone elongation is commenced by two implant distractors. Two distractors allow a better control of the vector of elongation. Grey rods represent the newly formed trabecular bone.

days, the mean rate of bone elongation per day was 0.81 mm, and the mean consolidation period was 79 days. Saulacic [33] reviewed 20 articles that described alveolar distraction osteogenesis. He showed a mean latency period of 7.26 days, a rate of bone elongation of 0.71 mm, and a consolidation period of 86 days.

We usually allow a four-day latency period after the insertion of the distraction devices and before initiation of bone elongation. The rate of distraction we use is 0.5 mm/day until the desirable length is acquired within the limitation of the device. Follow-up appointments include clinical examination and radiographic images. The consolidation period in which we leave the device as fixation for bone maturation is 90–120 days, after which the distraction devices are removed. Implants are placed 6 weeks post-removal of the device, although some advocate the immediate placement of the implants during device removal.

Controlling the vector of distraction

During the alveolar distraction process, three-dimensional vector control is a crucial factor in determining the planned movement and in maintaining precise evaluation of the desired direction of the distraction [44–46]. Owing to the curved architecture of the maxillary and mandibular alveolar ridge, especially along the intercanine arch span, the distractor is initially angulated appropriately, but accurate guidance of the vector's direction is limited. Consequently, alveolar ridge augmentation during distraction most often results in a straight and flat alveolar ridge structure rather than a curved one. The delicate distracted bone is also exposed to the molding forces exerted by the surrounding soft tissue matrix. In this way, the transported bone segment is forcefully pushed inward in a palatal or lingual direction during normal function of the buccinator muscle and due to palatal and lingual periosteal traction [44, 46, 47]. It is important to identify the direction of the newly regenerated bone early enough to avoid compromising the alveolar ridge augmentation results. In order to control the vector of creation of newly formed bone one can use teeth, if present, as anchorage to maintain a desirable vector. This approach can compromise existing teeth and can result in their movement and rotation [48].

Mommaerts and Laster developed a bidirectional distraction device [36] in which the bone is distracted vertically followed by correction in the buccal horizontal plane (Figure 22.2). Other methods for controlling the vector of distraction include usage of the antirelapse extension of the distractor located in its lower part or the use of control plates and screws. In case the vector was not maintained successfully, at the end of the consolidation period an osteotomy and correction of the vector of the newly regenerated bone can be performed.

We previously described a new method for controlling the vector of distraction using temporary anchorage devices (TADs) [44, 46]. TADs are fixed temporarily to the bone to enhance orthodontic anchorage and are removed after usage. Orthodontic elastics connect the TADs to the distraction device in the mandible or maxilla, thus minimizing unwanted components of the vector.

In case of severe bone deficiency in post-traumatic maxillary cases, a third procedure, Le Fort I advancement, might be needed following distraction osteogenesis in order to correct anterior–posterior (AP) maxillary bone projection and the interarch jaw relationship.

In summary, the distraction vector can be controlled by:
1 Usage of adjacent teeth.
2 TADs.
3 Control plates or an antirelapse extension plate connected to the basal plate of the extraosseous distractor.
4 At the end of the consolidation period by an osteotomy and correction of the vector of the regenerated bone.
5 In severe maxillary AP bone deficiency by an additional Le Fort I osteotomy and advancement.

Bone resorption and survival of implants inserted after distraction osteogenesis

Implants are usually placed in the newly formed bone 6 weeks post-removal of distraction devices. Pérez-Sayáns [49] showed minimal to no difference between bone resorption when placing implants in normal bone versus bone subjected to alveolar distraction osteogenesis, one and three years post-loading of the implants. Zwetyenga et al. [50] placed implants after a mean vertical alveolar distraction of 11.7 mm. They reported survival and success rates of 100% and 96.2%, respectively, within a mean follow-up of 62 months. Kim [51] showed a mean of 7.1 years follow-up of implant survival and success following a mean of 8.4 mm alveolar distraction. He demonstrated 97.3 and 92.7% survival and success rates, respectively.

The use of osteogenic molecules and stem cells

Bone morphogenetic protein (BMP) is known to play an important role in post-natal bone formation [52]. Our group showed in the past that injection of BMPs during the active bone elongation phase of distraction osteogenesis resulted in increased trabecular bone size and volume as well as an increased number of proliferating cells. We suggested that this shortened the consolidation period of DO allowing for earlier implant placement [53–55]. Other growth factors, such as deferoxamine, also showed potential for accelerating bone maturation. Through its ability to chelate iron, deferoxamine treatment results in the stimulation of hypoxia-inducible factor 1α (HIF-1α), which is inhibited by iron. HIF-1α stimulates the production of vascular endothelial growth factor (VEGF), resulting in increased angiogenesis in the wound and more robust bone formation.

In addition to growth factors, recently mesenchymal stem cells (MSCs) have been studied. Several experiments describe insertion of cells harvested from bone marrow into distraction sites with promising results in biomechanical tests and compact bone ratio [56].

Advantages of distraction osteogenesis [16, 57–59]

- Simultaneous expansion of both bone and soft tissue. There is no need for flap formation for primary closure, as it is needed in block bone grafting. This leads to a lower chance of soft tissue tension and bone exposure.
- Bone at the alveolar crest remains as cortical and mature bone. This is very important for primary stability of the dental implants. The implants are placed inside the mature lamellar cortical bone and not in the newly formed immature (woven) bone.
- The attached mucosa on the coronal side of the alveolar ridge remains intact. Vertical distraction osteogenesis provides the advantage of simultaneous distraction of bone and soft tissue,

while the original pre-operative attached mucosa remains intact at the crest.
- No donor site morbidity as it is common in autogenous block bone grafts.
- Minimal resorption of bone.
- Lower infection rate.
- Greater bone lengthening than other methods, thus reconstructing severe bone defects and allowing the insertion of longer dental implants.

The main advantage of alveolar distraction osteogenesis is the use of small distraction devices that gradually lengthen the bone and generate new bone at the distraction gap with no need for an autogenous bone graft with the associated donor site morbidity. A second major advantage is distraction of the surrounding soft tissue together with the transported bone segment called distraction histiogenesis.

Complications and disadvantages of alveolar distraction [25, 27, 41, 60–70]

Complications of distraction can be divided to intraoperative and post-operative.

Intraoperative complications of distraction osteogenesis include:
- Nerve injury that can be avoided by careful surgical flap elevation and carefully performed osteotomy.
- Fracture of the basal bone or transported bone. One should use proper well-maintained equipment and perform correct and accurate osteotomies.
- Adjacent tooth damage.

Post-operative complications, during bone elongation and consolidation:
- Misdirection of the transport segment. As discussed before, a major challenge in distraction osteogenesis is maintaining the proper vector of bone elongation. The different methods for controlling the vector of distraction were discussed above.
- Mechanical issues and fracture of the distraction device. At times the distraction device is prone to mechanical failure, as is any medical device. DO device functions under constant masticatory forces that contribute to its possible fracture and malfunction.
- Pain during distraction is possible and partially depends on the rate and extent of distraction. Pain management with medications is usually successful in these cases.
- Dehiscence of the soft tissue with exposure of the distraction device or bone is a known complication that might cause improper ossification and the need for the removal of the device.
- Occlusal interference due to the vector of bone elongation or rod location of the distraction device is possible and the position of the device has to be planned accordingly to avoid this complication.
- Resorption of the transport segment due to impaired vascular supply or physical pressure applied on the segment is possible and should be avoided by utilizing the proper surgical technique based on the applied surgical anatomy.
- Improper ossification and fibrotic tissue formation due to an inadequate rate of bone elongation, dehiscence of the distraction chamber, or infection are known complications. Adherence to the surgical protocol with an established rate of distraction is important.
- Relapse of bone formation, mostly due to masticatory forces opposing the direction of bone formation, improper ossification, or insufficient retention period. The literature shows 3–29% of bone relapse. Again, a proper surgical protocol can decrease the risk of a relapse.
- Paresthesia is a well-known and common complication of the surgery, but it is usually temporary with a careful surgical technique.
- Infection may develop due to dehiscence of the distraction device and can impair healing and proper ossification. Frequent post-operative examinations and antibiotic coverage can control the risk of infection.
- Fracture of the basal or transported bone during active distraction is rare. One should use proper well-maintained equipment.
- A disadvantage of the procedure is the need for a second operation for device removal prior to implant insertion. Some advocate insertion of dental implants during the device removal.

Mandibular fracture is the most severe intraoperative complication and requires an immediate surgical repositioning and osteosynthesis. Ugurlu [71] showed that the most common complication was undesirable bone movement, followed by mechanical problems.

Alveolar distraction osteogenesis is not applicable in the following cases:
- The transported bone is less than 6 mm in height.
- Presence of avascular transported bone with inadequate or lost lingual or palatal periosteal attachment to the segment.
- Significant horizontal alveolar bone defect. Thin transported bone might result in a fracture.

Case Report: Maxilla

The first case described is a post-traumatic vertical alveolar distraction of the deficient anterior maxillary bone. A 29-year-old patient with previous maxillofacial trauma resulting in avulsion and defect of anterior maxillary bone and teeth presented with a severe maxillary vertical bone deficiency (Figures 22.6a and 22.7a). A trapezoid osteotomy was created and two Track alveolar distraction devices (KLS Martin, Tuttlingen, Germany) were placed on each side of the osteotomy (Figures 22.6b and 22.7b). Elongation was commenced at a rate of 0.5 mm/day following a latency period of 4 days. A 13 mm vertical augmentation was obtained (Figures 22.6c and 22.7c). After a consolidation period of 3 months the distractor devices were removed and four endosseous root-form implants were placed, followed by successful prosthetic rehabilitation to full function and occlusion (Figures 22.6d and 22.7d).

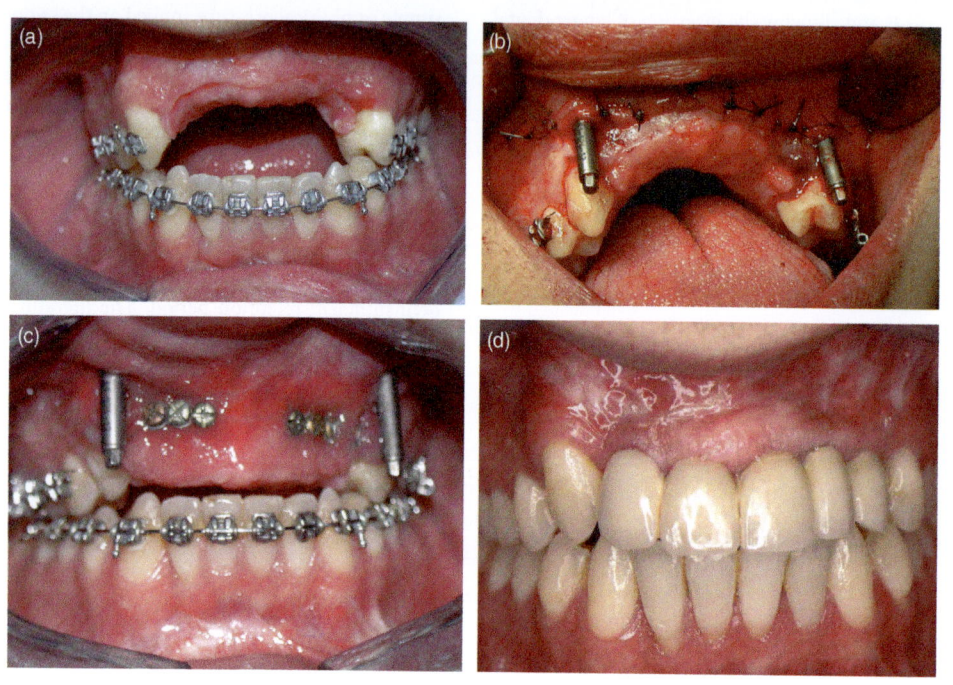

Figure 22.6 Clinical photos showing vertical alveolar distraction of the anterior maxilla in a trauma patient and rehabilitation. A 29-year-old patient presents with previous maxillofacial trauma resulting in avulsion of pre-maxillary bone and teeth. (a) Pre-operative maxillary vertical bone deficiency. (b) Placement of two distraction devices following a trapezoid osteotomy. (c) Vertical bone elongation after completion of alveolar distraction. (d) Distraction devices were removed, implants were placed, and the prosthetic rehabilitation can be observed. Source: Aizenbud 2012. Reproduced with permission from Elsevier [44].

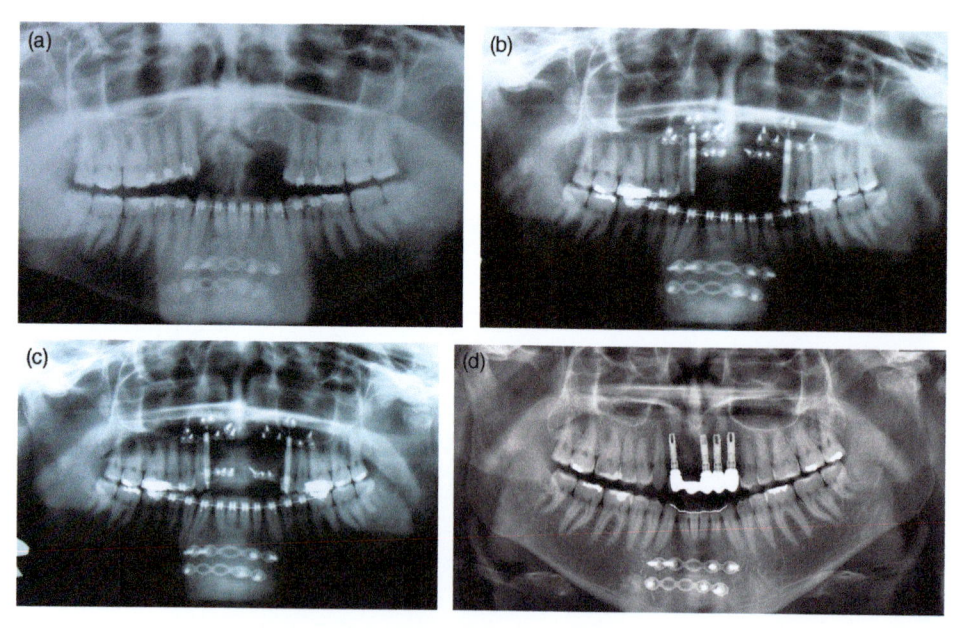

Figure 22.7 – Panoramic radiographs demonstrating vertical alveolar distraction of the anterior maxilla in a trauma patient and rehabilitation. Radiograph images of the same patient described in Figure 22.6. (a) Pre-operative maxillary vertical bone deficiency and loss of anterior maxillary teeth. (b) Two distraction devices can be observed, before commencement of vertical bone elongation. (c) Radiograph after 13 mm of vertical bone elongation. (d) Distraction devices were removed, implants were placed and the prosthetic rehabilitation can be observed with adequate crown–implant ratio. Source: Aizenbud 2012. Reproduced with permission from Elsevier [44].

Case Report: Mandible

The second case report described is a post-traumatic vertical alveolar distraction of the deficient posterior mandibular bone. A 25-year-old patient presented with a history of complex mid-face and mandible fractures resulting in a marked loss of alveolar bone and teeth in the left mandibular body (Figures 22.8a and 22.9a). Following removal of the mandibular reconstruction plate that was used to fixate mandibular fragments at the time of trauma, a trapezoid osteotomy was conducted in the left mandibular body and a Track alveolar distraction device (KLS Martin, Tuttlingen, Germany) was placed (Figure 22.9b). After a latency period of 4 days, gradual alveolar distraction was performed at a rate of 0.5 mm/day and 12 mm of vertical alveolar bone augmentation was obtained (Figures 22.8b and 22.9c). Following a consolidation period of 3 months, the distraction device was removed and three endosseous root-form 13 mm implants were placed (Figures 22.8c and 22.9d) on which successful prosthetic rehabilitation was performed to full function and occlusion (Figure 22.8d).

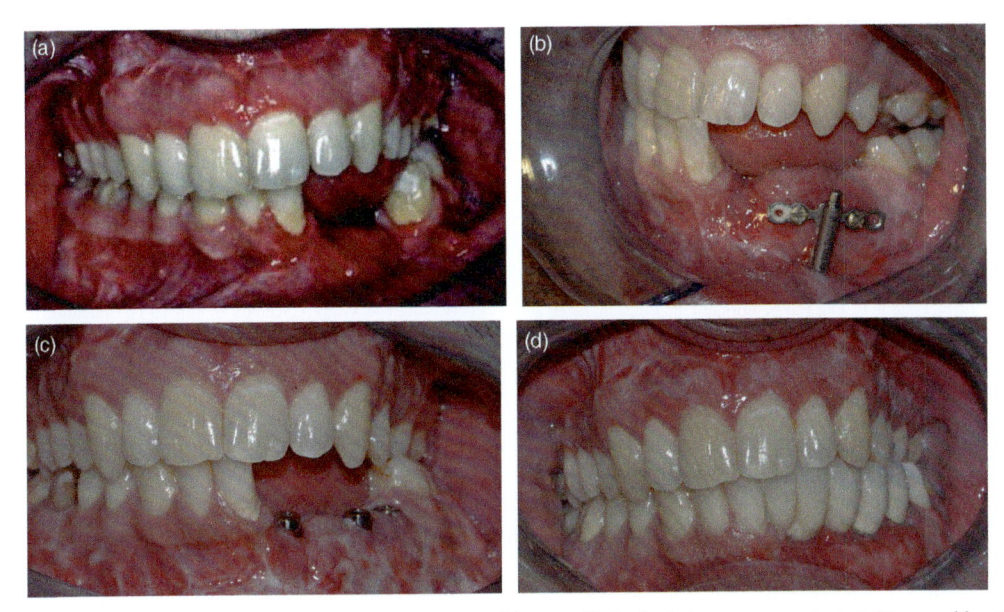

Figure 22.8 Clinical photos demonstrating vertical alveolar distraction of the mandibular body in a trauma patient. A 25-year-old patient presents with previous maxillofacial trauma resulting in a severe alveolar bone loss in the left mandibular body and avulsion of teeth. (a) Pre-operative mandibular vertical bone deficiency. (b) Vertical elongation of the alveolar bone by an extraosseous Track distraction device. (c) The distraction device was removed and three 13 mm root-form dental implants were placed. (d) Prosthetic rehabilitation was performed with adequate crown–implant ratio.

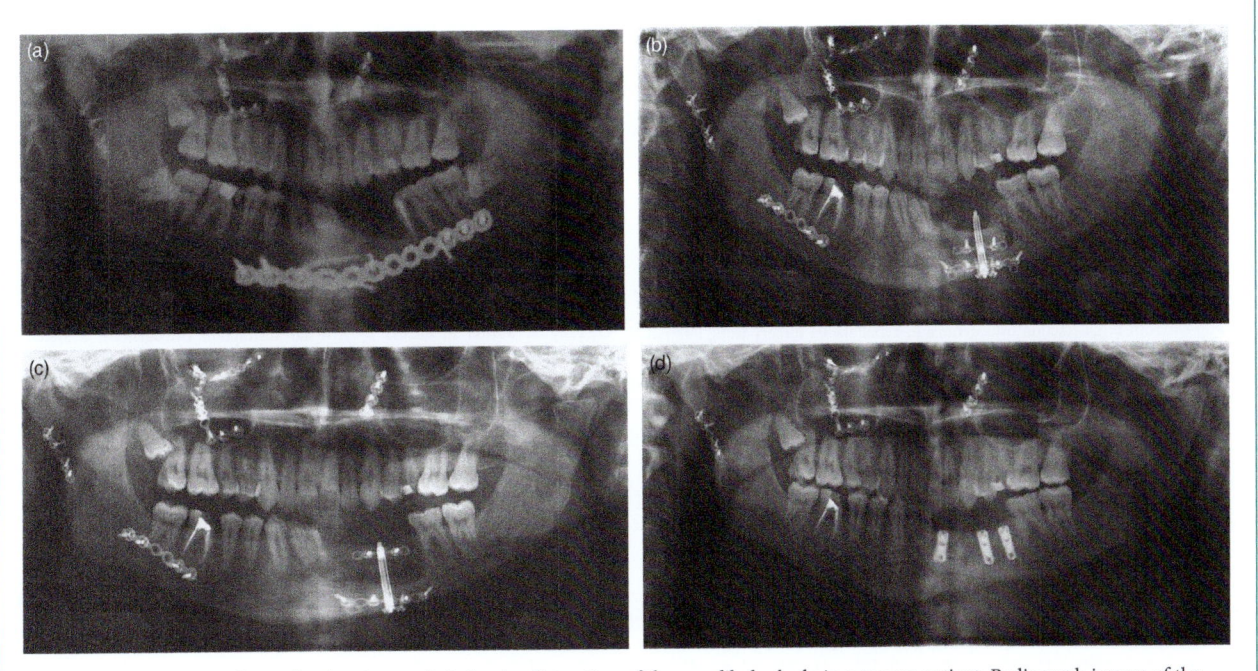

Figure 22.9 Panoramic radiographs showing vertical alveolar distraction of the mandibular body in a trauma patient. Radiograph images of the same patient described in Figure 22.8. (a) Post-traumatic panoramic X-ray demonstrates the alveolar bone deficiency on the left side. (b) The reconstruction plate was removed, followed by trapezoid osteotomy and placement of a distraction device. (c) Radiograph after 12 mm of vertical bone elongation. (d) Distraction devices were removed and three implants were placed.

Conclusion

Alveolar distraction osteogenesis is a procedure in which a segment of mature bone is transported in order to lengthen the alveolar crest for better implant anchorage, either for aesthetic purposes or functional prosthetic or occlusal requirements. The procedure offers an alternative method for bone reconstruction without donor site morbidity and sufficient stability of the final result.

In this chapter, we described different methods of alveolar distraction osteogenesis including advantages, disadvantages, and complications. One of the main challenges during the distraction process remains controlling the direction of the bone movement and prevention of complications. Alveolar distraction osteogenesis provides a method to regain both hard and soft tissue without additional bone grafting and is a useful choice in cases of medium to severe bone loss.

References

1. Alberktsson T, Dahl E, Enbom L, Engavall S, Enriquist B, Eriksson A, et al: Osseointegrated oral implants. A Swedish multicenter study of 8139 consecutively inserted Nobelpharma implants. *J Periodontol* 1988;59(5):287–296.
2. Tomasi C, Wennström J, Berglundh T: Longevity of teeth and implants – a systematic review. *J Oral Rehabil* 2008;35(1):23–32.
3. Milinkovic I, Cordaro L: Are there specific indications for the different alveolar bone augmentation procedures for implant placement? A systematic review. *Int J Oral Maxillofac Surg* 2014;43(5):606–625.
4. Ilizarov G: The tension-stress effect on the genesis and growth of tissues. Part I. The influence of stability of fixation and soft-tissue preservation. *Clin Orthop Relat Res* 1989;238:249–281.
5. Ilizarov G: The tension-stress effect on the genesis and growth of tissues. Part II. The influence of the rate and frequency of distraction. *Clin Orthop Relat Res* 1989;239:263–285.
6. Von Langenbeck B: About the pathologic length growth of long bones and its employment in surgical praxis. *Berl Klin Wochenschr* 1869;26:265.
7. Codivilla A: On the means of lengthening, in the lower limbs, the muscles and tissues which are shortened through deformity. *Am J Orthop Surg* 1905;2:353–369.
8. McCarthy J, Schreiber J, Karp N, Thorne C, Grayson B: Lengthening the human mandible by gradual distraction. *Plast Reconstr Surg* 1992;89(1):1–10.
9. Rachmiel A, Laufer D, Jackson I, Lewinson D: Midface membranous bone lengthening: a one-year histological and morphological follow-up of distraction osteogenesis. *Calcif Tissue Int* 1998;62(4):370–376.
10. Rachmiel A, Potparic Z, Jackson I, Sugihara T, Clayman L, Topf J, et al: Midface advancement by gradual distraction. *Br J Plast Surg* 1993;46(3):201–207.
11. Rachmiel A, Rozen N, Peled M, Lewinson D: Characterization of midface maxillary membranous bone formation during distraction osteogenesis. *Plast Reconstr Surg* 2002;109:1611–1620.
12. Jensen O: Alveolar segmental "sandwich" osteotomies for posterior edentulous mandibular sites for dental implants. *J Oral Maxillofac Surg* 2006;64(3):471–475.
13. Jensen O, Kuhlke L, Bedard J, White D: Alveolar segmental sandwich osteotomy for anterior maxillary vertical augmentation prior to implant placement. *J Oral Maxillofac Surg* 2006;64(2):290–296.
14. Chin M, Toth B: Distraction osteogenesis in maxillofacial surgery using internal devices: review of five cases. *J Oral Maxillofac Surg* 1996;54:45–53.
15. Hidding J, Lazar F, Zöller J: Initial outcome of vertical distraction osteogenesis of the atrophic alveolare ridge. *Mund Kiefer Gesichtschir* 1999;3(1):S79–83.
16. Rachmiel A, Srouji S, Peled M: Alveolar ridge augmentation by distraction osteogenesis. *Int J Oral Maxillofac Surg* 2001;30:510–517.
17. Polley J, Figueroa A: Management of severe maxillary deficiency in childhood and adolescence through distraction osteogenesis with an external, adjustable, rigid distraction device. *J Craniofac Surg* 1997;8(3):181–186.
18. Rachmiel A. Treatment of maxillary cleft palate: distraction osteogenesis versus orthognathic surgery – Part one: maxillary distraction. *J Oral Maxillofac Surg* 2007;65(4):753–757.
19. Rachmiel A, Aizenbud D, Peled M: Long-term results in maxillary deficiency using intraoral devices. *Int J Oral Maxillofac Surg* 2005;34(5):473–479.
20. Rachmiel A, Aizenbud D, Pillar G, Srouji S, Peled M: Bilateral mandibular distraction for patients with compromised airway analyzed by three-dimensional CT. *Int J Oral Maxillofac Surg* 2005;34:9–18.
21. Rachmiel A, Emodi O, Aizenbud D: Management of obstructive sleep apnea in pediatric craniofacial anomalies. *Ann Maxillofac Surg* 2012;2(2):111–115.
22. Rachmiel A, Emodi O, Rachmiel D, Aizenbud D: Internal mandibular distraction to relieve airway obstruction in children with severe micrognathia. *Int J Oral Maxillofac Surg* 2014;43(10):1176–1181.
23. Rachmiel A, Aizenbud D, Eleftheriou S, Peled M, Laufer D: Extraoral vs. intraoral distraction osteogenesis in the treatment of hemifacial microsomia. *Ann Plast Surg* 2000;45(4):386–394.
24. Rachmiel A, Manor R, Peled M, Laufer D: Intraoral distraction osteogenesis of the mandible in hemifacial microsomia. *J Oral Maxillofac Surg* 2001;59(7):728–733.
25. Chiapasco M, Romeo E, Casentini P, Rimondini L: Alveolar distraction osteogenesis vs. vertical guided bone regeneration for the correction of vertically deficient edentulous ridges: a 1–3-year prospective study on humans. *Clin Oral Implants Res* 2004;15:82–95.
26. Garcia-Garcia A, Somoza-Martin M, Gandara-Vila P, Saulacic N, Gandara-Rey J: Alveolar distraction before insertion of dental implants in the posterior mandible. *Br J Oral Maxillofac Surg* 2003;41:376–379.
27. Jensen O, Cockrell R, Kuhike L, Reed C: Anterior maxillary alveolar distraction osteogenesis: a prospective 5-year clinical study. *Int J Oral Maxillofac Implants* 2002;17:52–68.
28. Gaggl A, Schultes G, Karcher H: Vertical alveolar ridge distraction with prosthetic treatable distractors: a clinical investigation. *Int J Oral Maxillofac Implants* 2000;15:701–710.
29. Feichtinger M, Gaggl A, Schultes G, Karcher H: Evaluation of distraction implants for prosthetic treatment after vertical alveolar ridge distraction: a clinical investigation. *Int J Prosthodont* 2003;16:19–24.
30. Krenkel C, Grunert I: The Endo-Distractor for preimplant mandibular regeneration. *Rev Stomatol Chir Maxillofac* 2009;110(1):17–26.
31. Raghoebar G, Liem R, Vissink A: Vertical distraction of the severely resorbed edentulous mandible: a clinical, histological and electron microscopic study of 10 treated cases. *Clin Oral Implants Res* 2002;13:558–565.
32. Robiony M, Polini F, Costa F, Politi M: Osteogenesis distraction and plateletrich plasma for bone restoration of the severely atrophic mandible: preliminary results. *J Oral Maxillofac Surg* 2002;60:630–635.
33. Saulacic N, Iizuka T, Martin MS, Garcia AG: Alveolar distraction osteogenesis: a systematic review. *Int J Oral Maxillofac Surg* 2008;37:1–7.
34. Hwang S, Jung JG, Jung JU, Kyung S: Vertical alveolar bone distraction at molar region using lag screw principle. *J Oral Maxillofac Surg* 2004;62:787–794.
35. Kim S, Mitsugi M, Kim B: Simultaneous sinus lifting and alveolar distraction of the atrophic maxillary alveolus for implant placement: a preliminary report. *Implant Dent* 2005;14:344–348.
36. Jensen O, Ueda M, Laster Z, Mommaerts M, Rachmiel A: Alveolar distraction osteogenesis. *Selected Readings in Oral and Maxillofacial Surgery* 2002;10(4):1–48.
37. Laster Z, Rachmiel A, Jensen O: Alveolar width distraction osteogenesis for early implant placement. *J Oral Maxillofac Surg* 2005;63(12):1724–1730.
38. Laster Z, Reem Y, Nagler R: Horizontal alveolar ridge distraction in an edentulous patient. *J Oral Maxillofac Surg* 2011;69(2):502–506.
39. Gaggl A, Schultes G, Kärcher H: Distraction implants: a new operative technique for alveolar ridge augmentation. *J Craniomaxillofac Surg* 1999;27:214–221.
40. Gaggl A, Schultes G, Rainer H, Kärcher H: The transgingival approach for placement of distraction implants. *J Oral Maxillofac Surg* 2002;60:793–796.
41. McAllister B: Histologic and radiographic evidence of vertical ridge augmentation utilizing distraction osteogenesis: 10 consecutively placed distractors. *J Periodontol* 2001;72(12):1767–1779.
42. McAllister B, Gaffaney T: Distraction osteogenesis for vertical bone augmentation prior to oral implant reconstruction. *Periodontol 2000* 33:54–66.
43. Yang L, Suzuki E, Suzuki B: Alveolar distraction osteogenesis: a systematic literature review. *Med Dent J* 2014;34(3):289–300.
44. Aizenbud D, Hazan-Molina H, Cohen M, Rachmiel A: Combined orthodontic temporary anchorage devices and surgical management of the alveolar ridge augmentation using distraction osteogenesis. *J Oral Maxillofac Surg* 2012;70(8):1815–1826.
45. Grayson B, McCormick S, Santiago P, McCarthy J: Vector of device placement and trajectory of mandibular distraction. *J Craniofac Surg* 1997;8:473–480.
46. Rachmiel A, Emodi O, Gutmacher Z, Blumenfeld I, Aizenbud D: Oral and dental restoration of wide alveolar cleft using distraction osteogenesis and temporary anchorage devices. *J Craniomaxillofac Surg* 2013;41(8):728–734.
47. Shibuya Y, Takata N, Ishida S, Takeuchi J, Kobayashi M, Suzuki H, et al: Prevention of lingual inclination of the transport segment in vertical distraction osteogenesis in the mandible. *Implant Dent* 2012;21(5):374–378.
48. Herford A, Audia F: Maintaining vector control during alveolar distraction osteogenesis: a technical note. *Int J Oral Maxillofac Implants* 2004;19(5):758–762.
49. Pérez-Sayáns M, León-Camacho Mde L, Somoza-Martín J, Fernández-González B, Blanes-Vázquez-Gundín S, Gándara-Rey J, et al: Dental implants placed on bone

subjected to vertical alveolar distraction show the same performance as those placed on primitive bone. *Med Oral Patol Oral Cir Bucal* 2013;18(4):e686–692.
50 Zwetyenga N, Vidal N, Ella B, Siberchicot F, Emparanza A: Results of oral implant-supported prostheses after mandibular vertical alveolar ridge distraction: a propos of 54 sites. *Oral Surg Oral Med Oral Pathol Oral Radiol* 2012; 114(6):725–732.
51 Kim J, Cho M, Kim S, Kim M: Alveolar distraction osteogenesis versus autogenous onlay bone graft for vertical augmentation of severely atrophied alveolar ridges after 12 years of long-term follow-up. *Oral Surg Oral Med Oral Pathol Oral Radiol* 2013;116(5):540–549.
52 Chen D, Zhao M, Mundy G: Bone morphogenetic proteins. *Growth Factors* 2004; 22(4):233–241.
53 Rachmiel A, Aizenbud D, Peled M: Enhancement of bone formation by bone morphogenetic protein-2 during alveolar distraction: an experimental study in sheep. *J Periodontol* 2004;75(11):1524–1531.
54 Rachmiel A, Leiser Y: The molecular and cellular events that take place during craniofacial distraction osteogenesis. *Plast Reconstr Surg Glob Open* 2014;2(1):e98.
55 Yonezawa H, Harada K, Ikebe T, Shinohara M, Enomoto S: Effect of recombinant human bone morphogenetic protein-2 (rhBMP-2) on bone consolidation on distraction osteogenesis: a preliminary study in rabbit mandibles. *J Craniomaxillofac Surg* 2006;34(5):270–276.
56 Earley M, Butts S: Update on mandibular distraction osteogenesis. *Curr Opin Otolaryngol Head Neck Surg* 2014;22(4):276–283.
57 Chiapasco M, Lang N, Bosshardt D: Quality and quantity of bone following alveolar distraction osteogenesis in the human mandible. *Clin Oral Implants Res* 2006; 17(4):394–402.
58 Elo J, Herford A, Boyne P: Implant success in distracted bone versus autogenous bone-grafted sites. *J Oral Implantol* 2009;35(4):181–184.
59 Oda T, Sawaki Y, Ueda M: Alveolar ridge augmentation by distraction osteogenesis using titanium implants: an experimental study. *Int J Oral Maxillofac Surg* 1999; 28(2):151–156.
60 Enislidis G, Fock N, Ewers R: Distraction osteogenesis with subperiosteal devices in edentulous mandibles. *Br J Oral Maxillofac Surg* 2005;43(5):399–403.
61 Ettl T, Gerlach T, Schüsselbauer T, Gosau M, Reichert T, Driemel O: Bone resorption and complications in alveolar distraction osteogenesis. *Clin Oral Investig* 2010;15(5):481–489.
62 Froum S, Rosenberg E, Elian N, Tarnow D, Cho S: Distraction osteogenesis for ridge augmentation: prevention and treatment of complications. Thirty case reports. *Int J Periodontics Restorative Dent* 2008;28(4):337–345.
63 Günbay T, Koyuncu B, Akay M, Sipahi A, Tekin U: Results and complications of alveolar distraction osteogenesis to enhance vertical bone height. *Oral Surg Oral Med Oral Pathol Oral Radiol Endod* 2008;105(5):e7–13.
64 Klug C, Millesi-Schobel G, Millesi W, Watzinger F, Ewers R: Preprosthetic vertical distraction osteogenesis of the mandible using an L-shaped osteotomy and titanium membranes for guided bone regeneration. *J Oral Maxillofac Surg* 2001;59(11): 1302–1308.
65 Mazzonetto R, Serra E, Silva F, Ribeiro Torezan J: Clinical assessment of 40 patients subjected to alveolar distraction osteogenesis. *Implant Dent* 2005;14(2):149–153.
66 Polo W, Cury P, Sendyk W, Gromatzky A: Posterior mandibular alveolar distraction osteogenesis utilizing an extraosseous distractor: a prospective study. *J Periodontol* 2005;76:1463–1468.
67 Saulacić N, Somosa Martín M, de Los Angeles Leon Camacho M, García-García A: Complications in alveolar distraction osteogenesis: a clinical investigation. *J Oral Maxillofac Surg* 2007;65(2):267–274.
68 Saulacic N, Somoza-Martin M, Gándara-Vila P, Garcia-Garcia A: Relapse in alveolar distraction osteogenesis: an indication for overcorrection. *J Oral Maxillofac Surg* 2005;63(7):978–981.
69 Wolvius E, Scholtemeijer M, Weijland M, Hop W, van der Wal K: Complications and relapse in alveolar distraction osteogenesis in partially dentulous patients. *Int J Oral Maxillofac Surg* 2007;36(8):700–705.
70 Zaffe D, Bertoldi C, Palumbo C, Consolo U: Morphofunctional and clinical study on mandibular alveolar distraction osteogenesis. *Clin Oral Implants Res* 2002; 13(5):550–557.
71 Ugurlu F, Sener B, Dergin G, Garip H: Potential complications and precautions in vertical alveolar distraction osteogenesis: a retrospective study of 40 patients. *J Craniomaxillofac Surg* 2013;41(7):569–573.

CHAPTER 23

Management of Complications of Alveolar Distraction Osteogenesis Procedure

Stephanie J. Drew

Private Practice, The New York Center for Orthognathic and Maxillofacial Surgery, West Islip, New York
Stony Brook University Hospital and Hofstra Medical School, New York, USA

Introduction

Complications from distraction surgery can occur at any time during the treatment of these challenging patients. A time line from the initial evaluation, diagnosis, planning stages, execution of the surgical plan, and, finally, long-term complications should be noted (Figure 23.1). This time line approach is a way to break down sequences of treatment to find where things did not go as planned and to help prevent them in the future with better insight. References [1] to [15] provide the reader with an excellent review of complications reported.

Pre-operative complications

1. Failure to diagnose (properly)

Evaluation of the patient for distraction surgery begins with a thorough hard and soft tissue examination. The type of tissue overlying the defect as well as a history of radiation treatment in these areas will impact the overall predictability of healing from this surgery. When the tissue type is thin (thin gingival biotype), slowing down the rate of distraction may be necessary to prevent the leading transport disk edges from breaking through the tissues. Care should also be taken to make sure there are no sharp edges in these areas. If connective tissues will be needed it should be planned for later on as the vascularity of the graft may be challenged by the flap designs for distraction surgery if these flaps have not been given enough time to revascularize.

Hard tissue evaluation by computed tomography (CT) or cone beam CT (CBCT) is a must to allow planning and measurements to be done. Without a CT scan, an operator would be guessing at what the actual height and width of bone actually are. This tool will not only let you see how much bone is available but also where to place the osteotomies. Poor planning of transport disk size will often lead to loss of stability of the distractor and worse the whole transport disk due to devascularization of the segment. Proper planning at this stage will also allow you to see where to place the distractors to avoid vital structures such as the teeth roots, nerves or the sinus.

Failure to make a proper diagnosis is often a common issue. Distraction can lift up a thin piece of bone to get good height but onlay grafting will be needed at a second surgery to get the width necessary for fixture placement. Sequencing the onlay grafting first may also be a good choice, depending upon the soft tissues available for good wound healing.

Recognizing compliance issues for patients is very important here. If the patient cannot turn the distractor on his/her own, the disk will prematurely fuse. If he/she will turn too much or too fast the distraction chamber will fill with fibrous tissue and not bone. Thus, careful follow-up of this process is a must. Seeing these patients every 3–5 days during the actual distraction will give a surgeon more control over the process. If a patient refuses to turn the distractor, then the patient should be seen daily until the doctor completes distraction.

2. Failure to control the vector of distraction

Poor planning of the vector is another area in the pre-operative time slot that can lead to complications during the distraction period. If the vector is not correct, the bone will wind up in the wrong position (usually, too much to the palate or lingual side). Once this issue is recognized, several steps can take place to correct it (Figure 23.2). First the base plate can be repositioned and the disk can be manipulated while still attached to the upper moving plate. Not stripping the mucosa off the moving segment is important. The vector position can be accepted if it is not too far off and will not interfere with implant position. A CT scan and implant treatment planning software can help to monitor this issue.

3. Failure to execute proper planning of osteotomy

Osteotomy design is particularly important when thinking of how the segment will move and also of how it will impact the non-moving segment. When there is a small volume of bone left in the mandible (often with osteotomies with sharp angles where the vertical cuts meet the horizontal cuts), this may cause a point of weakness and predispose the patient to fracture of the inferior border of the mandible. In these cases, rounding the edges of where these osteotomies meet will decrease this risk of mandible fracture as long as there is enough bone to support the inferior border (typically, 10 mm of non-moving bone segment should be left intact).

Vertical Alveolar Ridge Augmentation in Implant Dentistry: A Surgical Manual, First Edition. Edited by Len Tolstunov.
© 2016 John Wiley & Sons, Inc. Published 2016 by John Wiley & Sons, Inc.

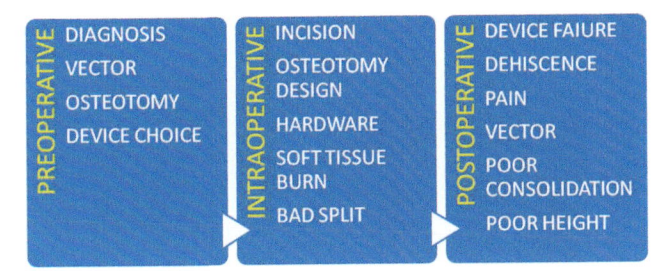

Figure 23.1 Time line of complications (pre-operative, intraoperative, and post-operative).

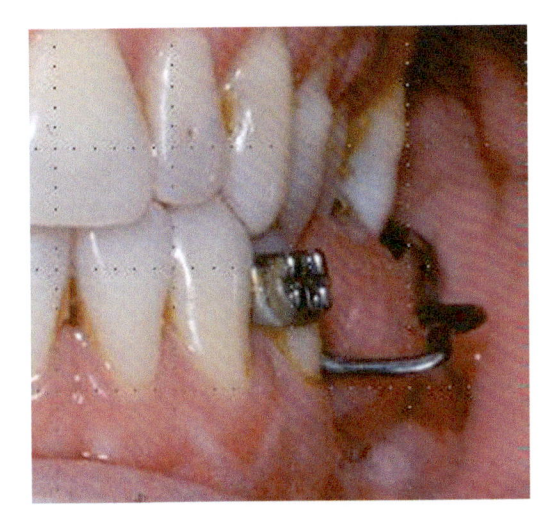

Figure 23.2 Orthodontic wire used to hold the distractor arm in position while lifting up the transport segment.

4. Choosing the wrong distractor

Hardware choices (picking the distractor) are made from knowing the distance needed to travel, the amount of bone volume of the transport disk and the basal non-moving bone for the base plate, space for the moving plate, and the ability to adjust it, if needed. If the wrong device is chosen, the result can be compromised and the needed required bone height might be too short. If the distraction rod is too long, it may interfere with the occlusion (Figure 23.3). The distractor may always be changed, if necessary. Given enough time for healing (consolidation), in the case of height deficiency, the upper part of the distractor can be unscrewed, the osteotomies can be recut, the distractor can be closed again, and the upper arm can be reattached lower than before; in this way the distractor can be opened again along the track and lifted to the desired position.

Intraoperative complications

1. Poor incision design

Flap design should be directed at avoiding vital anatomy while maintaining vascularity of the transport disk. Typically the incisions for distraction are placed in the unattached mucosa on the lateral aspect of the bone to keep the moving disk viable. If this mucosa is stripped off for access, it can easily become devascularized. The tissue can be extremely delicate and should be treated with care.

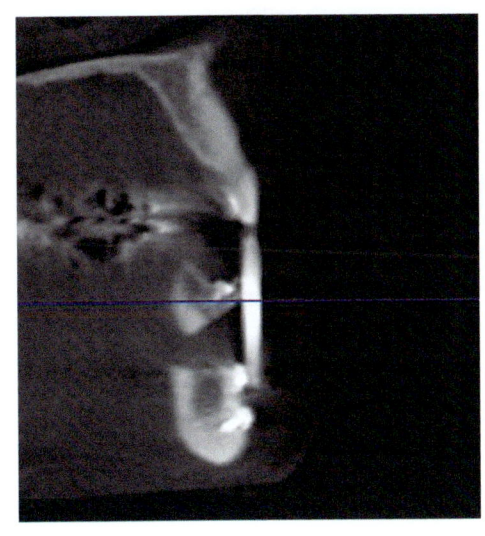

Figure 23.3 Distraction rod is under the tip of the incisor. This could damage the tooth as well as loosen the distractor.

2. Failed osteotomy

Poor osteotomy and "bad split" can happen with distraction surgery if the osteotomies are incomplete and one tries to separate the transport disk. There should only be minimal forces applied once these osteotomies are cut to separate it from the base. When this happens, the buccal plate usually separates from the medial portion of bone. It is advisable to stabilize this segment and abandon the distraction surgery. Let the bones heal and come back another time.

Also of concern is too much force, which can lead to a fracture of the basal bone, especially in the mandible. If the distractor cannot stabilize these fractures, they must be treated appropriately with rigid fixation or intermaxillary fixation, if indicated.

3. Hardware failure

Stripping of screws is a problem ("tight is good, too tight is busted"). Fingertight is the rule (Figure 23.4). These screws need to be retrieved later for placing implants. Failure of the device to move or fracture of the device may also occur. This is a mechanical device.

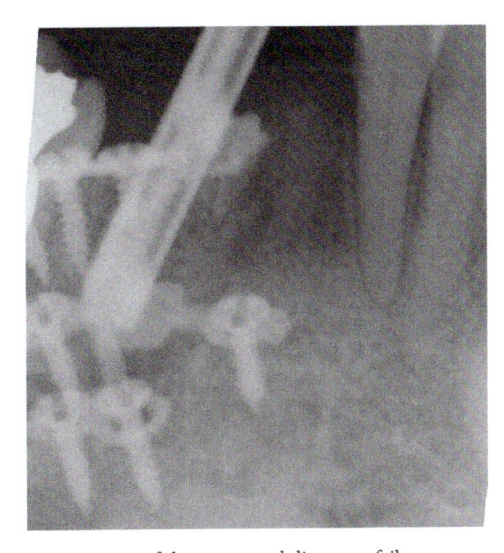

Figure 23.4 Loosening of the screws and distractor failure.

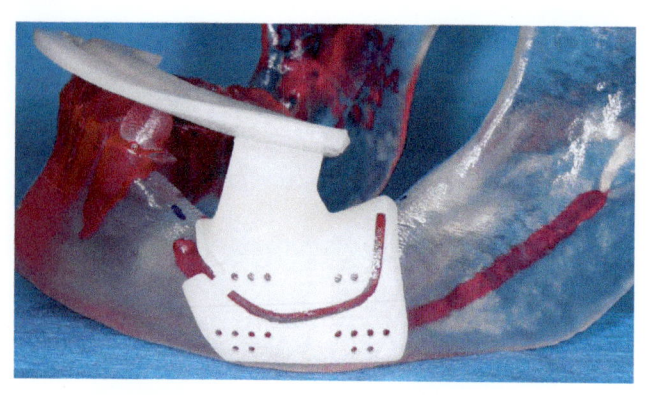

Figure 23.5 Cutting jig that can used for treatment planning and avoidance of complications of the distraction process.

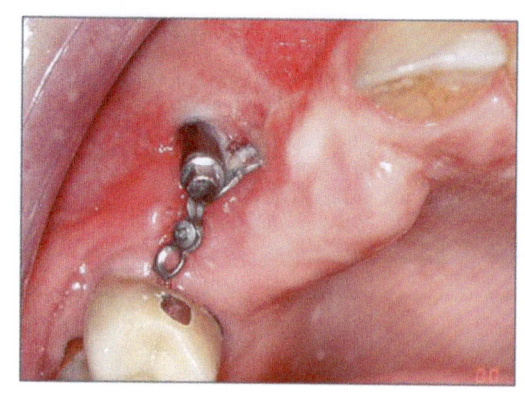

Figure 23.6 Exposure of the distractor arm plate. It might just be necessary to continue monitoring, improve hygiene of the device, and use chlorhexidine rinse.

It has moving parts that can fail or fracture. Since the titanium is so brittle, multiple bends of the arms can lead to stress fractures where they attach to the distractor body. The solder joint can also fracture if the device is not properly supported during the bending process.

4. Poor soft tissue management

Burning of tissue with a piezo knife is a significant problem for tissue vitality and wound healing. Though a precise and thin cut looks great on radiographs, the piezo knife itself can be challenging to use in thin cuts that are deep, like the horizontal cut of the transport disk segment. The blade heats up and can actually burn the palatal or lingual tissues. Consider cutting the initial cuts with a piezo knife and finishing with osteotomes similar to a segmental Le Fort osteotomy. Laceration of the lingual of palatal mucosa may occur. If it happened on the vertical cut it is not as critical as the horizontal cut. Laceration of the lingual or palatal soft tissue on the horizontal osteotomy can devascularize the segment. For the horizontal cut, an operator should allow at least two weeks for the soft tissue healing before activation of the device. If the segment does not move, a little gentle pressure through the original incision on the transport bone will loosen the segment. If that does not do, then the osteotomies need to be recut.

5. Bone osteotomies have the wrong shape, size, or are in the wrong place

There is another issue with a very thin cut. The transport disk bone needs room to move up. The bone can bind as it is moving up if the cuts are not divergent enough and too parallel. It is very unforgiving also if the vector is off. Opening the space a couple of millimeters will give the transport segment of bone some space. Bone cuts that are too close to teeth can lead to root damage due to devitalization or root section. Cutting guides (jigs) are a big help when there is a limited amount of space (Figure 23.5).

Post-operative complications

1. Device failure

There are two reasons why the device will not turn. First, the device is broken. Either the ring does not engage the screw or the plate is fractured off the moving disk. Second, the osteotomy is jammed. Again, this needs to be addressed before the segment consolidates. It can be freed up by widening the vertical osteotomies. The horizontal osteotomy is not typically the issue unless there is consolidation.

If the plates fracture off the distraction rod at the moving segment, the device needs to be replaced. If a part of the base plate fractures and the rod is still stable with the remainder of the support, it is possible to find a way to stabilize the rod superiorly with an occlusal splint or orthodontic wire and try to continue. If it remains unstable, then it is vital to change the device.

Screws can also loosen in the segments of either the moving disk or the base plate. If the device becomes unstable because of loose screws, it needs to be restabilized by new screws sometimes using the old screw holes [2].

2. Device dehiscence

As the leading edge of the transport disk rises, the tissue may dehisce over the titanium. As long as the device remains stable, treat this conservatively with good hygiene and chlorhexidine rinses (Figure 23.6).

3. Infection

As with any oral surgery, infection is a risk. This is especially true since the distractor is a foreign body protruding through the mucosa. Good oral hygiene is a must and chlorhexidine rinse is often administered perioperatively. A soft diet is important to prevent forces of mastication that can loosen the device.

4. Pain

After the initial inflammatory response, the patient typically should not complain of significant discomfort or pain. This is also true when turning the distraction screw. Pain in these cases during the distraction period may indicate infection or device failure or binding of the segments. Pain also may be an issue is if the sharp edge of the osteotomy on the moving segment is pushing through the mucosa.

5. Incorrect vector

There are several reasons why the vector is noted to be incorrect as the distraction device is being turned [12–14]. First, the original alignment was incorrect. Second, bound soft tissue on the medial surfaces (lingual or palatal) are tight and pulling the segment in this direction. Third, the device has failed.

In all cases the options to manage this complication would be to reposition the device by manual pressure under local anesthesia and then place a splint or orthodontic wire to stabilize the distraction rod. Second, the device can be removed and repositioned. If the device has to be repositioned, an operator should unscrew only the base plate from the bone, leaving the screws on the moving disk connected and tight. After this, the device will function as intended.

Post-consolidation complications

There is nothing more disappointing than not achieving a successful outcome. The distraction surgery itself could have moved the segment up but several other issues may interfere with proper implant placement.

1. Inadequate bone formation in the distraction chamber

Most of the time, this is not a complication. It takes a long time for the chamber to completely ossify. By 12 weeks post-distraction, the vertical edges should be well healed and the moving disk stabilized. It is important to remember that the area must be at least 50% calcified to see easily on a radiograph. Therefore, if the edges are beginning to heal, it is good to assume that the chamber will be filled in over more time. There is usually no need to delay placing of implants into the new bone after 4 months if it is confirmed as calcified on the radiograph.

If the width looks inadequate, the rod may have been turned too quickly. In this case, it almost looks like "pulled taffy." Since the disk above can heal on the vertical walls and this bone will consolidate over time, at the time of distractor removal additional bone such as allogeneic bone particles can be placed in onlay fashion to bulk out the site facial to the chamber. It is essential not to "clean" the new woven or soft bone out of the chamber; it will heal with more time.

2. Inadequate height (distraction)

Several reasons exist as to why inadequate bone height can happen at the completion of the distraction process [4, 5]. The first issue is the wrong choice of distractor rod height. Second, the moving disk piece binds up and prematurely consolidates. Third, the rotating pin was not turned all the way to meet the needs of the plan.

If this complication occurs, dental implants may wind up being in an inadequate vertical position relative to the prosthesis. The choice would be to accept the position or to recut the osteotomies and move the pieces up some more. If it is only a few millimeters, the other alveolar bone augmentation choices (described in this book) can be in order, like sandwich osteotomy. In this case, the patient will not have to go through another 3–4 months of distraction. Most of experts in different alveolar bone augmentation procedures agree on overcorrection to prevent primary or secondary bone loss (relapse). Overcorrection of distraction will bring more bone to allow for the resorption along the leading edge of the distraction segment [5].

The last issue is related to the implants placed into the distracted bone. It has been noted in some distraction cases that the bone around the implants may develop peri-implant bone resorption [10, 11].

Case Report

The patient had a distraction surgery done to move a two-tooth segment vertically after loss of bone height and width. The bone was cut with a piezo knife. A latency period was 7 days. The distraction started at a rate of 0.3 mm per day. Upon day 4 of distraction, the wound was noted to break down (Figure 23.7). The segment and the chamber were becoming exposed. The rate was slowed down to one turn per day and the wound kept clean with chlorhexidine rinses (Figure 23.8). The segment was lifted into the desired height and the mucosa eventually healed (Figure 23.9). The width, however, was deficient (Figure 23.10). The segment was allowed to heal, the distractor was removed, and the soft tissues were also allowed to heal. The width was then achieved with a block graft harvested from the ramus (Figure 23.11). The bone healed for 5 additional months prior to implant placement (Figures 23.12 to 23.14).

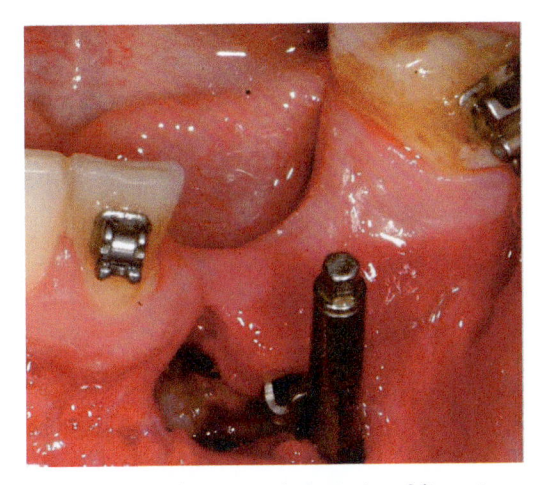

Figure 23.7 Wound dehiscence at the beginning of distraction.

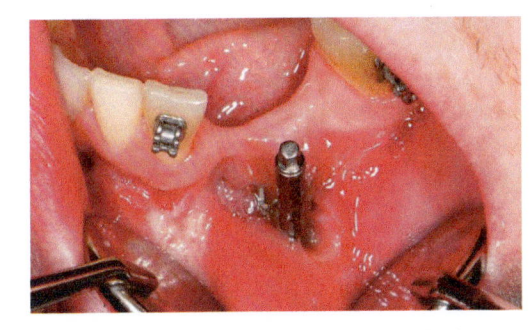

Figure 23.8 The distraction rate was decreased and the device was kept cleaned; the soft tissue healed and the bone moved up into the proper vertical position.

(continued)

(Continued)

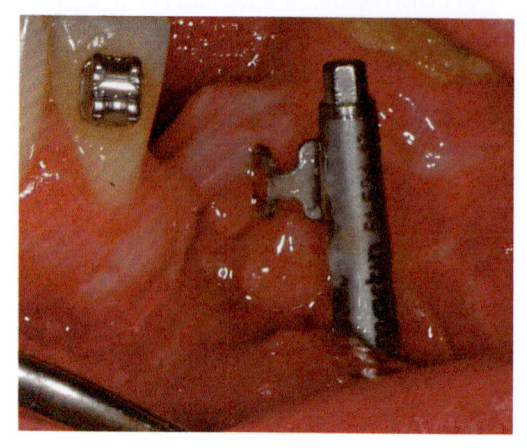

Figure 23.9 Although vertical bone height was achieved, there was not enough alveolar width for implant placement.

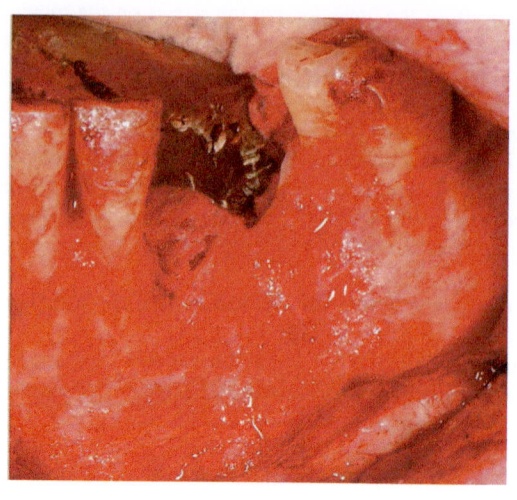

Figure 23.10 Deficient bone width after the distraction osteogenesis process and prior to block bone grafting.

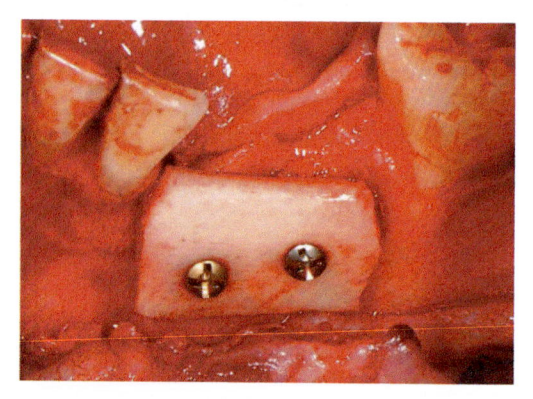

Figure 23.11 Block graft from the posterior mandible was fixated to improve the alveolar bone width.

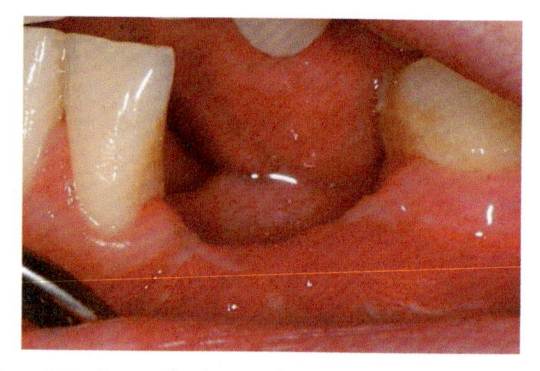

Figure 23.12 Bone and soft tissues healed over the grafted site.

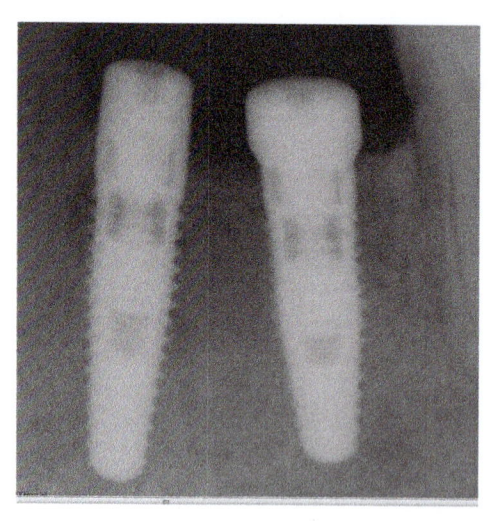

Figure 23.13 Radiograph demonstrating the two-implant placement.

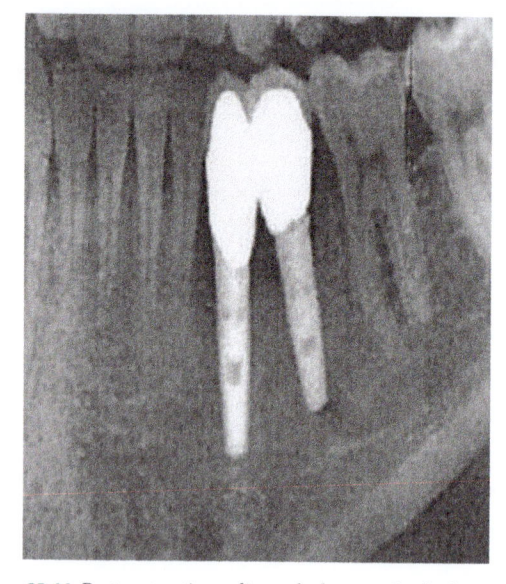

Figure 23.14 Post-restorative radiograph showing the final restoration.

Conclusion

The advents of three-dimensional planning with CBCT scans, stereolithic modeling, and the use of modern surgical tools like the piezo knife have improved distraction osteogenesis procedure and allowed more predictable outcomes. The use of morphologic classification described in 2004 by Garcia-Garcia et al. [15] of the distraction defects helped to decrease the complications associated with placing implants into the distracted sites. The system describes a classification of Type I for bone with no defect in the distraction chamber, Type II for having a good cortical rim with small concavity on the facial, Type III for a narrow rim and lateral bone concavity, and Type IV for having a bone bridge with no bone seen in the distraction chamber site. A subcategory D is used as a modifier when the transport disk is displaced lingually or palatally (for more details on this classification system please refer to Chapter 20 on Diagnosis and Treatment Planning in this section). The goal of following this classification system is to improve overall implant survival, which is the ultimate goal of distraction of the alveolus.

Distraction surgery is a very labor-intensive and technique-sensitive procedure. Mastering the small nuances of DO devices and the surgery takes time and practice. The surgery itself is not difficult, but the best results are only achieved with excellent planning and thorough control during the distraction process.

References

1. Gunbay T, Koyuncu BO, Akay MC, Sipahi A, Tekin U: Results and complications of alveolar distraction osteogenesis to enhance vertical bone height. Oral Surg Oral Med Oral Pathol Oral Radiol Endod 2008 May;105(5):7–13.
2. Muglali M, Inal S, Bas B, Bekcioglu B, Celebi N: Fixation of vertically distracted segment with dental implants after breakage of distraction device: case report. Oral Surg Oral Med Oral Pathol Oral Radiol Endod 2008 May:105(5):25–27.
3. Perdijk FB, Meijer GJ, Strijen PJ, Koole R: Complications in alveolar distraction osteogenesis of the atrophic mandible. Int J Oral Maxillofac Surg 2007 Oct;36(10):916–921.
4. Wolvius EB, Scholtemeijer M, Weijland M, Hop WE, van der Wal KG: Complications and relapse in alveolar distraction osteogeneis in partially dentulous patients. Int J Oral Maxillofac Surg 2007 Aug;36(8):700–705.
5. Saulacic N, Somoza-Martin M, Gandara-Vila P, Garcia-Garcia A: Relapse in alveolar distraction osteogenesis: an indication for over correction. Oral Maxillofac Surg 2005 Jul;63(7):978–981.
6. Enislidis G, Fock N, Millesi-Schogel G, Klug C, Wittwer G, Yerit K, Ewers R: Analysis of complications following alveolar distraction osteogenesis and implant placement in the partially edentulous mandible. Oral Surg Oral Med Oral Pathol Oral Radiol Endod 2005 Jul;100(1):25–30.
7. Garcia AG, Martin MS, Vila PG, Maceiras JL: Minor complications arising in alveolar distraction osteogenesis. J Oral Maxillofac Surg 2002 May;60(5):496–501.
8. Froum SJ, Rosenberg ES, Elian N, Tarnow D, Cho SC: Distraction osteogenesis for ridge augmentation: prevention and treatment of complications, thirty case reports. Int J Periodontics Restorative Dent 2008 Aug;28(4):337–345.
9. Perdijk FB, Meijer GJ, Soehardi A, Koole R: A lower border augmentation technique to allow implant placement after a bilateral mandibular fracture as a complication of vertical distraction osteogenesis; a case report. Int J Oral Maxillofac Surg 2013 Jul;42(7):897–900.
10. Ettl T, Gerlach T, Schusselbauer T, Gosau M, Reichert TE, Driemel O: Bone resorption and complications in alveolar distraction osteogenesis. Clin Oral Investig 2010 Oct;14(5):481–489.
11. Perez-Sayans M, Fernendez-Gonzalez B, Somoza-Martin M, Gandara-Rey JM, Garcia-Garcia A: Peri-implant bone resorption around implants placed in alveolar bone subjected to distraction osteogenesis. J Oral Maxillofac Surg 2008 Apr;66(4):787–790.
12. Oh H, Park HJ, Cho JY, Park YJ, Kook MS: Vector control of malpositioned segment during alveolar distraction osteogenesis by using rubber traction. J Oral Maxillofac Surg 2009 Mar;67(3):608–612.
13. Kilic E, Kilic K, Alkan A: Alternative method to reposition the dislocated transport segment during vertical alveolar distraction. J Oral Maxillofac Surg 2009 Oct;67(10):2306–2310.
14. Oncu E, Isik K, Alaaddinoglu EE, Ickan S: Combined use of alveolar distraction osteogenesis and segmental osteotomy in anterior vertical ridge augmentation. Int J Surg Case Rep 2015 Jan 28;8C:124–126.
15. Garcia-Garcia A, Somoza Martin M, Gadara Vila P, Gandara Rey JM: A preliminary morphologic classification of the alveolar ridge after distraction osteogenesis. J Oral Maxillofac Surg 2004 May;62(5):563–566.

SECTION V

Autogenous Block Bone Grafting for Vertical Alveolar Ridge Augmentation

CHAPTER 24
Vertical Alveolar Ridge Augmentation with Autogenous Block Grafts in Implant Dentistry

Vishtasb Broumand,[1] Arash Khojasteh,[2] and J. Marshall Green, III[3]

[1]Private Practice, Oral and Maxillofacial Surgery, Phoenix, Arizona, USA
Department of Oral and Maxillofacial Surgery, University of Florida College of Dentistry, Gainesville, Florida, USA
A.T. Still University, MD Anderson Cancer Center, Arizona School of Dentistry and Oral Health, Mesa, Arizona, USA
[2]Department of Oral and Maxillofacial Surgery, Dental Research Center, Dental School, Shahid Beheshti University of Medical Sciences, Tehran, Iran
[3]Lieutenant US Navy, Maxillofacial Oncology and Reconstructive Surgery, Division of Oral and Maxillofacial Surgery, University of Miami, Miller School of Medicine, Miami, Florida, USA

Introduction

Osseous defects of the maxillofacial region, prompting the investigation of autogenous bone harvest sites and advancement of grafting techniques, have long been a driving force in the clinical practice of surgeons focused on the head and neck region. More specifically the return of the maxilla and mandible to near anatomic shape and size for dental rehabilitation with endosseous implants is constantly an area of interest [1]. Defects of the maxilla and mandible often range from those associated with continuity defects to smaller localized losses of the alveolar bone proper. These osseous defects often are the result of cancer, pathologic processes, trauma, infection, or due to secondary edentulation and aging as a result of poor dental health [2]. To narrow the scope of discussion, focus will be given here only to the vertical augmentation of the maxillary and mandibular ridges.

The history of bone grafting is intertwined with conflict as many of the publications and advancements associated with this topic have been the direct result of armed conflicts such as World Wars I and II. While many of the techniques previously developed such as the block tibial harvest have fallen from use, these early pioneers paved the way out of an era where facial osseous defects often went unconstructed to today where bone grafts have developed into much more of a science. In this field autogenous bone has long proved to be the gold standard, but rapid developments in the understanding of bone physiology and growth have led to near equal if not superior results with no autogenous harvest required. While many of the alternatives to autogenous bone grafting have proven to be quite technique sensitive, the tried and true methods of block graft harvesting and subsequent vertical ridge augmentation within the scope of the oral and maxillofacial surgeon will be covered here in detail.

Optimal donor site depends on the volume and type of regenerated bone needed for the specific case. The following common non-vascular block bone harvests will be discussed: anterior and posterior ilium, ramus, chin, and cranium [3]. Selection of graft sites and their appropriate indications will be discussed in detail as well as techniques with various modifications such as interpositional bone grafting, cortical autogenous tenting and inferior alveolar nerve lateralization [4]. Caveats and various pitfalls in harvesting will be presented as well as incorporation of new modalities available to the surgeon, such as distraction osteogenesis and inferior alveolar nerve lateralization [5]. Novel approaches that apply concepts of tissue engineering such as bone morphogenetic protein and mesenchymal stem cells will be discussed as well [6].

Applied surgical anatomy, indications, contraindications, approaches, post-operative care, and complications as they relate to outcomes will be reviewed.

Recipient site classification and defect analysis

The focus of bone grafting studies has been mainly on improving the techniques and introducing novel augmentation materials to provide more promising outcomes. However, the variation among studies does not allow for a generalized conclusion on the effectiveness of the suggested protocols [7]. This inconsistency may be partly due to imprecise consideration of the properties of recipient sites within the study designs [8]. Morphological classification divided the jaw defects to the vertical, horizontal, and combined defects [9]. Khojasteh et al. presented their classification based on the importance of the vertical bone walls and width of the recipient site [8]. When the recipient site has two vertical walls it is Class "A," whereas with one vertical wall it is class "B," and without walls it is class "C." The second feature considered in the current classification is the width of the defect's base. Width site is divided to three groups: I: more than 5 mm; II: between 3 and 5 mm; III: less than 3 mm (Figure 24.1a and b).

Another potential factor affecting bone regeneration is the length of the edentulous span, which alters the surface area of a defect, hence influencing the degree of vascularization. Various studies have demarcated this factor by using terms such as localized or extensive ridge augmentation, though these have not been explicitly defined. Localized defects seem to pertain to missing teeth areas within a range of 1 to 6 teeth [10, 11]. while extensive augmentations often indicate a fully edentulous jaw [12].

Vertical Alveolar Ridge Augmentation in Implant Dentistry: A Surgical Manual, First Edition. Edited by Len Tolstunov.
© 2016 John Wiley & Sons, Inc. Published 2016 by John Wiley & Sons, Inc.

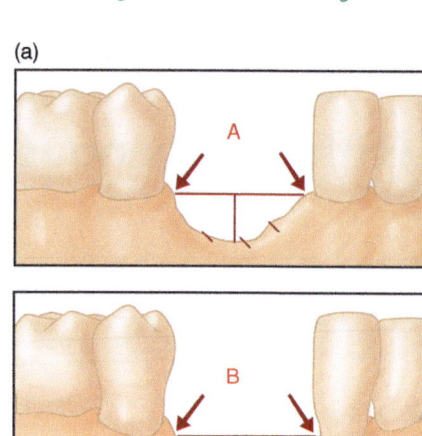

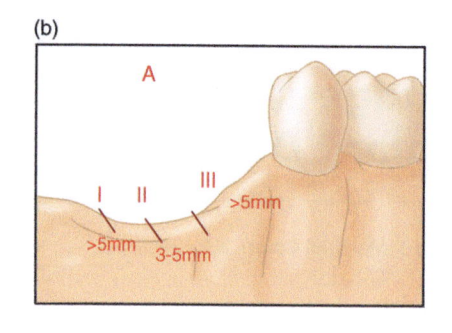

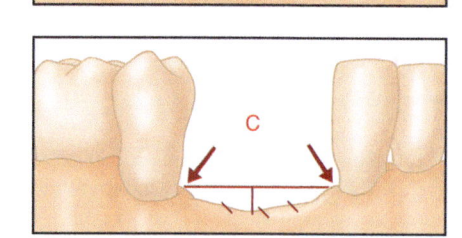

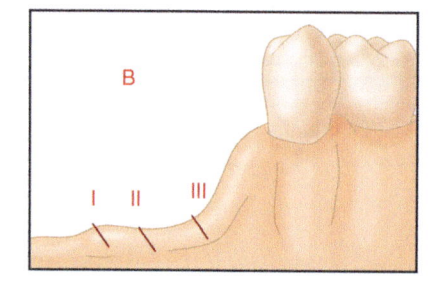

Figure 24.1 (a) Class A: two-wall defect, Class B: one-wall defect, Class C: defect with no surrounding bony walls. (b) Width of the defect's base: Class I: > 5mm, Class II: between 3mm and 5mm; Class III: < 3mm

Description of the technique: donor sites for block bone

Intraoral harvest
Ramus

Often definitive reconstruction of the maxillomandibular complex requires localized reconstruction of small horizontal or vertical defects. These are often associated with localized defects and desired implant restorations. When a small area of augmentation in a vertical or horizontal dimension is desired, the ramus is an obvious choice of primarily cortical bone stock. The amount of bone that can be harvested depends on the overall shape of the patient's mandible and the location of the mandibular canal. An average graft size ranges from 1 to 2 cm in length and 1 cm in height. A cone beam CT scanner can aid significantly in planning these surgeries due to the ability to appropriately identify not only the height but also the buncolingual position of the inferior alveolar canal in relation to the desired graft site. The benefits of this procedure are the proximity of the graft harvest site to the recipient site, low rate of post-operative complications, and familiarity with the anatomy associated with the procedure [13]. In contrast, the downsides of ramus harvest include a relatively small availability of bone and the rare potential for lip numbness following the procedure. Anesthesia can be achieved with local alone or i.v. sedation may provide additional benefit to the patient.

The surgical technique for a ramus block graft harvest entails an approach very similar to the removal of a full bone impacted wisdom tooth or the approach to a sagittal ramus osteotomy. After locating the external oblique ridge, which is the site of bone harvest, a local anesthesia can be injected with epinephrine to aid in hemostasis of the area. Surgical incision can be a sulcular design in the presence of adjacent teeth and include a distal release or can be placed laterally over the external oblique ridge in a vertical design. Incisions should be carried down through mucosa and subcutaneous tissues through the periosteum in a full-thickness fashion. This can be accomplished with a 15 blade or bovie cautery, which can aid in hemostasis. The periosteum can then be reflected using a 9 molt periosteal elevator. In the case of a thin mandibular ramus, exposure of the lingual cortex to gauge thickness may be beneficial. The graft should not extend more than half the width of the mandibular ramus. Osteotomy can be performed in two fashions: reciprocating saw and in postage stamp fashion with a 701 or 702 bur. These osteotomies should be performed through the cortex only especially as the vertical cuts are being made, as the nerve may be in close proximity in this region. Following this, small osteotomes can be used to deepen the osteotomies along the vertical and crestal aspects of the graft. The authors prefer to use a round bur at the inferior aspect of the block to weaken but not fully perforate the cortex and thus allow for an out-fracture without significant risk of nerve injury. Once the block begins to mobilize it can be out-fractured with an osteotome in the crestal osteotomy. The donor site edges should be smoothed with a bur or bone file, the site should be irrigated, and closed primarily with a resorbable suture. Some choose to place gel foam into the graft site prior to closure, which can further aid in hemostasis and does not appear to cause any detriment to healing. Patients can follow up in 1–2 weeks and saline mouth rinses may aid in healing. Post-operative antibiotics may be given based on practitioner preference if not provided in i.v. form during the procedure.

A representative case treated by ramus grafting in the area of a central incisor with simultaneous implant placements is illustrated by the photos and diagrams as follows (Figure 24.2). The grafted site was covered with allogeneic Dura Mater that was used as a barrier membrane [14].

Chin

An additional site of intraoral bone stock is the symphysis. This area can also provide a block of cortex with minimal cancellous marrow [13]. In the case of the symphysis, graft dimensions rarely extend beyond 2 cm in vertical height and 6 cm in length when extended across the mid-line. This block can be segmented into two

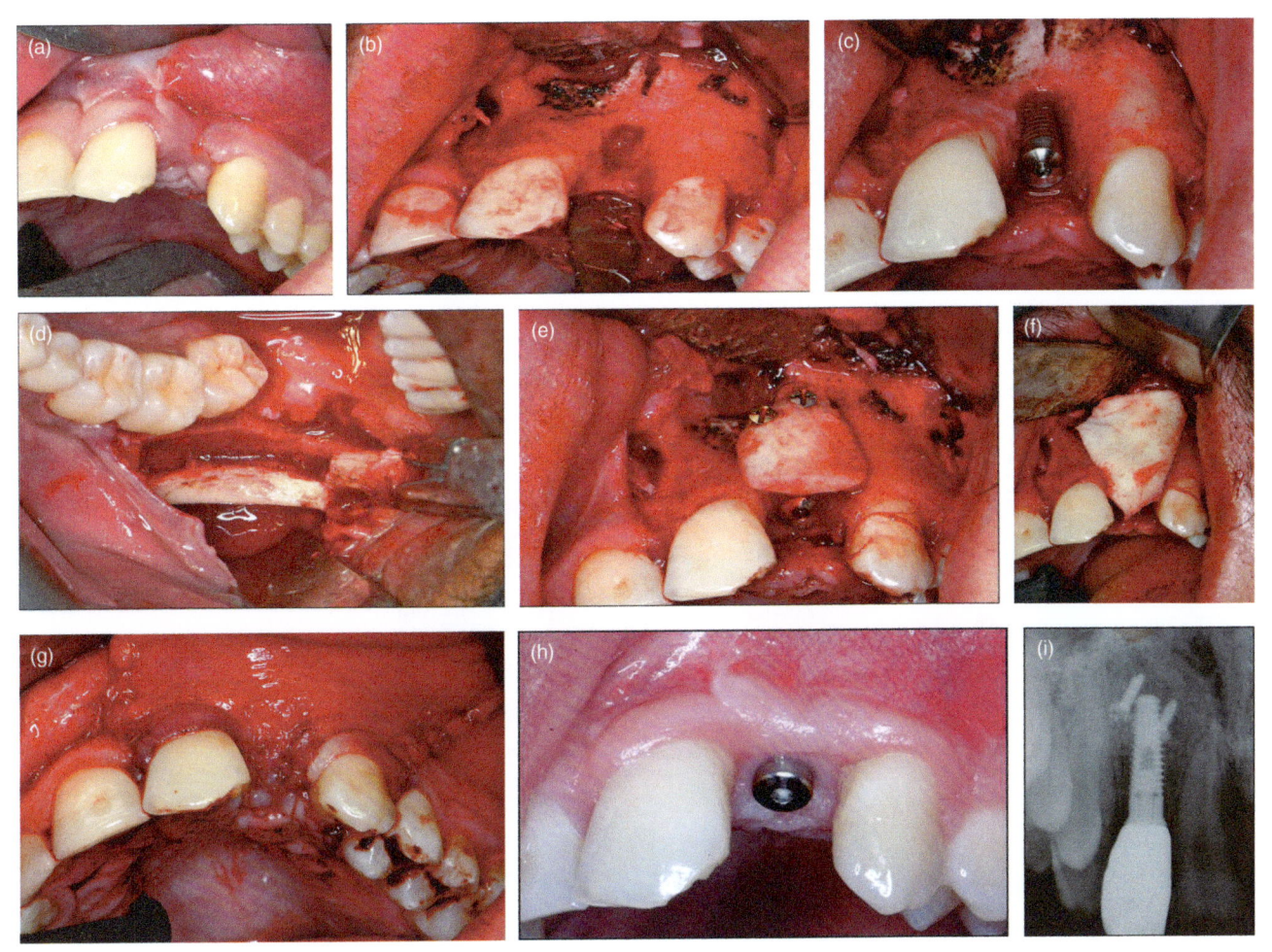

Figure 24.2 (a) Anterior maxillary defect with missing central incisor. (b to e) Osteotomy with immediate implant placement and onlay bone grafting from lateral ramus. (f and g) Implant site covered with allogeneic Dura and primary closure. (h and i) Healed graft and restoration after 6 months.

segments for bilateral applications. The benefits to this site of bone harvest include location within the oral cavity with the lack of a perceived donor site and a bone stock with a natural curvature. The potential downside of the symphyseal harvest is the lack of cancellous marrow, the possibility of post-operative numbness, and the relatively small bone stock available. Contraindications to use of the symphysis for bone harvest include previous radiation, excessive vertical bone loss from age or other preexisting conditions, and the presence of an alloplastic chin implant. In the authors' experience harvest of this graft can be accomplished under local anesthesia with regard to pain control, but repetitive osteotome use in this region can be disconcerting for the patient when an oral or IV sedative has not been planned.

In approaching the symphyseal bone harvest anesthesia can be obtained with bilateral mental nerve blocks and in addition local anesthesia can be deposited along the depth of the vestibule in this region for hemostasis. The incision is placed approximately 1 cm below the mucogingival junction from the distal of one canine to the other. This incision will protect not only the mental nerve, which is typically apical to the second molar, but also the labial branch, which lies just deep to the mucosa in this region. Upon identification of the labial branch laterally the incision can be deepened down to the periosteum. The mentalis muscle will be reflected inferiorly, ensuring that the attachment of the mental tubercles is left, as failure to preserve this attachment can lead to the colloquially labeled "witches chin." The superior tissues should also be reflected enough to visualize the form of the root apices through the thin buccal cortex. Beginning approximately 0.5 cm apical to the root tips of the incisors, the outline of the graft can be completed with a 701 or 702 bur. This cut should be performed at a slight angle to allow introduction of osteotomes into the site. The outline can be completed, remaining at least 5 mm anterior to the mental foramen if the dissection has been carried posterior to this extent and 1 cm above the inferior border. Alternative cutting instruments include the reciprocating saw or a piezoelectric instrument. After the cut has been sufficiently taken through the outer cortex, fine straight or curved osteotomes can be used to wedge out the bone blocks. Once the grafts have been harvested the defect can be left alone or an allogenic graft material may be used per the surgeon's preference. Closure should be completed in layers taking care to reapproximate the mentalis muscle. A chin pressure dressing as would be used in a genioplasty can be used in the post-operative setting to limit post-operative edema or hematoma formation. Other than paresthesia, which can occur, although usually only transiently, and ecchymosis, rare complications following this procedure can include hematoma, wound dehiscence, infection, and mandibular fracture. A representation of chin harvesting illustrated by photos and diagrams is given in Figure 24.3.

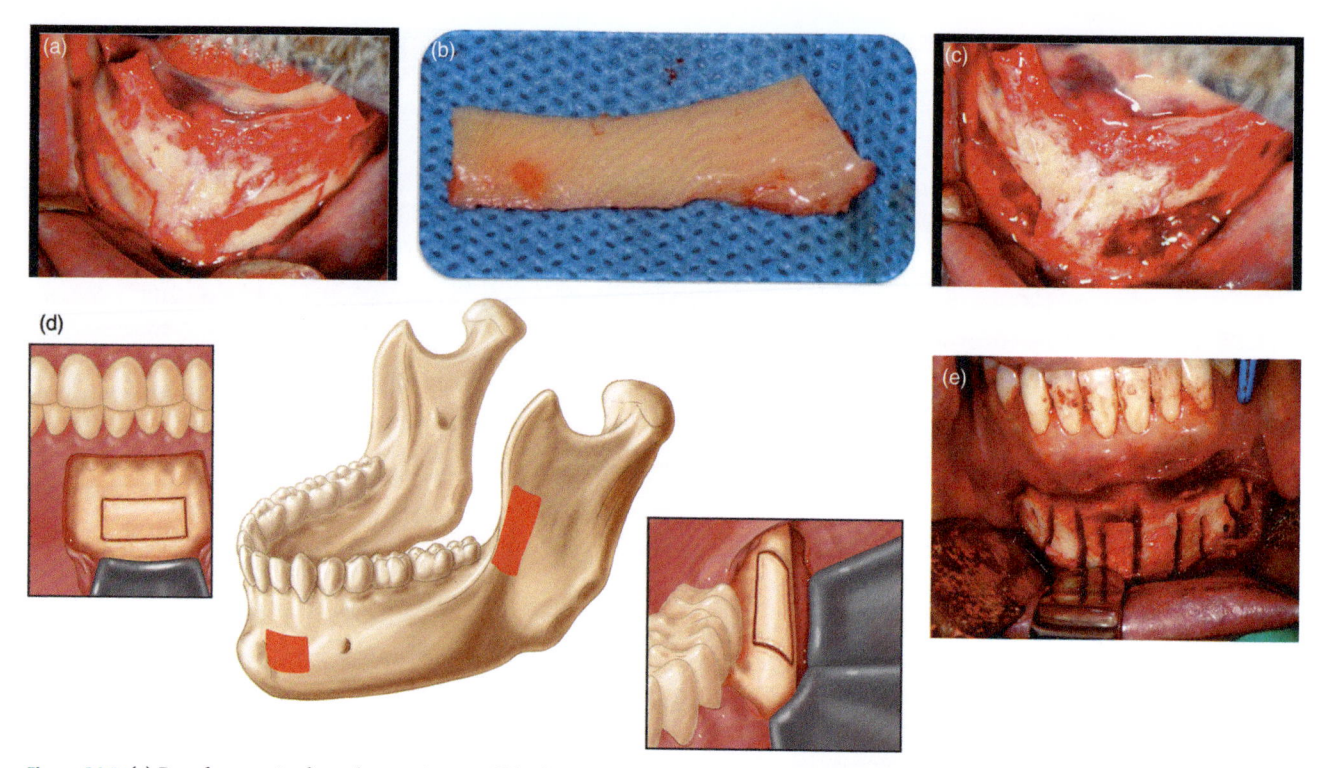

Figure 24.3 (a) Bone harvest site from the anterior mandible. (b) Onlay bone grafting harvested from mandible. (c) Remaining defect after harvest. (d) Schematic of multiple harvest sites. (e) Vertical variation of chin harvest. Illustrations by courtesy of Brittany King.

Extraoral harvest
Posterior iliac crest

The posterior iliac crest (PIC) has long been one of the most common and plentiful sources of autogenous bone for use in oral and maxillofacial surgery. It has been demonstrated that 100 to 150 ml of corticocancellous bone can be safely harvested from this region due to uniform thickness of the PIC. When compared to other harvest sites, the major advantage of the posterior iliac harvest is that it only involves the primary reflection of one muscle, the gluteus maximus, which is not primary to ambulation [15]. Many consider the PIC the gold standard in quantity and quality of bone graft material [16]. The bone stock available in the posterior ilium has been found to be highly osteogenic, osteoinductive, and osteoconductive. Due to the complex anatomy immediately approximating this region it is critical for the surgeon to know the anatomy of the posterior iliac region; however this region can be safely harvested with a zone of safety, as was reported by Xu et al. [15]. There are nearly zero exclusion criteria when considering the posterior iliac crest bone graft (PICBG) with only several relative contraindications or cautions: severely osteoporotic individuals, previous hip replacements, and retained hardware from previous femur fracture. The only known absolute contraindication to the authors is the confirmed presence of pelvic metastasis in the setting of metastatic disease. With the use of a proper surgical technique, the morbidity is minimal and the bone stock is unmatched for the oral and maxillofacial surgeon [17].

Perhaps the only downside of a PICBG is the time required to prone the patient and then return back to supine to complete the procedure. Patient positioning becomes critical for both the surgical and anesthetic team. The authors recommend the low prone jackknife position and a reverse flexion of approximately 210°, which provides superior access and identification of bony landmarks. The patient must have appropriate padding by the anesthetic team with the patient's head turned on its side with the endotracheal tube placed laterally without pressure to prevent pressure necrosis or in a neutral position with the use of a prone pillow. Arms are to be placed superiorly with shoulders abducted no greater than 90°, and care must be taken to lift the shoulder when bringing the arms from the sides to overhead to avoid dislocation. In addition to routine padding of all pressure points, bilateral small axillary rolls should be placed as well as a large pelvic roll positioned under the upper thigh just inferior to the anterior iliac crest. These aid in protecting the shoulders and supporting the pelvis, reducing intrathoracic and intra-abdominal pressures as well as avoiding compression of the vena cava. Hemodynamic variations in the prone position have been researched and care must be taken with the padding mentioned. Current reports do not appear to show variations in stroke volume or cardiac output, but a reduction in left ventricular volume and compliance has been documented. Furthermore, proper pelvic positioning is essential to raise the entire thoracic weight off the sternum and prevent excess pressure on the diaphragm, thereby avoiding decreased pulmonary compliance.

The surgical technique should consist of marking the spinal midline, posterior superior iliac spine, and posterior iliac crest. The triangular posterior tubercle of the ilium should be palpated and marked and a curvilinear incision of approximately 10 cm should be centered over this landmark and the posterior iliac crest. The area can be infiltrated with local anesthetic while sounding the iliac crest. The initial incision is started about 1 cm from the posterior superior iliac spine. Incision through skin and subcutaneous tissue can be performed with a 10 or 15 blade but the authors prefer a bovie cautery one through the dermis. Dissection should be taken down to the PIC where the fascial attachments of the internal oblique and gluteus maximus muscles are visible. These muscles must be released from the iliac crest sharply or with a bovie cautery. A Keyes periosteal elevator should then be used to reflect the periosteum and muscle inferiorly and laterally.

Approximately a 6 cm × 6 cm of bone should be exposed but dissection should not extend to the sciatic notch. A bovie cautery should be used to control bone perforators as inferior visualization can be difficult and blood loss can multiply. After identifying and exposing a 5 cm × 5 cm section of bone for harvest with a posterior hip retractor, a reciprocating saw should be used through the outer cortical bone, saving the inferior cut for last as is the authors' preference. Curved and straight osteotomes can then be used on the vertical and horizontal cuts as well as vertically through the marrow to the depth of the inferior cut. After the graft appears to loosen, the final osteotome pass should be from the most posterior superior point to the anterior inferior point, which will allow for easy outfracture. After securing the cortical block on the back table, cancellous bone can then be harvested with bone gouges (3/8 inch is recommended) and bone curettes. Once an adequate amount of bone has been harvested the authors recommend closure with Avitene, Microfibrillar bovine collagen, and a flat blake bulb suction in the defect. Vicryl sutures should be used to reapproximate the periosteal, muscular, subcutaneous layers. The skin can be closed with either suture or staples. The authors' preference of dressing is fluffs and microfoam tape held on with additional mastisol. Of note, the suction drain should exit laterally for patient comfort while in bed and should be removed after the patient has been ambulatory for at least 24 hours and drainage is less than 10 ml per 24 hours.

While this technique is quite straitforward and the only anatomical structures nearby are the cutaneous superior and middle cluneal nerves, more severe complications have been reported. The most commonly reported complication is formation of a seroma, which is treated by aspiration and a pressure dressing. Significant hemorrhage has been reported from transection of the superior gluteal artery, which is most likely from over aggressive dissection. In this scenario if local control is not possible, intervention radiology or even emergent laparotomy may be required to prevent exsanguination. As mentioned, nerve injury to the superior or middle cluneal nerves can cause dyesthesias and paresthesia of the buttocks, but this is rarely a complaint of the patient in the authors' experience. Also while damage to the sciatic nerve with associated lower extremity motor function compromise is possible, an overaggressive dissection of greater than 6–8 cm from the PIC would most likely be the cause. Pelvic fractures from harvest of the PIC is quite rare but is often associated with previous site surgery, severe osteoporosis, and osteotomy aberrations, with undermining of the posterior edge of the ilium. A representation of posterior iliac crest harvesting is illustrated by the photos and diagrams in Figure 24.4, with important anatomic landmarks illustrated as well.

Anterior iliac crest
The anterior iliac crest (AIC) has long been considered a mainstay of autogenous bone harvest for the oral and maxillofacial surgeon [18]. A source of cortical bone of up to 5 cm × 5 cm and 30–50 ml of uncompressed cancellous marrow can be harvested from this site. The anterior ilium has a plethora of osteoprogenitor cells, which allows for favorable bone growth as well as rapid revascularization. The AIC has been shown to have the highest cancellous bone-to-cortical bone ratio. Unlike the posterior hip with its superior bone quantity, the anterior iliac crest bone graft (AICBG) requires minimal repositioning for harvest. Often this area is prepped simultaneously at the beginning of the case and left draped under a three-quarter or split sheet until the appropriate time for harvest, with instruments set aside from the oral cavity for sterile use in this region.

The approach to the AIC is based on an understanding of the osseous and overlying soft tissue anatomy. The marrow of the AIC is mainly found in the anterior third of the iliac crest and is found 1 cm behind the anterior tubercle of the ilium. This region is usually located approximately 6 cm posterior to the anterior superior iliac spine (ASIS). This region is the thickest portion of the anterior crest. The most posterior boundary of the marrow compartment is actually 1–2 cm posterior to the tubercle and usually only extends 2 cm inferiorly from the iliac crest. The anterior inferior iliac spine (AIIS) lies inferior posterior to the ASIS and should not have been visualized during the routine approach to the AIC. Muscle attachments to the crest are most easily broken down into those approaching medially and those approaching laterally. Medial structures attaching to the AIC are the external and internal abdominal obliques, the transverses abdominis, the thoracodorsal fascia, the liliaceous muscle, the inguinal ligament (ASIS), and the sartorius (AIIS). The lateral attachments of the AIC are the tensor fascia muscle, the iliotibial tract, the gluteus medius, and the gluteus minimus. The nerves that course in this area are all sensory cutaneous and from anterior to posterior are the lateral femoral cutaneous, the subcostal, and the iliohypogastric. The most often affected is the iliohypogastric, which crosses over the area of the tubercle, which is often unavoidable. The subcostal nerve originates from T12 and courses over the tip of the ASIS. The lateral femoral cutaneous nerve courses medially between the psoas major and the medial edge of the iliacus. It is routinely under the inguinal ligament but is found on top of the crest in 2.5% of the population. When this nerve is injured a condition known as meralgia paresthetica can cause post-operative difficulties ranging from paresthesia to dyesthesia. The blood supply to the anterior ilium is provided mostly by perforators into the bone from the deep circumflex iliac artery, which courses on the medial aspect of the ilium from anterior to posterior and can be used to raise a vascularized osseous flap.

Surgical preparations should consist of a small bump or roll being placed under the supine positioned patient to elevate the iliac crest. Infiltration of 1% lidocaine with epi (1:100 000) may be placed at the planned incision site for local anesthesia and vasoconstriction. The overlying skin is pulled superiomedialy over the crest, preventing post-operative irritation of the incision by cloths or belts. A 4–6 cm incision should be used starting 2 cm posterior to the anterior superior spine and extending 1 cm posterior to the iliac tubercle. The authors prefer a blade on the skin with a bovie cautery beyond the dermis for hemostasis. The incision is carried through skin, a subcutaneous layer of fat, Scarpa's fascia, and through a deep fascial layer and periosteum. A subperiosteal reflection is then conducted in the medial direction to avoid dissection of the tensor fascia lata muscles laterally, which is known to create post-operative gait disturbances. Elevation of the iliacus muscle allows adequate access and visualization of the crest for retrieval of the graft. Osteotomies should be completed as described with the PIC, taking caution not to undermine the ASIS, which can lead to fracture if the anterior osteotomy is angled too anteriomedially. After harvest of the cortex and marrow as previously described, the wound should be explored for small bony and muscle bleeding points. Electrocautery can be used here to improve hemostasis prior to closure and any sharp bony edges should be smoothed. Once again hemostatic agents (thrombin, gelfoam, Avitene, bone wax) may be used if indicated. Multiple-layered closure should be completed by repositioning

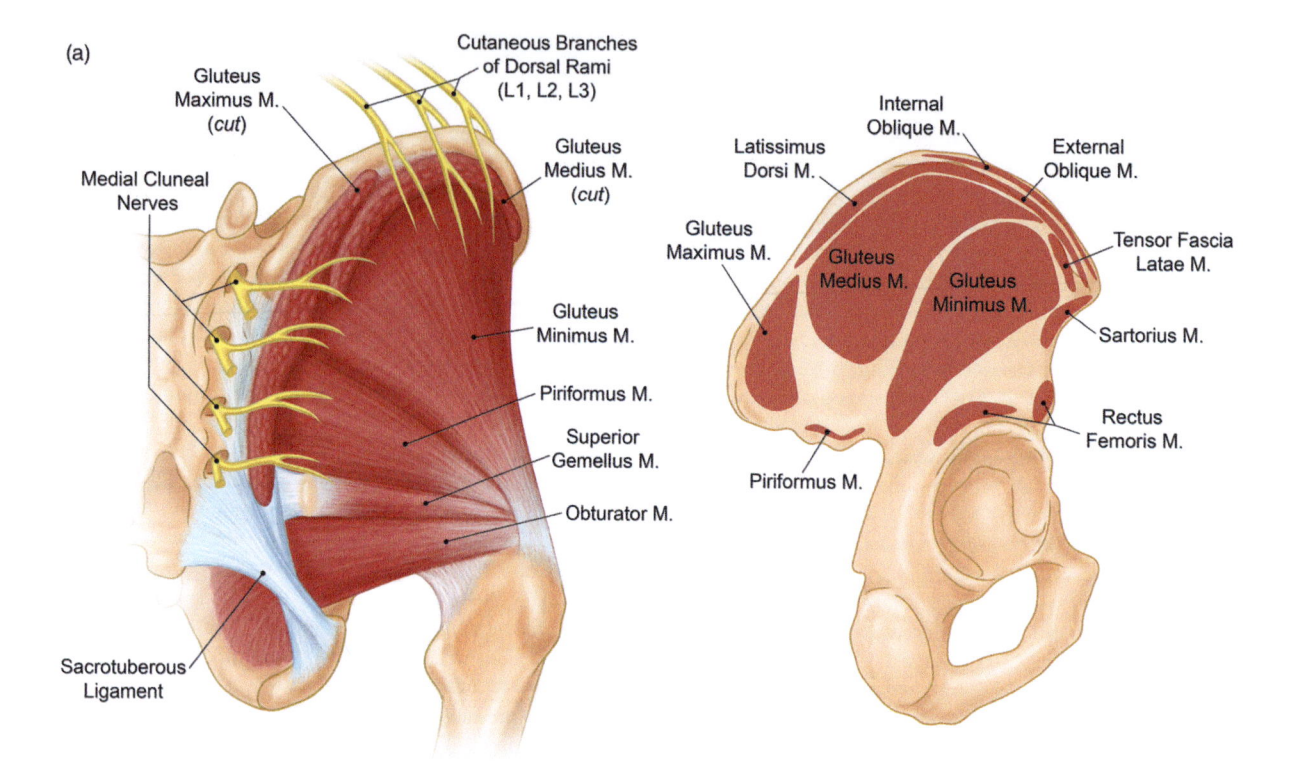

Figure 24.4 (a and b) Posterior Iliac crest harvesting with muscular attachments and cluneal nerves marked. The initial incision is started about 1 cm from the posterior superior iliac spine. (c) Exposure of the lateral ilium. (d) Reciprocating saw scores cortex. (e to h) Curved osteotome used to separate cortical bone from cancellous marrow (j and i) Block graft applied to the anterior maxilla with fixation screws to gain width and height. (k) Reconstructed with dental implants 9 months later.

muscle attachments to bone, followed by closure of fascial layers and then skin. The AIC may require a bulb suction drain but this should be left up to the surgeon's discretion, but should exit laterally if used.

In the post-operative period, if a suction drain is used it should be removed after the patient has been ambulatory for at least 24 hours and drainage is less than 10 ml per 24 hours. The most common complications associated with AICBG harvest are seroma formation, bruising, and gait disturbance associated with disturbance of the tensor fascia lata. As mentioned, major complications have been reported in small numbers to include fracture of the ilium, perforation of the peritoneum and/or bowel, infection, and sensory nerve damage. One must maintain the cartilaginous cap in children; therefore during the harvest the surgeon must either split or maintain it. A representation of anterior iliac crest harvesting is illustrated by photos and diagrams in Figure 24.5, with important anatomic landmarks also illustrated.

Calvarium

When a curvilinear bone graft is required with little to no cancellous bone, the split or full thickness calvarial bone should remain high on the list of bone stock available. The thin but formidable bone is excellent for grafting of the craniofacial skeleton, where curvature is the rule and not the exception. Harvested from the parietal region, posterior to the pinna, where the calvarium is thickest and a full thickness graft on average can yield 7–8 mm of width [19]. The use of full-thickness grafts is not routinely undertaken for elective cases and is often approached with a neurosurgical team when indicated.

Split thickness harvest, however, can safely provide excellent bone stock from this region for the oral and maxillofacial team. The bone from this region has shown exceptional resistance to resorption once reimplanted compared to other autogenous sources [20]. There are multiple other benefits of the calvarial bone harvest. With the exception of patients with significant alopecia, the incision is usually completely hidden within the hair, and additionally there are no significant functional disturbances associated with the procedure. Due to the native curvature of the calvarium in two dimensions, grafts from this region can fit perfectly into orbital floor defects, zygomatic fractures, and other curved structures of the craniofacial region, and even to cover large buccal wall defects around dental implants [21].

When considering a calvarial bone graft a computed tomography (CT) scan with fine cuts may aid in identifying the thickest areas for donor site selection. Contraindications to the procedure include previous trauma with an osseous defect, a history of metabolic bone disease, and radiation to the cranium. The only significant anatomical structures of interest are the superficial temporary artery, which can be ligated when encountered, and the superior sagittal sinus, which should be avoided by remaining 1–2 cm away from the sagittal suture as the sinus usually extends 5 mm to each side of the mid-line. The harvest should be kept superior to the temporal bone as well, as this area is known to be quite thin and prone to epidural hematomas associated with bone fractures. In preparation for surgery the scalp can be cleaned with a 4% povidone-iodine shampoo. Shaving the hair is rarely indicated and in females the hair can be lubricated and gathered into smaller braids with sterile

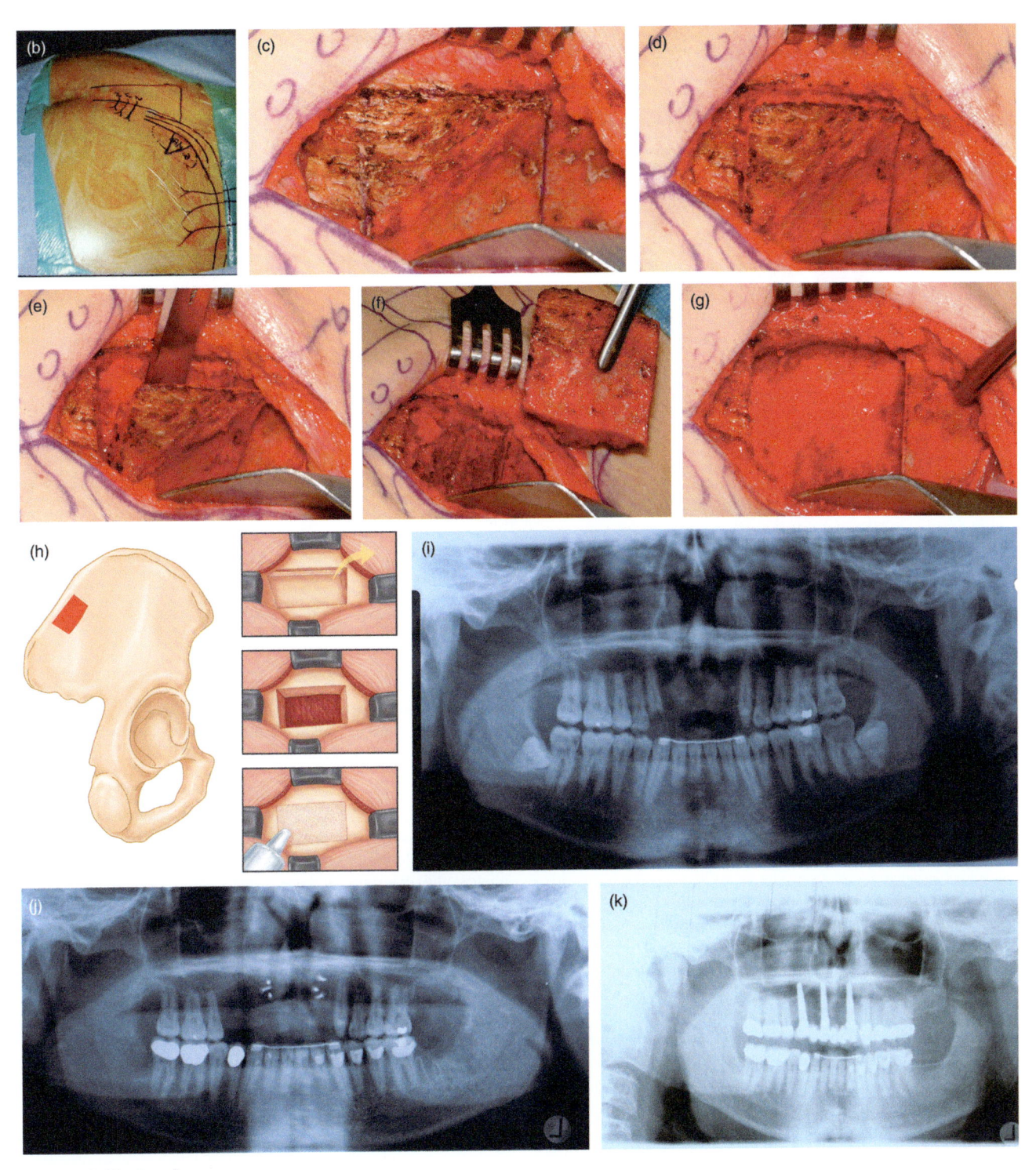

Figure 24.4 (*Continued*)

elastics or the cut fingers of a sterile glove. The anesthetic of choice should be a general endotracheal anesthetic and positioning can be accomplished with bilateral sandbags or a Mayfield head frame.

Once adequate sterility and exposure have been achieved the scalp should be incised following the direction of hair follicles sharply, dissecting through skin, subcutaneous tissue, galea aponeurotica, and loose connective tissue to the pericranium. Aggressive use of the bovie cautery is not recommended as this can cause alopecia. Raney clips or suture can be used to control bleeding at scalp margins although these clips can also result in alopecia if left in place for an extended period. After a subpericranial dissection exposing the parietal bone, a split or full-thickness graft can be harvested. In split thickness harvest the area of interest should be outlined with a fissure bur into the diploe. The use of an acrylic or barrel bur can aid in beveling the peripheral bone around the graft to facilitate insertion of osteotomes. Curved osteotomes can then be

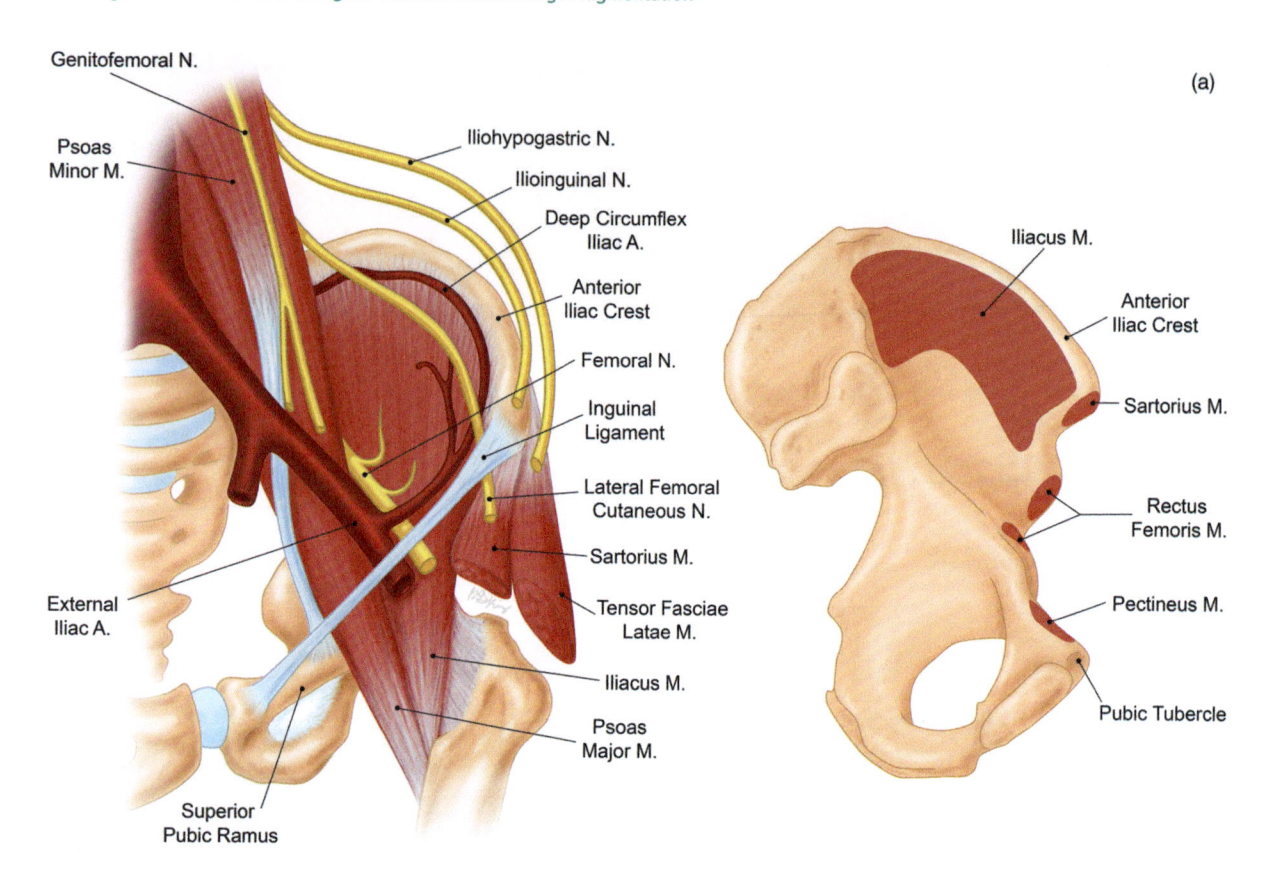

Figure 24.5 (a to c) Anterior iliac crest schematic and pictures illustrating sensory nerves in the region with muscle attachments. (d to g) Exposure of the medial surface of the iliac crest, reciprocating saw scores cortex, and curved osteotome used to separate cortical bone from cancellous marrow. (h to j) Maxillary defect at time of grafting and 12 months later with stable vertical and horizontal augmentation.

used in a circumferential fashion taking care not to elevate with the chisel, as this carries a risk of fracturing the inner table. Once adequately loosened the graft can be delivered and put on the back table for further manipulation. The defect itself can be filled with a bone cement or in larger harvests a titanium mesh. If a full-thickness graft is desired, a formal craniotomy is carried out and the inner table is perforated with 2–4 holes, followed by reflection of the Dura and cutting of the graft with a neurosurgical safe-sided saw. Full-thickness defects in this region can be filled with methyl methacrylate or a split calvarial graft. Prior to closure hemostasis can be achieved with bone wax, microfibular collagen, and bipolar diathermy or oxidized cellulose layered over the Dura in full-thickness harvests. Once hemostasis has been achieved closure should be completed in three layers; a drain is rarely indicated. A pressure dressing using fluffs, Kerlix, and Coban in a Barton pressure bandage fashion can provide a pressure dressing to the area.

In the post-operative setting the patient is monitored neurologically for 24 hours and the skin staples are left in place for a minimum of 7 days. If drains are placed they should be removed as soon as drainage has decreased to less than 10 ml in 24 hours. Complications associated with the procedure are rare and usually minor in nature but can be devastating. The more common complications include alopecia near the incision and hematoma formation. Other complications, although rare, may present when the inner table is perforated, including cerebrospinal fluid leak, extradural hematoma, and direct intracerebral trauma.

Furthermore, when foreign bodies are used in reconstruction an osteomyelitis can ensue in rare cases.

A representation of cranial bone harvesting is illustrated by the photos and diagrams in Figure 24.6, with important anatomic landmarks also illustrated.

Graft preparation and fixation
Bone grafting principles

Embryologically bone development may be classified as either intramembranous or endochondral. Intramembranous formation consists of direct ossification of the collagenous matrix and is evident in the genesis of the cranial vault, the facial skeleton, parts of the mandible, and clavicle. Endochondral bone formation involves a cartilaginous phase [22]. Weight-bearing bones and those terminating in joints, in addition to most of the cranial base, and a portion of the mandible have endochondral origins.

From a functional standpoint, osteoblasts in bone are responsible for laying down the organic matrix, which is then mineralized [23]. The organization of this matrix can take the form of either cortical or cancellous bone. Cortical bone is dense and is primarily responsible for bearing load and support. Cortical bone makes up about 80% of the skeleton by weight, and its functional units are known as osteons. Cancellous bone makes up about 20% of the skeleton by weight. The volume of cancellous bone, however, is generally greater than cortical bone as cancellous bone is highly porous. It takes on a honeycomb or trabecular structure. The primary function of cancellous bone is to produce bone marrow. Much of the cell population in bone resides in

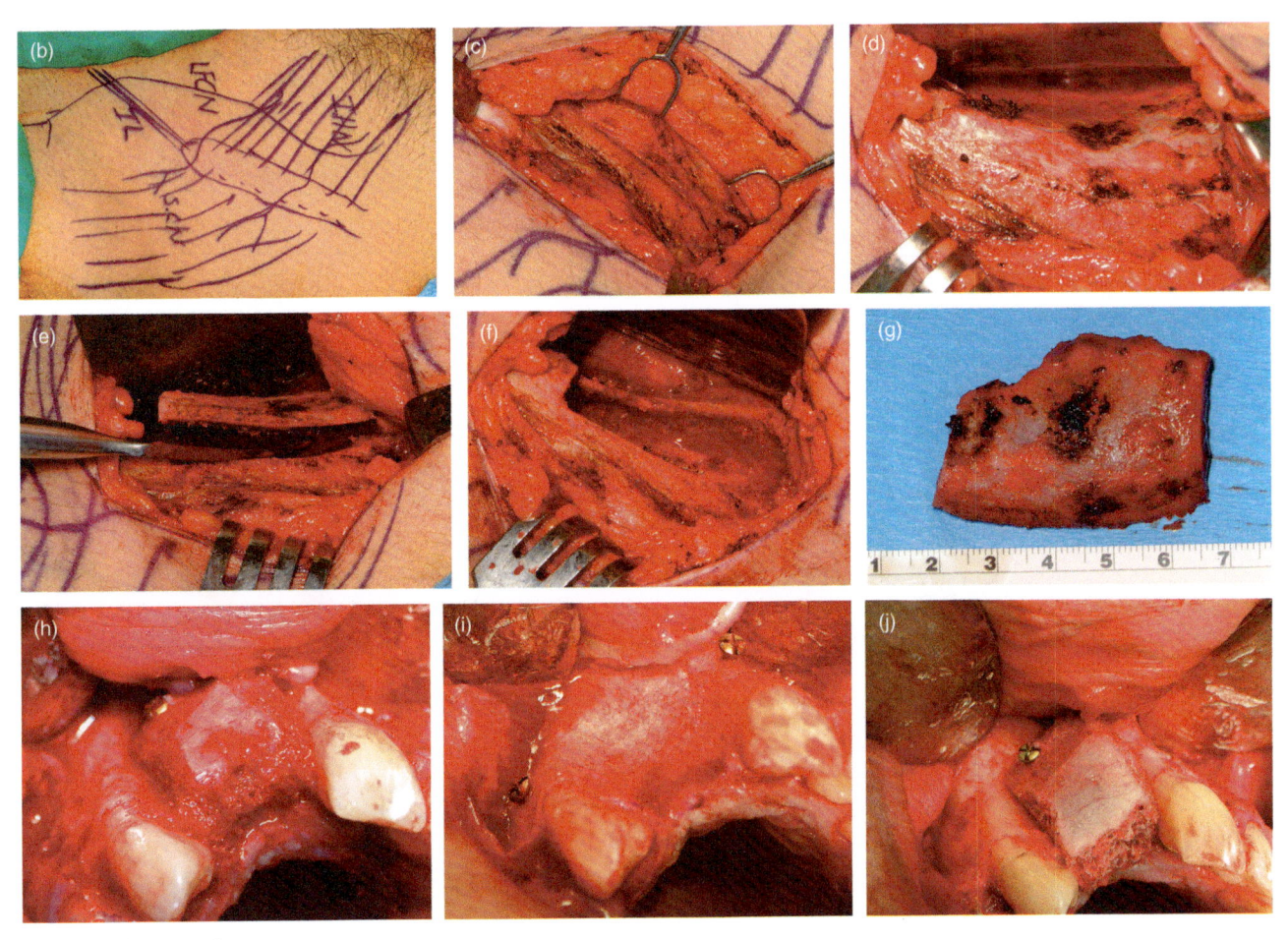

Figure 24.5 (*Continued*)

the marrow and the stem cells that give rise to osteoblasts originate in this marrow. Osteoblasts inhibit osteoclastic resorption via feedback mechanisms. As osteoblasts mature into osteocytes they lose the ability to inhibit osteoclastic activity, which leads to bone turnover and remodeling [24]. The systemic use of medications such as bisphosphonates or denosumab may affect osteoclastic activity and should be a consideration prior to placement of dental implants or other invasive surgical procedures [25]. In certain areas, cancellous bone is also responsible for carrying load.

The use of bone grafts has played an important role in oral and maxillofacial surgery since the early 1900s for reconstruction of a multitude of defects. Important properties to consider when evaluating grafting methods and materials include ostoegenesis, osteoinduction, and osteoinduction [26]. Other factors to consider are biocompatibility, availability, the ability to act as a matrix, mechanical stability, and of course surgeon preference. Types of bone grafting materials are autogenous, allogeneic, xenogeneic, and alloplastic, each with their own advantages and disadvantages.

The osteogenic potential is the ability to form new bone in a graft by transplanting viable endosteal osteoblasts. Osteoconduction is the ability of the graft to allow vascular and cellular invasion by the host site, which is generally adjacent bone, such as seen in a healing tooth extraction site. Osteoinduction is the ability of the graft to stimulate differentiation of mesenchymal cells into osteoblasts at the recipient site, such as seen with BMP. Bone may develop from one or a combination of these three mechanisms. The graft survives an initial harvest–transplant cycle because it contains endosteal osteoblast and marrow stem cells, which provide plasmatic circulation [27]. After a bone graft or upon reparative efforts of bone, such as a fracture or placement of a dental implant, bone healing is facilitated by entrapped platelets, which degranulate, releasing growth factors such as platelet-derived growth factors (PDGFs) and transforming growth factors (TGFs). Endothelial cells initiate capillary ingrowth as they bind PDGF. TGF-β1 stimulates endosteal osteoblasts and hematopoietic stem cell mitosis and osteoid production. Endosteal osteoblasts are especially abundant after autogenous grafting methods are employed. This comprises the inflammatory phase of bone healing.

The proliferative phase and revascularization are initiated as soon as the graft is placed, but capillary buds first appear and penetrate the graft by day three. Basic fibroblast growth factor (big) stimulates this angiogenesis. After the third day, locally induced macrophages synthesize growth factors and regulate bone healing. Complete vascularization of the graft occurs by the end of the second week. Osteoblasts from the transplanted bone begin depositing osteoid. Although revascularization is usually complete by day ten to fourteen it is dependent upon graft size/thickness and vascularity of the local tissue bed. Revascularization can be impeded by cortical bone, foreign body, or immunogenic response. By four months, bone graft integration is complete. The maturation phase is complete as the newly laid woven bone becomes lamellar bone due to function or in many cases upon loading of the dental implants.

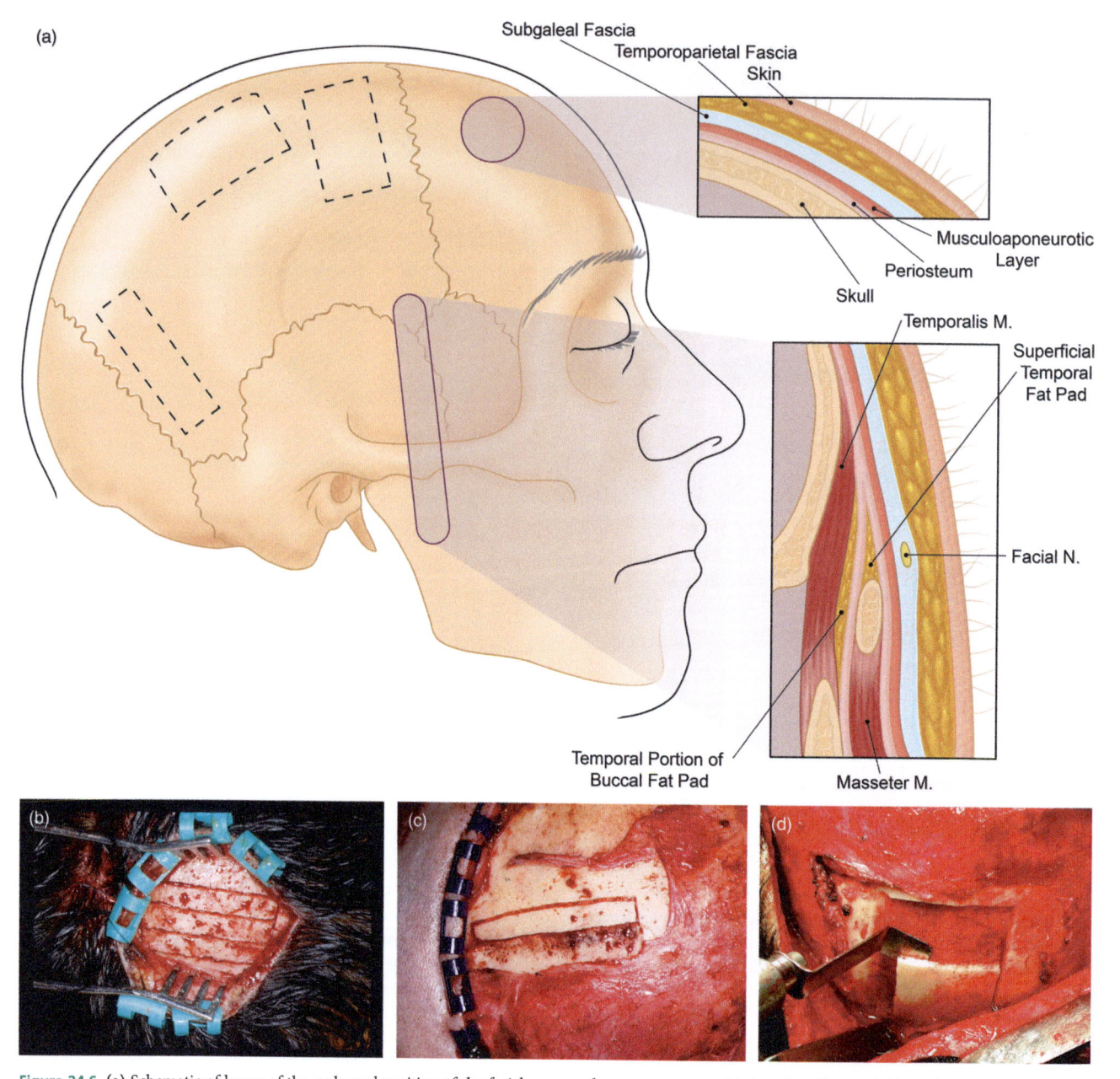

Figure 24.6 (a) Schematic of layers of the scalp and position of the facial nerve and numerous acceptable locations for cranial bone harvest. (b) Numerous blocks of cranial bone harvest for dentofacial or craniofacial reconstruction. (c) Harvest of strut of bone for nasal reconstruction. (d) Harvest of large cranial block with oscillating saw.

Bone grafting materials
Autogenous bone
Autogenous bone is the gold standard for bone regenerative grafting materials for several reasons, including transplanting live osseocompetent cells with the capability to support osteogenesis, osteoinduction, and osteoconduction. The downfall is the requirement for a donor site. The three forms of free bone grafts include cortical, cancellous, and corticocancellous grafts.

1. Cortical grafts. These grafts are able to withstand early mechanical forces, but they require more time to revascularize. Common donor sites include: cranium, iliac crest, ribs, mandibular symphysis, and the external oblique ridge.
2. Cancellous grafts. The advantage of cancellous grafts includes an apparent increase in healing rate. The most abundant supply can be harvested from the anterior or posterior iliac crest [28]. The only apparent disadvantage of autogenous cancellous grafts is their inability to provide mechanical stability and in general they tend to undergo more resorption [29].
3. Corticocancellous grafts. The advantages of the corticocancellous grafts are their ability to provide some mechanical stability and provide some increase in osteogenesis. Corticocancellous grafts do not have the ability to increase osteogenesis as much as cancellous grafts due to the layer of relatively non-porous cortical bone. Donor sites include the ribs, ilium, and skull.

Allogeneic bone
Allogeneic bone is non-vital, osseous tissue harvested from one individual and transferred to another of the same species [30].

Three forms of allogeneic bone include: fresh frozen, freeze-dried, and demineralized freeze-dried bone. The use of fresh frozen bone has recently gained more popularity in pre-implant reconstructive surgery, but it was rarely used in the past due to the concern related to transmission of disease [31].

Freeze-dried bone is osteoconductive, but it has no osteogenic or osteoinductive capabilities. Freeze-dried allogenic grafts are usually placed in conjunction with autogenous grafts.

Ademineralized freeze-dried allogeneic graft (DFDAG) lacks mechanical strength, but has osteoconductive and osteoinductive capabilities. Demineralizing the freeze-dried bone exposes the bone morphogenetic proteins, which have been shown to induce bone formation. Recent advances have incorporated the DBM into various carriers such as collagen or selected polymers.

Xenogeneic bone

Xenogeneic bone is osseous tissue that is harvested from one species, processed, and transferred to a different species. The most common graft of this type is bovine-derived bone. Its use was popular in the 1960s, but fell into disfavor after patients developed autoimmune diseases. The reintroduction of this product occurred in the 1990s after the development to further deproteinate the bone particles. This bone matrix is osteoconductive, without any osteoactive agents.

Alloplastic bone

Alloplastic bone is synthetic tissue that has been in clinical use in osseous regeneration. It may be classified as hydroxyapatite, ceramics, and polymers. These act as fillers primarily, and are eventually replaced by host bone, although this process may take up to 18–24 months.

Bone grafting techniques

Autogenous block grafting is considered as the "gold standard" for regeneration of atrophic jaws. The graft should be stabilized on the recipient bed by fixation screws or with simultaneous placement of dental implants. During the healing period, grafted bone is gradually replaced by new regeneration, which depends on revascularization from the recipient site [32]. Therefore, perforation of the recipient site is recommended to enhance angiogenesis and provide osteogenic cells [33]. On the other hand, an adequate primary stability would be achieved when dental implants are placed in block-augmented ridges in comparison to GBR techniques [34].

Block bone grafting by harvesting a piece of bone from either extraoral or intraoral donor sites allows three-dimensional reconstruction of defects with a complicated morphology. The main disadvantage of autogenous onlay block graft (OBG) is donor site morbidity [35]. Commercial allogeneic or xenogeneic blocks have been developed. Successful clinical application of these materials has been reported in the literature [36–38], but further studies are required to histologically prove new bone formation.

Secondary bone resorption is the main challenge in autogenous block grafting. The anterior iliac crest showed a range resorption between 20 and 92% in 10 years follow-up [39, 40]. The lateral ramus as an intraoral donor site showed 17.4% of bone resorption after 4–6 months of bone grafting [41].

Within the last two decades, different modifications to conventional augmentation methods have been brought into the literature. Merging with various concepts of guided bone regeneration (GBR) modifies onlay block bone grafting. For instance, after fixing block bone to the recipient site, bovine bone mineral or human mineral bone was applied to fill the gap and covered with resorbable or non-resorbable membrane [42] (Figure 24.7). Membrane usage showed better results in the amount of bone gain when used in vertical defects [43].

The three-dimensional reconstruction technique successfully applied the concept of exploiting high-strength cortical bone blocks for protection of particulate bone [44]. The efficacy of this concept was subsequently approved with the cortical tenting technique in which cortical blocks were tented over the particulate material to increase the ridge width [28]. In fact, thin cortical bone in this condition acts as an osteogenic membrane that provides a roof for a protected healing space. Lateral ramus and chin cortical bone are well adapted for the cortical autogenous tenting (CAT) technique (Figure 24.8). Harvested grafts were properly adapted to the recipient site and any sharp edges on the blocks were trimmed with a large round bur. Fixation screw holes were created in at least three sites on the lateral surface of the bone block using a drill. The cortical surface of the recipient bone was also perforated to expedite vascularization of the area to be regenerated. The bone block(s) were placed at least 3 to 4 mm from the vertically deficient site or buccal to the lateral surface of the horizontally deficient ridge. Fixation microscrews were tightened while a periosteal elevator was placed between the bone block and the recipient site to maintain the desired distance. Particulate bone substitute materials were used to fill the gap between the graft and the recipient site (Figure 24.9). When the cortical bone has a thickness more than 2 mm, a bone scraper is used to thin the bone. By gentle use of a wheel saw, the cortical piece could provide two thinned cortical layers, which are used in both the labial and lingual sides. The gap beneath the osteogenic roof when filled with the mixture of bone substitutes and autogenous particulate bone gave the best results [28].

In larger defects such as "B" or "C" defects multiple cortical autogenous tenting (mCAT) or bilateral CAT (biCAT) can help to provide proper implant positioning. In this way, a large piece of lateral ramus cortical bone (LRCB) is harvested, cut to 2–3 pieces, and tented both in the facial and lingual sides (Figures 24.10 to 24.12).

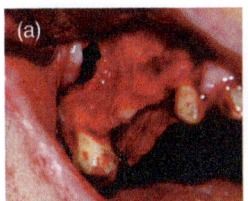

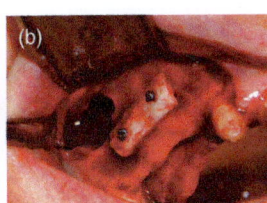

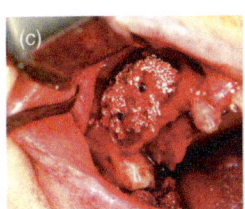

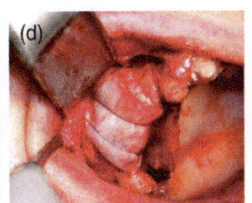

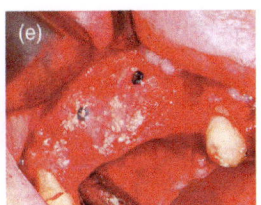

Figure 24.7 (a) "A III" defect. (b) Onlay bone grafting with lateral ramus. (c) Filling the gap with bovine bone mineral. (d) Covering with collagen membrane. (e) Bone healing after 5 months.

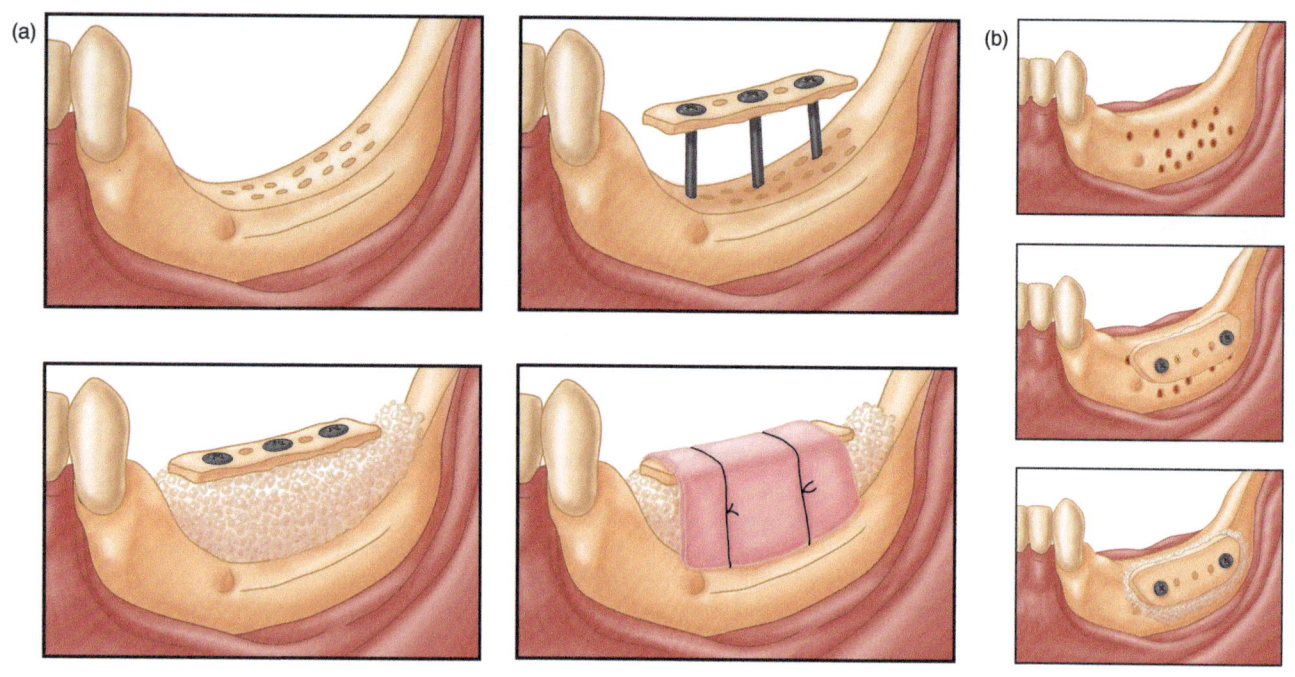

Figure 24.8 (a) Vertical and (b) horizontal CAT.

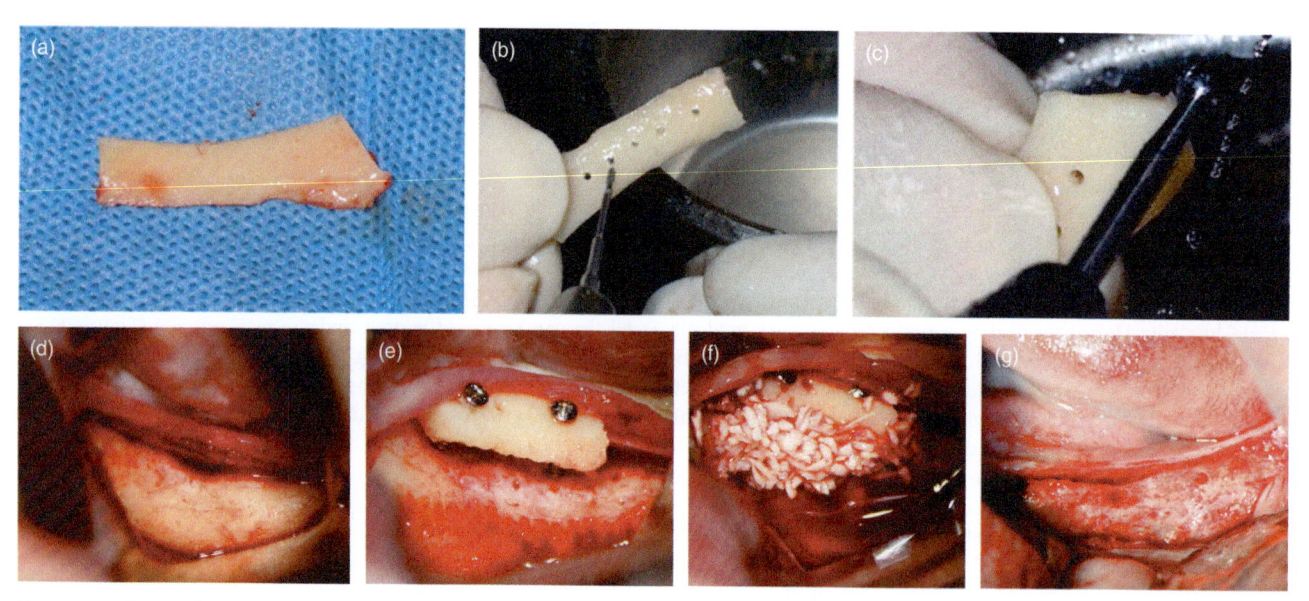

Figure 24.9 CAT in the posterior mandible. (a) Harvesting a large piece of lateral ramus cortical bone; (b) making drilling holes; (c) softening of rough edges of harvested bone; (d) "C" defect in posterior mandible; (e) cortical tenting with 3–4 mm distance; (f) filling the space with freeze-dried bone allograft; (g) bone healing after 6 months.

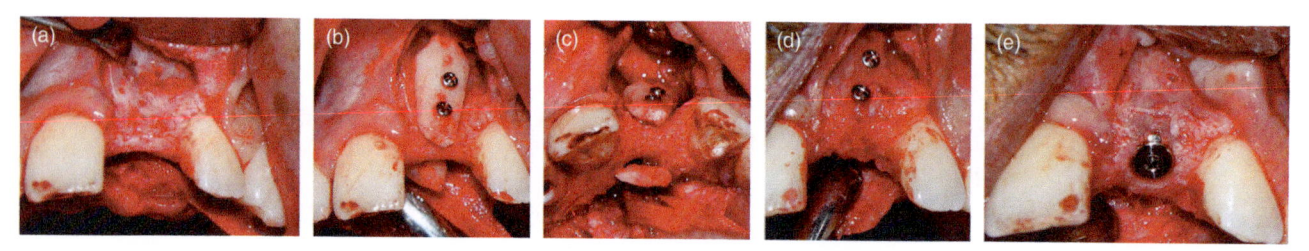

Figure 24.10 (a) Bilateral CTA in "A II" defect in anterior maxilla. LRCB tented with the distance of 2 mm both in the facial and lingual sides: (b) frontal view and (c) inferior view. (d) Bone healing following 5 months. (e) Implant placement in the grated bone.

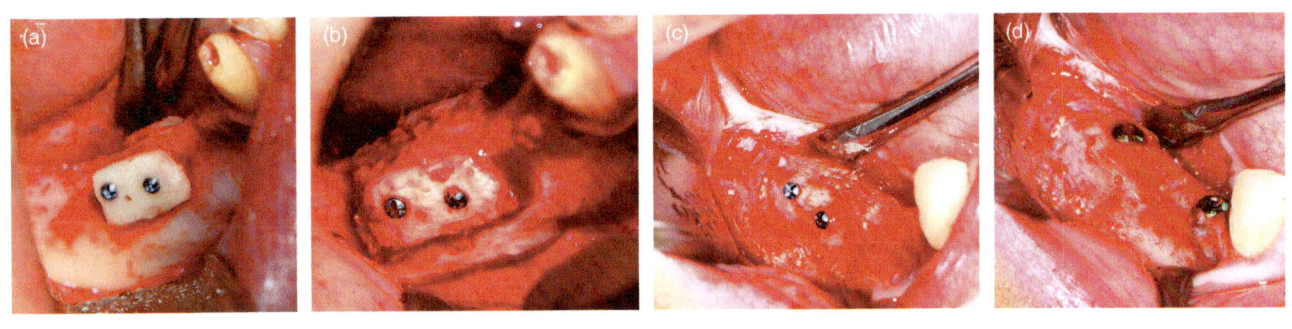

Figure 24.11 BiCAT in "BII" defect posterior mandible.

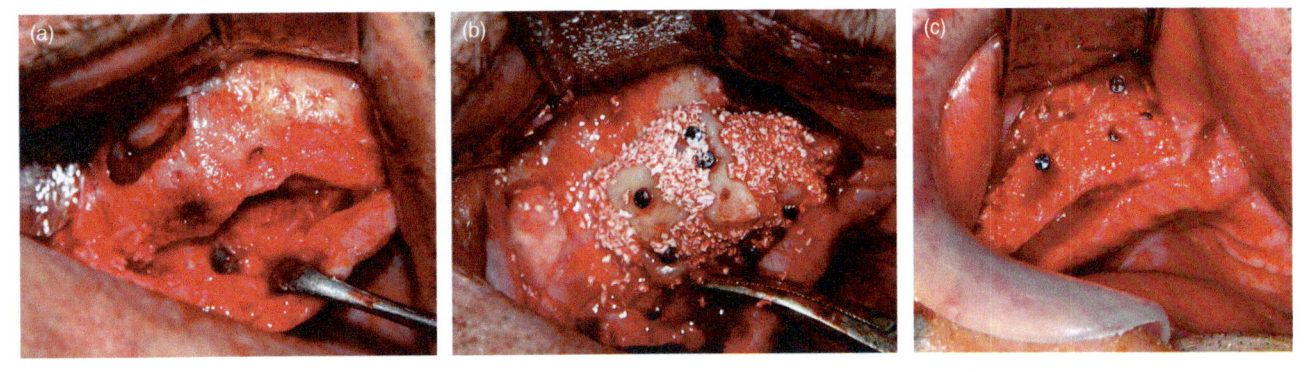

Figure 24.12 (a) Large "C" defects in the maxilla and (b) mCAT. (c) Filling the gap and bone healing after 6 months.

Prolonged treatment time, soft tissue complications, graft failure, and donor site morbidity make onlay block bone grafting a technique-sensitive procedure. Simultaneous placement of implants might be considered as a way to lessen the treatment period (Figure 24.13). While using a graft prior to implant therapy, complications such as graft exposure, infection, and total graft failure may result in implant failure [28] (Table 24.1).

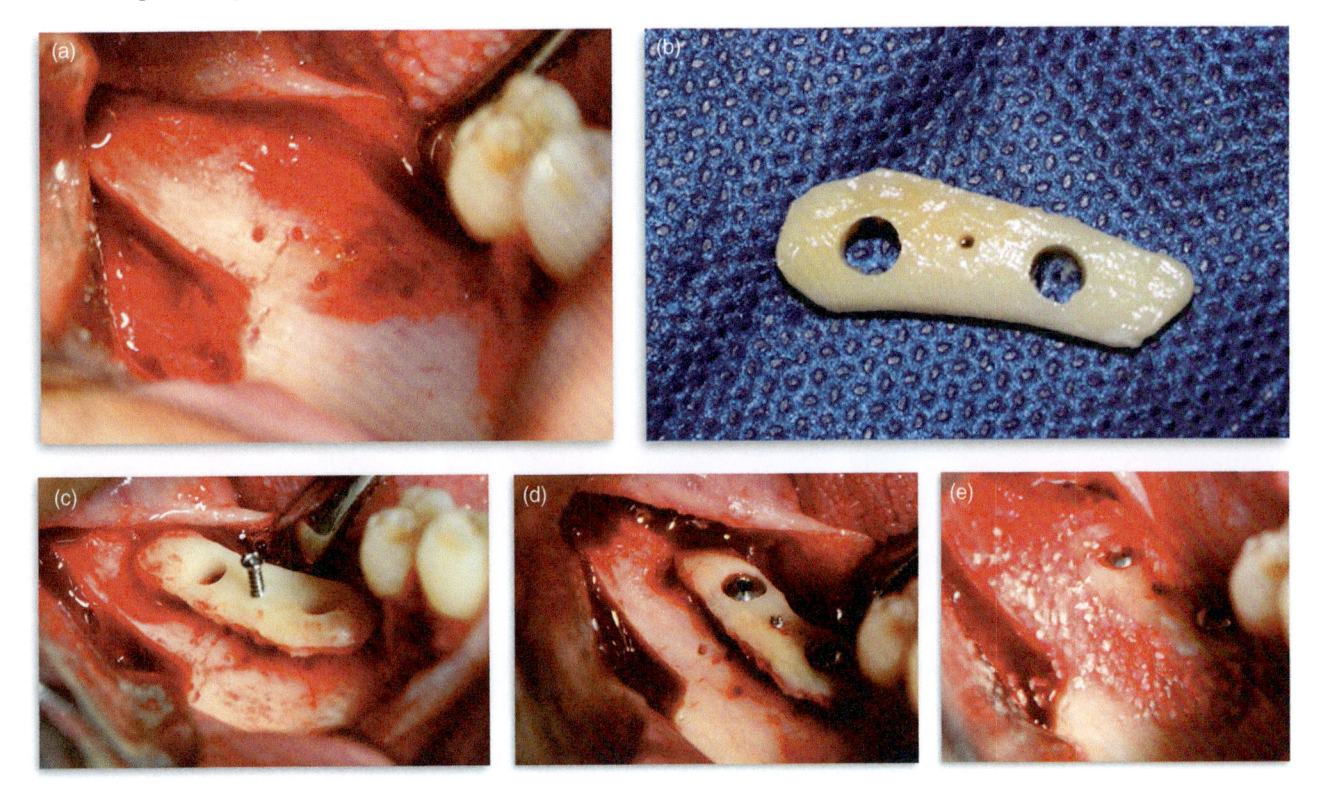

Figure 24.13 Simultaneous implant placement with CAT: (a) "B II" defect in posterior mandible; (b) predrilled LRCB; (c) CAT; (d) simultaneous implant placement; (e) filling the gap.

Table 24.1 Advantages and disadvantages of onlay block graft (OBG).

Advantages	Disadvantages
Simultaneous reconstruction of horizontal and vertical defects	Limited amount of bone gain (4–5 mm) Graft resorption
Applicable in defects with complicated morphology	Donor site • Limitations • Morbidity
Good primary stability of the implant	
	Time consuming • Two-stage surgery
	Bone graft failure may result in implant failure
	Soft tissue tension • Graft exposure • Peri-implantitis

Anatomic repositioning
Distraction osteogenesis

Distraction osteogenesis (DO), which was first developed to correct deformity of the limbs [45], is now a well-accepted technique for augmentation of atrophic ridges [46]. The biologic phenomenon during DO allows soft tissue extension as well as bone regeneration. Therefore, compared to other augmentation procedures more attached gingiva would be available with DO [47].

In an atrophic posterior mandible, DO is indicated for edentulous spans of three or more missing teeth when the vertical defect is more than 4 mm, and a minimum of 6–7 mm above IAN is available [46].

A relatively large amount of vertical bone gain has been reported using the DO technique [48]. In anterior maxillary vertical defects, where the level of gingiva is an important factor in the patient smile line, simultaneous distraction of bone and soft tissue can work well. Gradual segmental lengthening of the bone segment may need secondary augmentation to increase bone width (Figure 24.14).

Despite considerable vertical bone gain and a high survival rate of implants, DO has limited usage for augmentation of the atrophic posterior mandible due to its disadvantages [49] (Table 24.2). The most common complication is lingual inclination of the bone segment [50]. Other complications include relapse, tooth injury, nerve injury, distractor device failure, distraction chamber infection, fractures of distracted or basal bone, hypertrophic scarring, premature or delayed consolidation and fibrous non-union, temporomandibular joint injury, and soft tissue dehiscence [51, 52].

Inferior alveolar nerve lateralization

IAN transpositioning was first reported in 1987 as a part of pre-prosthetic treatment [53]. Transposition of inferior alveolar nerve allows simultaneous implant placement with longer length and high primary stability. Costly bone grafts and prolonged healing periods can be eliminated with this technique. Vestibular depth remained intact, as there is no augmentation in the underlying bone defect. However, it is a very technique-sensitive procedure and sensory dysfunction might happen. This complication is of a great significance as the procedure is primarily performed to preserve the IAN. The neurosensory dysethesia (NSD) following inferior alveolar nerve lateralization (IANL) includes but is not limited to anesthesia, paresthesia, hypoesthesia, a tingling sensation, and a burning sensation [54]. Fracture is an associated risk while transpositioning IAN as the crestal and lateral bone removal would weaken the mandible.

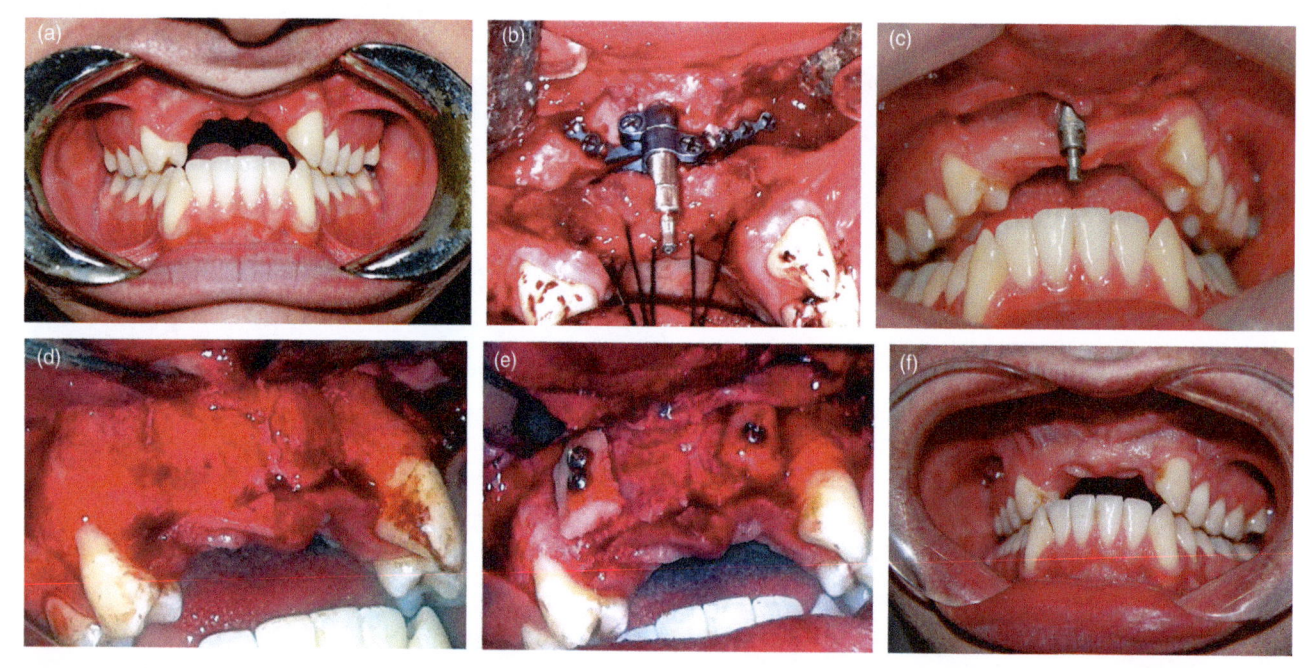

Figure 24.14 (a) Traumatic "C" defect in the anterior maxilla; (b) intraoral distraction device insertion; (c) 2 weeks after activation; (d) adequate bone height was present during device removal but the defect was changed from a "C" to a "A III" defect; (e) OBG with LRCP; (f) gingival profile after dental implant placement.

Table 24.2 Advantages and disadvantages of distraction osteogenesis (DO).

Advantages	Disadvantages
Considerable vertical bone gain	Technical sensitivity
Increase available in attached gingiva	Patient cooperation is necessary
Donor site morbidity is omitted	Improper movement of distracted segment
Less resorption	Could not be performed in defects with complicated morphology

Implant placement in the inferior cortex of the mandible for bicortical stabilization also would reduce the strength [55]. In cases with ridge atrophy and a large interarch space, without the augmentative procedure the height of the implant crown remains inevitably large with an unfavorable crown–implant ratio and a good emergence profile could not be obtained [56].

In the case of a limited interarch space, any augmentation may jeopardize prosthetic rehabilitation and nerve transposition can find its place as a suitable modality. However, a narrow basal bone or the presence of a jaw defect needs simultaneous augmentation [57] (Table 24.3).

According to the edentulous span length, two osteotomy techniques can be used. Nerve *lateralization*, which is IAN repositioning without mental nerve transpositioning or involvement of the mental foramen was performed when the edentulous area and alveolar ridge resorption did not include the premolars [58]. Nerve *distalization* that involves mental nerve and mental foramen (transpositioning of the mental neurovascular bundle and transection of the incisive nerve) with transposition of the IAN was performed when the edentulous area and ridge resorption included the premolar teeth [59].

Inferior alveolar nerve lateralization technique

- Nerve skeletonization. A crestal incision was made and then an anterior releasing incision was extended into the vestibular mucosa to allow good exposure of the mental foramen. After retracting the mucoperiosteal flap, the mental foramen was totally exposed and the dissection was extended towards the inferior border (Figure 24.15a).
- Lateral mandibular body osteotomy. The IAN pathway should be drawn on the lateral surface of the mandible with the tomographic evaluation. The lateral surface can be removed with a round bur or peizosurgical device (Figure 24.15b). Using the diamond burr helps to prevent damaging the IAN. When the mandible is "C III," even after nerve lateralization simultaneous vertical and horizontal augmentation is necessary. Therefore preservation of the thin cortical bone in the lateral side of the IAN should be considered. Four delicate osteotomy lines could remove the lateral cortical surface of IANL. The superior horizontal osteotomy line should be 5 mm away from the ridge crest, the inferior osteotomy line is placed inferior to the canal, and two vertical osteotomy lines are anterior and posterior to the deficient site (Figure 24.15c).
- Nerve relocation. When the osteotomy was finished, the neurovascular bundle inside the canal was freed and moved laterally using a nerve hook. Then a 10 mm wide gauze cord or elastic band was passed below the nerve trunk retracting it from the surgical site and decreasing nerve ischemic trauma. Nerve retraction was continued during drilling and implant insertion in order to reduce the risk of nerve damage. The nerve bundle should not be touched with any sharp instrument. A biangled curved round tip device helps to relocate the bundle (Figure 24.15d).
- Mental foramen osteotomy (optional). When removing a lateral cortex could not provide enough lateralization of the IAN, instead of cutting the incisive branch and distalization of the IAN, a peripheral mental osteotomy could be performed to locate the incisive branch. This can cause more mobilization and lateralization of the bundle. Protecting the incisive branch during nerve lateralization can reduce the risk of retrograde Wallerian degeneration of the IAN bundle. In order to do a safe incisive nerve lateralization, mental foramen peripheral osteotomy with anterior extension is necessary (Figure 24.15e). OBG and CAT with IANL can decrease fracture risk and enhance the prosthetic condition (Figure 24.15f).

Regenerative techniques in bone grafting
RhBMP-2

Discovered in 1965 by Dr. Marshall Urist, bone morphogenetic proteins (BMPs) are the only proteins known to induce new bone formation. Dr. Urist used the term "bone morphogenetic" in 1971 to describe the ability of these bone inductive factors to guide the modulation and differentiation of mesenchymal stem cells into bone and bone marrow cells [60]. BMPs have been shown to play a role in inducing bone formation during skeletal development and fracture repair. Over 20 BMPs have now been discovered. However, only a few of them appear to be osteoinductive and BMP-2 has gained popularity as an adjunct and in many cases an alternative to autogenous grafting. RhBMP-2 induces mesenchymal cells to differentiate into osteoblasts and stimulates the cascade of bone regeneration events, including chemotaxis, induction of pluripotent cells, and proliferation [61].

The application of BMP provides an unlimited supply of nonimmunogenic sterile protein that can induce de novo bone formation. The advantages of using BMP in the commercially available form of INFUSE® are shorter surgical time, avoidance of nerve damage, decreased risk of wound dehiscence, and possible infection. Acellular Type 1 bovine collagen sponges are the usual

Table 24.3 Advantages and disadvantages of inferior alveolar nerve lateralization (IANL).

Advantages	Disadvantages
Use of longer implants	Significant complications • Permanent neurosensory dysfunction • Mandibular fracture
Bone graft is not needed • Less morbidity	Technical sensitivity
Adequate primary stability • *Sometimes* bicortical anchorage	Complicated emergence profile in long interarch space
Time saving • One-stage surgery	Limited implant diameter in cases with horizontal defects
No reduction in vestibular depth • Reduces peri-implant disease	

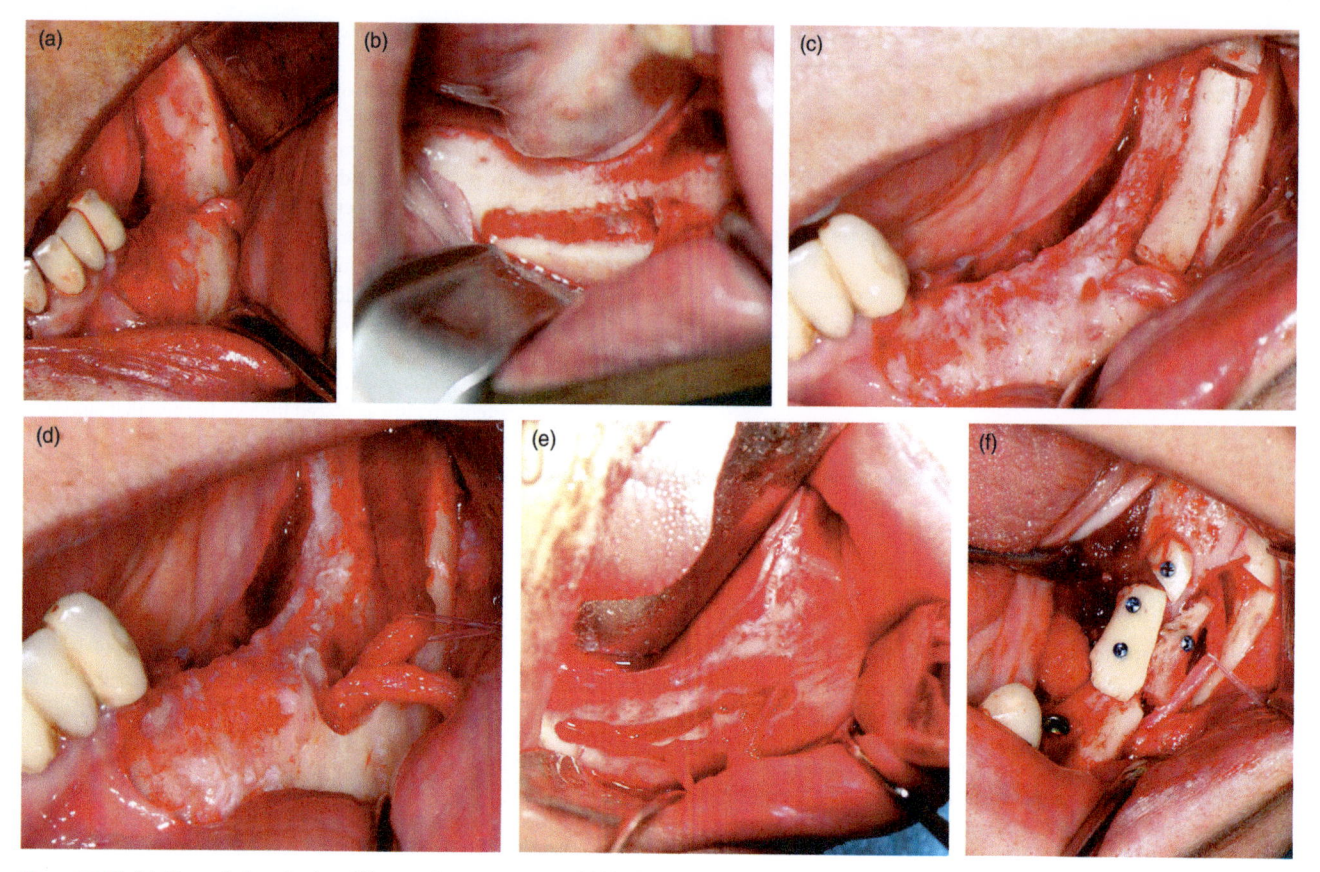

Figure 24.15 (a) Nerve skeletonization; (b) removing outer cortex; (c) block cortical window removal; (d) nerve relocation; (e) incisive branch lateralization; (f) simultaneous augmentation with lateral ramus block.

carriers that maintain the BMP in the graft site and are completely biodegradable.

BMP has very unique properties: it is synthesized inside the cell and acts extracellularly after it is secreted out of the cell. It has a very low molecular weight and it is non-collagenous and therefore not broken down by the enzymes that degrade collagen. It is composed of two small dimeric proteins in the form of two subunits linked by a special bond (disulfide bond).

The mechanism of bone formation is initially via chemotaxis and recruitment of cells. This causes proliferation of cells infiltrating from the periphery to undergo morphogenesis and new bone formation. Mesenchymal stem cells are recruited to the site by chemotaxis where they undergo cell division and increase in number. Mesenchymal stem cells differentiate ultimately into osteoblasts. Later, osteoblasts regulate the calcification of the callus. It also leads to vascular invasion and a robust angiogenic response, which is likely to be an indirect effect via induction of VEGF in BMP responsive cells. Newly formed woven bone remodels into trabecular bone and increases in vascularity as it matures. BMPs are an integral part of natural bone formation and the fracture healing response [62]. The osteogenic process is different between BMP-2 and autogenous bone graft [63].

INFUSE® bone graft contains this recombinant human BMP-2. INFUSE® bone graft is an iliac crest bone graft replacement. The kits include two components, rhBMP-2 and the absorbable collagen sponge (ACS). The active ingredient is rhBMP-2, which is reconstituted with the included sterile water at a fixed concentration of 1.5 mg/ml. The concentration of rhBMP-2 is very important in effectively inducing new bone formation. The protein in highly pure and is the inductive component within INFUSE® bone graft.

The absorbable collagen sponge (ACS) is the carrier and delivery agent that maintains local concentration of rhBMP-2 and induces new bone growth at the surgical site. The ACS is the osteoconductive component found within INFUSE® bone graft. Over time, it is remodeled and replaced with host bone. Goals of the surgical procedure are to extract tooth and debride soft tissue, gain access to cells (perforate cortical plates), implant enough material to fill the defect site, and achieve tension-free wound closure.

Histologically the rhBMP-2/ACS induced bone contained a vascular marrow space, had a moderate degree of new trabecular bone formed, which contained both woven (initial) bone and lamellar (mature) bone, and a higher proportion of osteoblasts than osteoclasts was seen, which was consistent with overall bone growth. There was little to no histological evidence of inflammation. The collagen carrier acts as a pre-implantation matrix. As the sponge degrades the chemotactic effects of BMP-2 attract mesenchymal stem cells, which migrate to where the bone is formed. During the migration stem cells differentiate to osteoblasts. These osteoblasts condense into a cluster and release osteoid unmineralized bone matrix to form a woven bone island. The osteoblasts form new bone bridges that connect all the individual woven islands into a woven trabecular network as the island is then mineralized to complete the process of de novo bone formation as

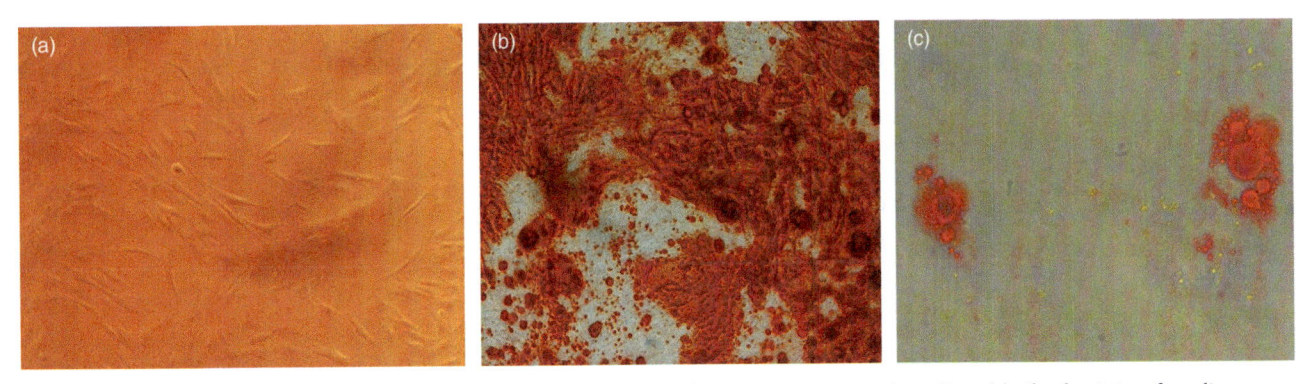

Figure 24.16 (a) Stellate adherent MSCs under light microscopy; (b) Alizarin red staining in an osteogenic medium; (c) oil red staining after adipose differentiation.

Table 24.4 Different genes expressed by mesenchymal stem cells.

Cell lineage	Genes
Osteogenic differentiation	Osteopontin, Collagen I
Chondrogenic differentiation	Decorin, Collagen II
Adipogenic differentiation	LPL, PPARG2

the woven bone becomes lamellar bone through remodeling. The entire marrow area is very rich in spindle-shaped stem cells and vascularity. No collagen matrix was detected at 6 months to 1 year post-operative. Studies have found no significant difference in implant survival either by patient or by implant between the autograft and INFUSE® bone graft groups over 2 years post-prosthesis placement [64].

Mesenchymal stem cells

The traditional triad of tissue engineering attempts to replicate the intrinsic properties of autograft reconstruction. Bone tissue engineering requires a combination of osteogenic cells, three-dimensional (3D) scaffolds, and osteogenesis-inducing factors to produce a mature bone structure. Some studies have shown promising outcomes for cell-based approaches in bone regeneration; however, the best technique for reproducing bone in defective regions is still controversial [65].

The most important advantage of tissue engineering over autogenous grafting is that tissue-engineered bone is produced in an *ex vivo* context that avoids the drawbacks of autograft donor morbidity and availability. Mesenchymal stem cells (MSCs) fulfill these essential criteria. One of the original studies that introduced MSCs dates to the 1960s, when Friedenstein et al. isolated a population of cells from bone marrow that formed colonies and differentiated into osteoblasts [66].

Adult stem cells derived from bone marrow (BMSCs) are most commonly used for bone regeneration purposes. Yet, seeking for more accessible sources of stem cells with limited morbidity, adult stem cells derived from other tissues such as adipose tissue and dental and periodontal tissues were also examined [67]. MSCs are adherent stellate like cells and should prove their multipotentiality *in vitro*. Differentiation staining with Alizarin Red (osteogenic differentiation), Oil Red (adipose differentiation), and Toluidine Blue (cartilage differentiation) (Figure 24.16) or RT-PCR for the gene expression can demonstrate multipotentiality of MSCs [68, 69] (Table 24.4). On the molecular level, MSCs can be identified based

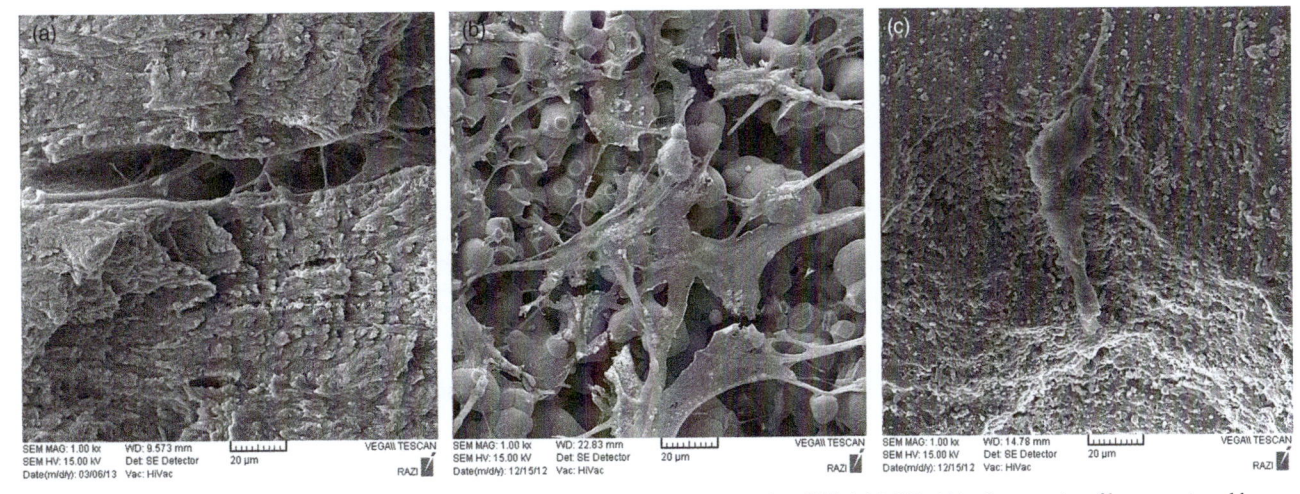

Figure 24.17 Morphologic characteristics of the MSCs when cultured on different types of scaffold. (a) MSC within the porosity of human mineral bone (allograft); (b) wide multipod MSCs on β-TCP; (c) long thin MSCs on bovine bone mineral.

on positivity for several tissue markers, such as CD90, CD105, CD44, CD29, CD160, and CD119, and negativity for others, such as CD14, CD45, CD34, and CD11 [70].

Synthetic or natural scaffolds can be used for delivery of the MSCs to bone defects. An incubation period of 24 to 48 hours is necessary for appropriate cell lodgment. Cell entrapment could be detected within the pores of the scaffold. Morphological characteristics of MSCs can be influenced by type of scaffold (Figure 24.17). Cell delivery methods, incubation period, presence of adhesive agents, possible use of growth factor, genetic modification, and, most importantly, defect size can affect treatment outcome of bone tissue engineering. In our studies with the same methods of cell delivery synthetic scaffold showed better results in bone healing (Table 24.5).

Table 24.5 Cell therapy for bone regeneration.

Author(s) and year	Study model	Scaffold	Stem cell	Growth factor	Sample size	Defect size and location	Tests	Results
Khojasteh et al. (2008) [68]	Rat	A: NBBM B: β-TCP	BMMSCs	PRP	11	5 mm in diameter Calvari defect in parietal bone	HMMA	Bone Formation after 6 w: A + PRP: 1.27 mm A + BMMSCs: 1.44 mm B + PRP: 1.21 mm B + BMMSCs: 2.53 mm
Behnia et al. (2013) [88]	Rabbit	Nano silica gel/HA (nHA)	BMMSCs	PRGF	8	8 mm in diameter Parietal bone	HMMA	After 12 w nHA: 32.53% nHA + PRGF: 39.74% nHA + MSCs: 39.11% nHA + PRGF + MSCs: 44.55%
Behnia et al. (2012) [87]	Rabbit	FDBA	BMMSCs	PRGF	8	8 mm in diameter Parietal bone	HMMA	After 12 w FDBA: 20.31% FDBA + PRGF: 28.44% FDBA + MSCs: 31.33% FDBA + PRGF + MSCs: 37.21%
Khojasteh et al. (2013) [86]	Rabbit	Particulate allogenic bone	BMMSCs	Fibrin glue	5	Tibial bone	HMMA	-2.09 mm Mean amount of vertical bone length after 2 m -28.5 64.5% new supra crestal trabecular bone formation
Eslaminejad et al. (2008) [85]	Dog	HA/TCP NBBM	BMMSCs	–	4	Masseter muscle	HMMA	Ectopic bone formation after 2 m HA/TCP: 29.12% NBBM: 23.55%
Jafarian et al. (2008) [84]	Dog	HA/TCP NBBM	BMMSCs	–	4	10 mm through defect in mandible	HMMA	Percentage of bone fill after 6 w HA/TCP + MSCs: 65.78% NBBM + MSCs: 50.31% HA/TCP: 44.90% NBBM: 36.83%
Khojasteh et al. (2013) [69]	Dog	PCL-TCP	BMMSCs	–	4	20 mm × 10 mm × 10 mm Posterior mandibular	HMMA	After 2 m -48.63% Lamellar Bone -24.1% Remaining scaffold
Khojasteh et al. (2013) [83]	Dog	FDMBB	BMMSCs	PDGF	4	25 mm × 10 mm Mandible	HMMA μCT	New bone after 8 w FDMBB + MSCs: 21.38% FDMBB + MSCs + PDGF: 26.63% FDMBB + MSCs: 8.20% FDMBB + MSCs + PDGF: 10.34%
Shayesteh et al. (2008) [71]	Human	HA/TCP	BMMSCs	–	7	Patients required sinus lift	HMMA RG	-41.34% newly bone formation (3 m) -The mean of the initial bone height was 2.25 mm, initial grafted sinus height (SBH1) was 12.08 mm (3 m), and secondary bone height after 1 year (SBH2) was 10.83 mm
Behnia et al. (2009) [72]	Human	DBM/ CaSO$_4$	BMMSCs	–	2	Unilateral alveolar cleft	Panoramic and intraoral inspection and palpation CT	-Integrity of nasal floor -*34.5% the mean postoperative defect of patient 1 (4 m) *25.6% the mean postoperative defect of patient 2 (4 m)
Behnia et al. (2012) [73]	Human	HA/TCP	BMMSCs	PDGF	4	Anterior maxillary cleft	CBCT	-51.3% mean fill of the bone defect (3 m)

BMMSC: bone marrow mesenchymal stem cell; HMMA: histomorphometric analysis; m: month; w: week; CT: computed tomography, PRP: platelet-rich plasma; PRGF: platelet-released growth factors; PDGF: platelet-derived growth factor; CBCT: cone beam computed tomography, RG: radiography; NBBM: natural bovine bone mineral; DBM: demineralized bone mineral, HA: hydroxylapatite; TCP: tricalcium phosphate, FDBA: freeze dried bone allograft; PCL: polycaprolactone; FDMBB: freeze-dried mineral bone block.

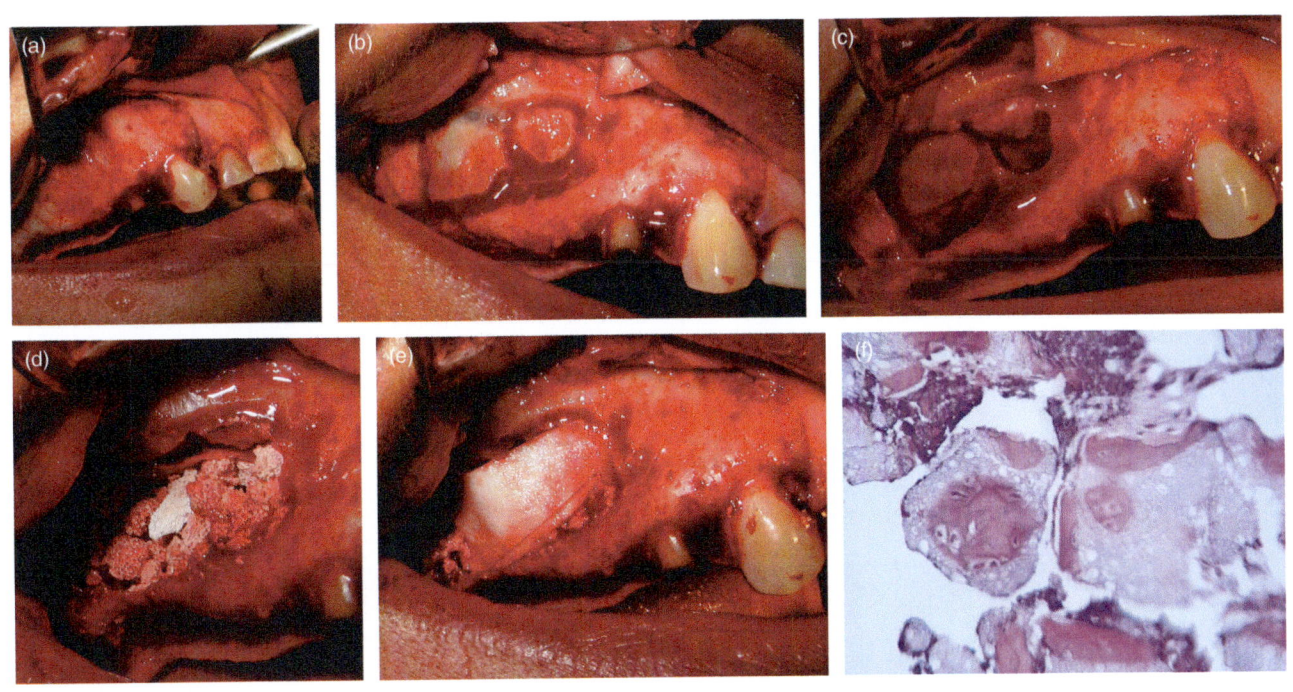

Figure 24.18 Bone marrow derived MSCs cultured on HA/TCP biphasic scaffolds for maxillary sinus augmentation. Reproduced by permission of Elsevier from Shayesteh YS, Khojasteh A, Soleimani M, Alikhasi M, Khoshzaban A, Ahmadbeigi A: Sinus augmentation using human mesenchymal stem cells loaded into a [beta]-tricalcium phosphate/hydroxyapatite scaffold. Source: Shayesteh et al 2008 [71]. Reproduced with permission from Elsevier.

Bone marrow derived MSCs for human sinus augmentation resulted in 41% of new bone formation after 3 months [71] (Figure 24.18), whereas alveolar cleft defects when treated with MSCs showed a range of 25.6 to 34.5% of new bone formation [72] (Figure 24.19). Adding platelet rich in growth factors to MCSs as an adhesive agent and replacing demineralized bone mineral by biphasic scaffolds increased the amount of bone formation in alveolar cleft defects by up to 52% [73].

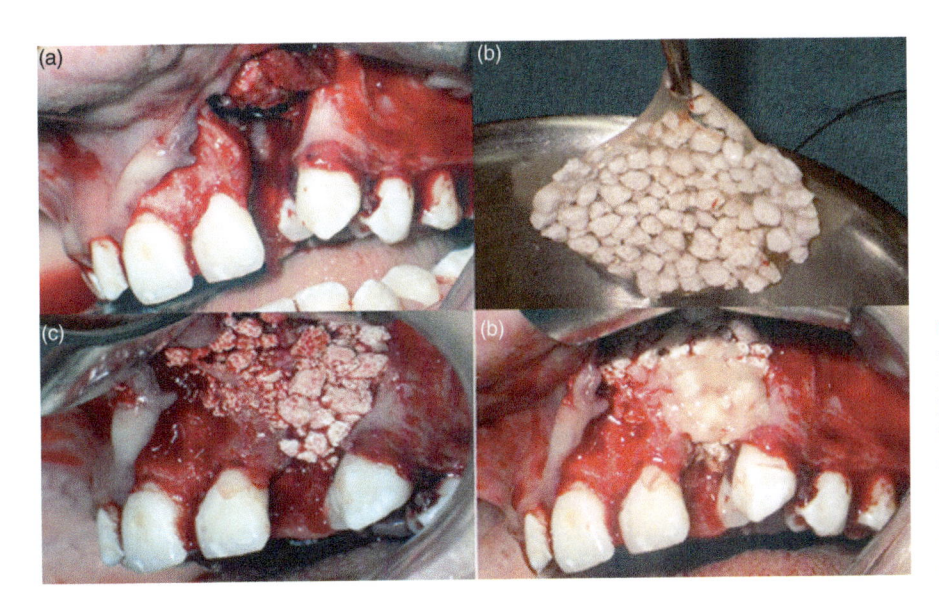

Figure 24.19 MSCs loaded on HA/TCP for the treatment of alveolar cleft defects. Reproduced by permission of Elsevier from Behnia H, Khojasteh A, Soleimani M, Tehranchi A, Atashi A: Repair of alveolar cleft defect with mesenchymal stem cells and platelet derived growth factors: a preliminary report. Source: Behnia et al 2012 [73]. Reproduced with permission from Elsevier.

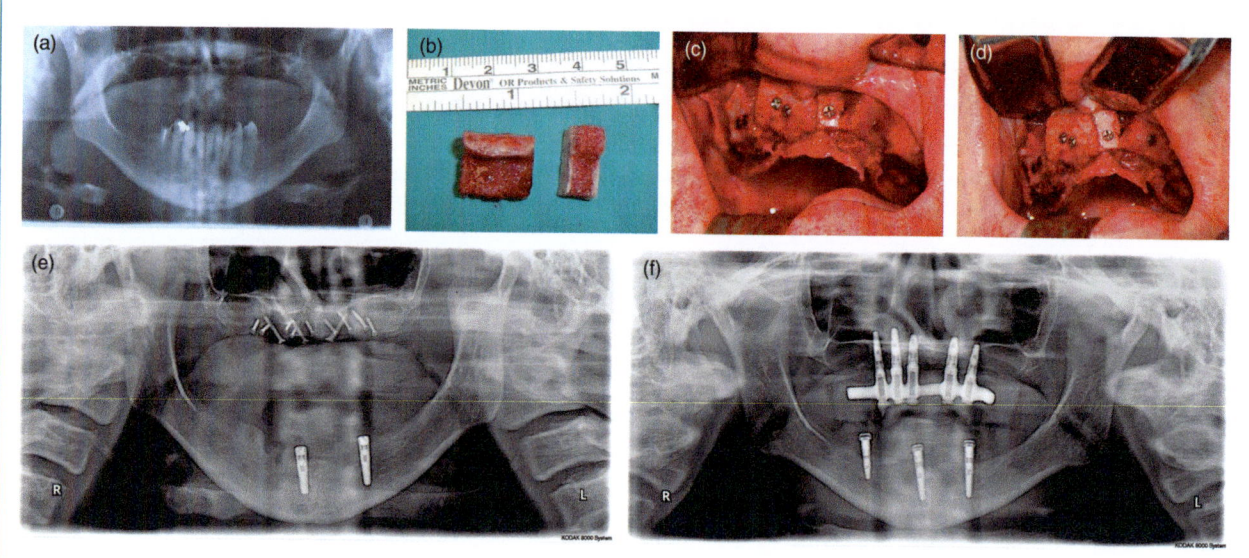

Case reports

The representative case treated by anterior iliac crest bone grafting for vertical ridge augmentation is shown in Figure 24.20. A 65-year-old female with a severely resorbed knife-edge maxillary anterior ridge undergoes reconstruction with autogenous posterior iliac crest block grafting and cortical fixation screws. She undergoes reconstruction with placement of mandibular and future maxillary implants after vertical and horizontal reconstruction.

The representative case treated by BMP-2 is introduced as shown in Figure 24.21. A 63-year-old female with a severely resorbed knife-edge maxillary anterior ridge undergoes *simultaneous* reconstruction of the deficient alveolar ridge with rhBMP-2/ACS plus a demineralized freeze-dried allogeneic corticocancellous graft with immediate placement of four maxillary implants. A titanium mesh is used as a space maintainer, which is removed after 9 months while uncovering the dental implants [74]. Alternatively, a resorbable poly-D-L-lactide mesh can be used as a spacer, which may require use of a water bath [75]. Mucosal inflammation was not observed around the implants or the mesh, but significant edema can be observed around the grafted site, which patients should be warned about [76].

The representative case treated by tibial bone grafting for vertical ridge augmentation is shown in the anterior mandible with simultaneous placement of three mandibular implants as a modification of the "Tent Pole" technique described by Carlson and Marx [29] (Figure 24.22). A 65-year-old male with a severely atrophic mandible (less than 6 mm in height) undergoes reconstruction with an autogenous tibial bone for vertical and horizontal augmentation. The implants serve as a scaffold to prevent loss of graft during healing of the bone. After a period of six months the dental implants are uncovered with a stable gain of 8 mm of mandibular height. The final restoration is a bar-retained mandibular denture.

The representative case is treated by a Le Fort I osteotomy and block bone harvested from the anterior iliac crest for an extensive maxillary reconstruction (Figure 24.23). A buccal fat pad is used to harvest and culture MSCs and bovine bone mineral is used to deliver third passage cultured cells to the operating room. Gaps are filled with loaded scaffolds and a collagen membrane is used to cover the grafted tissue with collagen membrane. Healing of the bone graft is observed after 6 months.

Figure 24.20 The representative case treated by anterior iliac crest bone grafting for vertical ridge augmentation is shown. (a) A 65-year-old female with a severely resorbed knife-edge maxillary anterior ridge undergoes reconstruction with (b) autogenous posterior iliac crest block grafting and (c to e) cortical fixation screws. (f) She undergoes reconstruction with placement of mandibular and future maxillary implants after vertical and horizontal reconstruction.

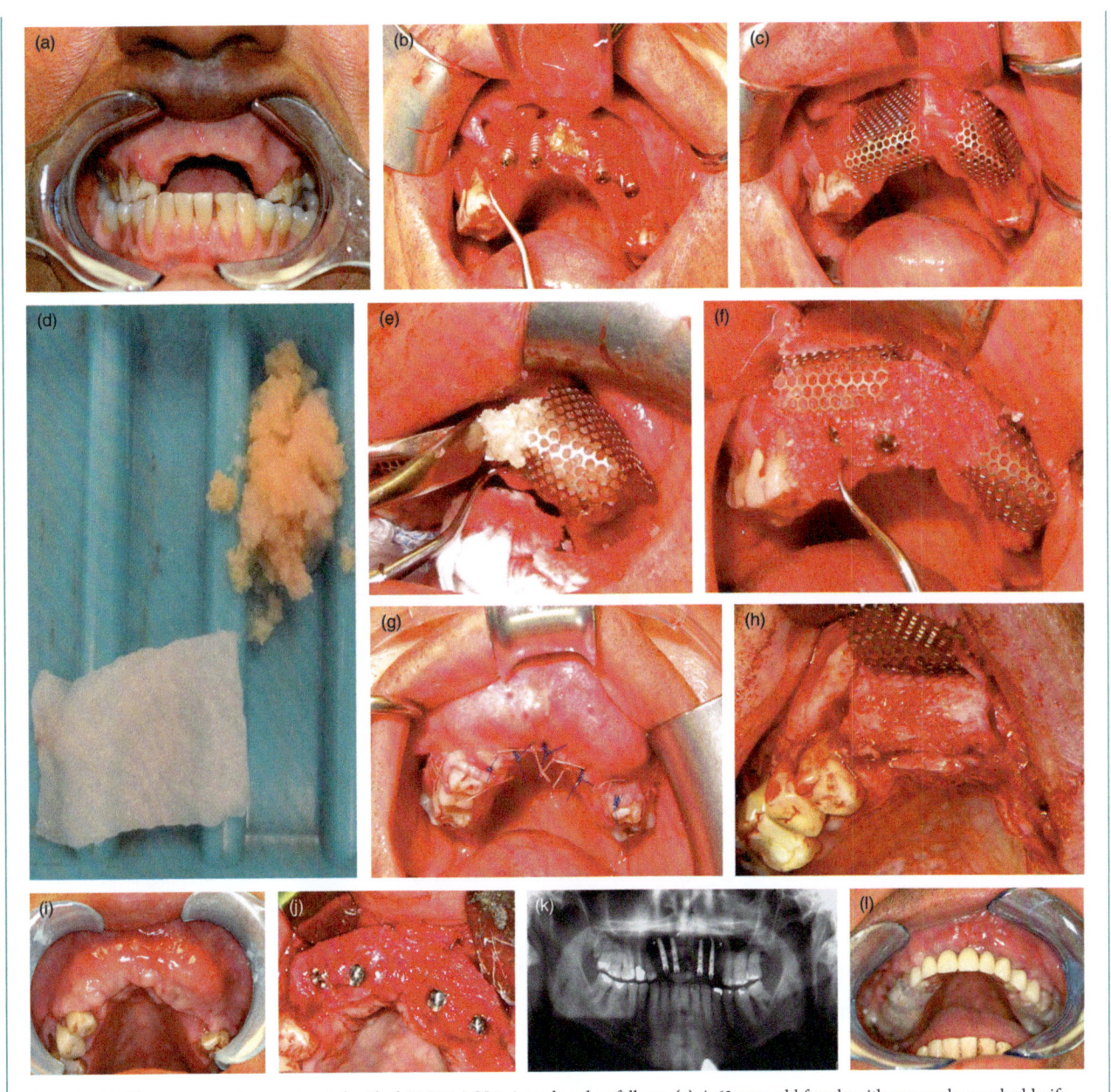

Figure 24.21 The representative case treated with rhBMP2-ACS is introduced as follows. **(a)** A 63-year-old female with a severely resorbed knife-edge maxillary anterior ridge **(c)** undergoes reconstruction with rhBMP-2/ACS and a demineralized freeze-dried allogeneic corticocancellous graft. **(b)** She undergoes simultaneous reconstruction placement of maxillary implants. **(c to f)** A titanium mesh is used as a space maintainer, which is removed after 9 months **(h to j)** while uncovering the dental implants **(k and l)** Restoration after dental implant placement is performed after 9 months. **(m to o)** Diagrams depicting the mode of action of BMP. Source: Michael Peleg DDS, Professor of Surgery, University of Miami School of Medicine, Miami, FL. Reproduced with permission from Michael Peleg.

(continued)

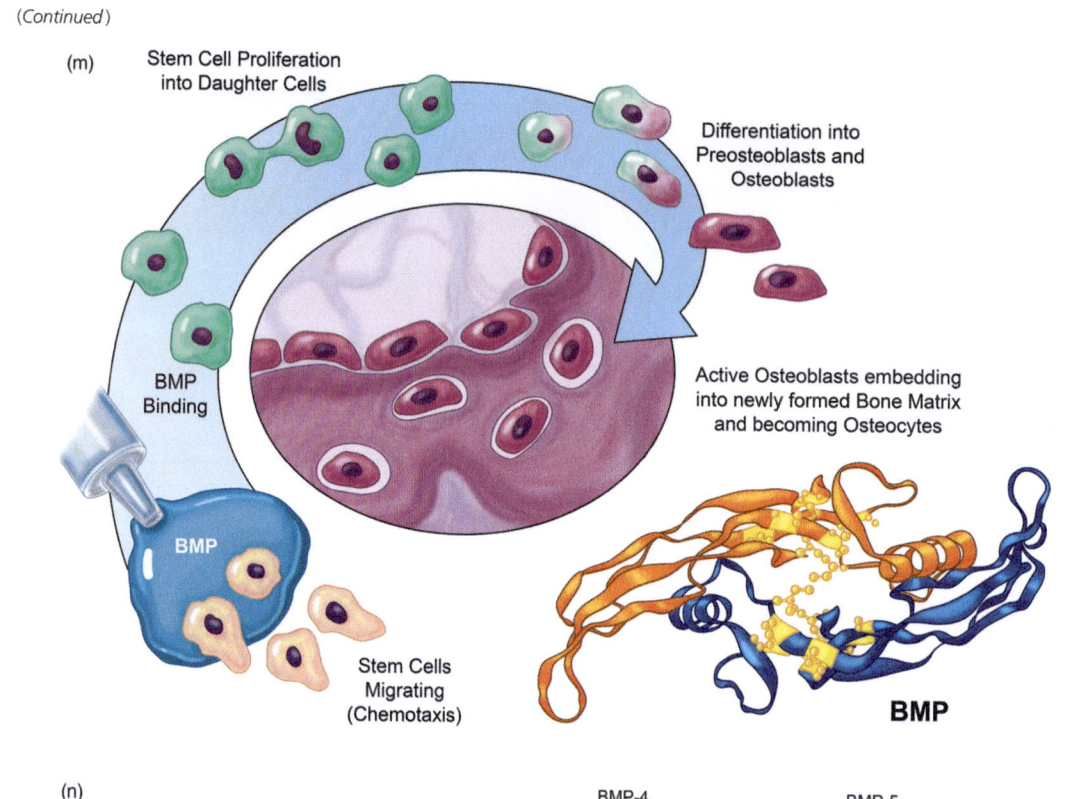

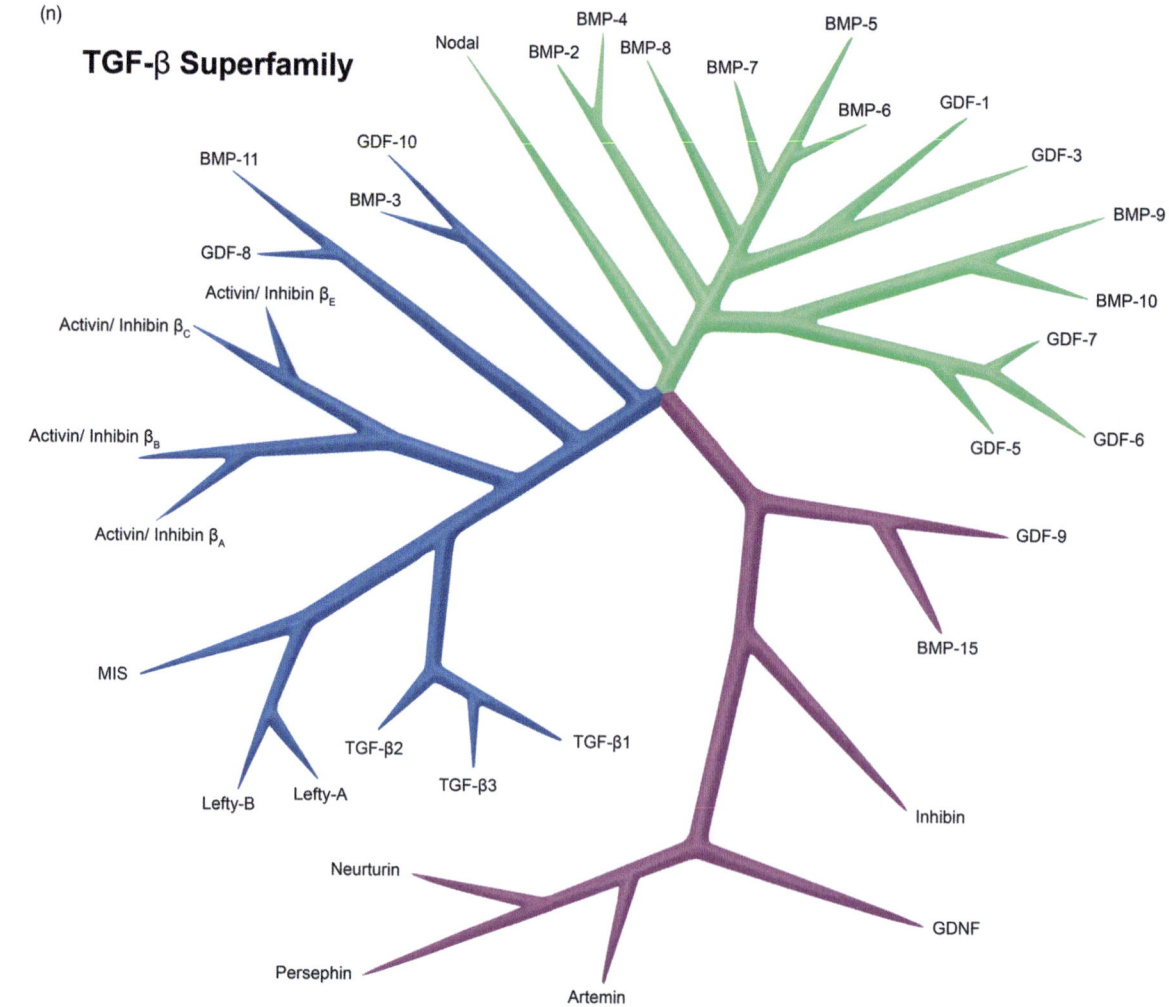

Figure 24.21 (*Continued*)

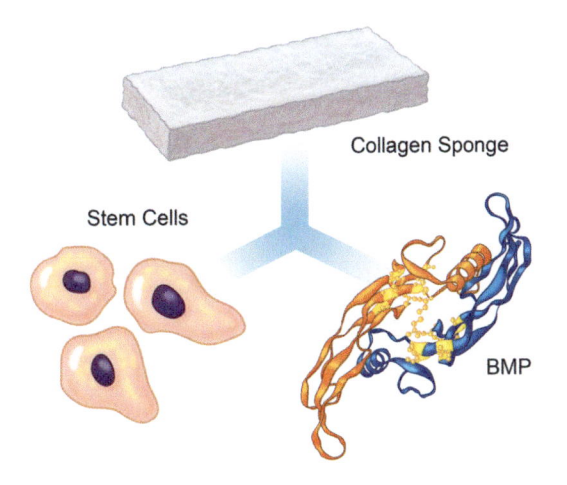

Figure 24.21 (*Continued*)

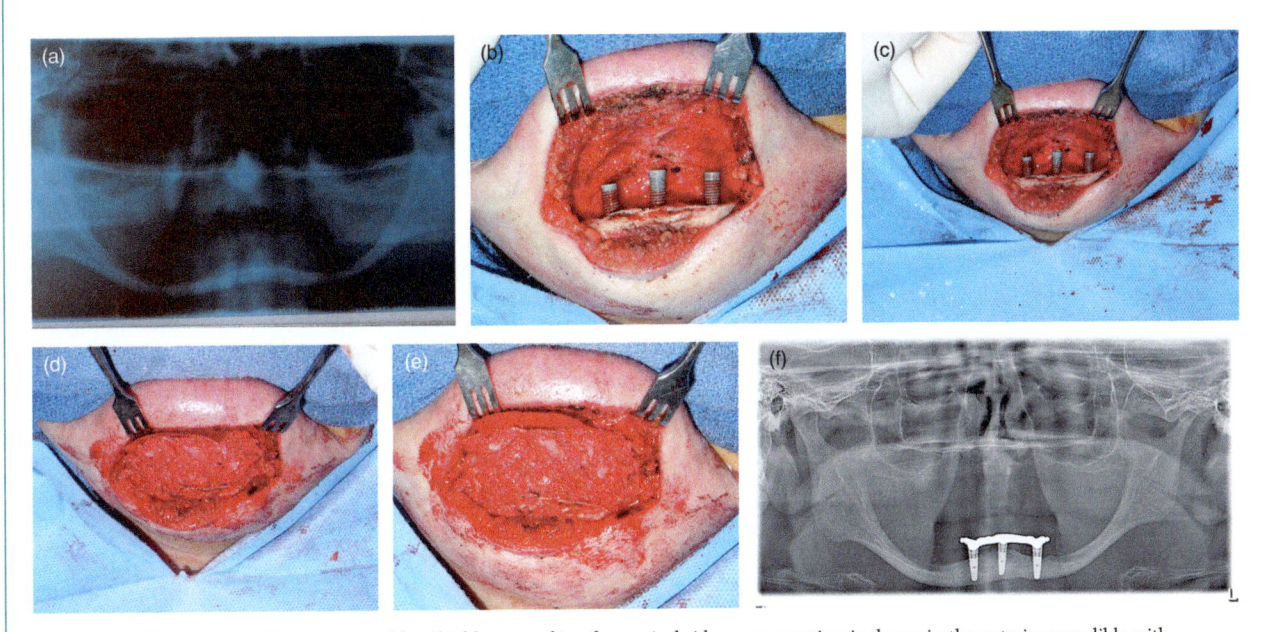

Figure 24.22 The representative case treated by tibial bone grafting for vertical ridge augmentation is shown in the anterior mandible with simultaneous placement of three mandibular implants as a modification of the "Tent Pole" technique described by Carlson and Marx [29]. A 65-year-old male with a severely atrophic mandible (less than 6 mm in height) undergoes reconstruction with autogenous tibial bone for vertical and horizontal augmentation. The implants act as a scaffold to prevent loss of graft. After a period of 6 months the dental implants are uncovered with a stable gain of 8 mm of mandibular height. The final restoration is a bar-retained mandibular denture.

(*continued*)

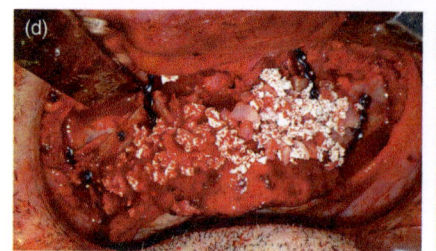

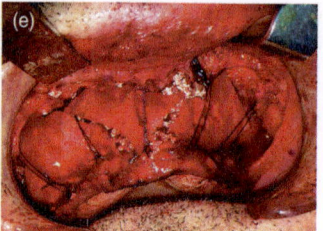

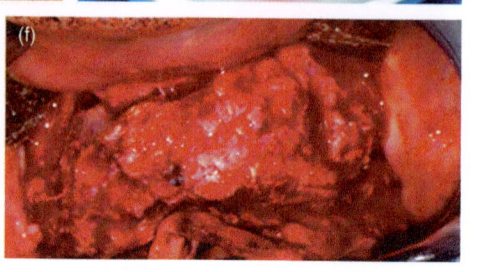

Figure 24.23 (a) Le Fort I osteotomy and block bone harvested from anterior iliac crest for an extensive maxillary reconstruction. (b) Buccal fat pad used to harvest and culture MSCS. (c) Bovine bone mineral used to deliver third passage cultured cells to the operating room. (d) Filling the gap with loaded scaffolds. (e) Covering the grafted tissue with collagen membrane. (f) Bone healing after 6 months.

Discussion

When considering the option for reconstruction of the partially or completely edentulous patient with inadequate bone, the surgeon must establish a plan to take the patient from his/her current state to a fully functional restoration in a restoratively driven (pre-prosthetic) manner. Understanding all stages of this surgical–restorative implant process is critical to obtaining an ideal outcome.

When asking a colleague or even reminiscing on one's own practice it is all too often clear that clinical practice closely mirrors one's training. The focus and purpose of this chapter is to remind the practitioner that there are many surgical ways and varieties of surgical techniques to obtain an ideal result. The collective authors here would encourage the reader to think beyond how they may have been trained and consider employing new and various techniques that they may not have previously considered.

The approaches discussed here can be broken down into two larger categories and then further subdivided from there. Initially, the first decision must be made to decide whether to use the patient's own bone stock by its manipulation or to focus on augmentation. Manipulation of existing bone would include techniques discussed here, such as distraction osteogenesis, inferior alveolar nerve lateralization, as well as others discussed in other chapters of this book, such as ridge-splitting, etc. Augmentation, as discussed in this chapter, can take on many forms. The variety of autogenous harvests described can be used as indicated based on the desired graft size and consistency. When the decision has been made to avoid autogenous harvest, multiple other options exist, such as rhBMP-2, mesenchymal stem cells, allogeneic bone, xenogeneic bone, and alloplastic bone substitutes. It is the authors' collective opinion that by utilizing bone science tissue engineering grafts can rival or even surmount the results of autogenous bone grafting.

With the constant advancements that are being made in the understanding of bone science and the clinical applications of these findings, we hope all readers are encouraged through the discussion here and the cases presented to broaden their collective toolbox of surgical techniques when addressing complex osseous defects of the maxillofacial region.

Conclusion

The oral and maxillofacial surgeon is commonly faced with the task of hard tissue reconstruction for the following indications: jaw atrophy with associated dental implant rehabilitation, benign and cancer ablated defects, and extensive craniofacial fracture repair [77]. Reconstruction of hard tissue defects in the oral and maxillofacial region has made use of recent technological advances and tissue engineering. *Vertical ridge augmentation* has always posed a challenge even to the skilled surgeon. Although cancellous cellular marrow transfer still represents the gold standard for successful grafting and bone formation in oral and maxillofacial reconstruction, the use of many novel techniques and advances in science have lessened the need for autogenous grafting with decreased morbidity, operating room time, and cost [78]. In this chapter, the authors have reviewed the more common types of non-vascular autogenous block bone grafting techniques based on their clinical expertise employed in oral and maxillofacial surgery.

The issue to consider when formulating a proper surgical plan and appropriate donor site to reconstruct the maxillofacial defects is the recognition that there is both a horizontal and vertical deficiency of bone. Traditionally, vertical ridge augmentation has posed a clinical challenge that can be overcome by topics reviewed by the authors in this chapter. Prosthetic implant treatment should ultimately help determine the most effective surgical plan and type and amount of bone needed.

Implant osseointegration is determined by the de novo bone regeneration at the bone–implant surface [79]. The ideal osseointegration takes place in native bone with cortical components and trabecular vascular and marrow components. Predictable osseointegration also takes place with autogenous grafts that heal by osteoconduction and osteoinduction, as well as with BMP engineered de novo regenerated bone [80]. In many cases BMP usage has completely replaced autogenous grafting [81]. BMP is unique in its mechanism of bone induction, which includes several phases: chemotaxis, recruitment, proliferation, morphogenesis, and differentiation followed by calcification and maturation.

Bone fillers such as xenografts and alloplasts result in less than ideal vertical and horizontal bone regeneration as they conduct bone regeneration yet leave inert residual particles that may impede osseointegration as the implants are not completely placed in vital bone [82].

Disclaimer

The views expressed in this chapter are those of the authors and do not necessarily reflect the official policy or position of the Department of the Navy, Department of Defense, or the United States Government.

References

1. Nevins M, Mellonig J: Enhancement of the damaged edentulous ridge to receive dental implants: a combination of allograft and Gore Tex membrane. *Int J Periodont Rest Dent* 1992;**12**:97–111.
2. Fonseca RJ: Reconstruction of the maxillofacial cancer patient, Chapter 15. In: *Oral and Maxillofacial Surgery*, vol. 7. Saunders, 2000, pp. 366–369.
3. Yates D, Brockhoff II HC, Finn R, Phillips C: Comparison of intraoral harvest sites for corticocancellous bone grafts. *J Oral Maxillofac Surg* 2013;**71**(3):497–504.
4. Jensen O: Alveolar segmental "sandwich" osteotomies for posterior edentulous mandibular sites for dental implants. *J Oral Maxillofac Surg* 2006;**64**:471–475.
5. Jenson OT, Block M: Alveolar modification by distraction osteogenesis. *Atlas Oral Maxillofacial Surg Clin N Am* 2008;**16**:185–214.
6. Ueda M, et al: Tissue engineering: applications for maxillofacial surgery. *Material Sciences and Engineering*, 2000;**13**:7–14.
7. Rocchietta I, Fontana F, Simion M: Clinical outcomes of vertical bone augmentation to enable dental implant placement: a systematic review. *J Clin Periodontol* 2008;**35**:203–215.
8. Khojasteh A, Morad G, Behnia H: Clinical importance of recipient site characteristics for vertical ridge augmentation: a systematic review of literature and proposal of a classification. *J Oral Implantol* 2013;**39**:386–398.
9. Tinti C, Parma-Benfenati S: Clinical classification of bone defects concerning the placement of dental implants. *Int J Periodontics Restorative Dent* 2003;**23**:147–155.
10. Jensen SS, Terheyden H: Bone augmentation procedures in localized defects in the alveolar ridge: clinical results with different bone grafts and bone-substitute materials. *Int J Oral Maxillofac Implants* 2009;**24**(Suppl):218–236.
11. Proussaefs P, Lozada J: Use of titanium mesh for staged localized alveolar ridge augmentation: clinical and histologic–histomorphometric evaluation. *J Oral Implantol* 2006;**32**:237–247.
12. Iizuka T, Smolka W, Hallermann W, Mericske-Stern R: Extensive augmentation of the alveolar ridge using autogenous calvarial split bone grafts for dental rehabilitation. *Clin Oral Implants Res* 2004;**15**:607–615.
13. Schwartz-Arad D, Levin L, Sigal L: Surgical success of intraoral autogenous block onlay bone grafting for alveolar ridge augmentation. *Implant Dentistry* 2005;**14**:131–138.
14. Heller AL, Heller RL: Soft tissue management techniques for implant dentistry: a clinical guide. *J Oral Implantol* 2000;**26**:91–103.
15. Xu R, Ebraheim NA, Yeasting RA, Jackson WT: Anatomic considerations for posterior iliac bone harvesting. *Spine* 1966;**21**:1017–1020.
16. Colterjohn NR, Bednar DA: Procurement of bone graft from the iliac crest. *Journal of Bone and Joint Surgery*, 1997;**79**:756–759.
17. Kolomvos N, Iatrou I, Theologie-Lygidakis N, Tzerbos F, Schoinohoriti O: Iliac crest morbidity following maxillofacial bone grafting in children: a clinical and radiographic prospective study. *J Cranio-Maxillofacial Surgery* 2010;**38**(4):293–302.
18. Ahlmann E, Patzakis M, Roidis N, Shepherd L, Holtom P: Comparison of anterior and posterior iliac crest bone grafts in terms of harvest-site morbidity and functional outcomes. *Journal of Bone and Joint Surgery* 2002;**84**:716–720.
19. Bruno BJ, Gustafson PA: Cranial bone harvest, grafting: a choice for maxillofacial reconstruction. *AORN Journal* 1994 Jan;**59**(1):242–251.
20. Iizuka T, Smolka W, Hallermann W, Mericske-Stern R: Extensive augmentation of the alveolar ridge using autogenous calvarial split bone grafts for dental rehabilitation. *Clin Oral Implants Res* 2004;**15**:607–615.
21. Gutta R, Waite PD: Cranial bone grafting and simultaneous implants: a submental technique to reconstruct the atrophic mandible. *British Journal of Oral and Maxillofacial Surgery* 2008 Sep;**46**(6):477–479.
22. Davis WB: The development of the bones of the face. Original Research Article. *International Journal of Orthodontia* 1917 Oct;**3**(10):567–596.
23. Naidich TP, Blaser SI, Lien RJ, Mclone DG, Fatterpekar GM, Bauer BS: Embryology and congenital lesions of the midface, Chapter 1. In: *Head and Neck Imaging*, 5th edn, vol. I, 2011, pp. 3–97.
24. Marx RE, Sawatari Y, Fortin M, Broumand V: Bisphosphonate-induced exposed bone (osteonecrosis/osteopetrosis) of the jaws: risk factors, recognition, prevention, and treatment. Original Research Article. *J Oral Maxillo Surg* 2005;**63**(11):1567–1575.
25. Broumand V, Marx RE: M623: risk factors, recognition, prevention, treatment of bisphosphonate-induced osteonecrosis of the jaws. *J Oral Maxillo Surg* 2006;**64**(9 Suppl):96.
26. Marx RE: Clinical application of bone biology to mandibular and maxillary reconstruction. *Clin Plast Surg* 1994;**21**:377–392.
27. Roden RD: Principles of bone grafting: a review article. *Oral and Maxillofacial Surgery Clinics of North America* 2010;**22**(3):295–300.
28. Khojasteh A, Behnia H, Shayesteh YS, et al: Localized bone augmentation with cortical bone blocks tented over different particulate bone substitutes: a retrospective study. *J Oral Maxillofac Implants* 2012;**27**:1481–1493.
29. Carlson ER, Marx RE: Mandibular reconstruction using cancellous cellular bone grafts. *J Oral Maxillofac Surg* 1996;**54**:889–897.
30. Araujo PP, Oliveira KP, Montenegro SC, Carreiro AF, Silva JS, Germano AR: Block allograft for reconstruction of alveolar bone ridge in implantology: a systematic review. *Implant Dent* 2013;**22**:304–308.
31. Rodella LF, Favero G, Labanca M: Biomaterials in maxillofacial surgery: membranes and grafts. *Int J Biomed Sci* 2011;**7**:81–88.
32. Burchardt H, Enneking WF: Transplantation of bone. *Surg Clin North Am* 1978;**58**:403–427.
33. Pikos MA: Block autografts for localized ridge augmentation: Part II. The posterior mandible. *Implant Dent* 2000;**9**:67–75.
34. Ozkan Y, Ozcan M, Varol A, Akoglu B, Ucankale M, Basa S: Resonance frequency analysis assessment of implant stability in labial onlay grafted posterior mandibles: a pilot clinical study. *Int J Oral Maxillofac Implants* 2007;**22**:235–242.
35. Scheerlinck LM, Muradin MS, van der Bilt A, Meijer GJ, Koole R, Van Cann EM: Donor site complications in bone grafting: comparison of iliac crest, calvarial, and mandibular ramus bone. *Int J Oral Maxillofac Implants* 2013;**28**:222–227.
36. Araujo PP, Oliveira KP, Montenegro SC, Carreiro AF, Silva JS, Germano AR: Block allograft for reconstruction of alveolar bone ridge in implantology: a systematic review. *Implant Dent* 2013;**22**:304–308.
37. Waasdorp J, Reynolds MA: Allogeneic bone onlay grafts for alveolar ridge augmentation: a systematic review. *Int J Oral Maxillofac Implants* 2010;**25**:525–531.
38. Simion M, Rocchietta I, Dellavia C: Three-dimensional ridge augmentation with xenograft and recombinant human platelet-derived growth factor-BB in humans: report of two cases. *Int J Periodontics Restorative Dent* 2007;**27**:109–115.
39. Baker RD, Connole PW, Davis WH, et al: Long-term results of alveolar ridge augmentation. *J Oral Surg* 1979;**37**:486.
40. Sbordone C, Toti P, Guidetti F, Califano L, Santoro A, Sbordone L: Volume changes of iliac crest autogenous bone grafts after vertical and horizontal alveolar ridge augmentation of atrophic maxillas and mandibles: a 6-year computerized tomographic follow-up. *J Oral Maxillofac Surg* 2012;**70**(11):2559–2565.
41. Proussaefs P, Lozada J: The use of intraorally harvested autogenous block grafts for vertical alveolar ridge augmentation: a human study. *Int J Periodontics Restorative Dent* 2005 Aug;**25**(4):351–363.
42. von Arx T, Buser D: Horizontal ridge augmentation using autogenous block grafts and the guided bone regeneration technique with collagen membranes: a clinical study with 42 patients. *Clin Oral Implants Res* 2006;**17**:359–366.
43. Khojasteh A, Soheilifar S, Mohajerani H, Nowzari H: The effectiveness of barrier membranes on bone regeneration in localized bony defects: a systematic review. *Int J Oral Maxillofac Implants* 2013 Jul–Aug;**28**(4):1076–1089.

44. Khoury F, Khoury C: Mandibular bone block grafts: diagnosis, instrumentation, harvesting technique and surgical procedures. In: Khoury F, Antoun H, Missika P (eds.), Bone Augmentation in Oral Implantology. Quintessence Publishing Co., Chicago, IL, 2007, pp. 169–183.
45. Codivilla A: The classic: on the means of lengthening, in the lower limbs, the muscles and tissues which are shortened through deformity. 1904. *Clin Orthop Relat Res* 2008 Dec;**466**(12):2903–2909. doi: 10.1007/s11999-008-0518-7. Epub 2008 Sep 27.
46. McAllister BS, Haghighat K: Bone augmentation techniques. *J Periodontol* 2007;**78**:377–396.
47. Artzi Z, Tal H, Moses O, Kozlovsky A: Mucosal considerations for osseointegrated implants. *J Prosthet Dent* 1993;**70**:427–432.
48. Bianchi A, Felice P, Lizio G, Marchetti C: Alveolar distraction osteogenesis versus inlay bone grafting in posterior mandibular atrophy: a prospective study. *Oral Surg Oral Med Oral Pathol Oral Radiol Endod* 2008;**105**:282–292.
49. Laster Z, Rachmiel A, Jensen OT: Alveolar width distraction osteogenesis for early implant placement. *J Oral Maxillofac Surg* 2005;**63**:1724–1730.
50. Rocchietta I, Fontana F, Simion M: Clinical outcomes of vertical bone augmentation to enable dental implant placement: a systematic review. *J Clin Periodontol* 2008;**35**:203–215.
51. Chiapasco M, Casentini P, Zaniboni M: Bone augmentation procedures in implant dentistry. *Int J Oral Maxillofac Implants* 2009;**24**(Suppl):237–259.
52. Master DL, Hanson PR, Gosain AK: Complications of mandibular distraction osteogenesis. *J Craniofac Surg* 2010;**21**:1565–1570.
53. Jensen O, Nock D: Inferior alveolar nerve repositioning in conjunction with placement of osseointegrated implants: a case report. *Oral Surg Oral Med Oral Pathol* 1987;**63**:263–268.
54. Lorean A, Kablan F, Mazor Z, Mijiritsky E, Russe P, Barbu H, Levin L: Inferior alveolar nerve transposition and reposition for dental implant placement in edentulous or partially edentulous mandibles: a multicenter retrospective study. *Int J Oral Maxillofac Surg* 2013;**42**:656–659.
55. Karlis V, Bae RD, Glickman RS: Mandibular fracture as a complication of inferior alveolar nerve transposition and placement of endosseous implants: a case report. *Implant Dent* 2003;**12**:211–216.
56. Norton MR: Multiple single-tooth implant restorations in the posterior jaws: maintenance of marginal bone levels with reference to the implant-abutment microgap. *Int J Oral Maxillofac Implants* 2006;**21**:777–784.
57. Khojasteh A, Hassani A, Motamedian SR, Saadat S, Alikhasi M: Cortical bone augmentation versus nerve lateralization for treatment of atrophic posterior mandible: a retrospective study and review of literature. *Clin Impl Dent Relat Res* 2015 Jun 17. doi: 10.1111/cid.12317. [Epub ahead of print].
58. Babbush CA: Transpositioning and repositioning the inferior alveolar and mental nerves in conjunction with endosteal implant reconstruction. *Periodontol 2000* 1998;**17**:183–190.
59. Vasconcelos Jde A, Avila GB, Ribeiro JC, et al: Inferior alveolar nerve transposition with involvement of the mental foramen for implant placement. *Med Oral Pathol Oral Cir Bucal* 2008;**13**:E722-725.
60. Urist MR: Bone: formation by autoinduction. *Science* 1965;**150**:893.
61. Postlethwaite AE, Raghow R, Stricklin G, Ballou L, Sampath TK: Osteogenic protein-1, a bone morphogenic protein member of the TGF-beta superfamily, shares chemotactic but not fibrogenic properties with TGF-beta. *J Cell Physiol* 1994;**161**:562–570.
62. Lynch SE, et al: *Tissue Engineering*. Chicago: Quintessence Publishing Co., Chicago, IL, 2008.
63. Li XJ, Boyne P, Lilly L, Spagnoli DB: Different osteogenic pathways between rhBMP-2/ACS and autogenous bone graft in 190 maxillary sinus floor augmentation surgeries. *J Oral Maxillofac Surg* 2007;**65**(9 Suppl 2):36.
64. Triplett G, Nevins M, Marx RE: Pivotal, randomized, parallel evaluation of recombinant human bone morphogenetic protein-2/absorbable collagen sponge and autogenous bone graft for maxillary sinus floor augmentation. *J Oral Maxillofac Surg* 2009;**67**:9.
65. Khojasteh A, Behnia H, Dashti SG, Stevens M: Current trends in mesenchymal stem cell application in bone augmentation: a review of the literature. *J Oral Maxillofac Surg* 2012;**70**:972–982.
66. Friedenstein AJ, Gorskaja JF, Kulagina NN: Fibroblast precursors in normal and irradiated mouse hematopoietic organs. *Expl Hematol* 1976;**4**:267.
67. Morad G, Kheiri L, Khojasteh A: Dental pulp stem cells for *in vivo* bone regeneration: a systematic review of literature. *Arch Oral Biol* 2013 Dec;**58**(12):1818–1827.
68. Khojasteh A, Eslaminejad MB, Nazarian H: Mesenchymal stem cells enhance bone regeneration in rat calvarial critical size defects more than platelete-rich plasma. *Oral Surg Oral Med Oral Pathol Oral Radiol Endod* 2008;**106**:356–363.
69. Khojasteh A, Behnia H, Hosseini S, Dehghan MM, Mashhadi Abbas F, Abbasnia P: The effect of PCL-TCP scaffold loaded with mesenchymal stem cells on vertical bone augmentation in dog mandible: a preliminary report. *J Biomed Mater Res B Appl Biomater* 2013;**101**:848–854.
70. El Tamer MK, Reis RL: Progenitor and stem cells for bone and cartilage regeneration. *J Tissue Eng Regen Med* 2009;**3**:327.
71. Shayesteh YS, Khojasteh A, Soleimani M, Alikhasi M, Khoshzaban A, Ahmadbeigi A: Sinus augmentation using human mesenchymal stem cells loaded into a [beta]-tricalcium phosphate/hydroxyapatite scaffold. *Oral Surg Oral Med Oral Pathol Oral Radiol Endod* 2008;**106**:203–209.
72. Behnia H, Khojasteh A, Soleimani M, Tehranchi A, Khoshzaban A, Keshel SH, et al: Secondary repair of alveolar clefts using human mesenchymal stem cells. *Oral Surg Oral Med Oral Pathol Oral Radiol Endod* 2009;**108**:e1-6.
73. Behnia H, Khojasteh A, Soleimani M, Tehranchi A, Atashi A: Repair of alveolar cleft defect with mesenchymal stem cells and platelet derived growth factors: a preliminary report. *J Craniomaxillofac Surg* 2012;**40**:2–7.
74. Louis P: Vertical ridge augmentation using titanium mesh. *Oral Maxillofacial Surg Clin N Am* 2010;**22**:353–368.
75. Burger BW: Use of ultrasound-activated resorbable oly-D-L-lactide pins (Sonic-Pins) and foil panels (Resorb-X) for horizontal bone augmentation of the maxillary and mandibular alveolar ridges. *J Oral Maxillofac Surg* 2010 Jul;**68**(7):1656–1661.
76. Louis PJ, Gutta R, Naief S: Reconstruction of the maxilla and mandible with particulate bone graft and titanium mesh for implant placement. *J Oral Maxillofac Surg* 2008;**66**(2):235–245.
77. Davies JE, Ajami E, Moineddin R, Mendes VC: The roles of different scale ranges of surface implant topography on the stability of the bone/implant interface. *Biomaterials* 2013;**34**(14):3535–3546.
78. Pogrel MA, Podlesh S, Anthony J, et al: A comparison of vascularized and nonvascularized bone grafts for reconstruction of mandibular continuity defects. *J Oral Maxillofac Surg* 1997;**55**:1200.
79. Rowan M, Lee D, Pi-Anfruns J, Shiffler P, Aghaloo T, Moy PK: Mechanical versus biological stability of immediate and delayed implant placement using resonance frequency analysis. *J Oral Maxillo Surg* 2015;**73**(2):253–257.
80. Liu Y, Enggist L, Kuffer AF, Buser D, Hunziker EB: The influence of BMP-2 and its mode of delivery on the osteoconductivity of implant surfaces during the early phase of osseointegration, *Biomaterials* 2007;**28**(16):2677–2686.
81. Dahlin C, Linde A, Gottlow J, Nyman S: Healing of bone defects by guided tissue regeneration. *Plast Reconstr Surg* 1988;**81**:672–676.
82. Steflik DE, Corpe RS, Lake FT, Young TR, Sisk AL, Parr GR, et al: Ultrastructural analyses of the attachment (bonding) zone between bone and implanted biomaterials. *J Biomed Mater Res* 1998;**39**:611–620.
83. Khojasteh A, Dashti SG, Dehghan MM, Behnia H, Abbasnia P, Morad G: The osteoregenerative effects of platelet-derived growth factor BB cotransplanted with mesenchymal stem cells, loaded on freeze-dried mineral bone block: a pilot study in dog mandible. *J Biomed Mater Res B Appl Biomater* 2014 Nov;**102**(8):1771–1778.
84. Jafarian M, Eslaminejad MB, Khojasteh A, Mashhadi Abbas F, Dehghan MM, Hassanizadeh R, Houshmand B: Marrow-derived mesenchymal stem cells – directed bone regeneration in the dog mandible: a comparison between biphasic calcium phosphate and natural bone mineral. *Oral Surg Oral Med Oral Pathol Oral Radiol Endod* 2008 May;**105**(5):e14–24.
85. Eslaminejad MB, Jafarian M, Khojasteh A, Mashhadi Abbas F, Dehghan MM, Hassanizadeh R, Houshmand B: *In vivo* bone formation by canine mesenchymal stem cells loaded onto HA/TCP scaffolds: qualitative and quantitative analysis. *Yakhteh* 2008;**10**(3):205–212.
86. Khojasteh A, Eslaminejad MB, Nazarian H, Morad G, Dashti SG, Behnia H, Stevens M: Vertical bone augmentation with simultaneous implant placement using particulate mineralized bone and mesenchymal stem cells: a preliminary study in rabbit. *J Oral Implantol* 2013 Feb;**39**(1):3–13.
87. Behnia H, Khoshzaban A, Zarinfar M, Mashhadiabbas F, Bahraminasab V, Khojasteh A: Histological evaluation of regeneration in rabbit calvarial bone defects using demineralized bone matrix, mesenchymal stem cells and platelet rich in growth factors. *J Dent Sch* 2012;**30**(3):143–154.
88. Behnia H, Khojasteh A, Kiani MT, Khoshzaban A, Mashhadi Abbas F, Bashtar M, Dashti SG: Bone regeneration with a combination of nanocrystalline hydroxyapatite silica gel, platelet-rich growth factor, and mesenchymal stem cells: a histologic study in rabbit calvaria. *Oral Surg Oral Med Oral Pathol Oral Radiol* 2013 Feb;**115**(2):e7–15.

SECTION VI

Free Bone Flaps and Osseointegrated Implants for Mandibular and Maxillary Alveolar Bone Reconstruction

CHAPTER 25

Mandibular and Maxillary Alveolar Bone Reconstruction with Free Bone Flaps and Osseointegrated Implants

Edward I. Chang and Matthew M. Hanasono

Department of Plastic Surgery, The University of Texas MD Anderson Cancer Center, Houston, Texas, USA

Introduction

Head and neck reconstruction has witnessed tremendous advances over the years with the emergence of free tissue transfer replacing the archaic "waltzing" flap and supplanting pedicle flaps with improvement in patient function and overall cosmesis [1, 2]. A number of different flaps have now been described giving reconstructive microsurgeons an abundance of donor site options that can be tailored to any particular defect [3–5]. Soft tissue defects can be reconstructed with a myriad of different flaps depending on the size and location of the defect while bony defects can also be reconstructed with a variety of osteocutaneous free flaps [6–8]. Since its description by Hidalgo, the free fibula osteocutaneous flap has become one of the workhorse flaps for mandible reconstruction and serves as the foundation for optimizing form and function in reconstruction of the craniofacial skeleton [9–12]. However, while the use of vascularized bone flaps is generally considered the most optimal way to reconstruct the mandible, advanced training is necessary to minimize complications and maximize flap survival and patient outcomes.

Fibula free flap

The fibula osteocutaneous flap is probably the most frequently used choice for mandibular reconstruction. The fibula is primarily an ankle stabilizer and provides the origin for several muscles of the lower leg, but is expendable provided the distal bone, extending 5 to 7 cm above the lateral malleolus, is spared. Generally, a 22 to 25 cm segment of fibula bone may be harvested in the adult patient, permitting reconstruction of near-total mandibular defects. Further, the benefit of harvesting a cutaneous skin paddle with the fibula bone allows for reconstruction of composite soft tissue and mucosal defects as many mandibular defects involve some component of the intraoral lining, tongue, or mucosa.

The vascular supply of the fibula free flap is the peroneal artery and vein. It is important to examine both lower extremities and palpate for dorsalis pedis and posterior tibial pulses pre-operatively. A patient with findings consistent with arterial insufficiency or venous stasis may not be a candidate for a fibula free flap. In addition to pathologic conditions, it is important to rule out the possibility of peroneal arteria magna; an anatomic variant where the peroneal artery is the dominant arterial inflow to the distal lower extremity. When the peripheral arteries are not palpable or the circulation to the lower extremity is questionable, additional studies, such as conventional, magnetic resonance, or computed tomographic angiography, may be necessary.

The choice of leg is based on the anticipated side of the recipient blood vessels and expected need for an extra- or intraoral lining. In general, we prefer to use the leg that is contralateral to the side of the recipient blood vessels for mandibular reconstruction when an intraoral lining is needed. For maxillary reconstruction, the ipsilateral leg is used to orient the skin paddle to close the palatal mucosal defect. The flap is typically oriented so the pedicle is on the lingual side, to minimize external compression and allow plate placement on the lateral aspect of the fibula.

Osteotomies may be completed while the flap is left *in situ* or during the inset of the flap into the defect. Performing the osteotomies while the pedicle is still attached has the advantage of minimizing ischemia time. Also, any injuries to the pedicle can be identified well in advance of revascularization, an advantage that is perhaps most important when rigid fixation and skin paddle inset are performed prior to the microvascular anastomosis. Other surgeons prefer to perform osteotomies after the pedicle is divided due to increased freedom of movement, potentially avoiding traction injury to the pedicle blood vessels.

We prefer to use a locking titanium reconstruction plate to secure the osteotomized fibula to the remaining native mandibular segments. In recent years, lower profile hardware has resulted in decreased rates of plate exposure. Some surgeons have had success using miniplates, which allow for fine adjustments to the final shape of the reconstructed mandible, while locking reconstruction plates are considered to possess superior stability and are able to tolerate higher loads.

In certain cases, a double-barrel approach to mandibular reconstruction is used to increase bony height. In this technique, reconstruction proceeds in the usual manner but the distal portion of the fibula is turned back 180 degrees on to the proximal fibula to add additional height to more closely approximate the height of the normal dentulous mandible. We reserve use of the double-barrel technique for anterior mandibular defects, as the normal height of the mandible is greater in this region. Laterally, the width of a single fibular segment closely approximates the height of the native mandible. When a single width of fibula is used, we prefer to align

---

Vertical Alveolar Ridge Augmentation in Implant Dentistry: A Surgical Manual, First Edition. Edited by Len Tolstunov.
© 2016 John Wiley & Sons, Inc. Published 2016 by John Wiley & Sons, Inc.

the fibula with the lower border of the mandible, rather than the alveolus, in order to achieve the best possible external contour.

Malocclusion following mandibular reconstruction may also occur. Whenever possible, the mandible is pre-plated prior to mandibular resection so that the reconstruction can be designed to maintain the spatial orientation of the native mandible. When pre-plating is not feasible due to an expansile tumor, pathologic fracture, or prior resection, use of an external fixator can be considered. More recently, use of computer planning and rapid prototype modeling has helped improve outcomes, particularly when pre-plating is not feasible.

Free fibula osteocutaneous flap harvest technique

Harvesting the free fibula osteocutaneous flap has undergone substantial modification and advancements since its original description. The use of pre-operative imaging has also played a significant role in flap design, in particular the skin paddle, in order to be able to harvest a flap for reconstruction of composite mandibulectomy defects [9]. Harvesting the flap under tourniquet control facilitates flap harvest with a bloodless field and allows for precise identification of perforators and dissection of the main pedicle. The design of the flap should take into account preservation of approximately 5 to 7 cm of the proximal and distal fibula in order to preserve function of the ankle joint and avoid injury to the peroneal nerve, which crosses the neck of the fibula, respectively (Figure 25.1).

A line from the fibular head to the lateral malleolus marks the central line to orient the skin paddle [13]. Based on prior anatomic studies, we have reliably identified a perforator that lies approximately one-third the distance from the fibular head to the lateral malleolus. While this is a reliable perforator, it may not always arise from the main peroneal vessels, which may preclude its utility for resurfacing an intraoral defect, but has been described for use in through-and-through defects [14]. There are three additional reliable perforators that are routinely located approximately one-half, two-thirds, and three-quarters the distance from the fibular head to the lateral malleolus, which we have termed perforators A, B, and C for the sake of simplicity. A hand-held Doppler ultrasound probe can be used to verify the location of these perforators, or a limited anterior incision will allow direct visualization of the perforators prior to committing to the final skin paddle design (Figure 25.2).

Once the perforators have been visualized, the fibula bone is harvested. Briefly, the peroneus longus muscle is detached from the fibula periosteum until the anterior septum is seen, which is incised, exposing the muscles in the anterior compartment. These muscles are also detached from the fibula, paying careful attention to identify and prevent injury to the anterior tibial neurovascular bundle. Once the anterior musculature is released from the fibula, the interosseous membrane is visualized.

At this time, dissecting right angle clamps can be used to circumscribe the fibula both proximally and distally, again paying careful attention not to damage the main peroneal pedicle. The distal and proximal osteotomies are performed, and the interosseous membrane can then be released allowing the fibula to be retracted from the leg (Figure 25.3). The distal personal vessels are identified and ligated, and the dissection of the posterior compartment muscles proceeds from a distal to proximal direction until the entire fibula is released and the peroneal vessels dissected to the tibial-peroneal trunk, which marks the limit of the proximal dissection.

At this point, the skin paddle design is finalized based on the size of the defect and exact locations of the perforators. The posterior incision is made and the soleus muscle is separated from the posterior septum and flexor hallucis longus muscle, taking care to carefully dissect and release the cutaneous perforator blood vessels from the soleus muscle, which may require ligation of small side branches that enter and supply the muscle (Figure 25.4). At this point the entire fibula osteocutaneous flap has been dissected and the tourniquet is released (Figure 25.5). Attention should be paid to

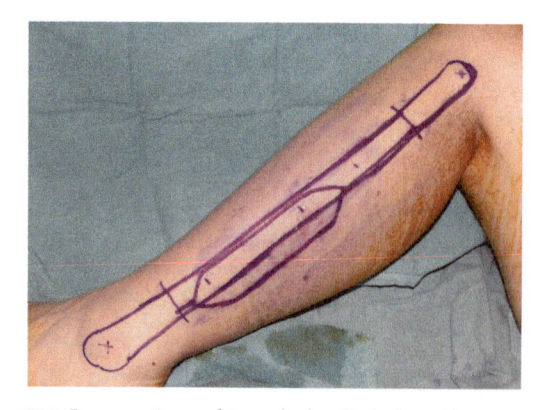

Figure 25.1 Pre-operative markings of a free fibula flap with preservation of 5–6 cm of proximal and distal fibula and anticipated skin paddle.

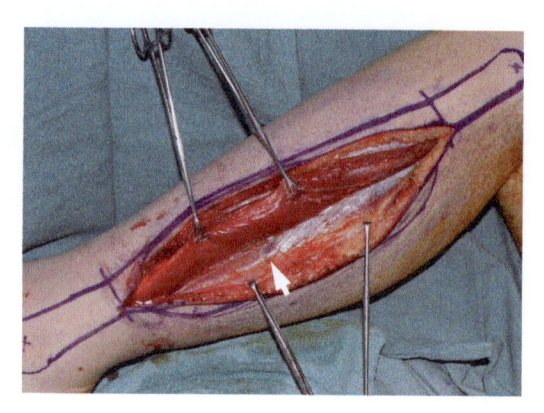

Figure 25.2 Anterior incision with identification of a large septocutaneous perforator (white arrow) that can be used to perfuse the skin paddle.

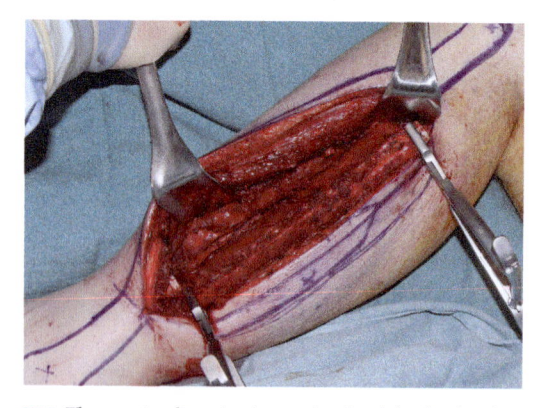

Figure 25.3 The anterior dissection is completed and the distal and proximal osteotomies have been completed allowing release of the interosseus membrane so the fibula can be retracted from the leg, allowing for the pedicle and posterior dissection.

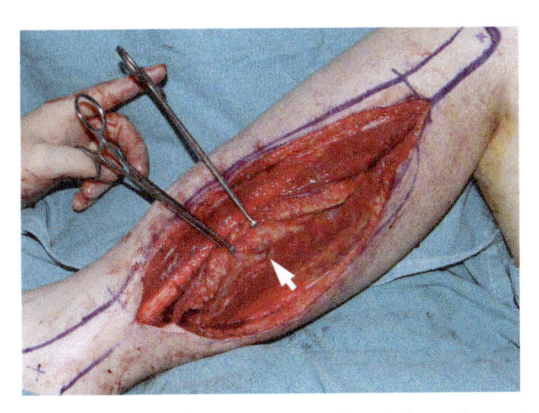

Figure 25.4 The posterior skin incision is made and the perforator is identified from the posterior approach (white arrow).

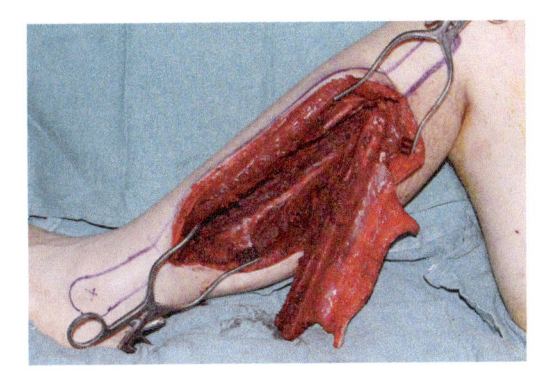

Figure 25.5 The entire fibula is now free and the tourniquet is released with excellent perfusion of the fibula, muscle, and skin paddle.

make certain the flap and skin paddle are well perfused and that the toes are perfused as well with normal capillary refill.

Osteotomy and plating

The osteotomies to contour the fibula to resemble the mandible or maxilla can be performed *in situ* in order to minimize the ischemia time or can be performed after rendering the flap ischemic to improve the freedom to perform the osteotomies (Figure 25.6). Of critical importance is protection of the main pedicle when performing the osteotomies. The number of osteotomies is dictated by the extent of the defect and a template can be created from the native mandible or maxilla. If the native mandible or maxilla is not available secondary to severe trauma or distortion from an exophytic tumor, cephalometric guidelines exist that can help guide the dimensions of the bony construct [15]. Alternatively, the use of three-dimensional medical models created using computer-assisted design (CAD) software can also be useful in these circumstances. The use of the technology is rapidly advancing and growing in popularity as cutting guides can be manufactured for the mandible and maxilla as well as the fibula that coincide with each other. Further, custom-engineered or prefabricated titanium plates can be made to the precise anticipated defect and reconstruction [16–18].

Osseointegrated dental implants

Given the primary objective of restoring form and function, the use of vascularized bone flaps, such as the fibula, allows for the potential of dental rehabilitation. The fibula provides sufficient bone stock to support dental implants, which can be placed at the time of reconstruction or in a second stage with comparable outcomes and implant survival [19, 20]. In general, we prefer placing the implants at a second stage after bony healing of flap to the mandible or maxilla is complete. Primary placement needs to be very precise and there is a risk not only of damaging the blood supply to the flap but also misplacement such that the angulation of implants makes it difficult for loading an abutment and retaining prosthesis.

Our protocol for secondary implant placement is to wait 6 months (no sooner than 4 months) for osteotomies to heal. Imaging prior to implant placement, including computed tomography (CT) or panoramic radiograph, is also recommended; however, bony healing often lags behind radiographic studies, with some areas of lucency at the osteotomy sites, but complete healing is usually observed by 4 months. The implant placement is usually done in coordination with the microvascular surgeon. Prior to implant placement, titanium hardware may need to be removed to accommodate the implants. At the same time, skin flaps are thinned of subcutaneous fat, and in some cases completely removed, leaving only periosteum, which is allowed to spontaneously remucosalize or covered with a skin graft.

A thin layer of tissue between the bone and the eventual dental prosthesis is usually desirable due to limitations of abutment length and need to leave sufficient room for the prosthesis. Implants are usually given at least 3 months to undergo osseointegration prior to uncovering and abutment placement rather than loaded immediately. Skin flaps can undergo additional thinning at the time of implant uncovering and abutment placement if necessary.

One of the greatest controversies surrounding the placement of dental implants in the cancer patient is the impact of radiation therapy on long-term implant survival. Some studies have demonstrated increased risk for complications while other studies have demonstrated equivalent outcomes when implants were placed into radiated bone compared to non-radiated bone [21–23]. In general, we prefer to reserve implant-based dental rehabilitation for use in a non-radiated patient; however, we have demonstrated successful dental rehabilitation even in patients who have received postoperative radiation therapy [24]. Some authors feel that hyperbaric oxygen therapy prior to implant placement can reduce the risk of implant failure or bone fracture in irradiated patients, but outcomes data supporting this practice is still preliminary.

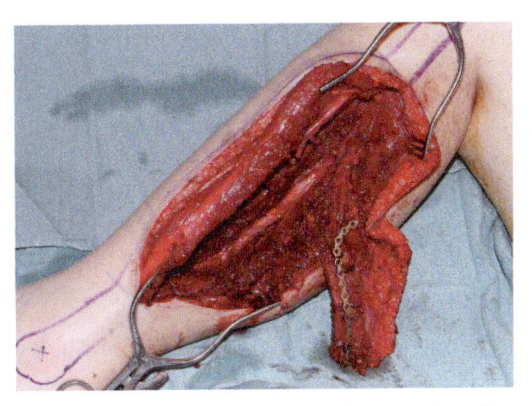

Figure 25.6 The osteotomies and subsequent plating can be performed *in situ* while the flap is still attached and perfused by the main peroneal vessels.

Case Report 1

A 68-year-old man with a history of tonsillar squamous cell carcinoma treated with prior radiation presents with worsening jaw pain, trismus, and weight loss. The patient was found to have a pathologic fracture secondary to osteoradionecrosis (Figure 25.7) and was taken to the operating room for an extensive composite resection and reconstruction with a double skin paddle free fibula flap from the contralateral leg (Figure 25.8). The proximal skin paddle was used for external skin resurfacing while the distal skin paddle was used for the intraoral defect. One osteotomy was necessary in order to restore the contour of the native mandible. The anastomoses were completed to the facial artery and the common facial vein.

The patient recovered uneventfully and underwent a revision of the intraoral skin paddle to debulk the flap and subsequent placement of dental implants 14 months following the initial reconstruction (Figure 25.9). Five Astra dental implants were placed (1 × 4 mm and 4 × 5 mm implants) and allowed to integrate prior to unroofing and placement of the abutments 3 months after the implant placement (Figure 25.10). The patient was fitted with his prosthesis with some minor adjustments as well as fitted for a maxillary denture.

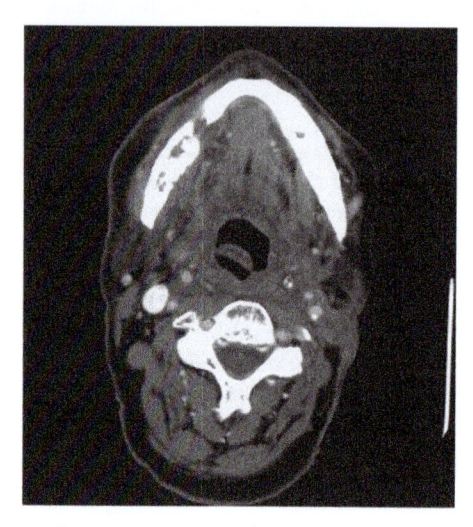

Figure 25.7 Pre-operative CT scan demonstrated osteoradionecrosis of the mandible with a pathologic fracture.

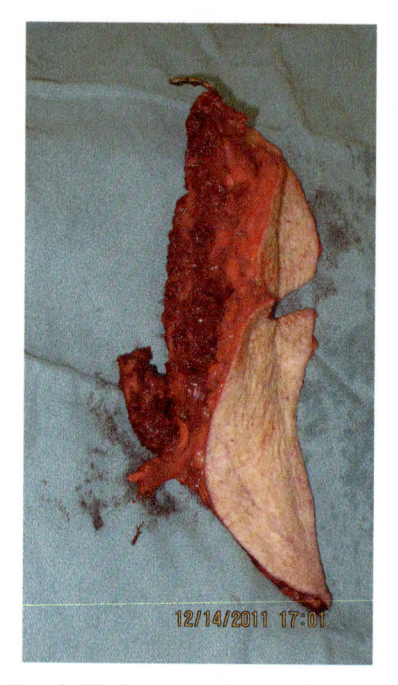

Figure 25.8 Free double skin paddle fibula flap harvested with *in situ* osteotomy with titanium plating.

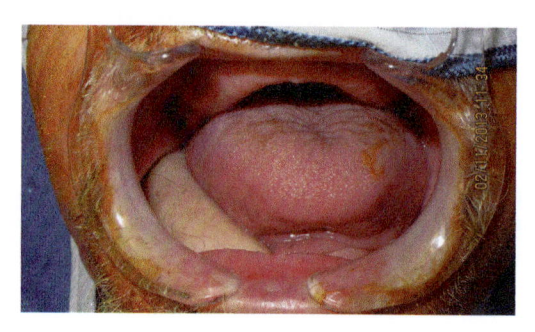

Figure 25.9 Post-operative photo prior to flap debulking and placing of dental implants.

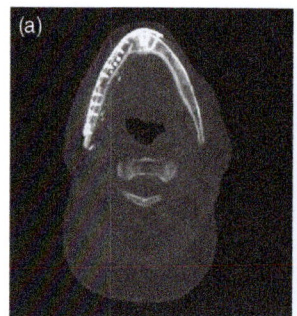

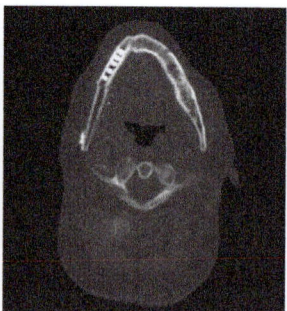

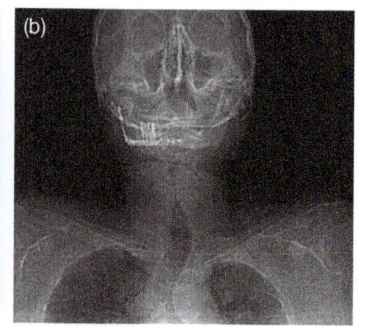

Figure 25.10 Post-operative CT scans and scanning view demonstrating integration of dental implants on (a) axial view and (b) scanning anterior–posterior view.

Given the prior radiation injury and subsequent osteoradionecrosis, the patient needed vascularized osteocutaneous reconstruction of the anticipated composite defect to maximize and optimize his post-operative quality of life [25]. Given the need for both external and intraoral soft tissue as well as bone, we opted to use a free fibula osteocutaneous free flap with two skin paddles rather than other osteocutaneous flaps. An iliac crest would have been limited in pedicle length and would not have afforded design of a second skin island to resurface the neck. While a pectoralis flap could have been used for neck coverage, we prefer to reserve the pectoralis flap for salvage situations as the flap can tether the neck and limit a patient's range of motion. While a chimeric free scapular flap would also have been a viable option, it would require a change in position and potentially a skin graft to cover the muscle, which would increase the ischemia time and operative time with a less ideal cosmetic result.

For the majority of composite defects involving only an intraoral defect, we prefer to use the contralateral leg so the pedicle can be oriented as previously described. However, in the setting when there is a through-and-through defect, two perforators are necessary to supply two skin paddles that can be moved independently of each other. A proximal perforator is ideal for these defects as the proximal skin island would lie close to the anastomosis and provides coverage for the vessels to resurface the neck. The use of the proximal perforator obviates the need for a second set of recipient vessels, which can be challenging in a previously radiated and operated neck with depleted vessels. In such circumstances, the use of vein grafts may be necessary to reach alternate recipient vessels to supply a second free flap. The distal skin paddle is used for the intraoral defect as the distal skin is generally thinner and more suitable for mucosal lining than the proximal skin, which tends to be thicker.

Post-operative swelling typically takes a minimum of 3 months to resolve, but in general we recommend delaying any revisions for a minimum of 6 months in the setting of prior radiation. During the thinning and debulking process, care should be taken to avoid injuring the perforator to the skin paddle and is best coordinated with the dental specialists to optimize exposure of the bone for precise placement of the osseointegrated implants and preservation of the vascularity of the skin island.

Case Report 2

A 45-year-old man presented with a hemangioendothelioma of the hard palate and left maxillary sinus. He underwent resection of his entire hard palate and left maxillary sinus, sparing the orbital floor (Figure 25.11). A fibula osteocutaneous free flap was harvested from the left leg and used for immediate reconstruction (Figure 25.12). Three closing wedge osteotomies were required to restore the left anterior maxillary wall as well as the bilateral anterior alveolar arch. The fibula free flap was anchored to the right maxilla and left zygoma with 1.5 mm thick titanium reconstruction plates (Figure 25.13). The skin paddle of the fibula flap was sutured circumferentially to the buccal and labial mucosa and to the cut edge of the soft palate. The microvascular anastomoses were performed to the left facial artery and vein via saphenous vein grafts because the pedicle of the fibula free flap, which was approximately 6 cm long in this case, was not long enough to reach.

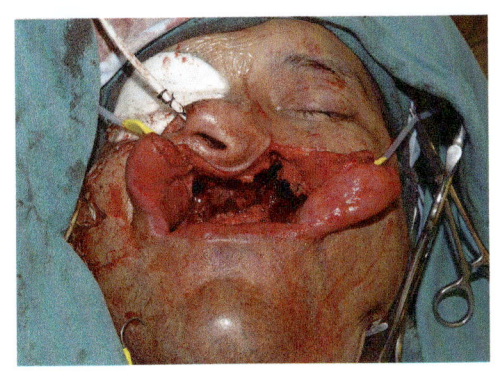

Figure 25.11 Surgical defect following left total and right partial maxillectomy. The entire hard palate has been removed.

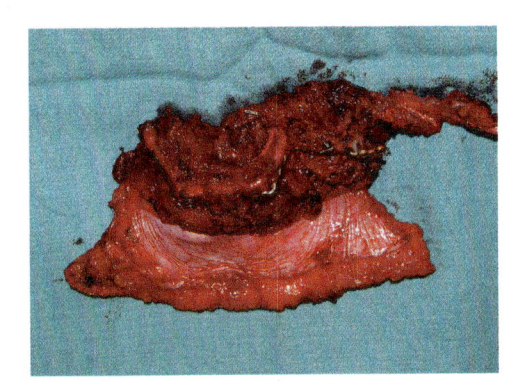

Figure 25.12 Fibula osteocutaneous free flap after three closing wedge osteotomies and rigid fixation with titanium reconstruction plates.

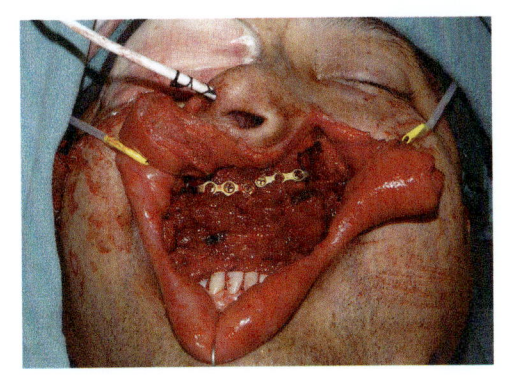

Figure 25.13 Inset of the fibula osteocutaneous free flap to restore the bilateral maxillary defect. The skin paddle of the free flap is used to close the oral cavity defect.

(continued)

(Continued)

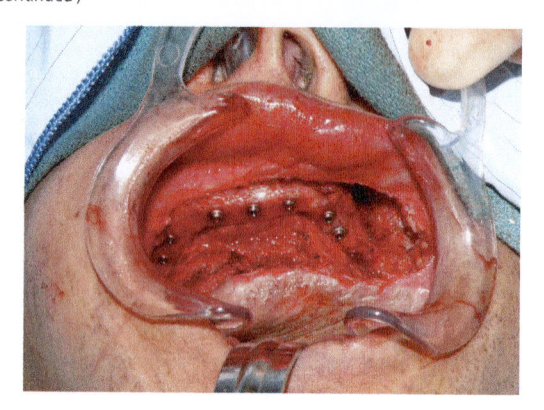

Figure 25.14 After adequate bony healing of the fibula free flap, the flap is re-exposed, the titanium hardware is removed, and osseointegrated implants are placed. The skin paddle is judiciously thinned by removing subcutaneous fat to allow space for a future dental prosthesis.

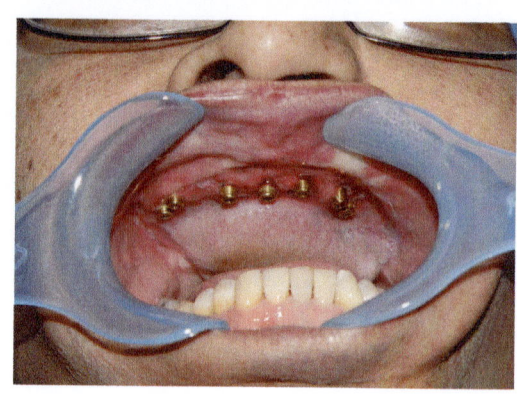

Figure 25.15 After waiting for osseointegration of the implants, the implants are uncovered, cover screws are removed, and abutments are placed.

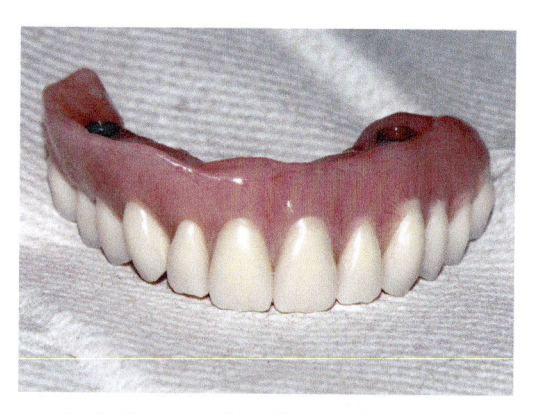

Figure 25.16 Implant retained maxillary prosthesis.

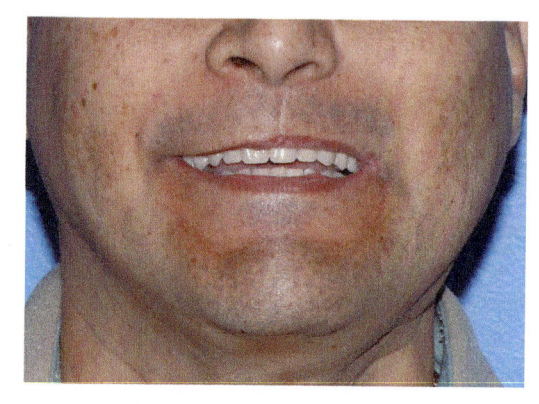

Figure 25.17 Final appearance following fibula free flap reconstruction and dental rehabilitation with an implant retained prosthesis.

Eight months following his initial operation, all hardware was removed, including screws and the reconstruction plates, by making an incision between the labial and buccal mucosa and the fibula free flap skin paddle. During the same surgery, seven osseointegrated implants, ranging from 9 to 11 mm in length and 3.55 to 4.05 mm in diameter based on the height and thickness of the fibula bone, were placed (Figure 25.14). Cover screws were placed over the implants and the skin paddle was closed over the implants and bone after thinning it by trimming the subcutaneous fat to a thickness of about 1–1.5 mm with scissors. Three months later, the implants were uncovered and Locator abutments were placed into the implants after removing the cover screws (Figure 25.15). The prosthesis was delivered several weeks later (Figure 25.16) with an acceptable result (Figure 25.17).

Such an extensive defect would have been difficult to manage with an obturator as there were no teeth remaining to stabilize the prosthesis. A soft tissue free flap or pedicled flap would not have been appropriate as they would not adequately restore his mid-facial projection, causing retrusion of his mid-face and loss of support for his nose. The fibula free flap was selected as a source of vascularized bone because of the length and complex shape of the defect. Multiple osteotomies were required to restore the curved shape of the anterior mid-face and alveolar arch. Note that the orientation of the flap was such that it was harvested from the same side as the microvascular anastomoses so that the skin paddle could be used to close the oral defect. The nasal side of the bone and skin flap mucosalized spontaneously. The bone was harvested with about 0.5–1.0 cm of muscle attached to the periosteum, to encourage spontaneous mucosal healing.

As mentioned above, we usually wait 6 months from the time of fibula reconstruction to hardware removal and osseointegrated implant placement. When plate removal would require extensive dissection, we opt to only remove screws and, occasionally, cut and remove only portions of the plate beneath the incision, rather than perform extensive undermining of already well-healed tissues. A fissure cut burr can cut through a 1.5 to 2.0 mm reconstruction plate without damaging the fibula bone. Thinning must be performed cautiously if the skin paddle has been irradiated, as wound healing problems following thinning are not uncommon and may result in bone and implant exposure. In non-irradiated patients with a very thick skin paddle, we occasionally remove the skin paddle and skin graft the underlying periosteum and scar tissue.

Discussion

The risks of microvascular free flaps include anastomotic or pedicle thrombosis, flap failure, infection, fistula, non-union or mal-union, and donor site complications with overall success rates higher than 95% in experienced hands. As with all microvascular free flaps, clinical examination and close monitoring is the gold standard for detecting flap compromise. In our experience, mal-union or non-union is exceedingly rare, given their high degree of vascularity.

In a series of 157 consecutive patients, we observed donor site complications following fibula free flap harvest in 31%, including skin graft loss (15%), cellulitis (10%), wound dehiscence (8%), and abscess (1%), with some patients having more than one complication [26].

There were no significant differences in the complication rates observed between patients who underwent donor site repair by primary closure or skin grafting. Long-term morbidities occurred in 17% of patients and included leg weakness (8%), ankle instability (4%), great toe flexion contracture (9%), and decreased ankle mobility (12%). All patients eventually returned to their pre-operative level of ambulatory activity with the vast majority achieving normal mobility within 3 to 6 months following surgery.

The fibula osteocutaneous free flap is the most commonly used free bone flap based on its many desirable characteristics. The vascular pedicle diameter of the fibula is generous, which helps make the microvascular anastomosis straightforward, the bone length is adequate for near-total mandibular reconstruction, the bone thickness is satisfactory for osseointegrated implant placement, the skin paddle is reliable, and the donor site morbidity is acceptable. Other bone free flap options include the iliac crest, scapula, and radial forearm osseous/osteocutaneous free flaps and may occasionally be selected in patients who are not good candidates for a fibula free flap or who have already previously had a fibula free flap and require another bony reconstruction.

The iliac crest free flap provides a generous amount of cortical and cancellous bone for mandibular reconstruction. The deep circumflex iliac vessels comprise the vascular pedicle of the iliac crest free flap and demonstrate consistent anatomy, reasonable length (8 to 10 cm), and appropriate vessel diameter (2 to 3 mm) for microsurgical application. The blood supply of the iliac crest bone flap is robust, incorporating both nutrient perforators and periosteal vessels, allowing the flap to tolerate multiple osteotomies. The bone stock reliably accommodates osseointegrated dental implants.

The flap may be harvested as a bone-only flap or with an associated skin and/or muscle paddle for reconstruction of composite defects. The skin paddle, which is nourished by several perforators arising from the deep circumflex iliac vessels, may be as wide as 9 to 12 cm in some patients and still allow the donor site to be closed primarily. Previously, osteocutaneous iliac crest free flaps included harvesting a cuff of external oblique muscle, internal oblique muscle, and transversalis fascia with the skin paddle, but in recent years perforator dissection has been more common, resulting in a less bulky soft tissue component.

The donor site, while hidden in clothing, may result in a contour deformity and/or hernia, a complication that may be ameliorated by careful closure techniques and harvest of a split flap. Gait abnormalities have also been reported. Harvesting the bone flap as a split-cortical flap decreases the morbidity by preserving hip contour, minimizing gait disturbances, and providing better support for the abdominal viscera resulting in a decreased risk for hernia. Due to difficulty in flap dissection and risk for post-operative donor site hernias, this flap is relatively contraindicated in obese patients.

The *scapular free flap* is another alternative for mandibular reconstruction. The scapula flap is usually based on the circumflex scapular artery. The length of the pedicle can be increased 4 to 5 cm by including the more proximal subscapular vessels. The bone may be harvested from either the lateral or the medial edge of the scapula. The lateral scapular bone flap has the shorter vascular pedicle but is usually preferred because the bone is thicker than the medial bone flap, which is particularly important if osseointegrated implant placement is to be attempted. Approximately 10 to 14 cm of linear bone may be harvested from either the lateral or medial aspect of the scapula.

A skin paddle, based on a cutaneous branch of the circumflex scapular artery, can be harvested with the osseous portion of the flap if needed. For larger defects, a chimeric flap utilizing the subscapular regional blood supply can be harvested to include a scapular or parascapular skin paddle and the latissimus dorsi (with or without an overlying skin paddle) and serratus anterior muscles. The potential configurations are numerous.

A major disadvantage of the scapular bone, regardless of whether it is harvested from the medial or lateral edge, is that it is often quite thin and does not consistently provide enough bone stock for osseointegrated implant placement. The location of the scapula makes it very difficult to perform a two-teamed approach for harvesting the flap and preparation of the recipient site and may require a change in position, thereby increasing the operative time as well. Patients may note a degree of shoulder stiffness and limited abduction following flap harvest.

The radial forearm fasciocutaneous free flap is a workhorse flap with thin, pliable skin and is indicated for head and neck reconstruction. This flap can also be designed as an osteocutaneous flap by inclusion of the anterior (volar) cortex of the radius. Up to 14 cm and 50% of unicortical radius nourished by periosteal branches from the radial artery may be harvested for selected osseous defects. However, the use of the osteocutaneous radial forearm free flap is typically not a first line option due to the limited thickness of the bone, which may be harvested without disturbing the structural mechanics of the hand and the risk for radial bone fracture in the forearm after harvest. Osseointegrated implant placement in the radial bone flap has occasionally been accomplished, but, in most cases, the bone obtained with this technique without destabilizing the forearm is too thin to stably accommodate implants.

The donor site morbidity following the harvest of an osteocutaneous radial forearm free flap can be significant. Tendon rupture, carpal tunnel syndrome, and a significantly weakened extremity have been reported. A radius fracture is estimated to occur about 15% of the time, and some surgeons recommend prophylactically plating the radius at the time of flap harvest.

Conclusions

For sizable segmental mandibular or maxillary defects, reconstruction with vascularized bone free flaps is indicated. The fibula osteocutaneous free flap is usually the first choice because of its ample length, ability to tolerate multiple shaping osteotomies, inclusion of a skin paddle for mucosal wound closure, and good bone stock for osseointegrated implants. We favor delayed implant placement with simultaneous titanium hardware removal and skin paddle revision, although others have successfully placed implants primarily. Other options include the iliac crest, scapula, and radial forearm osteocutaneous free flaps, in order of decreasing ability, to accommodate osseointegrated implants based on bone thickness and height.

References

1. Hanasono MM, Friel MT, Klem C, et al: Impact of reconstructive microsurgery in patients with advanced oral cavity cancers. *Head Neck* 2009;31:1289–1296.
2. Hanasono MM, Matros E, Disa JJ: Important aspects of head and neck reconstruction. *Plast Reconstr Surg* 2014;134(6):968e–980e.
3. Yu P, Chang EI, Selber JC, Hanasono MM: Perforator patterns of the ulnar artery perforator flap. *Plast Reconstr Surg* 2012;129(1):213–220.
4. Lin SJ, Rabie A, Yu P: Designing the anterolateral thigh flap without preoperative Doppler or imaging. *J Reconstr Microsurg* 2010;26(1):67–72.

5 Disa JJ, Pusic AL, Hidalgo DH, Cordeiro PG: Simplifying microvascular head and neck reconstruction: a rational approach to donor site selection. Ann Plast Surg 2001;47(4):385–389.
6 Chim H, Salgado CJ, Mardini S, Chen HC: Reconstruction of mandibular defects. Semin Plast Surg 2010;24(2):188–197.
7 Smith RB, Henstrom DK, Karnell LH, et al: Scapula osteocutaneous free flap reconstruction of the head and neck: impact of flap choice on surgical and medical complications. Head Neck 2007;29(5):446–452.
8 Kim JH, Rosenthal EL, Ellis T, Wax MK: Radial forearm osteocutaneous free flap in maxillofacial and oromandibular reconstructions. Laryngoscope 2005;115(9):1697–1701.
9 Garvey PB, Chang EI, Selber JC, Skoracki RJ, Madewell JE, Liu J, Yu P, Hanasono MM: A prospective study of preoperative computed tomographic angiographic mapping of free fibula osteocutaneous flaps for head and neck reconstruction. Plast Reconstr Surg 2012;130(4):541e–549e.
10 Hidalgo DA: Fibula free flap: a new method of mandible reconstruction. Plast Reconstr Surg 1989;84(1):71–79.
11 Hidalgo DA: Aesthetic improvements in free-flap mandible reconstruction. Plast Reconstr Surg 1991;88(4):574–585.
12 Zlotolow IM, Huryn JM, Piro JD, Lenchewski E, Hidalgo DA: Osseointegrated implants and functional prosthetic rehabilitation in microvascular fibula free flap reconstructed mandibles. Am J Surg 1992;164(6):677–681.
13 Yu P, Chang EI, Hanasono MM: Design of a reliable skin paddle for the fibula osteocutaneous flap: perforator anatomy revisited. Plast Reconstr Surg 2011;128(2):440–446.
14 Potter JK, Lee MR, Oxford L, Wong C, Saint-Cyr M: Proximal peroneal perforator in dual-skin paddle configuration of fibula free flap for composite oral reconstruction. Plast Reconstr Surg 2014;133(6):1485–1492.
15 Chang EI, Clemens MW, Garvey PB, Skoracki RJ, Hanasono MM: Cephalometric analysis for microvascular head and neck reconstruction. Head Neck 2012;34:1607–1614.
16 Roser SM, Ramachandra S, Blair H, Grist W, Carlson GW, Christensen AM, Weimer KA, Steed MB: The accuracy of virtual surgical planning in free fibula mandibular reconstruction: comparison of planned and final results. J Oral Maxillofac Surg 2010;68(11):2824–2832.
17 Hanasono MM, Skoracki RJ: Computer-assisted design and rapid prototype modeling in microvascular mandible reconstruction. Laryngoscope 2013;123(3):597–604.
18 Gil RS, Roig AM, Obispo CA, Morla A, Pagès CM, Perez JL: Surgical planning and microvascular reconstruction of the mandible with a fibular flap using computer-aided design, rapid prototype modelling, and precontoured titanium reconstruction plates: a prospective study. Br J Oral Maxillofac Surg 2015;53(1):49–53.
19 Schepers RH, Raghoebar GM, Vissink A, Lahoda LU, Van der Meer WJ, Roodenburg JL, Reintsema H, Witjes MJ: Fully 3-dimensional digitally planned reconstruction of a mandible with a free vascularized fibula and immediate placement of an implant-supported prosthetic construction. Head Neck 2013;35(4):E109–114.
20 Avraham T, Franco P, Brecht LE, Ceradini DJ, Saadeh PB, Hirsch DL, Levine JP: Functional outcomes of virtually planned free fibula flap reconstruction of the mandible. Plast Reconstr Surg 2014;134(4):628e–634e.
21 Doll C, Nack C, Raguse JD, Stricker A, Duttenhoefer F, Nelson K, Nahles S: Survival analysis of dental implants and implant-retained prostheses in oral cancer patients up to 20 years. Clin Oral Investig 2015 Jul;19(6):1347–1352.
22 Chrcanovic BR, Albrektsson T, Wennerberg A: Dental implants in irradiated versus non-irradiated patients: a meta-analysis. Head Neck. Epub Nov 2014.
23 Schiegnitz E, Al-Nawas B, Kämmerer PW, Grötz KA: Oral rehabilitation with dental implants in irradiated patients: a meta-analysis on implant survival. Clin Oral Investig. 2014;18(3):687–698.
24 Ch'ng S, Skoracki RJ, Selber JC, Yu P, Martin JW, Hofstede TM, Chambers MS, Liu J, Hanasono MM: Osseointegrated implant based dental rehabilitation in head and neck reconstruction patients. Head Neck. Epub Dec 2014.
25 Chang EI, Leon P, Hoffman WY, Schmidt BL: Quality of life for patients requiring surgical resection and reconstruction for mandibular osteoradionecrosis: 10-year experience at the University of California San Francisco. Head Neck 2012;34(2):207–212.
26 Momoh AO, Yu P, Skoracki RJ, Liu S, Feng L, Hanasono MM: A prospective cohort study of fibula free flap donor-site morbidity in 157 consecutive patients. Plast Reconstr Surg 2011;128:714–720.

SECTION VII

Soft Tissue Grafting for Implant Site Development

CHAPTER 26

Soft Tissue Grafting for Implant Site Development: Diagnosis and Treatment Planning

Georgios A. Kotsakis,[1] Suheil Boutros,[2] and Andreas L. Ioannou[3]

[1]University of Washington, Department of Periodontics, Seattle, Washington, USA
[2]Private Practice, Limited to Periodontics and Implants Surgery, Grand Blanc, Michigan, USA
[3]Department of Development and Surgical Sciences, Division of Periodontology, University of Minnesota, Minneapolis, Minnesota, USA

Introduction

Although bone osseointegration is very important, long-term success in implant dentistry depends on achievement of a stable and long-lasting soft tissue profile prior, during, and after implant insertion. A stable and esthetic soft tissue profile includes buccal soft tissue and interproximal papillae. Adjunctive procedures may be necessary to complement the surgical preparation of the implant site or to modify an existing implant to achieve an esthetic restoration.

In contemporary oral implantology where crown-down (prosthetically driven) treatment planning is an emerging concept, the initial diagnostic setup or the temporary restoration are used to assess the need for further ridge augmentation with hard or soft tissue graft or for modification of the position of the gingival margin. Inadequate dimensions of the soft tissue profile around dental implant restorations can result in esthetic and functional complications, such as poor oral hygiene, visual and phonetic discrepancies, and susceptibility for soft tissue recession and its progression [1]. Figures 26.1 and 26.2 demonstrate normal gingival and bone levels around an implant on the clinical and radiographic images. Figure 26.3 shows buccal gingival recession around an implant.

It is vital for the implant function and esthetics to achieve ideal soft tissue contours, volume, and color around dental implants [2]. To better assess the esthetic success of implant treatment Fürhauser et al. (2005) [3] developed a pink esthetic score (PES) for evaluating soft tissue characteristics around dental implants, assessing the soft tissue profile and pink esthetics as those relate to dental implant restorations [4]. The PES reproducibly evaluates dental peri-implant soft tissue around single-tooth dental implants by evaluating seven variables in comparison to a natural reference tooth: the mesial papilla, the distal papilla, the soft-tissue level, the soft-tissue contour, the alveolar process deficiency, the soft-tissue color, and the texture [3]. The PES as well as other soft tissue indices are gaining increasing acceptance for the assessment of implant success beyond simply evaluating osseointegration [4].

Plaque accumulation [5], oral hygiene habits [5], subcrestal or supracrestal position of the dental implant [6], crown profile, and distance between implants or between implants and teeth may have a negative effect on the esthetic and functional result of a dental implant restoration [7]. All these factors must be taken into account during every step of treatment planning, implant placement, and placement of the implant retained restoration to avoid any soft tissue discrepancies around the dental implant. This chapter will discuss the indications and contraindications for soft tissue grafting around dental implants and the rationale behind treatment planning of these cases.

Indications

Practically every surgery for the placement of dental implants requires some kind of soft tissue periodontal plastic surgery to a different extent, to address already established soft tissue discrepancies or to avoid and minimize the risk for future ones [8]. The indications for soft tissue grafting around dental implants are presented in Table 26.1.

Bone and soft tissue deficiency – absence of the papilla (Figure 26.4)

Following tooth extraction, there is a reduction in the soft and hard tissue volume in comparison to neighboring dentate sites [9, 10]. The discrepancy is more evident in single implant sites where an unesthetic concavity forms between the edentulous site and the root prominences of neighboring teeth. Ridge (bone) preservation (grafting) procedures are often employed to counter this resorptive phenomenon at the time of extraction. Ridge resorption can be limited to the point where implant placement is feasible 4–6 months post-extraction, but resorption cannot be completely prevented [11]. However, in esthetic cases the remaining ridge resorption causes an abrupt transition from the implant site to the root eminence of adjacent sites and demands periodontal soft tissue grafting procedures to attain an esthetically pleasing outcome [8]. As mentioned

---

Vertical Alveolar Ridge Augmentation in Implant Dentistry: A Surgical Manual, First Edition. Edited by Len Tolstunov.
© 2016 John Wiley & Sons, Inc. Published 2016 by John Wiley & Sons, Inc.

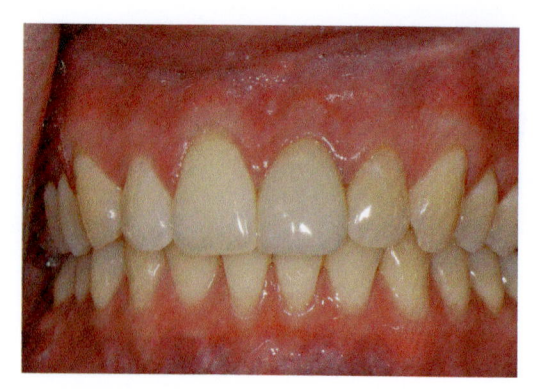

Figure 26.1 Maxillary left central incisor has been rehabilitated with a dental implant with healthy peri-implant soft tissues.

Table 26.1 Indications for soft tissue grafting around implants.

- Ridge and soft tissue deficiencies – papilla absence
- Lack of keratinized tissue
- Thin biotype and/or color discrepancies
- Rescue procedures

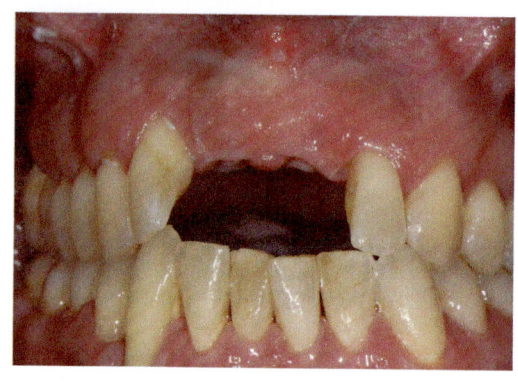

Figure 26.4 Severe vertical and horizontal bone loss in the edentulous region. Note the recession on the adjacent teeth that further complicates treatment planning and increases complexity of treatment in this case.

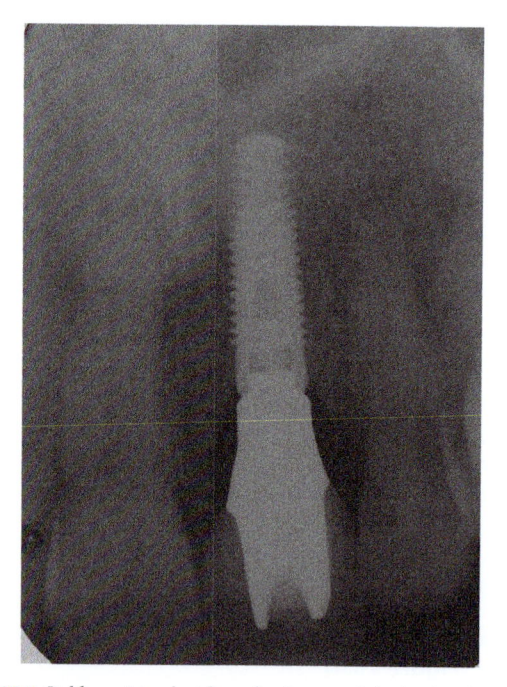

Figure 26.2 Stable peri-implant bone levels around the implant in Figure 26.1.

above, the use of a soft tissue graft, like subepithelial connective tissue graft, to *augment* deficient gingiva in dental implant sites in these cases is based on the premise that after a tooth has been extracted both the hard and the soft tissues change in form and quantity.

Lack of keratinized tissue

The importance of keratinized tissue (KT) around natural teeth and dental implants continues to be controversial (Figure 26.5). A classic periodontal study by Lang and Loe examined the relationship between the width of keratinized tissue and tissue health [12]. They reported that over 80% of tooth sites with a minimum of 2 mm of KT, and at least 1 mm of it attached, was recommended for maintenance of tissue health around teeth. In a similar study Kennedy et al. exemplified the importance of plaque control in

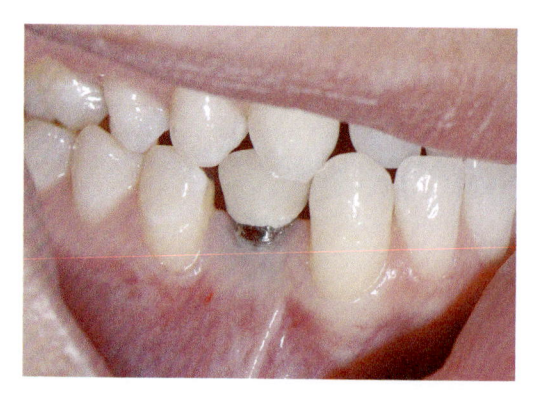

Figure 26.3 Recession around an implant that causes an esthetic concern for the patient.

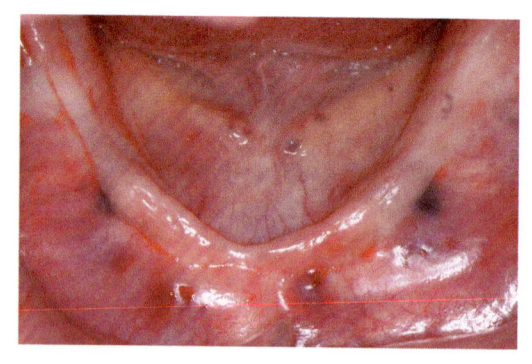

Figure 26.5 Lack of keratinized gingiva in the edentulous mandible. The lack of keratinized tissue can be managed either at the pre-implant stage or at the second stage. If the incision design during implant placement adequately divides the residual keratinized tissue between the lingual and buccal sides of the healing abutments, further soft tissue grafting may be avoided.

cases of a lack of KT [13]. In a cohort of patients lacking attached KT, the chance of recession was 20% under poor plaque control, while tissue loss was not noted in subjects with wide zones of attached tissue despite gingival inflammation [13]. In the dental implant literature, Adell et al. [14] and Albrektsson et al. [15] indicated that smooth titanium implants placed entirely in alveolar mucosa yielded similar survival rates to those placed within keratinized mucosa. Nonetheless, direct comparisons in the attachment apparatus between teeth and dental implants should be viewed conservatively due to the distinct differences between the two structures on a histological level [15]. Peri-implant and periodontal tissues appear to differ in their resistance to bacterial inflammation. Supracrestal collagen fibers around dental implants are oriented in a parallel "cuff" circumferentially to the implant platform, rather than the perpendicular configuration encountered in the dentoalveolar complex. The peri-implant cuff may have a weaker mechanical attachment when compared to the periodontal attachment around teeth.

Bouri et al. found that the mean plaque index score, bleeding on probing, and radiographic bone loss were significantly higher in implants with narrow (<2 mm) KT than broad KT (>2 mm) and concluded that increased width of keratinized mucosa (>2 mm) around dental implants is associated with lower mean alveolar bone loss and improved indices of soft tissue health [16]. However, when evaluating the entire body of literature, Esposito et al. [17] in a systematic review concluded that there was insufficient evidence to invariably recommend keratinized tissue augmentation around dental implants to maintain tissue health. In clinical reality, when there is a lack of KT, clinicians are called upon to make a decision about whether to augment the zone of KT at a site based on evidence literature, the individual dental history, the unique clinical characteristics of the site being treated, and their previous clinical experience. Greenstein and Cavallaro [18] have recommended the following indications for augmentation of KT:

- Chronically inflamed sites, despite maintenance therapy and oral hygiene instructions.
- Ongoing loss of clinical attachment, recession, and bone loss, regardless of maintenance therapy and appropriate oral hygiene.
- Soreness during brushing, even despite the appearance of tissue health.
- History of periodontitis and recessions.
- Non-compliance with periodic maintenance visits.
- Unsatisfactory esthetics.

Thin biotype and color discrepancies

The long-term stability of pink esthetics around dental implant prostheses has been strongly associated with adequate peri-implant soft tissue thickness (Figure 26.6). The thickness of the peri-implant gingiva (gingival biotype) is usually empirically defined during probing based on whether the probe shows through the gingival pocket or not [19]. When a thin biotype is diagnosed, a subepithelial soft tissue graft can be used to prevent potential future recession of the facial mucosa margin with possible permeation of a gray color from the dental implant on its buccal side.

Rescue procedures

Every surgical procedure carries with it a level of risk for adverse events. Adequate pre-operative treatment planning minimizes such risks, but when esthetic complications arise, periodontal surgical procedures can be employed as rescue procedures. A "rescue procedure" is used to manage esthetic complications associated

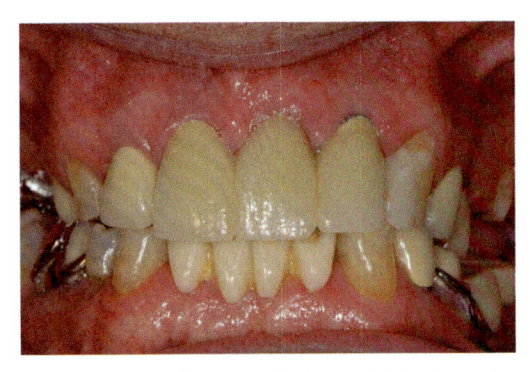

Figure 26.6 Thin gingival biotype resulted in metal showing on the maxillary left incisor implant.

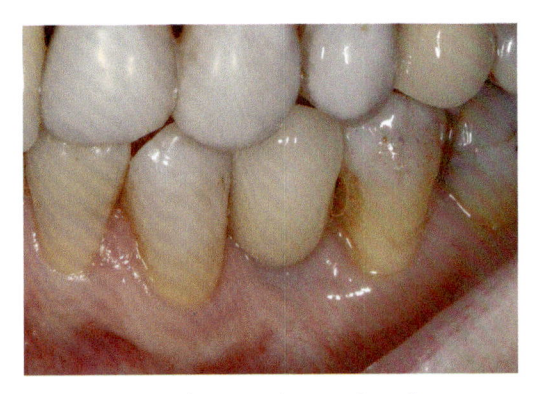

Figure 26.7 Connective soft tissue graft was performed as a rescue procedure to cover the titanium abutment in the thin biotype case.

with dental implants (Figure 26.7). Labial inclination of implants and/or buccal implant placement contribute to thin soft tissue, which may lead to the gray shade of the implant structure, showing through the tissue, recession, and exposure of the titanium implant neck for an inharmonious emergence profile of the implant-supported restoration. These complications produce an unpleasant appearance of the smile [20]. Soft tissue grafting following implant placement is easy and a minimally invasive technique that can be used to correct complications associated with soft-tissue color mismatch to a level below clinical perception [21].

Tooth extraction – implant site development

When a tooth is extracted with the purpose of being replaced with a dental implant restoration, implant site development needs to be planned before extraction. One fundamental consideration is that the *gingival level before tooth extraction influences the mucosal zenith of the implant restoration*. If the gingival facial margin is ideal, the final implant restoration has an excellent prognosis, especially in a patient with a thick gingiva biotype. However, if the facial gingival margin position is not ideal due to pre-existing attachment loss because of periodontal disease or aggressive oral hygiene methods, the future mucosal margin level will have a questionable prognosis unless soft tissue grafting is performed to correct the pre-existing level during the tooth extraction and implant site development phase. Bone grafting of the extraction socket at the time of tooth extraction does not correct problems of the soft tissue, such as the gingival margin location. In these cases adjunctive soft tissue grafting procedures are needed to facilitate an ideal esthetic dental implant restoration (Table 26.2).

Table 26.2 Implant site development during a tooth extraction.

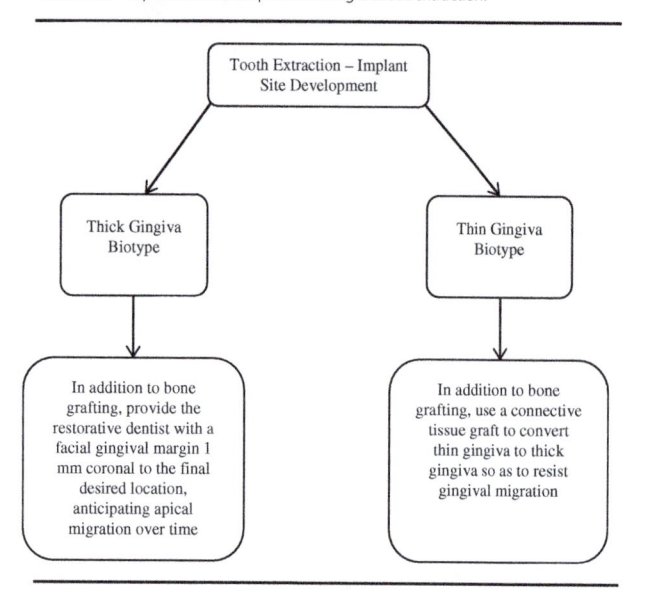

```
                Tooth Extraction – Implant
                    Site Development
                    /              \
          Thick Gingiva         Thin Gingiva
             Biotype              Biotype
                |                    |
    In addition to bone      In addition to bone
    grafting, provide the    grafting, use a connective
    restorative dentist with a  tissue graft to convert
    facial gingival margin 1    thin gingiva to thick
    mm coronal to the final     gingiva so as to resist
    desired location,           gingival migration
    anticipating apical
    migration over time
```

Table 26.3 Contraindications for soft tissue grafting around implants.

- Medical conditions (uncontrolled diabetes, etc.)
- Collagen disorders
- Smoking
- Anatomical considerations (greater palatine artery)

Contraindications

As in all types of periodontal surgery, general and specific contraindications apply to the use of soft tissue grafting techniques around dental implants (Table 26.3). General contraindications are any medical condition that may pose a threat to the patient in general or the patient's recovery and healing after surgery, such as uncontrolled diabetes. Any uncontrolled or unstable medical condition is considered an absolute contraindication for elective procedures, such as periodontal plastic surgery. Medical conditions associated with connective tissue disorders, such as erosive lichen planus and pemphigoid, may pose a risk to the viability of the soft tissue graft placed on a recipient bed that exhibits a pathologic healing mechanism. There is no published evidence to support the use of this technique in such cases. Nonetheless, there is no concrete data either to support that connective tissue disorders are an absolute contraindication for soft tisue grafting procedures [2].

A key factor for the success of soft tissue grafting procedures is revascularization of the graft. Smoking has a strong peripheral, local vasoconstrictive effect that can have deleterious sequelae on the survival of the grafted soft tissue and may lead to necrosis of the soft tissue graft and subsequent failure of the procedure. Failure of these procedures in smokers could also be attributed to the negative effect that smoking has in the adherence of the fibroblasts and the immune response [22]. Pre-operative assessment during treatment planning must identify patients who smoke, and the surgeon must inform the patient of the potential adverse effects associated with smoking. The surgeon must put effort into having the patient participate in a smoking cessation program prior to any surgery.

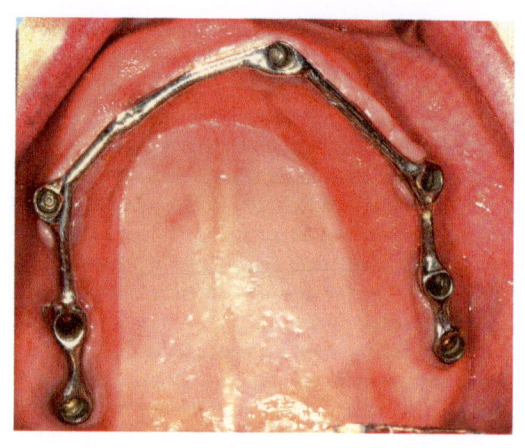

Figure 26.8 Insufficient palatal tissue for donor site harvesting. In such cases, either the tuberosity or allogeneic soft tissue matrix can be utilized to accommodate the need for soft tissue grafting.

However, in clinical reality, this is not always an option. Cessation of the smoking habit pre-operatively and adherence to a smoke-free period during the critical stages of initial revascularization should be the minimum precautions taken before subjecting a smoker to soft tissue grafting procedures.

Finally, local anatomical factors can also limit patient selection for soft tissue grafting around dental implants. Insufficient soft tissue for harvesting in the donor site (hard palate, maxillary tuberosity), proximity with anatomical structures, such as the greater palatine artery, may pose a relative contraindication for periodontal soft tissue surgery (Figure 26.8). In such cases, either the maxillary tuberosity or allogeneic soft tissue matrix can be utilized to accommodate the need for soft tissue grafting.

Diagnosis and treatment planning

Periodontal plastic surgical procedures aim to prevent or correct anatomical, developmental, traumatic, or plaque-induced defects of the tissue, alveolar mucosa, or bone around natural teeth and dental implants. The advancements achieved in implant dentistry thus far have dictated a transition of the aim of dental implant therapy from "implant survival" to "implant success." Even though osseointegration is the main goal of implant dentistry, long-term success in implant dentistry is supported by the achievement of a stable, esthetic result, which includes an intact soft tissue profile around the dental implant. The term "implant success" not only encompasses functional osseointegration but also extends to include soft and hard tissue integration of the tooth replacement in esthetic harmony with the remaining dentition. Successful bony integration of an implant does not ensure patient satisfaction. Soft-tissue health and esthetics are critical to the patient's perception of a successful restoration. Patients expect not only the ability to function with their implants long term but also to have reasonable esthetic results. In that direction, the straightforward, advanced, and complex (SAC) classification was developed to aid patient-driven clinical decision making and to help minimize complications based on the experience level of the clinician and the potential difficulty of the treated implant site [23]. The SAC classification has both restorative and surgical categories that use a normative classification system, which can be influenced by modifying factors based on the individual clinical situation. One factor that can influence the SAC grading is the esthetic risk assessment (ERA) analysis, as proposed by the International Team for Implantology (ITI) [24].

The ERA is a pre-treatment assessment tool that assesses clinical risk indicators to determine the predictability of achieving an esthetic result versus the risk for complications [24, 25]. In order to establish a trust relationship between the surgeon and the patient and to set reasonable expectations regarding the treatment outcome, esthetic risk factors should be addressed directly with the patient before the initiation of treatment. At the initial consultation, collection of information using an ERA form might be helpful to prevent complications and to establish patient's expectations. The overall goal of pre-operative risk assessment is to identify patients who may be in high risk for a negative outcome or treatment complications (i.e., persons with thin biotype, smokers, and others). The more high-risk categories that the patient falls into, the more sophisticated surgical and restorative planning might be required to achieve a favorable and predictable outcome. Nonetheless, in clinical reality some cases of implant placement in the esthetic zone with unsatisfactory esthetic results may arise. In those cases, there is an important clinical dilemma: can soft tissue grafting enhance, or even restore, the esthetic outcome of implant therapy? In these cases, the patient must know what the surgical limitations are and set realistic expectations before starting the treatment.

Table 26.4 Soft tissue considerations – key factors for success.

Level of clinical attachment on adjacent teeth to support papillary height
Thickness of the coronal soft tissue margin to ensure a proper emergence profile
Thickness of labial soft tissue to simulate root eminence and prevent transillumination of underlying metallic structure
Position of the mucogingival junction and amount of keratinized tissue in relation to the mucosal margin of the planned restoration
Symmetry of the mucosal margin in relation to adjacent teeth
Color and texture of the mucosa
Presence of scars from previous surgical procedures

Prior to intraoral examination, it is of the utmost importance for the clinician to evaluate the patient's smile line and the lip line. Many clinicians underestimate the importance of extraoral examination, resulting in inadequate treatment planning and consequently poor implant restoration esthetics.

Table 26.5 Protocol for implant site development. Modified from Ioannou et al. [8].

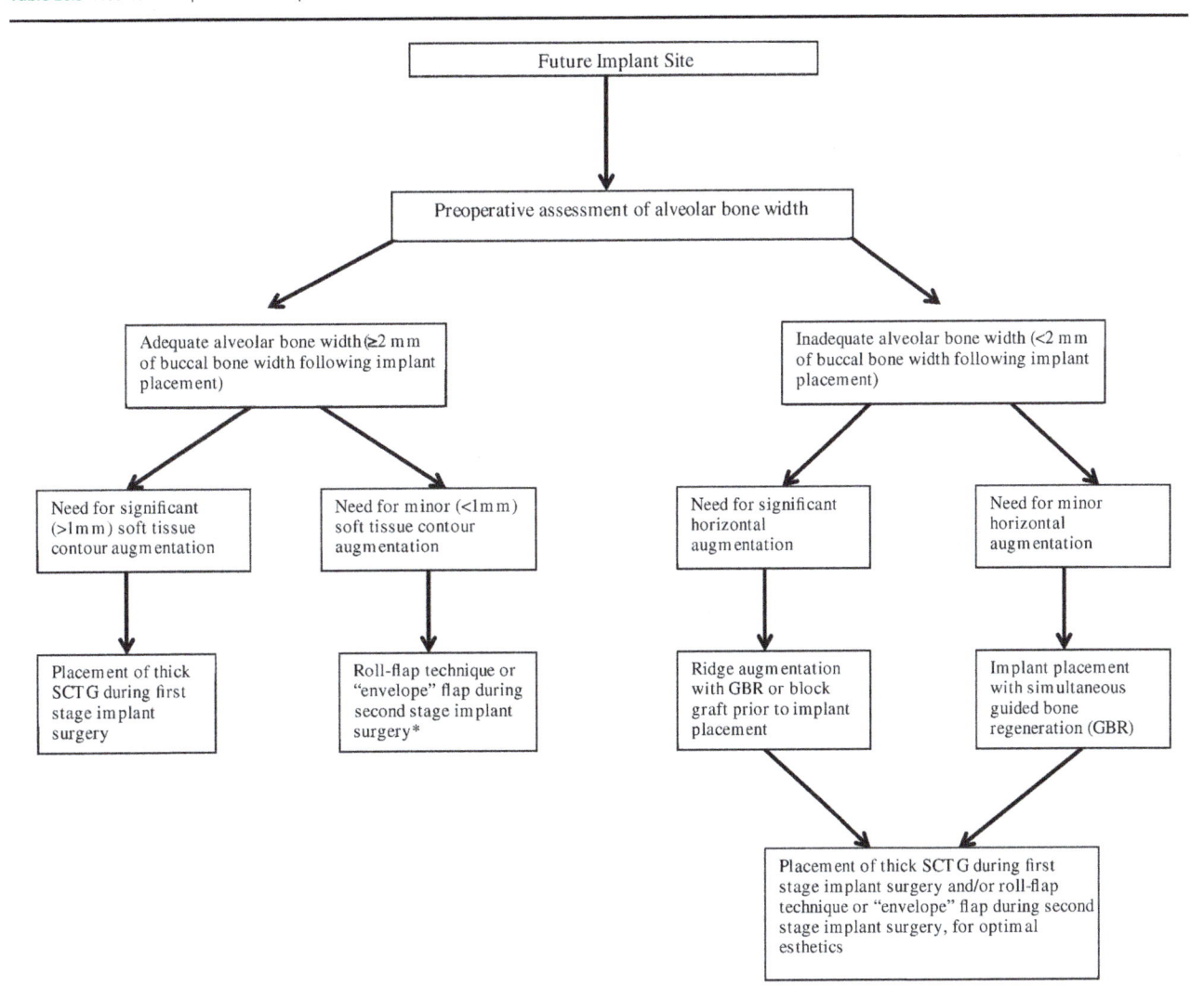

```
                        Future Implant Site
                                │
                                ▼
                Preoperative assessment of alveolar bone width
                ┌───────────────┴───────────────┐
                ▼                               ▼
    Adequate alveolar bone width       Inadequate alveolar bone width
    (≥2 mm of buccal bone width        (<2 mm of buccal bone width
    following implant placement)       following implant placement)
        ┌───────┴───────┐                   ┌───────┴───────┐
        ▼               ▼                   ▼               ▼
    Need for        Need for minor      Need for        Need for minor
    significant     (<1mm) soft         significant     horizontal
    (>1mm) soft     tissue contour      horizontal      augmentation
    tissue contour  augmentation        augmentation
    augmentation
        ▼               ▼                   ▼               ▼
    Placement of    Roll-flap           Ridge           Implant placement
    thick SCTG      technique or        augmentation    with simultaneous
    during first    "envelope" flap     with GBR or     guided bone
    stage implant   during second       block graft     regeneration (GBR)
    surgery         stage implant       prior to implant
                    surgery*            placement
                                            └───────┬───────┘
                                                    ▼
                                    Placement of thick SCTG during first
                                    stage implant surgery and/or roll-flap
                                    technique or "envelope" flap during second
                                    stage implant surgery, for optimal
                                    esthetics
```

During the intraoral examination of the patient it is necessary to pay attention to specific anatomic and restorative characteristics (Table 26.4). After the intraoral examination has revealed characteristics that would benefit from an adjunctive soft tissue graft procedure, the specific soft tissue grafting procedure can be performed to correct the soft tissue discrepancies or to modify the soft tissue profile, resulting in symmetry and esthetic harmony of the smile. These soft tissue procedures can take place at any stage before, during, or after the implant site development and placement. Nevertheless, the benefit of a single surgical procedure combining soft tissue grafting with bone grafting procedures should weigh the increased complexity and risk for adverse events when performing multiple procedures simultaneously.

Soft tissue grafting around dental implants should be employed only if it serves a specific purpose and can improve or sustain the functional or/and esthetic role of the dental implant (Table 26.5). That is, soft tissue grafting around dental implants or for implant site development should take place if it can provide a natural emergence profile for the restoration through healthy peri-implant gingiva, create a labial profile resembling the root eminence, support papillae, fill interdental embrasures, and hide the restorative components of the restoration. The long-term stability of pink esthetics around dental implant restorations has been strongly correlated with an adequate soft tissue thickness around the dental implant [26, 27].

When a thin biotype is diagnosed, a subepithelial connective tissue graft or a free gingival graft can be used to prevent potential long-term recession of the facial mucosa margin [28]. Factors that should be considered when evaluating the need for soft tissue grafting include the level of clinical attachment on adjacent teeth to support papillary height, the thickness of the coronal soft tissue margin to ensure a proper emergence profile, thickness of labial soft tissue to simulate root eminence and prevent transillumination of an underlying metallic structure, and finally the position of the mucogingival junction and amount of keratinized tissue so as to blend harmoniously with that of the adjacent teeth (Table 26.4).

Conclusion

Correct diagnosis and careful treatment planning before any implant procedure are of great importance for a functional and esthetic outcome leading to a long-term success of the dental implant prosthesis and for patient satisfaction. Soft tissue grafting around dental implants prior to, during, or after the implant placement can make the difference and facilitate success in implant dentistry by fulfilling both functional and esthetics success criteria. The next chapter will discuss different types of soft tissue grafts and the timing and techniques for soft tissue augmentation.

References

1 Kotsakis GA, Maragout T, Ioannou AL, Romanos G, Hinrichs JE: Prevalence of maxillary midline papillae recession and association with interdental smile line: a cross-sectional study. *Int J Periodontics Restorative Dent* 2014 Feb;**34**(Suppl): s81–s87.
2 Hinrichs JE, Kotsakis GA, Lareau D: Soft tissue augmentation surgery for dental implants. In: Kademami D,. Tiwanqa P (eds.), *Atlas of Oral and Maxillofacial Surgery*, Chapter 27, 1st edn. Elsevier, 2015.
3 Fürhauser R, Florescu D, Benesch T, Haas R, Mailath G, Watzek G: Evaluation of soft tissue around single-tooth implant crowns: the pink esthetic score. *Clin Oral Implants Res* 2005;**16**(6):639–644.
4 Jemt T: Regeneration of gingival papillae after single implant treatment. *Int J Periodontics Restorative Dent* 1997;**17**:326–333.
5 Abrahamsson I, Berglundh T, Lindhe J: Soft tissue response to plaque formation at different implant systems. A comparative study in the dog. *Clin Oral Implants Res* 1998;**9**:73–79.
6 Tarnow D, Elian N, Fletcher P, Froum S, Magner A, Cho SC, et al: Vertical distance from the crest of bone to the height of the interproximal papilla between adjacent implants. *J Periodontol* 2003;**74**:1785–1788.
7 Tarnow DP, Cho S, Wallace SS: The effect of inter-implant distance on the height of inter-implant bone crest. *J Periodontol* 2000;**71**:546–549.
8 Ioannou A, Kotsakis G, McHale M, Lareau DE, Hinrichs JE, Romanos GE: Soft tissue surgical procedures for optimizing anterior implant esthetics. *Int J Dentistry* 2015;**2015**:740–764.
9 Schropp L, Wentzel A, Kostopoulos L, Karring T: Bone healing and soft tissue contour changes following single-tooth extraction: a clinical and radiographic 12-month prospective study. *Int J Periodontics Restorative Dent* 2003;**23**:313.
10 Kotsakis GA, Chrepa V, Marcou N, Prasad H, Hinrichs J: Flapless alveolar ridge preservation utilizing the "socket-plug" technique: clinical technique and review of the literature. *J Oral Implantol* 2014 Dec;**40**(6):690–698.
11 Kotsakis GA, Salama M, Chrepa V, Hinrichs J, Gaillard P: A randomized, blinded, controlled clinical study of particulate anorganic bovine bone mineral and calcium phosphosilicate putty bone substitutes for alveolar ridge preservation. *Int J Oral Maxillofac Implants* 2014 Jan-Feb;**29**(1):141–151.
12 Lang NP, Loe H: The relationship between the width of keratinized gingiva and gingival health. *J Periodontol* 1972;**43**:623–627.
13 Kennedy J, Bird W, Palanis K, et al: A longitudinal evaluation of varying widths of attached gingiva. *J Clin Periodontol* 1985;**12**(8):667–675.
14 Adell R, Lekholm U, Rockler B, Brånemark PI, Lindhe J, Eriksson B, Sbordone L: Marginal tissue reactions at osseointegrated titanium fixtures (I). A 3-year longitudinal prospective study. *Int J Oral Maxillofac Surg* 1986 Feb;**15**(1):39–52.
15 Albrektsson T, Abrahamsson I, Berglundh T, Glantz PO, Lindhe J: The mucosal attachment at different abutments. An experimental study in dogs. *J Clin Periodontol* 1998 Sep;**25**(9):721–727.
16 Bouri A Jr, Bissada N, Al-Zahrani MS, Faddoul F, Nouneh I: Width of keratinized gingiva and the health status of the supporting tissues around dental implants. *Int J Oral Maxillofac Implants* 2008 Mar-Apr;**23**(2):323–326.
17 Esposito M, Grusovin, M, Maghaireh H, Coulthard P, Worthington HV: Interventions for replacing missing teeth: management of soft tissues for dental implants. *Cochrane Database Syst Rev* 2007 Jul;**18**(3):CD006697.
18 Greenstein G, Cavallaro J: The clinical significance of keratinized gingiva around dental implants. *Compend Contin Educ Dent* 2011 Oct;**32**(8):24–31; quiz 32, 34. Review.
19 Kan JY, Morimoto T, Rungcharassaeng K, Roe P, Smith DH: Gingival biotype assessment in the esthetic zone: visual versus direct measurement. *Int J Periodontics Restorative Dent* 2010 Jun;**30**(3):237–243.
20 Al-Sabbagh M: Implants in the esthetic zone. *Dent Clin North Am* 2006 Jul;**50** (3):391–407, vi. Review.
21 Happe A, Stimmelmayr M, Schlee M, Rothamel D: Surgical management of peri-implant soft tissue color mismatch caused by shine-through effects of restorative materials: one-year follow-up. *Int J Periodontics Restorative Dent* 2013 Jan;**33** (1):81–88.
22 Tipton DA, Dabbous M: Effects of nicotine on proliferation and extracellular matrix production of human gingival fibroblasts *in vitro*. *J Periodontol* 1995;**66**:1056.
23 Dawson A, Chen S: *The SAC Classification in Implant Dentistry*. Quintessence, Berlin, 2009.
24 Buser D, Martin W, Belser UC: Optimizing esthetics for implant restoration in the anterior maxilla: anatomic and surgical considerations. *Int J Oral Maxillofac Implants* 2004;**19**(Suppl):43–61.
25 Levine RA, Nack G: Team treatment planning for the replacement of esthetic zone teeth with dental implants. *Compend Contin Educ Dent* 2011;**32**:44–50.
26 Geurs NC, Vassilopoulis P, Reddy MS: Soft tissue considerations in implant site development. *Oral Maxillofac Surg Clin North Am* 2010 Aug;**22**(3):387–405.
27 Fu JH, Lee A, Wang HL: Influence of tissue biotype on implant esthetics. *Int J Oral Maxillofac Implants* 2011 May-Jun;**26**(3):499–508.
28 Kan JY, Rungcharassaeng K, Lozada JL, Zimmerman G: Facial gingival tissue stability following immediate placement and provisionalization of maxillary anterior single implants: a 2- to 8-year follow-up. *Int J Oral Maxillofac Implants* 2011 Jan-Feb;**26**(1):179–187.

CHAPTER 27
Soft Tissue Grafting Techniques in Implant Dentistry

Suheil Boutros[1] and Georgios A. Kotsakis[2]

[1]Private Practice, Limited to Periodontics and Implants Surgery, Grand Blanc, Michigan, USA
[2]University of Washington, Department of Periodontics, Seattle, Washington, USA

Introduction

Patient satisfaction with implant treatment is largely dependent on the harmonious incorporation of the implant prosthesis with the remaining dentition. The previous chapter discussed the indications for use of soft tissue grafting procedures around an implant that range from correction of mucogingival defects to enhancement of the alveolar ridge contour or even rescue procedures [1]. Peri-implant plastic surgery soft tissue grafting procedures represent a versatile family of techniques that differ depending on the timing of the procedure and the type of soft tissue graft that is utilized [2].

Autogenous epithelized palatal grafts or free gingival grafts (FGGs) for root coverage were first introduced in the early 1960s and since then have been employed by numerous clinicians to provide functional results of increasing the zone of keratinized gingiva and gaining coverage of exposed roots [3, 4]. The use of FGGs is very widespread due to their high predictability; nonetheless the color match of the tissues is less than esthetic due to the lighter and more opaque color of the palatal tissue color as compared with the buccal gingiva, thus limiting their application in areas where esthetics are important.

The subepithelial connective tissue graft (SCTG) as described by Langer and Langer [5] has a better color match and the donor site has less morbidity. Both the FGG and SCTG require adequate donor tissue, which might be a challenge in large multiple tooth defects or in patients that are hesitant in having a second surgical donor site. These concerns have addressed the use of the acelluar dermal matrix (ADM) [6] for treatment of recession around natural teeth and mucosal defects with a porcine collagen matrix (Mucograft) [7] and tissue engineered bilayered cell therapy [8].

Types of soft tissue grafts

Free gingival graft (FGG)

Historically, free gingival grafts (FGGs) first paved the way for periodontal plastic surgery procedures [9]. Periodontal plastic surgery procedures are performed to correct or eliminate anatomic, developmental, or traumatic deformities of the gingiva and alveolar mucosa. Bjorn described a technique of autogenous tissue harvesting in a presentation abstract where he procured thin gingival grafts containing the epithelium and lamina propria to treat areas of the dentition that had loss of attached keratinized tissue due to periodontitis [9]. Since then, the FGG has been used for every periodontal plastic surgery procedure in the oral cavity both around teeth and implants with consistent results. The healing cascade following the placement of an FGG on a recipient soft tissue bed has been thoroughly characterized and graft integration has been found to occur through a phase of (1) plasmatic circulation, (2) vascular invasion, (3) connective tissue attachment and bridging of vessels, and (4) connective tissue maturation [10, 11].

The main limitation in the use of FGGs is the esthetic incorporation of graft with the adjacent soft tissues. It has been well established that the donor site characteristics dictate the phenotype of the transplanted tissue [12]. Thus, the healed FGG frequently resemble palatal tissue, which is the most common area for harvesting of FGGs, and do not blend in well with the adjacent tissue in terms of color and texture. In addition, characteristics of the palatal tissue, such as rugae, will be maintained in the transplanted tissue indefinitely and should be removed during harvesting to allow more esthetic graft incorporation [13]. Despite its esthetic shortcomings, the FGG is a very predictable method for increasing keratinized tissue. When performed within its limitations this is a very reliable technique that can be utilized to increase the zone of keratinized tissue prior to advanced grafting procedures, such as vertical ridge augmentation, in order to ascertain proper flap management and secure primary closure or as a rescue procedure around implants with limited keratinized tissue width. The most common donor site of the FGG is the highly keratinized palate. The color and shade of the augmented recipient site often do not provide an ideal match with the adjacent soft tissue, but the palate provides a large surface area of keratinized tissue that allows procuring large grafts prior to vertical and horizontal bone augmentation or for the increase of keratinized tissue around multiple implants. Alternative donor sites include the maxillary tuberosity or edentulous regions. These areas can only provide a limited volume of FGG, but are advantageous in terms of color and texture.

Subepithelial connective tissue graft (SCTG) with coronally advanced flap (CAF)

SCTG procedures have been successfully used for many years for the management of recession and soft tissue defects around natural teeth and for augmenting alveolar ridge contours [14]. SCTG grafts may have some limitations when attempting to graft and achieve coverage of a non-vital implant surface since the soft

---

Vertical Alveolar Ridge Augmentation in Implant Dentistry: A Surgical Manual, First Edition. Edited by Len Tolstunov.
© 2016 John Wiley & Sons, Inc. Published 2016 by John Wiley & Sons, Inc.

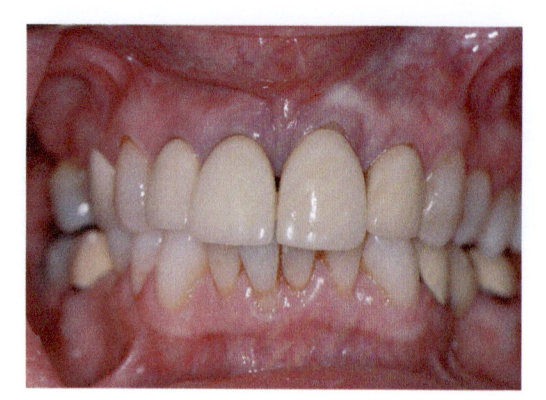

Figure 27.1 Severe periodontal disease around the two maxillary central incisors.

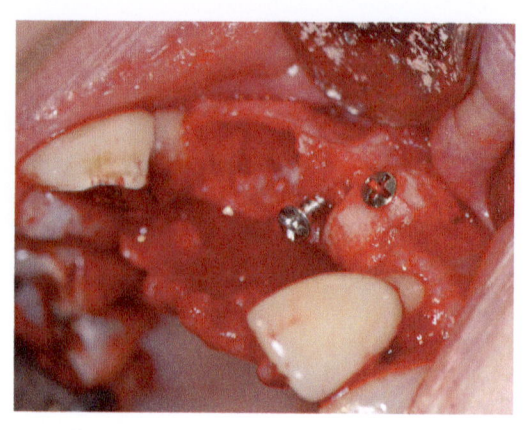

Figure 27.3 Allogeneic block graft along with a tenting screw for vertical bone augmentation.

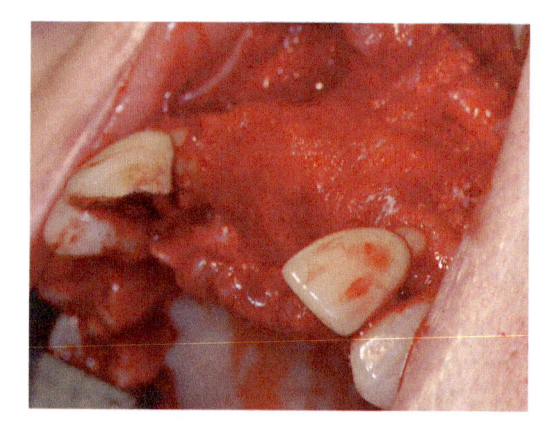

Figure 27.4 Collagen membrane for GBR.

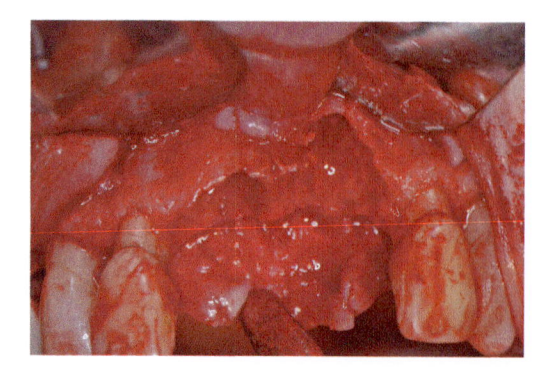

Figure 27.2 Severe bone loss following the extraction of the maxillary incisors.

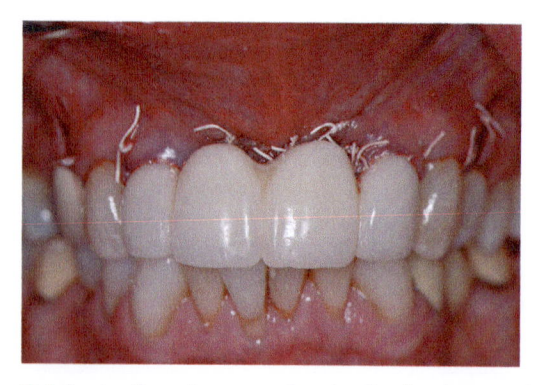

Figure 27.5 Scoring the periosteum and tension free flap closure with an e-PTFE suture.

tissue around the implant does not respond in the same manner as a natural tooth. Nonetheless, SCTG, when indicated and properly used, can provide stable and significant gains in soft tissue volume and contour that can enhance the esthetic outcome of deficient implant sites.

The evolution of soft tissue grafts came with the subepithelial connective tissue graft (SCTG). SCTGs initially were conceived as FGGs without the epithelial component (referred to as "free connective tissue grafts" by Edel [15] and were introduced in an effort to increase the esthetic incorporation of the soft tissue graft to the adjacent tissues. Langer and Calagna [16] and later Langer and Langer [5] contributed to the widespread use of the SCTG in contemporary periodontology by introducing this epithelium-free graft underneath a partial thickness flap to exploit the blood supply from the underlying periosteum and the overlaying connective tissue of the flap. This bilaminar blood supply is a key component for the predictability of SCTG techniques and the increased root coverage associated with this technique [5]. An additional advantage of SCTGs is that there is no need for retention of the epithelium. Thus, graft harvesting can be a closed wound procedure that minimizes patient discomfort and risk for bleeding (Figures 27.1 to 27.16).

Despite these advancements there are always patients who are hesitant to undergo autogenous tissue harvesting or are medically compromised and there is a need to minimize invasiveness of surgical procedures. For such cases, acellular dermal connective tissue grafts (ADCTs) have been introduced in the market. These skin allografts are screened and processed in tissue banks to ensure no antigenicity and all cellular content is removed while maintaining the biochemical components of the matrix [17]. Thus, ADCT functions as a three-dimensional scaffold for connective tissue regeneration. Clinical results have shown promising results in the short term, although an active debate exists on whether recession coverage with ADCT is more prone to relapse in the long term [18].

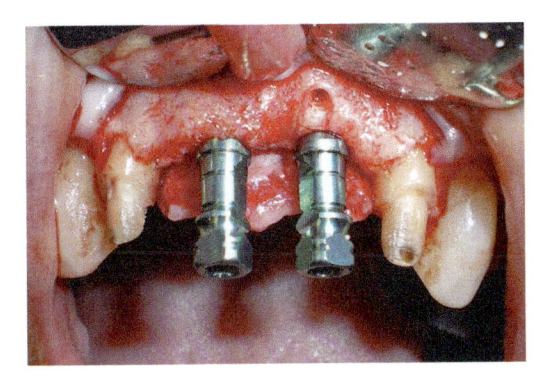

Figure 27.6 Implant placement six months following ridge augmentation.

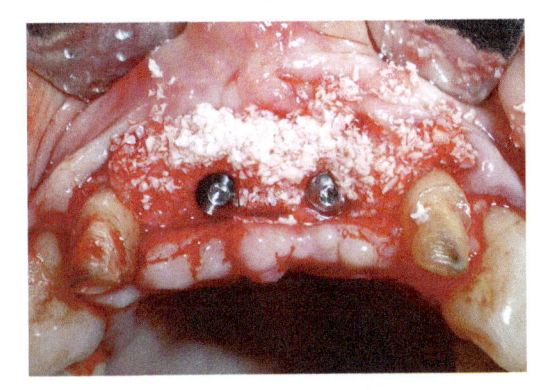

Figure 27.7 Bovine bone at the time of placement to enhance bone augmentation.

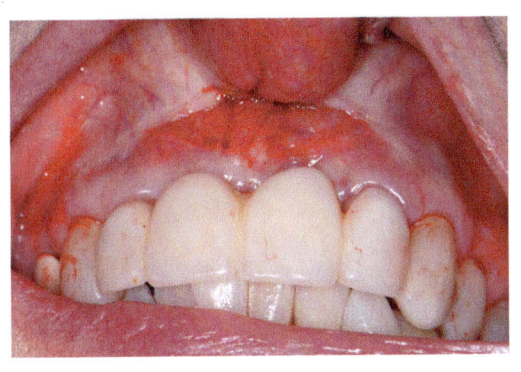

Figure 27.8 Frenectomy to correct a deficient vestibule.

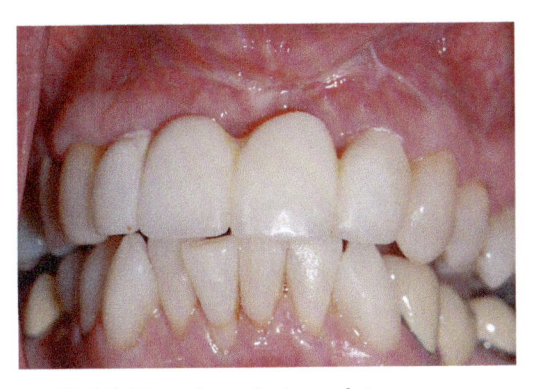

Figure 27.9 Healed ridge at the implant second stage.

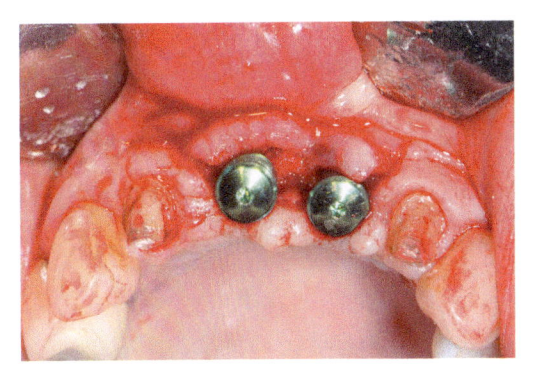

Figure 27.10 For the placement of the CTG either a split- or a full-thickness flap can be utilized with comparable success. In this case a split-thickness flap was designed by positioning the blade crestally almost parallel to the periosteum and proceeding with sharp dissection until approximately the level of the mucogingival junction. The crestal incision was connected with two releasing incisions to facilitate space maintenance for placement of the graft. Clinical image shows placement of the healing abutments and the recipient site prepared for CTG positioning.

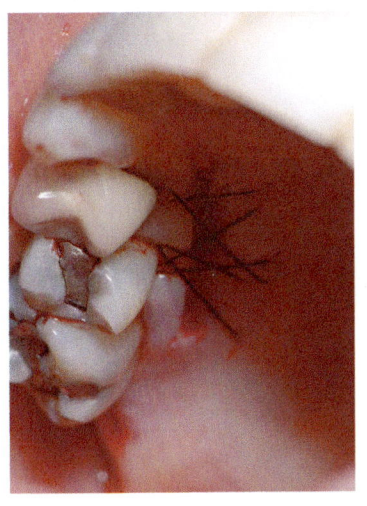

Figure 27.11 For the palatal harvest a linear incision is utilized at a distance of at least 3 mm from the palatal marginal gingiva of the adjacent teeth to avoid iatrogenic marginal tissue recession. A 15c or 12d blade is utilized to trace an incision perpendicular to the periosteum and the same blade is then turned parallel to the periosteum to separate the CTG from the overlying epithelium. This technique avoids a large open wound associated with FGG harvesting. The clinical image shows a palatal donor site with a collagen wound dressing for hemostasis.

Pedicle flap

When there is a large amount of keratinized gingiva on the adjacent area, it is possible to use a connective tissue pedicle rather than a free connective tissue graft. The advantage of using a pedicle flap is to preserve vascularization, which is critical for the graft survival and helps in reducing graft shrinkage. The other advantage of the pedicle flap is great color match and with a single incision approach it eliminates the need for a donor site and the risk of complications. A partial thickness flap is recommended on the adjacent area and then the base of the flap is freed by scoring the periosteum, allowing the rotation of the flap to be tension free. After preparing the recipient bed, the pedicle flap is rolled into the buccal pouch and

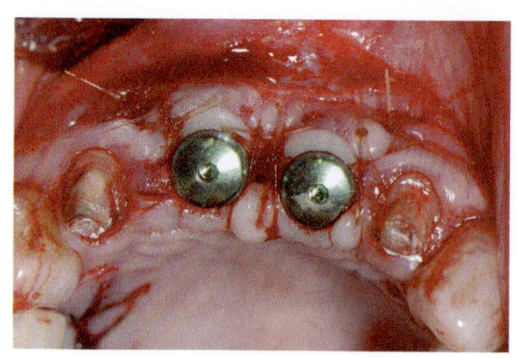

Figure 27.12 Following harvesting, the CTG is trimmed and adapted to the recipient bed and secured with periosteal sutures at the base of the split-thickness flap. Subsequently the overlying flap is repositioned to completely cover the CTG and support its vascularization. In this case, the CTG was performed during second stage surgery, thus combined with an apically repositioned flap. Note that the sutures placed on the vertical incisions with the appropriate direction facilitate appropriate positioning of the flap at the desired apical position.

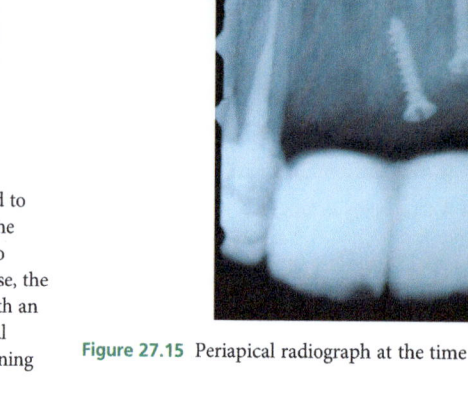

Figure 27.15 Periapical radiograph at the time of bone augmentation.

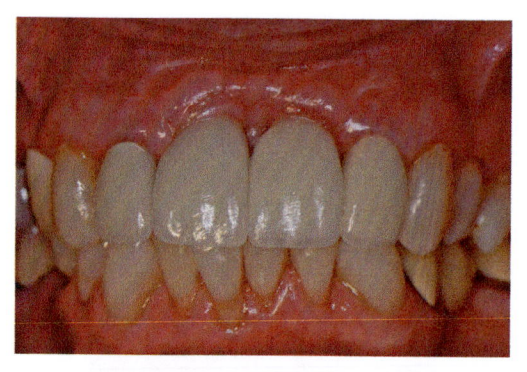

Figure 27.13 Final restoration one year post-augmentation.

secured with an internal sling suture. The palatal interdental is sutured with single interrupted sutures [19] (Figures 27.17 to 27.23). If more keratinized gingiva is needed in thin biotype cases, then a free connective tissue graft might be indicated in addition to the pedicle flap.

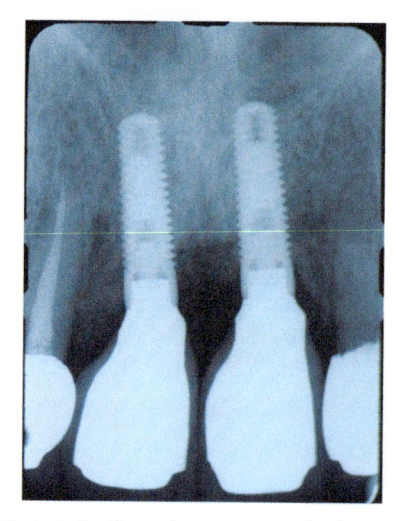

Figure 27.16 Periapical radiograph one year post-loading.

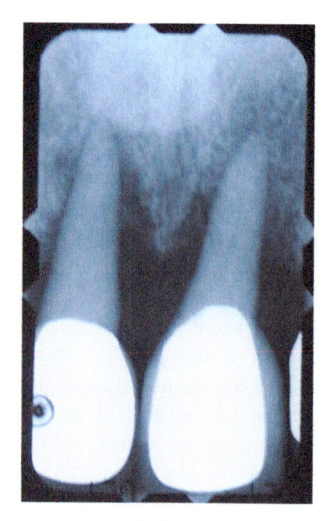

Figure 27.14 Pre-operative periapical radiograph.

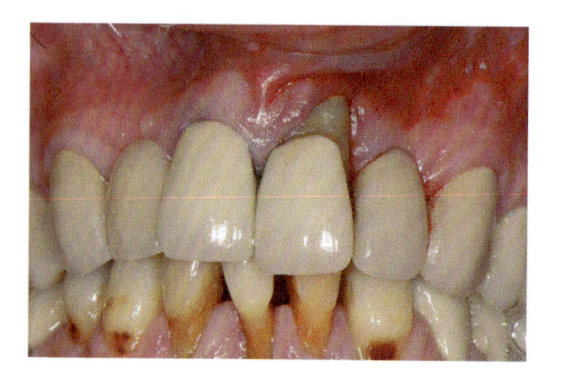

Figure 27.17 Severe recession resulted from failed root canal therapy.

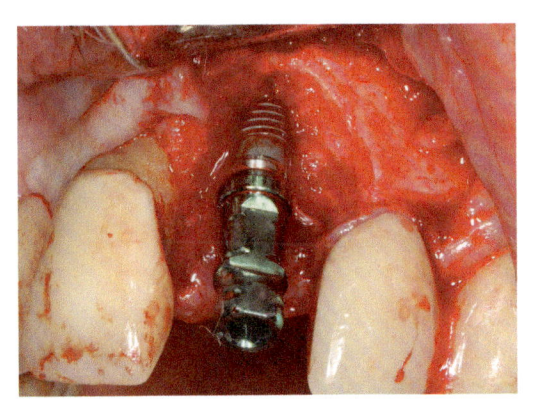

Figure 27.18 Immediate implant placement in the extraction socket.

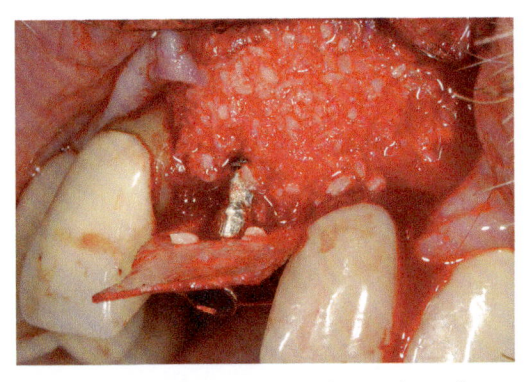

Figure 27.19 Temporary abutment along with cortical cancellous mineralized allograft.

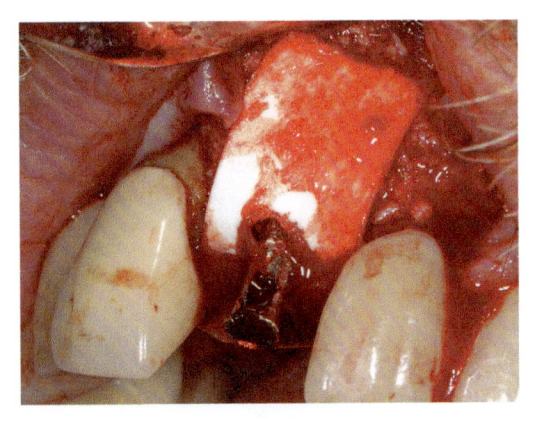

Figure 27.20 Resorbable collagen membrane for GBR.

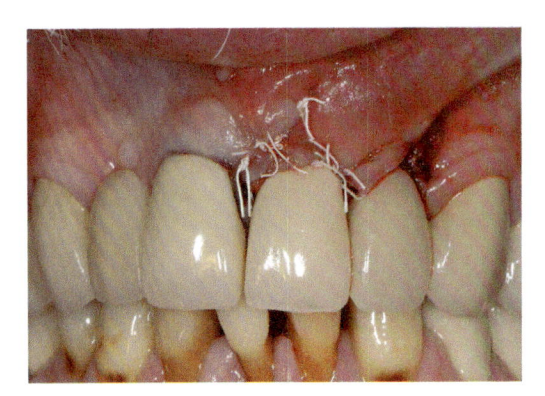

Figure 27.21 Tension-free partial thickness lateral pedicle flap to cover the augmented site.

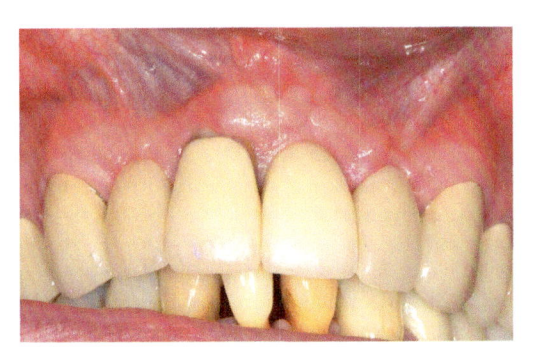

Figure 27.22 One year following augmentation.

Figure 27.23 Stable bone level one year post-implant loading.

Allograft and coronally advanced flap

The acellular dermal matrix (ADM) graft can be used as an alternative to autogenous FGG or SCTG to augment the facial soft tissue around dental implants. The recipient bed is prepared by performing a partial thickness flap so that the flap can be advanced passively over the ADM. The dermis graft is secured to the surgical bed and then the coronally advanced pedicle flap is raised to cover the dermis; coverage of the ADM is crucial for the augmentation success.

Timing for soft tissue grafting

Timing for soft tissue grafting is a factor that largely affects both the selection of the grafting technique as well as the predictability of the outcome. The ideal situation arises when the hard and soft tissue profile of the area are ideal prior to implant placement. In clinical

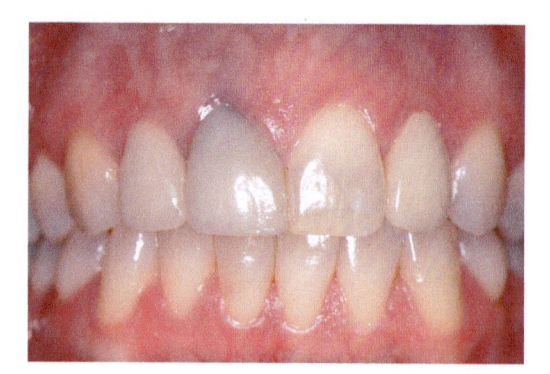

Figure 27.24 Failed endodontic therapy on the right maxillary central incisor.

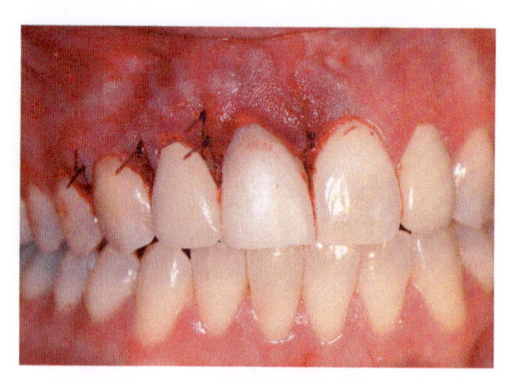

Figure 27.26 Flap closure with an immediate non-occluding restoration.

practice this scenario rarely occurs after tooth extraction due to the resorptive cascade of events, which is referred to as ridge resorption [20]. The intervention to augment soft tissue at the time of extraction allows the time from extraction to implant uncovering to evaluate healing and decide whether additional intervention is required. On the other hand, accelerated protocols that involve extraction, immediate implant placement with hard and soft-tissue grafting, and immediate loading minimize treatment time and response to patient needs for timely rehabilitation, but have the inherent risk of not giving the operator the opportunity to perform a surgical revision.

In healed sites, soft tissue augmentation can take place either during implant placement or during second stage surgery [2]. Although the predictability of both treatment strategies is comparable [17], in the case of significant tissue profile deficiencies soft tissue augmentation simultaneously with implant placement can allow for additional tissue grafting during second stage surgery, if needed, but not vice versa [2]. Additionally, SCTG can also be utilized for pontic site development in lieu of vertical augmentation. Exploiting the bilaminar blood supply offered by pouch procedures, SCTG can provide minimally invasive alternatives to bone grafting for vertical augmentation in pontic sites [21].

Lastly, soft tissue grafting procedures play a key role as "rescue" procedures in implant dentistry. When an implant in function demonstrates esthetic problems related to recession, tissue discoloration, or lack of keratinized tissue, soft tissue grafting can be employed to solve these problems and enhance long-term implant treatment success [2]. Nonetheless, when soft tissue grafting techniques are utilized as rescue procedures clinicians and patients should have moderate expectations (Figures 27.24 to 27.33).

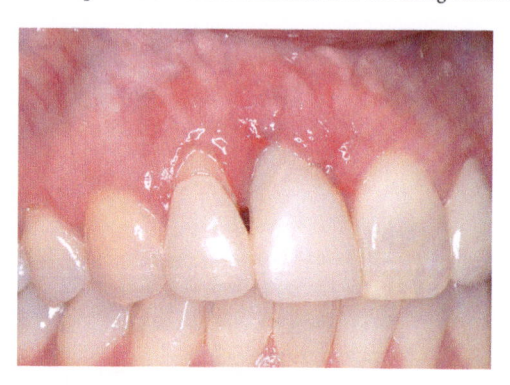

Figure 27.27 Recession on the implant and the adjacent natural tooth.

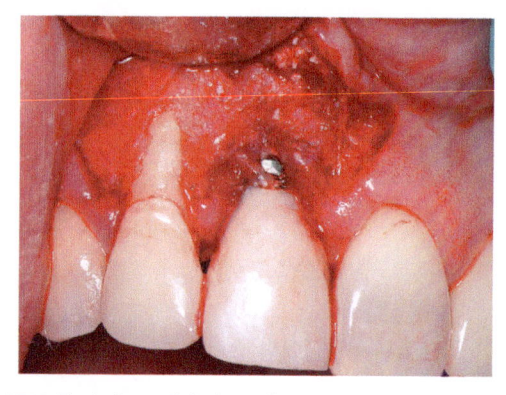

Figure 27.28 Typical partial thickness flap in preparation for a connective tissue graft. Note that the incisions are traced at the base of the papillae and subsequently the papillae are de-epithelized with a blade or a sharpened curette for a connective tissue to connective tissue attachment.

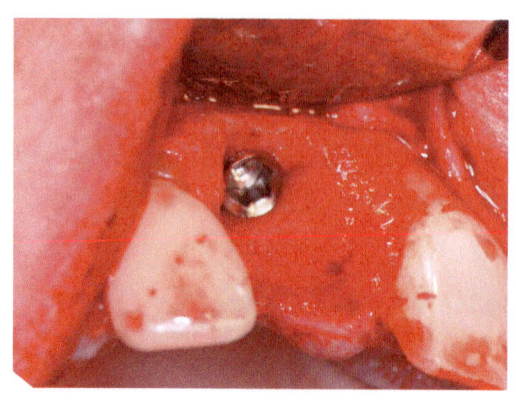

Figure 27.25 Implant placement with a flap approach.

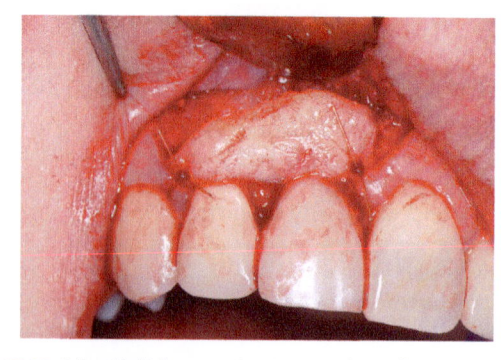

Figure 27.29 Subepithelial connective tissue graft as a "rescue procedure." The CTG is stabilized laterally with resorbable suture material and the single interrupted technique. Frequently periosteal suspension sutures are utilized to further immobilize the graft.

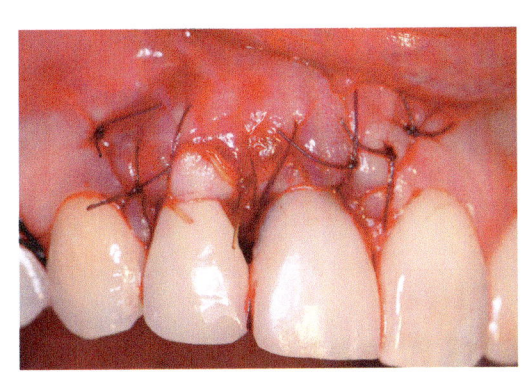

Figure 27.30 Coronally advanced pedicle flap to cover the connective tissue graft. In this case semisubmersion of the CTG was elected. As a rule of thumb, if two-thirds of the CTG are covered by the overlaying flap, the remaining one-third can be left partially exposed and still be successfully integrated [5].

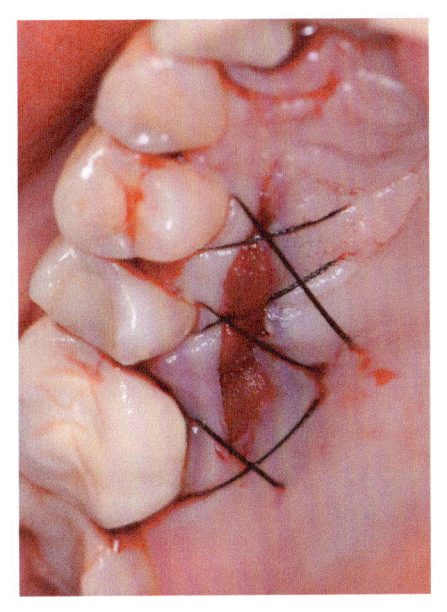

Figure 27.31 Palatal donor site managed with a mattress suture to minimize bleeding and necrosis.

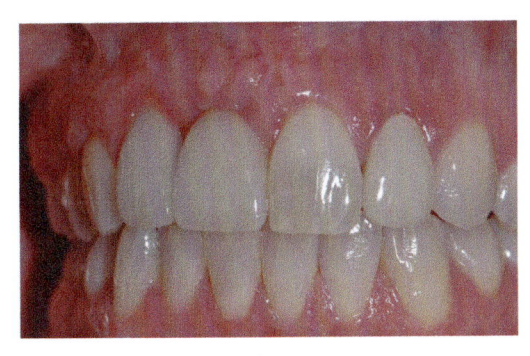

Figure 27.32 One year following soft tissue augmentation.

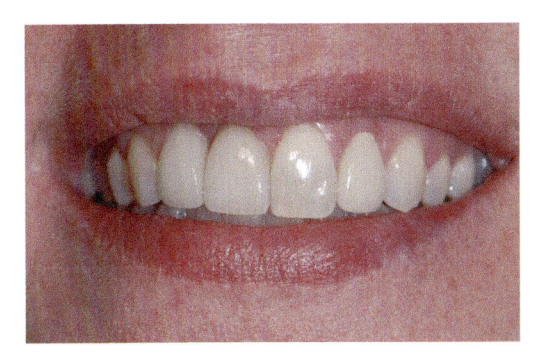

Figure 27.33 High lip line with an esthetic outcome.

Soft tissue augmentation prior to implant placement

Evaluation of the site needs to be analyzed on a case-by-case basis for soft tissue augmentation. Consideration for soft tissue augmentation would be based on the quantity and quality of the keratinized gingiva present, which may be reflected as a thin or thick gingival biotype. A minimum of 3 mm of keratinized gingiva in the esthetic zone is recommended to allow for the biological width to reform with a minimum thickness of 2 mm. Soft tissue augmentation can be performed at the time of tooth extraction, in healed sited prior to ridge augmentation, simultaneously with implant placement (stage 1) and at the implant stage 2 (placement of healing abutments).

At the time of the extraction

The main goals when treating the extraction socket in the esthetic zone is to preserve as much as possible existing soft and hard tissue volume. To effectively limit the loss of the thin buccal plate, the avoidance of a buccal gingival flap is recommended for socket preservation procedures. At the time of extraction and socket preservation, considerations need to be made as to the fate of soft tissues in the area and the need to augment the future implant site. The concept of augmenting keratinized tissue in the extraction site was initiated by Landsberg and Bichacho [22], who described a modified ridge preservation technique called "socket seal surgery." In this technique, both bone and soft tissue grafting is done prior to implant placement. Following atraumatic extractions and bone grafting of the extraction socket with the appropriate bone graft biomaterials [4] a free gingival graft is obtained from the palate to function as a seal and prevent washout of the graft and contribute to clot stability (Figures 27.34 to 27.37). Although the epithelial

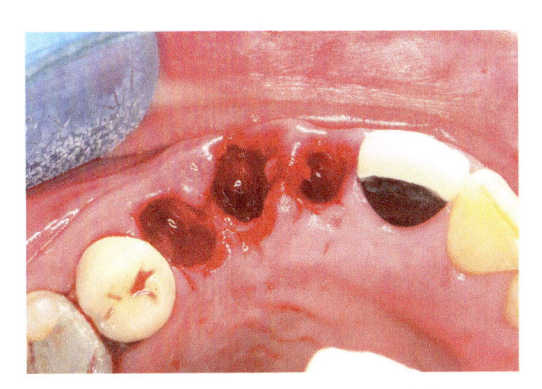

Figure 27.34 Upper right maxillary view immediately following atraumatic extraction of three adjacent teeth.

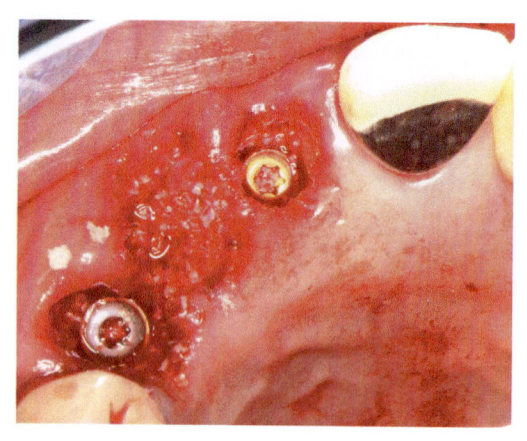

Figure 27.35 Immediate placement of maxillary right lateral and first premolar implants with subsequent grafting of the horizontal buccal gap and canine socket with anorganic bovine bone mineral for long-term preservation of tissue contours.

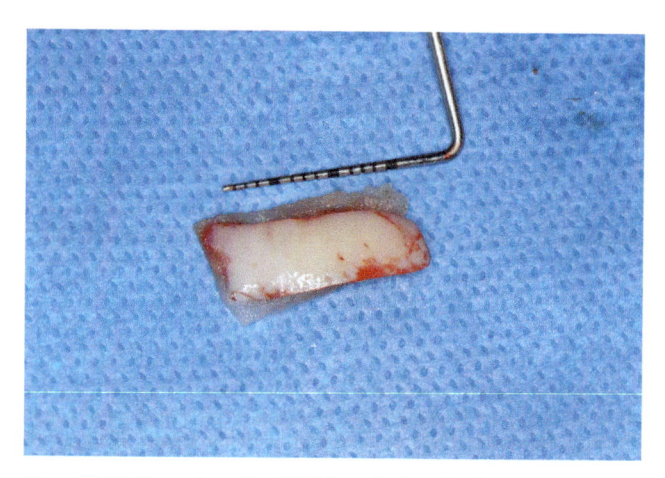

Figure 27.36 Harvesting of an FGG from the lateral palate to perform the socket seal technique. Note that the collagen tape behind the FGG has been trimmed according to its dimensions as a template.

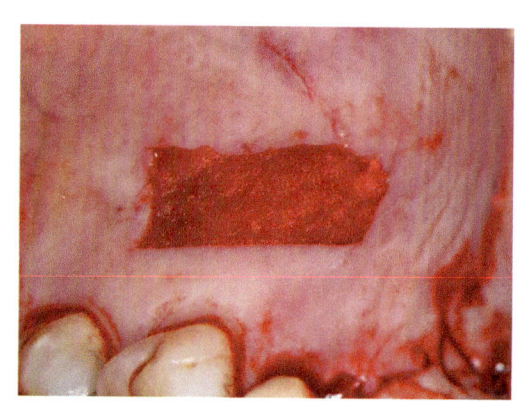

Figure 27.37 Placement of the Colla-Tape to the palatal donor site to minimize post-operative bleeding and facilitate healing.

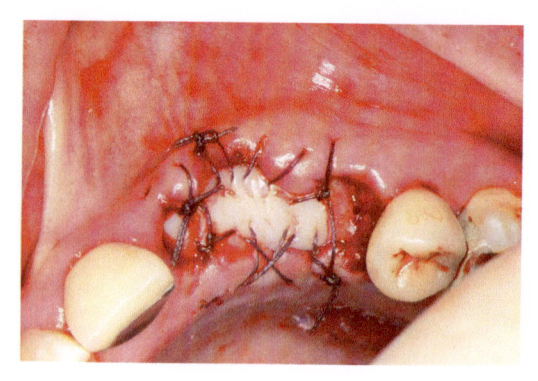

Figure 27.38 Suturing of the FGG on the sites to contain the graft.

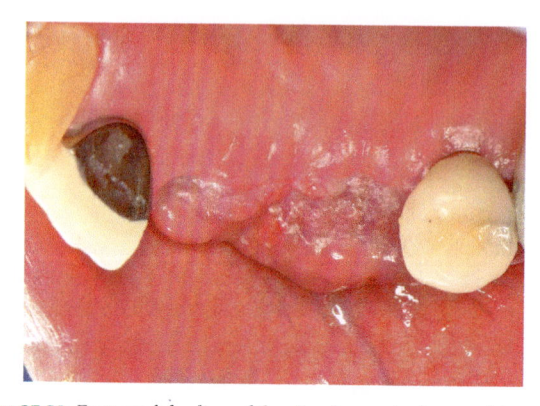

Figure 27.39 Four-week healing of the site, demonstrating partial incorporation of the graft with areas of fibrinoid that are characteristic of partial graft necrosis, as expected with this technique.

portion of the graft will undergo partial necrosis due to the poor blood supply derived from the grafted sockets, the newly formed tissue will share the keratinized tissue phenotype [23] (Figures 27.38 to 27.39). This technique is particularly useful in the anterior region, since the FGG is positioned at the occlusal aspect of the ridge and in most cases will not compromise the peri-implant esthetics while providing a broad zone of keratinized tissue that can often be combined with a simple "tissue-punch" type of second stage surgery (Figures 27.40 and 27.41). The use of palatal epithelized free tissue graft as a socket seal for good adaptation of the tissue graft to the soft tissue of the socket has documented success.

In healed sites prior to ridge augmentation

Abrams et al. [24] studied the prevalence of anterior ridge deformities in partially edentulous patients and reported the presence of defects in 91% of cases. Seibert [25, 26] categorized ridge defect in three categories:
1 Class I: buccolingual loss of tissue with normal ridge height in the apicocoronal dimension.

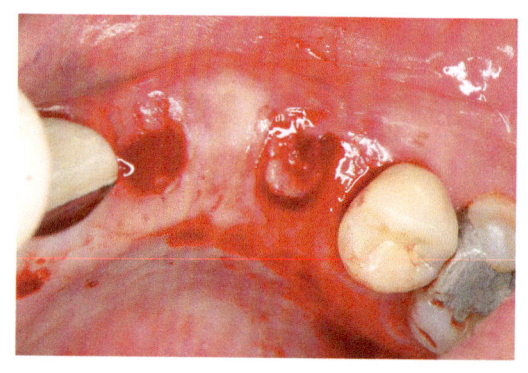

Figure 27.40 Second stage appointment at 4-month post-placement. Based on the ample zone of KT a tissue "punch" approach is indicated in this case.

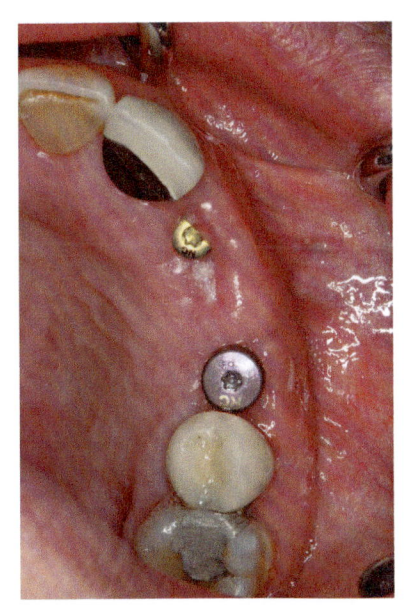

Figure 27.41 Healing following second stage surgery. Note the broad zone of KT and favorable tissue contours. The lateral incisor's healing abutment was intentionally selected for semisubmerged healing to gain keratinized tissue height.

2 Class II: apicocoronal loss of tissue with normal ridge width in a buccolingual dimension.
3 Class III: combined buccolingual and apicocoronal loss of tissue resulting in loss of normal ridge height and width (Figures 27.42 and 27.43).

Class I defects can be frequently treated in a single procedure but classes II and III defects may require more than one procedure to accomplish the goal of ridge reconstruction. The prevalence of defects were evaluated by Abams et al. [24] in partially edentulous patients, the most prevalent being class III (55.8%) followed by class I (32.8%), with class II (2.9%) being the least detected clinically.

In extreme cases of vertical and horizontal bone loss where ridge augmentation is planned, soft tissue augmentation might be indicated prior to bone augmentation (Figures 27.44 to 27.57). In cases of block grafting, since primary closure is a key factor, increasing the amount and the thickness of the keratinized mucosa prior to bone augmentation might be a prerequisite for success. In other cases of significant alveolar ridge atrophy, the simultaneous soft tissue augmentation at the same time of implant placement will allow sufficient healing time to properly assess the site during second stage surgery. Consequently, if additional soft tissue augmentation is needed, it can be performed at second stage surgery.

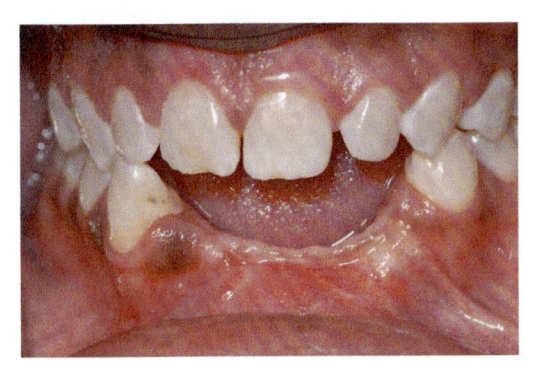

Figure 27.42 Severe bone resorption that resulted from trauma.

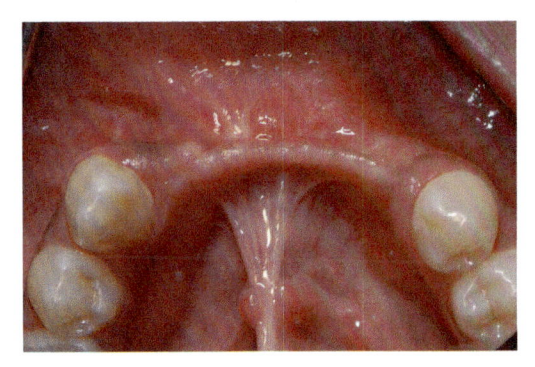

Figure 27.43 Horizontal and vertical deficiency (Seibert Class III).

Soft tissue augmentation simultaneously with implant placement

Considerations need to be made on a case-by-case, site-by-site basis using the esthetic risk assessment (ERA) analysis as a guide to decide the need to augment at the time of implant placement with soft and/or hard tissue (Figures 27.58 and 27.59).

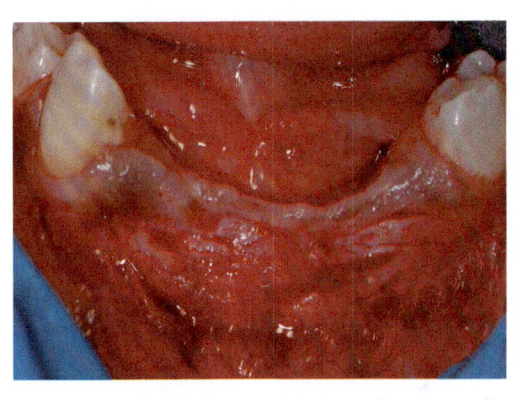

Figure 27.44 Surgical bed using a partial-thickness flap, leaving the periosteum intact. A blade is utilized to initiate a linear split-thickness incision at the mucogingival junction. The split-thickness flap is elevated with sharp dissection to the desired vestibular extension. The remaining keratinized epithelium is de-epithelized with the same blade or a sharp curette until bleeding is evident.

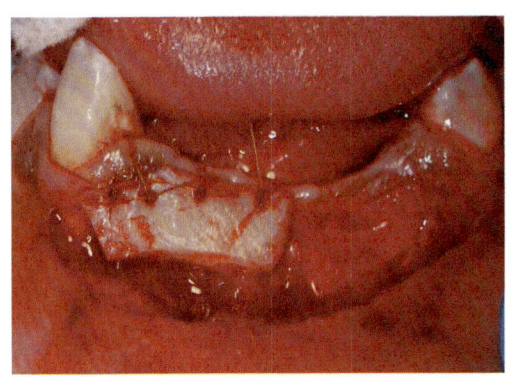

Figure 27.45 The FGGs are positioned in place and first sutured to the epithelium that exists coronally to the mucogingival junction. Clinical image showing the first of the two FGGs sutured coronally.

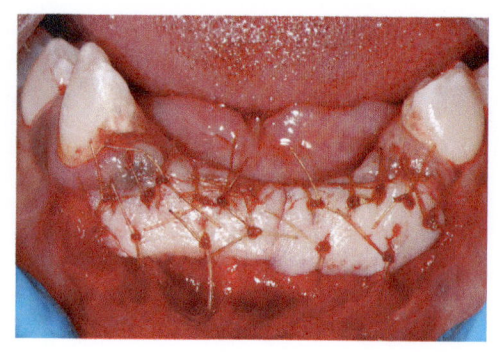

Figure 27.46 Then, the second FGG is sutured to the first graft and secured by suturing it to the periosteum. Overall there are four series of sutures; (1) to the coronal zone of keratinized tissue; (2) between the two FGGs; (3) laterally to the remaining keratinized tissue; and (4) to the underlying periosteum.

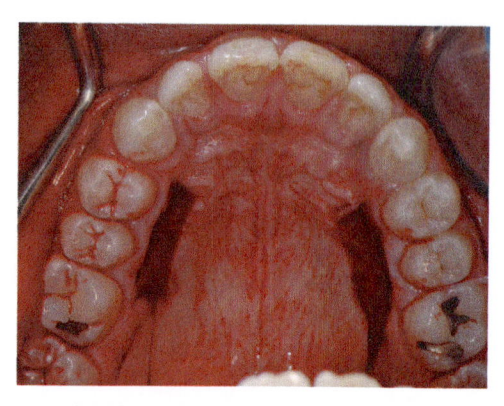

Figure 27.47 Bilateral palatal donor sites; the donor is managed by applying collagen wound dressing.

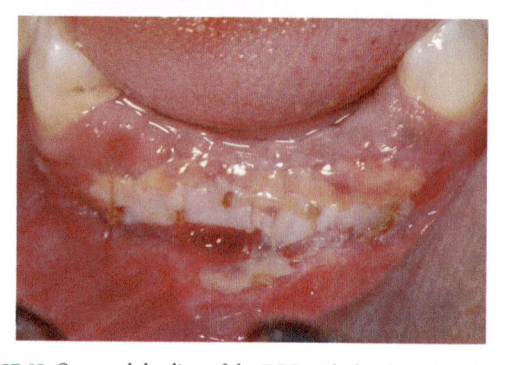

Figure 27.48 One week healing of the FGG with the chromic gut sutures still intact. Revascularization of the graft is evident.

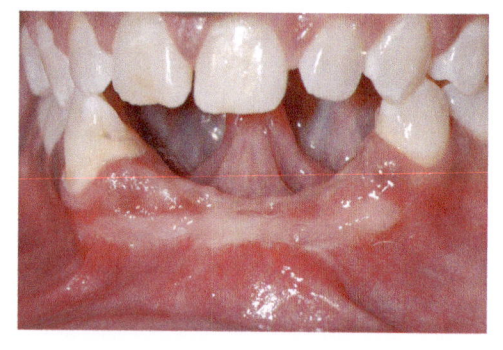

Figure 27.49 Three months healing of FGG with color discrepancy from the native gingiva.

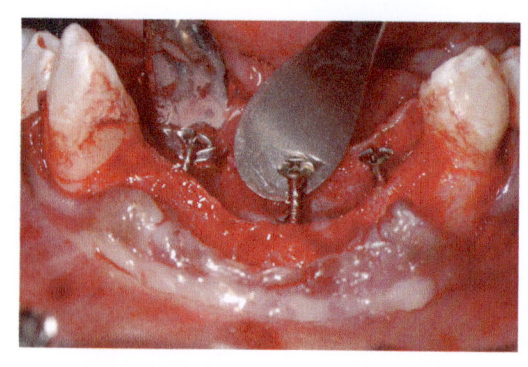

Figure 27.50 Tenting screws for space maintenance during vertical augmentation.

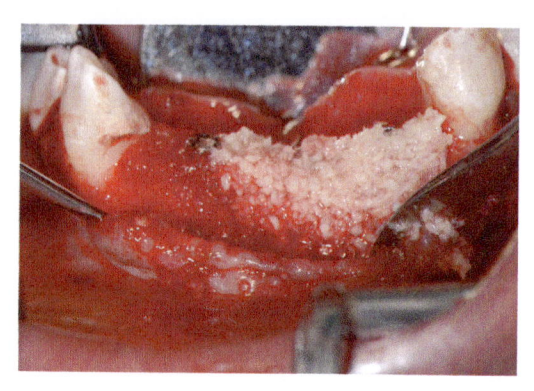

Figure 27.51 Mineralized allograft along with mineralized bone matrix.

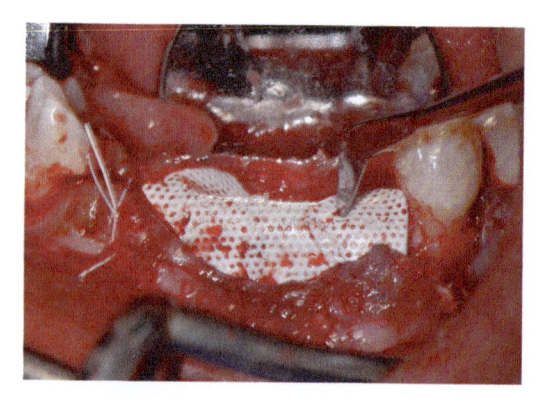

Figure 27.52 Titanium reinforced dense-polytetrafluoroethylene (d-PTFE) membrane for vertical ridge augmentation.

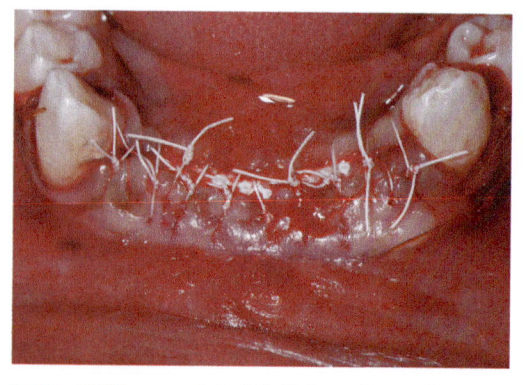

Figure 27.53 e-PTFE suture of the full-thickness flap to allow primary closure over the membrane.

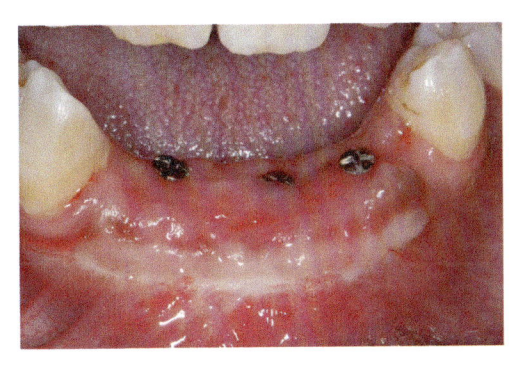

Figure 27.54 Six months following augmentation with the thick band of keratinized gingiva. The heads of the tenting screws can often be seen to "poke" through the tissue and are managed with daily local chlorhexidine application by the patient.

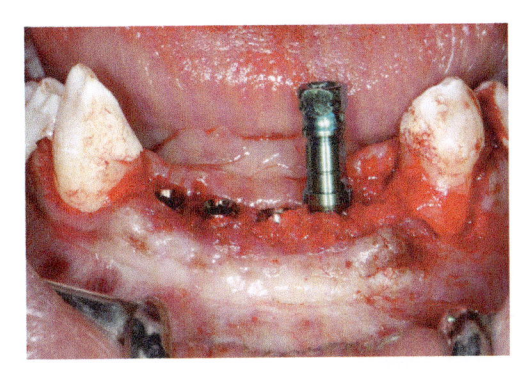

Figure 27.55 Full-thickness flap at the time of implant placements in augmented bone and soft tissue.

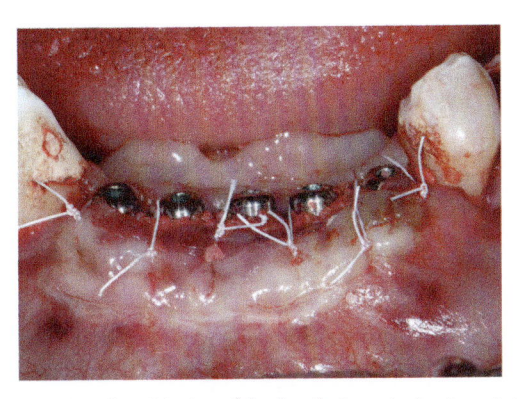

Figure 27.56 Apical positioning of the flap during suturing to maintain all the augmented KT.

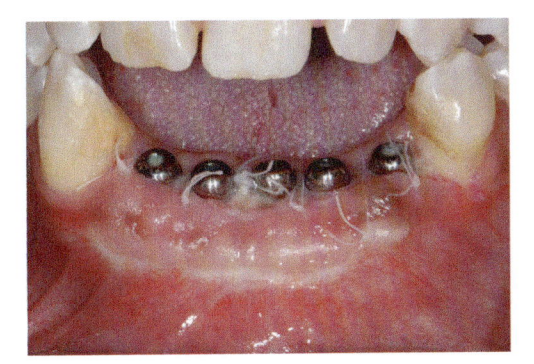

Figure 27.57 Two weeks healing following implant placements with thick and wide KG.

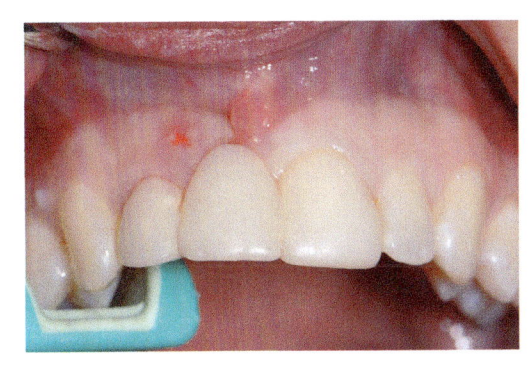

Figure 27.58 Pre-operative prominent frenum and ridge deficiency. The mucogingival defect and associated altered ridge contours necessitate the use of soft tissue grafting for augmentation of the site. Pre-operative risk assessment allows that to be communicated to the patient promptly.

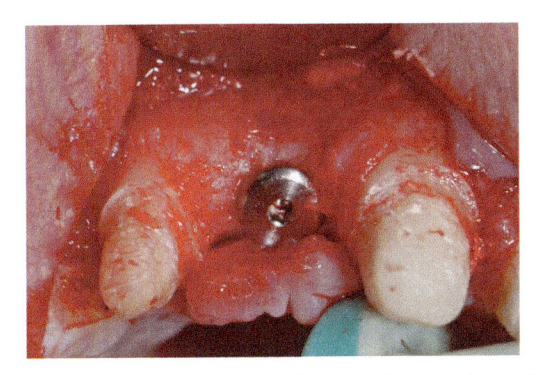

Figure 27.59 Clinical image at implant placement showing adequate bone dimensions for implant placement but residual facial concavity that can be adequately augmented with soft tissue grafting for esthetics.

SCTG procedures have been successfully used for many years for the management of recession and soft tissue defects around natural teeth and for augmenting alveolar ridge contours. SCTG grafts may have some limitations when attempting to graft and achieve coverage of a non-vital implant surface since the soft tissue around the implant does not respond in the same manner as a natural tooth. There has recently been a debate on the ideal donor site for CTG harvesting. Although traditionally the lateral palate has been recommended due to the large volume of donor tissue that can be harvested, tuberosity grafts are gaining popularity. The reason is the high quality of dense connective tissue that can be procured from the tuberosity versus the large portion of adipose tissue that follows the connective tissue obtained from the palate [1] (Figures 27.60 to 27.63).

Nonetheless, SCTG, when indicated and properly used, can provide stable and significant gains in soft tissue volume and contour that can enhance the esthetic outcome of deficient implant sites (Figures 27.64 to 27.67).

Soft tissue augmentation at the second implant stage

Soft tissue augmentation can be performed simultaneously with implant placement and/or at second stage surgery. There is no evidence in the literature to support any advantage of simultaneous soft tissue augmentation over augmentation during second stage surgery. Both treatment modalities have been shown to lead to

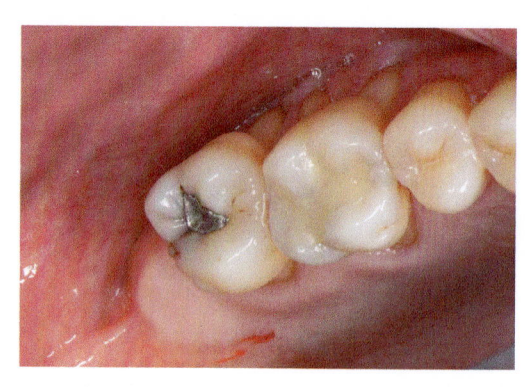

Figure 27.60 Clinical image of the tuberosity arc. The tuberosity harvest incision design resembles that of a linear wedge incision as performed in traditional periodontal surgery. A linear incision is traced from the mucogingival junction distal to the tuberosity to the distal line angle of the second molar (if present). Source: Hinrichs et al 2015 [1]. Reproduced with permission from Elsevier.

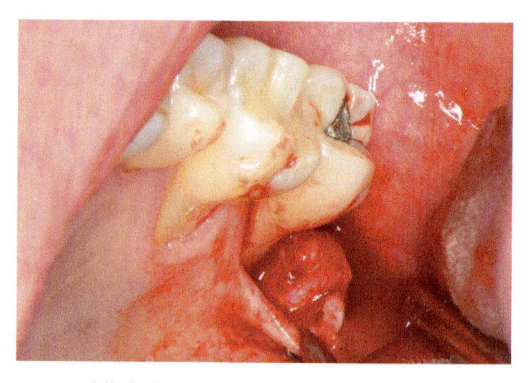

Figure 27.61 A full-thickness flap is raised and extended into the sulcus of the most distal tooth if needed. Then a blade is utilized for a split thickness incision in order to separate the tuberosity connective tissue from the palatal flap. Care is taken to leave only a thin layer of palatal epithelium to obtain as much CT as possible.

better esthetics and increased soft tissue thickness [27]. While the need for keratinized gingiva (KG) around a "functional" implant is still a contentious subject, it has been shown clinically that the development of KG around an implant/restorative interface will enhance the long-term health of the bone and soft tissue surrounding an implant [28].

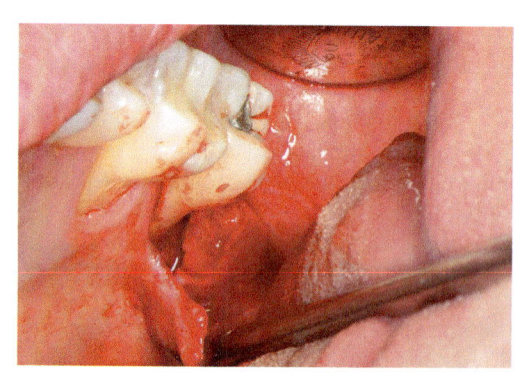

Figure 27.62 Tuberosity CTG following complete separation from the palatal flap. At this point the CTG is only held by the crestal periosteum and can be easily separated with a periosteal elevator.

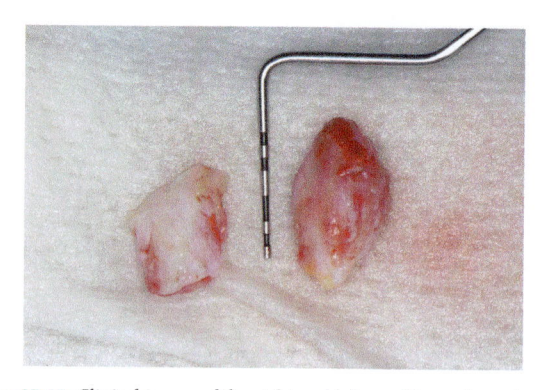

Figure 27.63 Clinical image of the right and left maxillary tuberosity harvests.

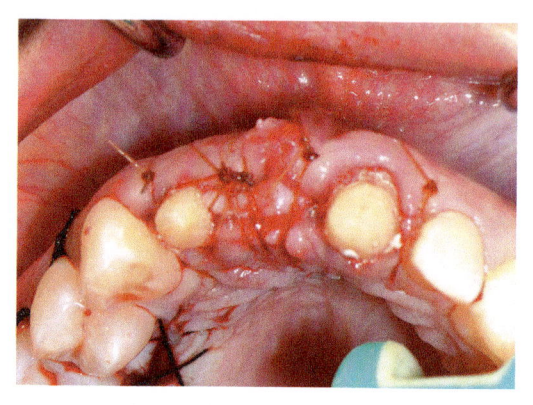

Figure 27.64 Bovine bone graft and a connective tissue graft at the time of implant placement.

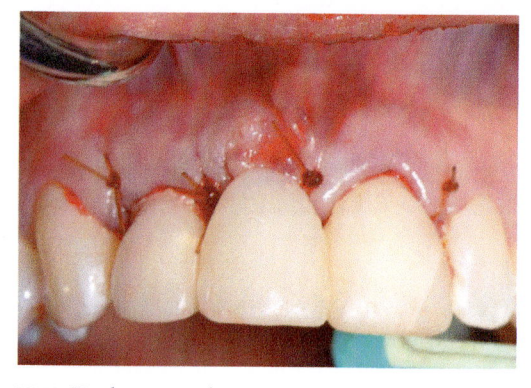

Figure 27.65 Fixed provisional restoration at the time of augmentation.

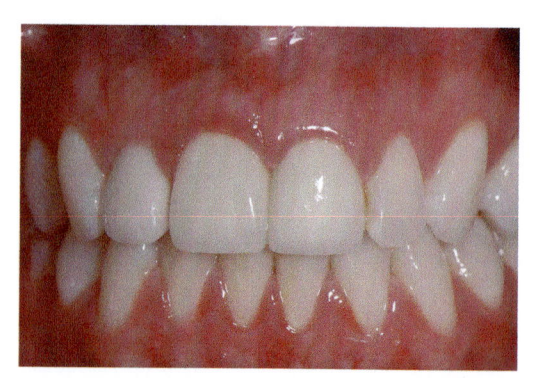

Figure 27.66 Final restoration one year following implant placement

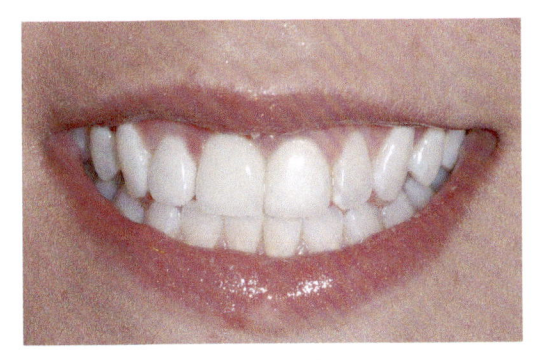

Figure 27.67 High lip line showing the esthetic restoration.

Where there is inadequate KG around an implant, less than 1 mm thick and 1 mm wide, enhancement should be considered. While soft tissue augmentation may be performed at various stages of implant therapy, prior to, during, or after the implant placement, the most advantageous time to consider soft tissue augmentation is at implant uncovering on a two-stage, submerged approach. Although a single stage approach may be feasible and predictable, the need for soft tissue augmentation may, in some cases, make treatment better suited to a two-stage approach. When uncovering an implant at a second stage surgery, several surgical approaches are available depending on the width and thickness of the KG. The preservation of existing KG requires a careful surgical approach that can result in enhancement or the contraction of the soft tissue.

Punch technique

When there is adequate KG of at least 1 mm and there is no need to build up buccal thickness, a circular incision of the same implant diameter can be done to remove the tissue. This could be done using a scalpel, rotary tissue punch, or a regular tissue punch (Figure 27.40).

Roll flap

If an adequate KG is present on the buccal but there is a need to enhance thickness, a roll flap uncovering can be used. A U-shaped full-thickness incision is made on the palatal and interproximal margins of the implant. The flap is de-epithelialized and a pouch is created on the buccal and the de-epithelialized pedicle is rolled into the pouch and secured with an internal sling suture and single interrupted sutures are placed around the healing abutment to secure the buccal tissue [29] (Figures 27.68 to 27.73).

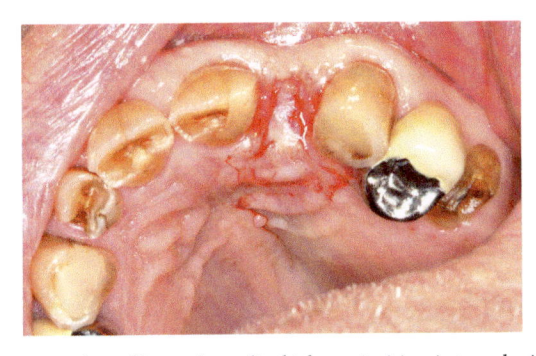

Figure 27.68 A papilla sparing split-thickness incision is traced with a microblade or with the tip of a 12d blade. The split-thickness flap should be as thin as possible to leave a generous amount of underlying CT for the roll flap. Alternatively, the epithelium can be scraped off and discarded.

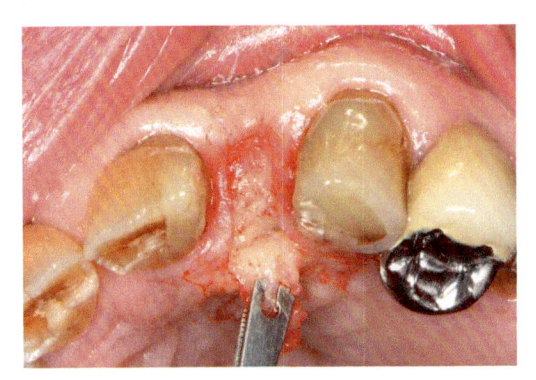

Figure 27.69 Following elevation of the split-thickness flap carrying the epithelium the exposed CT that will be rolled inwards is visible.

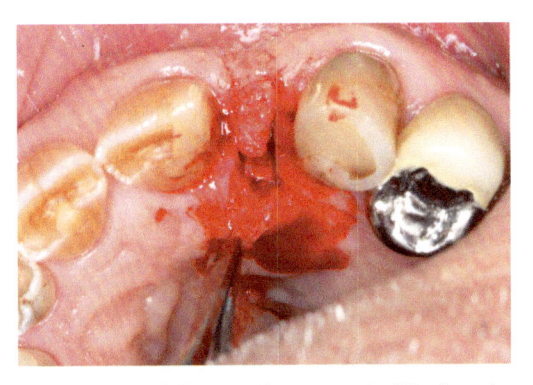

Figure 27.70 A periosteal elevator with a narrow tip (Woodson elevator) is utilized to release the CTG from the underlying periosteum so that the only remaining connection of the CTG is with the facial soft tissue. Subsequently, the same instrument is utilized to "tunnel" the facial tissue and create a pouch for inversion of the roll flap.

Tissue preservation technique

This is a very common approach in the mandible. If there is an inadequate band of KG where it is less than 4 mm, this thin band of KG can be split in half by placing the incision more lingually. Next, a buccal and lingual reflection of the flap is performed and the flap margins are repositioned buccally 2–3 mm from the implant healing

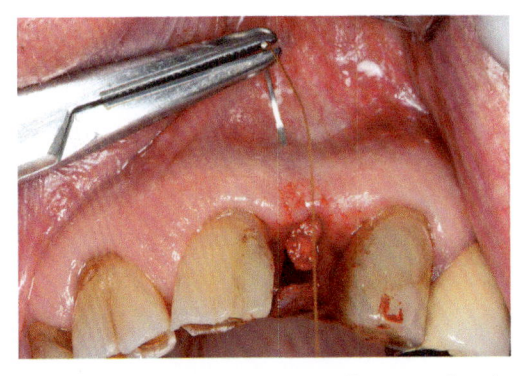

Figure 27.71 A resorbable suture on a PS3 needle is inserted on the apex of the facial tissue and exited through the crestal opening adjacent to the cover screw of the implant. It is then utilized to grab the coronal end of the released connective tissue and then slid back through the same route to exit adjacent to the entry point. In this way the CT is forced to roll inwards in the created pouch and enhance the facial tissue contours.

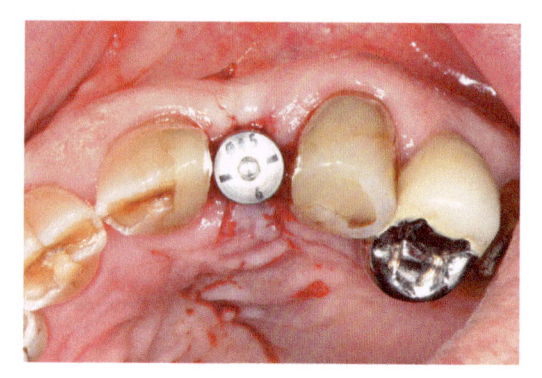

Figure 27.72 Occlusal view showing the abutment connection after rolling of the flap. Note the thick soft tissue profile facially following the roll flap procedure.

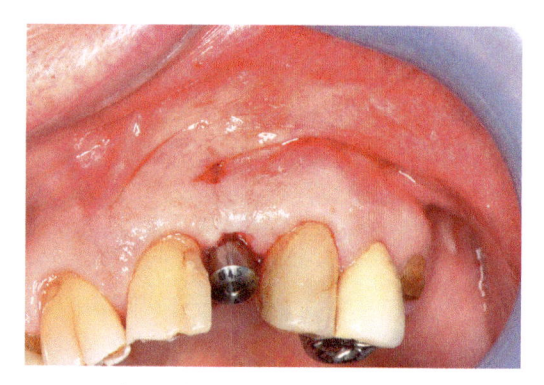

Figure 27.73 Facial view showing a single suture at the apical region of the implant site and maintenance of papillae due to the incision design.

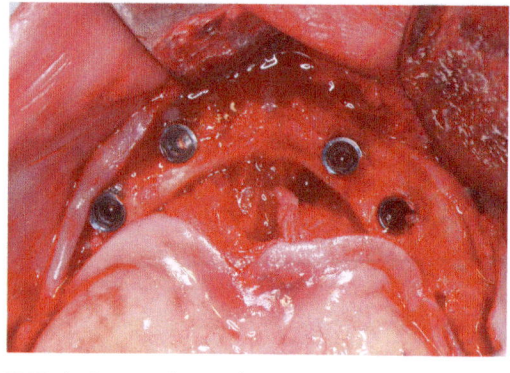

Figure 27.75 At the second stage, the incision was lingual and the KG was split in half.

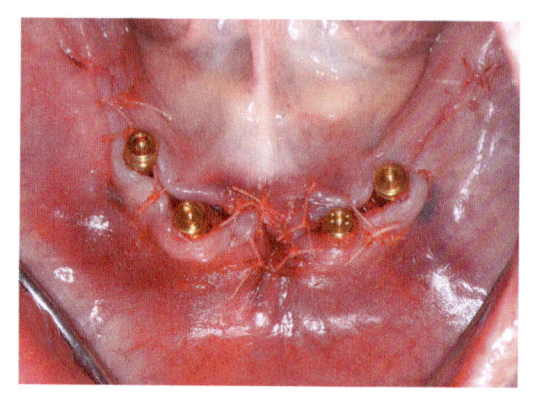

Figure 27.76 Buccal repositioning of the KG using a mattress Vicryl suture.

abutment. Healing by secondary intention will result in increased thickness of the KG [19] (Figures 27.74 to 27.77).

Free connective tissue graft

When a large amount of tissue augmentation is needed, a free connective tissue (CT) graft can be harvested from the palate or the maxillary tuberosity. The connective tissue graft (CTG) is placed under a partial-thickness or full-thickness buccal flap, as described by Kan et al. [30]. The graft must be immobilized with internal periosteal sutures or cross mattress sutures prior to flap closure. If the frenum has a low position, a frenectomy should be performed before suturing the CT graft.

Rescue procedures

Every surgical procedure carries a level of risk with it. Adequate preoperative treatment planning minimizes such risks, but when esthetic complications arise periodontal surgical procedures can be employed as rescue procedures. Soft tissue grafting can also be utilized as a "rescue procedure" to manage esthetic complications following implant restoration. Labial inclination, buccal implant placement, or the use of a wide diameter implant can contribute to a thin tissue biotype or a thin buccal bone that may lead to recession, permeation of gray from the implant structure through the tissue,

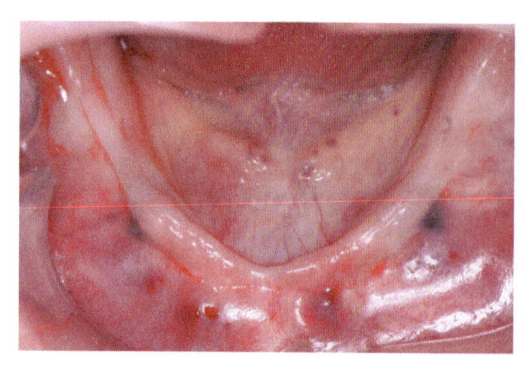

Figure 27.74 Thin keratinized gingiva in a thin biotype case.

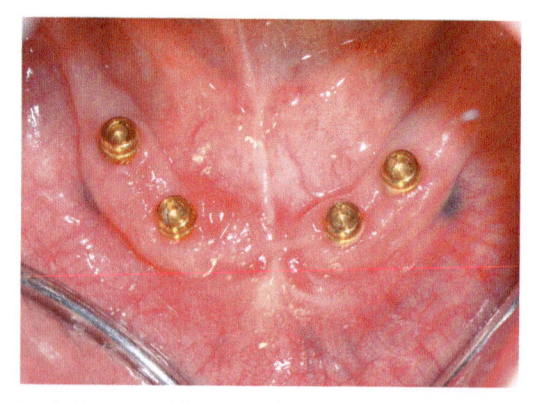

Figure 27.77 Two years following implant placements with healthy keratinized gingiva that allows the maintenance and function of the implants.

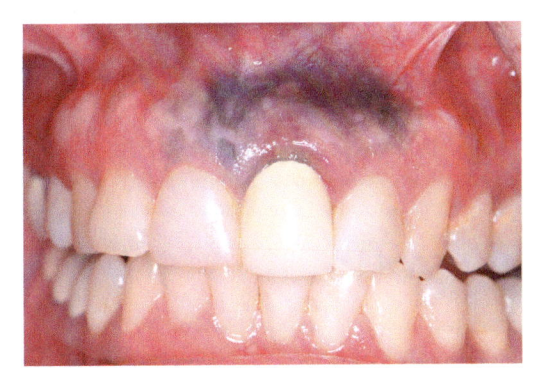

Figure 27.78 Failed endodontic therapy with an amalgam tattoo.

and exposure of the implant neck, all of which contribute to an inharmonious emergence profile of the implant restoration and a compromised appearance of the patient's smile [31].

The use of an autogenous free gingival graft (FGG) in mucogingival surgeries predates any other type of tissue grafts. FGGs are considered a reliable and effective approach for augmenting peri-implant soft tissue defects and are most often used to increase the amount of KT around an implant. FGGs are the gold standard in cases when an increase in keratinized tissue is desired. Nonetheless, the FGG has a non-esthetic result, contradicting the initial purpose of the procedure. FGG is indicated to increase the KG tissue and is recommended as a "rescue" procedure to cover exposed implant threads (Figures 27.78 to 27.87).

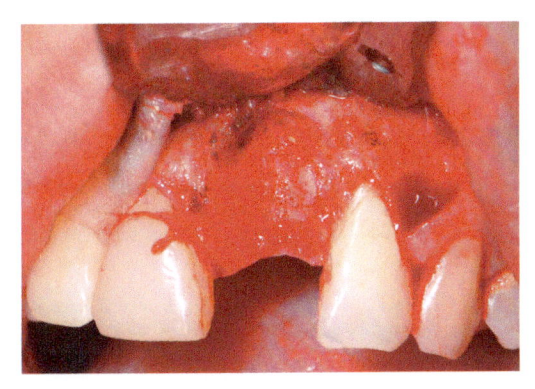

Figure 27.79 Severe bone loss following the extraction.

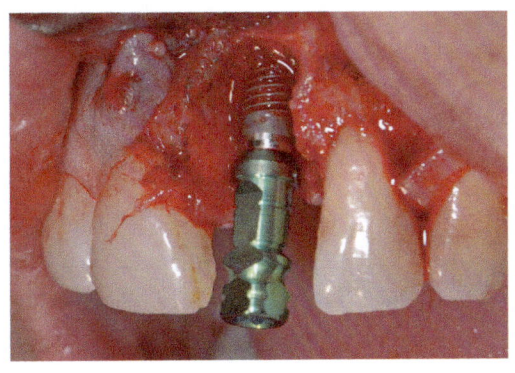

Figure 27.80 Implant placed 3 mm below the adjacent teeth line of CEJ.

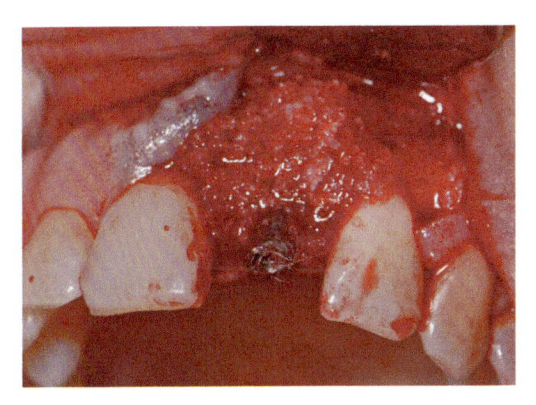

Figure 27.81 Mineralized cancellous allograft for GBR.

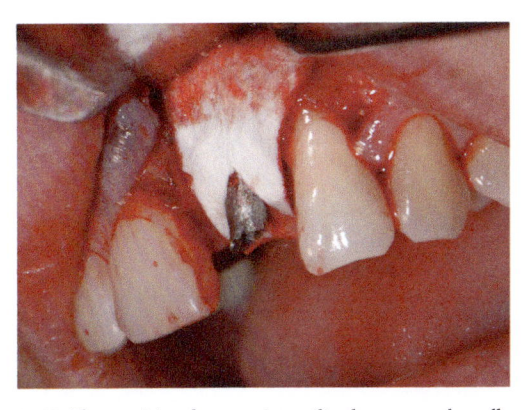

Figure 27.82 The provisional restoration utilized to secure the collagen membrane

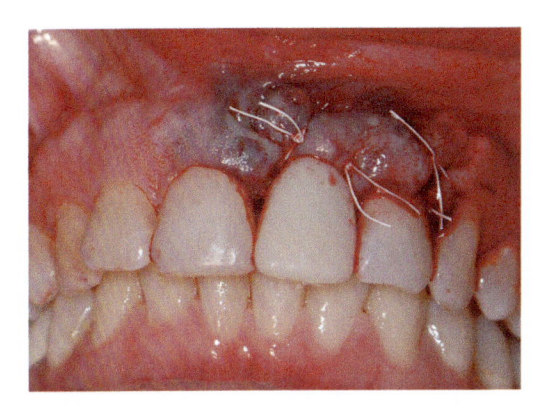

Figure 27.83 Non-occluding provisional and primary flap closure with an e-PTFE suture.

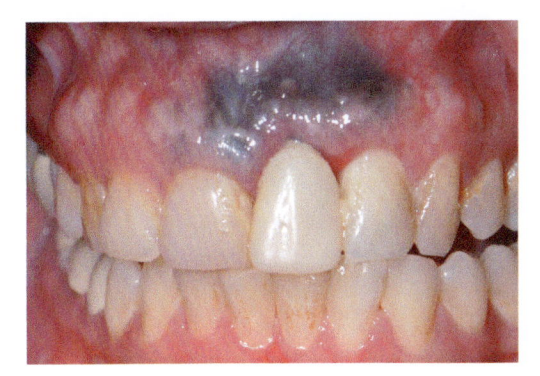

Figure 27.84 Six months following an implant placement with an unesthetic tattoo.

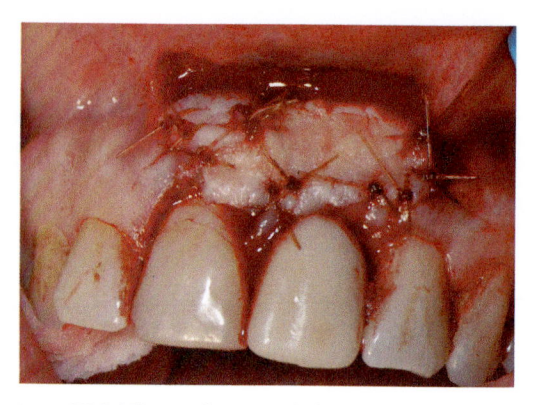

Figure 27.85 FGG following the removal of the tattoo to enhance esthetics.

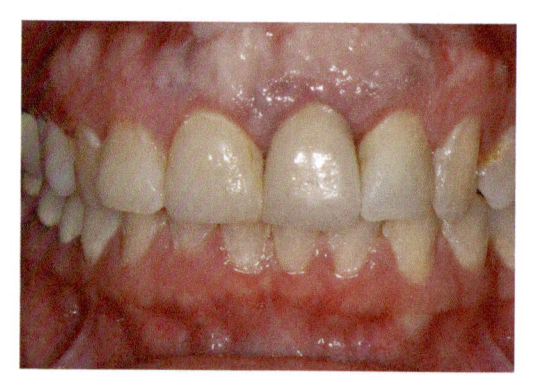

Figure 27.86 One year following soft tissue augmentation.

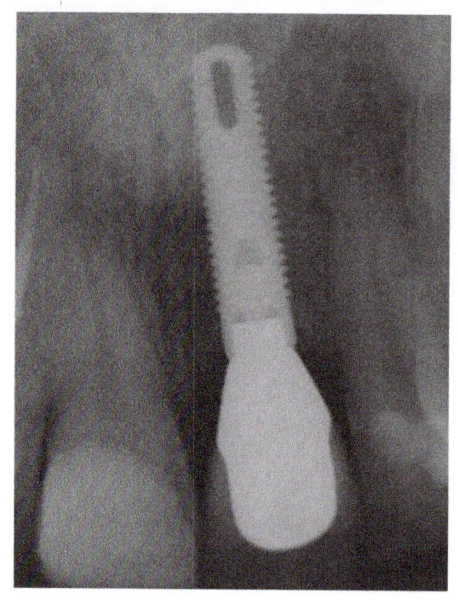

Figure 27.87 Stable bone level one year post-loading.

Conclusion

It is evident that a large breadth of techniques is available for soft tissue augmentation in implant dentistry and only the knowledge of the clinician and his or her skills puts limits on what can be accomplished. These techniques usually involve manipulation of vascular autogenous flaps (e.g., rotated pedicle flap) or free soft tissue grafts that either retain the epithelial component (FGG) or not (CTG). As a general rule the timing of the intervention for soft tissue grafting determines the predictability of the technique, with earlier interventions being much more predictable than late ones (i.e., rescue procedures). In conclusion, in this modern era of esthetic implant dentistry where esthetic factors are key determinants of implant success and patient satisfaction, advanced periodontal plastic surgery procedures must be part of the armamentarium of every implant surgeon.

References

1 Hinrichs JE, Kotsakis GA, Lareau, D: Soft tissue augmentation surgery for dental implants, Chapter 27. In: Kademami D, Tiwana P (eds.), *Atlas of Oral and Maxillofacial Surgery*, 1st edn. Elsevier, 2015.
2 Ioannou A, Kotsakis G, McHale M, Lareau DE, Hinrichs JE, Romanos GE: Soft tissue surgical procedures for optimizing anterior implant esthetics. *Int J Dentistry* 2015;**2015**:740–764.
3 Matter, J: Free gingival grafts for the treatment of gingival recession. *J Clin Periodontol*, 1982;**9**:103–114.
4 Holbrook T, Ochsenbein C: Complete coverage of the denuded root surface with a one stage gingival graft. *Int J Periodontics Restorative Dent* 1983;**3**:8–27.
5 Langer B, Langer L: Subepithelial connective tissue graft technique for root coverage. *J Periodontol* 1985;**56**:715–720.
6 Harris RJ: Clinical evaluation of 3 techniques to augment keratinzed tissue without root coverage. *J Periodontol* 2001;**72**:932–938.
7 Cardaropoli D, Tamagnone L, Roffredo A, Gaveglio L: Treatment of gingival recession defects using coronally advanced flap with a porcine collagen matrix compared to coronally advanced flap with connective tissue graft: a randomized controlled clinical trial. *J Periodontol* 2012;**83**:321–328.
8 McGuie MK, Scheyer ET, Nunn ME, Lavin PT: A pilot study to evaluate a tissue-engineered bilayered cell therapy as an alternative to tissue from the palate. *J Periodontol* 2008;**79**:1847–1856.
9 Bjorn H: Free transplantation of gingival propria. *Sven Tandlak Tidskr* 1963;**55**:684–689.
10 Sullivan HC, Atkins JH: Free autogenous gingival grafts. I. Principles of successful grafting. *Periodontics* 1968;**6**:121–129.
11 Gargiulo AW, Arrocha R: Histo-clinical evaluation of free gingival grafts. *Periodontics* 1967;**5**:285–291.
12 Karring T, Lang NP, Loe H: The role of gingival connective tissue in determining epithelial differentiation. *Journal of Periodontal Research* 1975;**10**:1–11.
13 Breault LG, Fowler EB, Billman MA: Retained free gingival graft rugae: a 9-year case report. *Journal of Periodontology* 1999;**70**:438–440.
14 Nemcovsky CE, Artzi Z, Tal H, Kozlovsky A, Moses O: A multicenter comparative study of two root coverage procedures: coronally advanced flap with addition of enamel matrix proteins and subpedicle connective tissue graft. *Journal of Periodontology* 2004;**75**:600–607.
15 Edel A: Clinical evaluation of free connective tissue grafts used to increase the width of keratinised gingiva. *Journal of Clinical Periodontology* 1974;**1**:185–196.
16 Langer B, Calagna LJ: The subepithelial connective tissue graft. A new approach to the enhancement of anterior cosmetics. *The International Journal of Periodontics and Restorative Dentistry* 1982;**2**:22–33.
17 Harris RJ: A comparative study of root coverage obtained with an acellular dermal matrix versus a connective tissue graft: results of 107 recession defects in 50 consecutively treated patients. *The International Journal of Periodontics and Restorative Dentistry* 2000;**20**:51–59.
18 Harris RJ: A short-term and long-term comparison of root coverage with an acellular dermal matrix and a subepithelial graft. *Journal of Periodontology* 2004;**75**:734–743.
19 Sclar A: *Soft Tissue Esthetic Considerations in Implant Dentistry*. Quintessence Publishing Co., Chicago, IL, 2003, p. 165.
20 Kotsakis G, Chrepa V, Marcou N, Prasad H, Hinrichs J: Flapless alveolar ridge preservation utilizing the "socket-plug" technique: clinical technique and review of the literature. *The Journal of Oral Implantology* 2014;**40**:690–698.
21 Langer B, Calagna L: The subepithelial connective tissue graft. *The Journal of Prosthetic Dentistry* 1980;**44**:363–367.
22 Landsberg CJ, Bichacho N: A modified surgical/prosthetic approach for optimal single implant supported crown. Part I – The socket seal surgery. *Pract Periodontics Aesthet Dent* 1994;**6**:11–17.

23 Tal H: Autogenous masticatory mucosal grafts in extraction socket seal procedures: a comparison between sockets grafted with demineralized freeze-dried bone and deproteinized bovine bone mineral. *Clinical Oral Implants Research* 1999;**10**:289–296.
24 Abrams H, Kopczyk R, Kaplan A: Incidence of anterior ridge deformities in partially edentulous patients. *J Prosthet Dent* 2004;**57**:191–194.
25 Siebert JS: Reconstruction of deformed partially edentulous ridges using full thickness onlay grafts. I. Technique and wound healing. *Compendium Contin Educ Dent* 1983;**4**:437–453.
26 Siebert JS: Reconstruction of deformed partially edentulous ridges using full thickness onlay grafts. II. Prosthetic/periodontal interrelationships. *Compendium Contin Educ Dent* 1983;**4**:549–562.
27 Esposito M, Maghaireh M, Grusovin G, Ziounas I, Worthington H: Soft tissue management for dental implants: what are the most effective techniques? A Cochrane systemic review. *European Journal of Oral Implantology* 2012;**5**:221–238.
28 Block MS, Kent JN.: Factors associated with soft and hard tissue compromise of endosseous implants. *J Oral Maxillofac Surg* 1990;**48**(11):1153–1160.
29 Barone R, Clauser C, Prato GP: Localized soft tissue ridge augmentation at phase 2 implant therapy. A case report. *Int J Periodontics Rest Dent* 1999;**19**:141–145.
30 Kan JY, Rungcharassaeng K, Lozada JL: Bilaminar subepethilial connective tissue grafts for implant placement and provisonalization in the esthetic zone. *J Calif Dent Assoc* 2005;**33**(11):865–871.
31 Goldberg PV, Higginbottom FL, Wilson TG: Periodontal considerations in restorative and implant therapy. *Periodontology 2000* 2001;**25**(1):100–109.

CHAPTER 28

Management of Complications Associated with Soft Tissue Grafting in Implant Dentistry

Fawad Javed,[1] Suheil Boutros,[2] and Georgios A. Kotsakis[3]

[1]Division of General Dentistry, Eastman Institute for Oral Health, University of Rochester, New York, USA
[2]Private Practice, Limited to Periodontics and Implants Surgery, Grand Blanc, Michigan, USA
[3]Department of Periodontics, University of Washington, Seattle, Washington, USA

Introduction

Esthetics is a major requisite of all dental treatment plans, especially in the maxillary arch. The subepithelial connective tissue graft, also referred to as a soft tissue graft (STG), is a periodontal plastic surgical procedure that was introduced nearly four decades ago, mainly for root coverage procedures [1, 2].

Dental implants are a contemporary alternative for the conventional fixed and removable dental prosthesis, such as bridges and dentures, for the replacement of missing teeth. The inevitable remodeling of alveolar ridge dimensions, which follows every tooth extraction, necessitates significant implant site development to predictably and esthetically place an implant in a site that has undergone reduction in tissue volume in comparison to neighboring dentate sites [3, 4]. In cases with vertical and horizontal bone loss, implant placement, esthetics, and their long-term survival may challenge clinicians. In addition, a thin tissue biotype is usually associated with a labial and/or buccal inclination of implants [5]. Therefore, almost every implant that is placed in the esthetic region constitutes an indication for soft tissue grafting as an integral part of implant site development [6, 7]. Failure to restore the soft tissue volume may result in the *implant* showing under the soft *tissue* as a *grey* shadow, or peri-implant soft tissue recession, which may expose the neck of the titanium implant and initiate a cascade of unfavorable events. For the correction of esthetic deformities and restoration of the mucosal zenith to the ideal vertical position, STG can be a treatment of choice [8, 9].

Although the effectiveness of STG procedures in the correction of esthetics related to dental implants cannot be disregarded, there are a number of complications that can be encountered. Common complications that can occur due to the placement of STG around implants include destabilization of the STG, excessive bleeding, pus discharge, soft tissue infection, edema, and impaired healing of the donor and/or recipient site/s. This chapter describes the aforementioned complications and addresses their management.

Complications

Destabilization of the graft

A common complication associated with STG is their destabilization at the recipient site.

Mobility of the STG prevents the establishment of microcirculation between the recipient site and the graft [10]. In this case, failure is practically inevitable. Thus, clinicians should confirm the stabilization of the graft with adequate suturing. This is especially true for a free gingival graft utilized for the increase of keratinized tissue width during implant site development. A straightforward clinical approach is to utilize the blunt side of a periosteal elevator and apply slight horizontal pressure to the graft following suturing. If noticeable mobility is present, suturing should be revised prior to discharging the patient (Figure 28.1). Furthermore, active hemorrhage after graft fixation prevents the formation of the clot, which also contributes to destabilization of the graft.

It has been recommended that once the soft tissue graft from the donor site has been harvested, it should be trimmed to be slightly smaller than the intended dimensions of the recipient site. This allows immobilization of the graft and suturing of the cover flap without unwanted engagement of the underlying graft. As mentioned before, it is also essential for the clinician to verify the stability of the STG by palpating the graft with a periodontal probe or a narrow periosteal elevator. In situations where the graft either dislodges or mobilizes following palpation, it must be restabilized using additional sutures. Figure 28.2 demonstrates infection at the recipient site after harvesting of the palatal CTG to improve thickness of the tissue on the buccal side of the implant and hide grey color through the thin buccal gingiva. The graft was not attached securely and became destabilized and, due to mobility and lack of adherence to surrounding tissues, proper microcirculation was not established and the graft did not heal (was rejected). The wound had to be reopened and debrided 2 weeks later with removal of the graft (Figure 28.3).

Vertical Alveolar Ridge Augmentation in Implant Dentistry: A Surgical Manual, First Edition. Edited by Len Tolstunov.
© 2016 John Wiley & Sons, Inc. Published 2016 by John Wiley & Sons, Inc.

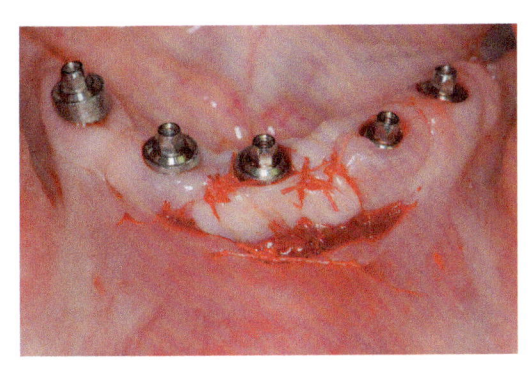

Figure 28.1 Illustration of basic sutures to retain FGG on to the recipient bed. Additional strapping sutures are highly advised to prevent mobility of the graft during tissue contraction.

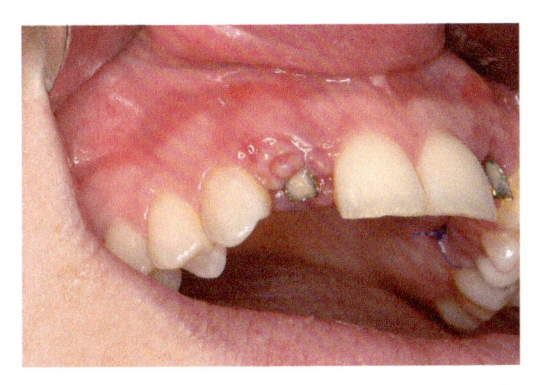

Figure 28.2 Illustration of the infected CTG at the recipient site due to graft destabilization and mobility. Source: G. Kotsakis, University of Washington, Seattle, WA. Reproduced with permission from G. Kotsakis.

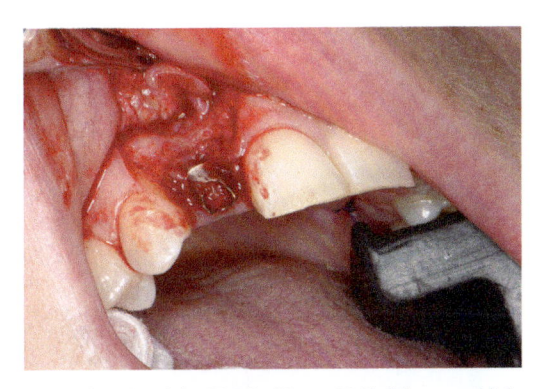

Figure 28.3 Infected mobile CTG (in Figure 28.2) did not establish proper microcirculation from the surrounding tissues at the recipient site and had to be removed 2 weeks post-operatively. Source: G. Kotsakis, University of Washington, Seattle, WA. Reproduced with permission from G. Kotsakis.

Infection and necrosis of the graft

Both local and systemic factors have been associated with infection and necrosis of the STG. As a general rule, it is known that the outcomes of oral surgical interventions are less predictable in patients with systemic conditions, such as poorly controlled diabetes mellitus or among tobacco smokers [11, 12]. Smoking can have a detrimental effect on the survival of grafted soft tissue, primarily by producing gingival vasoconstriction that often results in necrosis of the STG [13]. A controlled clinical trial that specifically addressed the effect of active smoking on graft vascularization following periodontal plastic surgical procedures with STG found that following healing the grafted tissue demonstrated significantly lower blood vessel density in smokers than non-smokers [13]. This difference in vascularization was translated into compromised clinical success, with grafts in smokers achieving almost 25% less root coverage than in non-smokers [13].

Likewise, persistent hyperglycemia in diabetic patients can compromise soft tissue healing. Although the pathologic mechanism has not been completely elucidated, hyperglycemia has been associated with increased formation and accumulation of advanced glycation end products in periodontal tissues that jeopardize soft tissue healing [14–16]. Moreover, the increased oxidative stress in periodontal tissues of hyperglycemic patients has also been associated with poor healing and tissue response [17–21]. Not all diabetic patients respond unfavorably to implant treatment. A systematic review concluded that diabetics that are within the normoglycemic range demonstrate a similar healing response to that of healthy patients [11]. Nonetheless, there is limited information on patients that have poor diabetic control. The limited available studies report an increased incidence of soft tissue complications with glycated hemoglobin test (HbA1c) greater than 8.0% [22].

Therefore, patients' habits and medical history must be reviewed pre-operatively in order to avoid complications during surgery. Pre-operative assessment of patients' habits is an effective means to identify potential candidates for STG procedures and persons who may be in increased risk for complications. Clinicians should also educate patients about the deleterious effects of chronic hyperglycemia and smoking on healing and overall health. The hyperglycemic patient should be encouraged to maintain optimal glycemic levels, which would facilitate the healing of the placed STG and good communication with the attending physician is necessary. Similarly, smokers should be encouraged to pursue tobacco cessation and access to such programs should be provided. At a minimum, a tobacco "holiday" period should be discussed. Although there are no clinical guidelines, empirically it is often recommended to abstain from smoking for at least one week pre-operatively and two weeks post-operatively.

In the case of post-operative complications that are associated with infection, amoxicillin is the treatment of choice for patients who are not allergic to penicillin. However, in individuals with a medical history of penicillin allergy, clindamycin may be prescribed as an alternative medication. Prophylactic antibiotics may also be appropriate for immunocompromised persons, such as those with poorly controlled diabetes mellitus.

Patient education regarding regular oral hygiene, glycemic maintenance, and abstaining from habits such as tobacco smoking may also help in the survival and success of the STG. Survival of the STG depends on the maintenance of vascular supply. Therefore, the extent of surgical trauma should be kept at a minimum and the graft should remain immobilized to prevent the "tearing" of delicate blood vessels that will ideally invade the graft during the healing phase. Such measures may prevent necrosis of the STG.

Excessive bleeding

During harvesting of a soft tissue graft (STG), the most dreaded operative risk is the occurrence of hemorrhage. Excessive bleeding can occur in some STG procedures as a consequence of local anatomical causes, such as damage to the greater (major) palatine artery. Many clinicians suggest palpation of the greater palatine artery at the point where it exits the greater palatine foramen; however, palpation of the foramen provides little information about

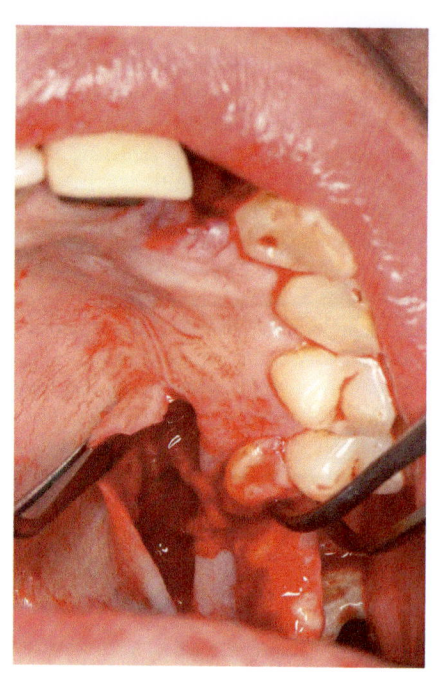

Figure 28.4 Intraoperative view of the greater palatine artery at the apical extent of the STG. Source: Dr. George Kotsakis, University of Washington, Seattle, WA. Reproduced with permission from Dr. George Kotsakis.

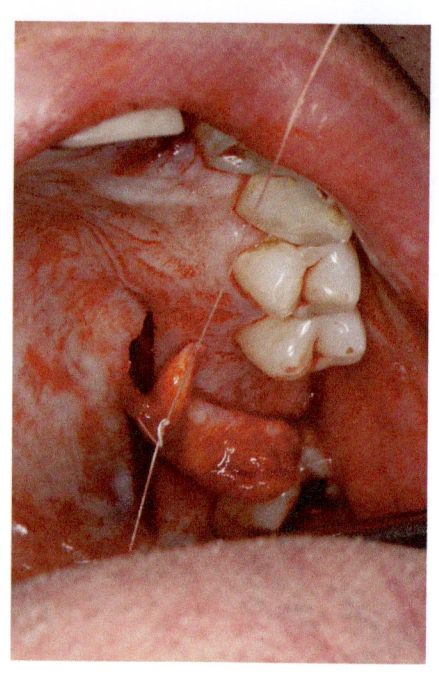

Figure 28.5 Ligating sutures are placed mesially and distally of the exposed vessel to prevent hemorrhage, if traumatized. This approach is much more predictable than attempting to ligate a hemorrhaging vessel with reduced visibility. Source: Dr. George Kotsakis, University of Washington, Seattle, WA. Reproduced with permission from Dr. George Kotsakis.

the course the vessel traverses in the palate [23]. Therefore, surgeons must be aware of the physiologic anatomy and individual variations to minimize the risk of unintentional damage to the greater palatine artery. Reiser et al. assessed palatal donor sites in a cadaver study and concluded that the location and course of the greater palatine artery varies according to the shape and size of the palatal vault [24]. When they categorized donors according to "high," "average," or "shallow" palate they found that the artery was located at 7 mm, 12 mm, or 17 mm, respectively, from the cementoenamel junction of the first maxillary molar [24]. Nonetheless, even when these clinical guidelines are considered the individual variations in the course of the greater palatine artery should be considered. The following case report describes the management of excessive hemorrhage that occurred during harvesting of an STG from a patient.

A 56-year-old white male patient was referred for extraction of a maxillary central incisor and implant site development utilizing soft and hard tissue grafting. The patient was a smoker and the self-reported medical history indicated no current or previous systemic disease. Extraoral and intraoral exams demonstrated normal findings and assessment of the palate revealed an average palatal vault. The patient consented to tooth extraction, ridge preservation with freeze-dried allograft, and soft tissue augmentation with a subepithelial connective tissue graft obtained from the lateral palate with a single-incision deep harvest [23]. Following local anesthesia, tooth extraction was performed atraumatically and a linear incision was initiated in the left lateral palate to procure the STG. The greater palatine artery was assumed to be located at the junction of the vertical and horizontal walls of the palatal vault; however, during the harvesting of the STG, the greater palatine artery was visible at the apical extent of the STG (Figure 28.4). This complication was managed by ligating the artery with 4–0 resorbable sutures to avoid excessive bleeding in case of vessel damage during manipulations (Figure 28.5). Additionally, a local anesthetic with 1:100 000 concentration of epinephrine was utilized for infiltrations in the area to induce vasoconstriction. A 15c blade was then utilized to carefully dissect the STG from the vessel with the ligating sutures in place to manage a potential adverse event (Figure 28.6). The STG was successfully separated and the flap was closed with a single interrupted and cross-mattress suturing technique (Figure 28.7). The patient was informed of the complication and a protective clear

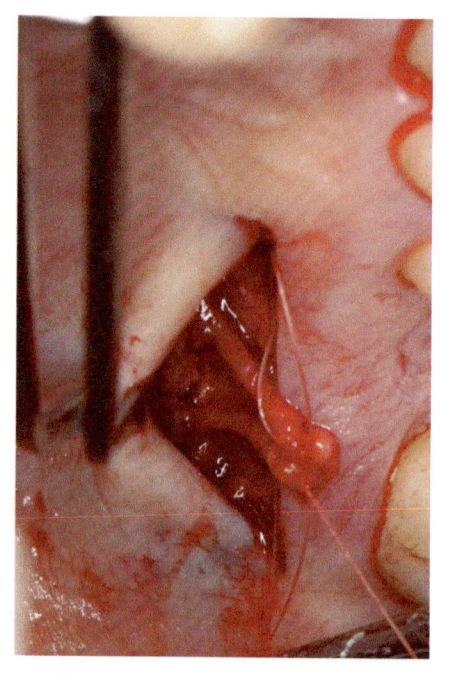

Figure 28.6 Vessel with the ligating sutures intact after procuring the STG. Image by courtesy of Dr. George Kotsakis, Minneapolis, MN, USA.

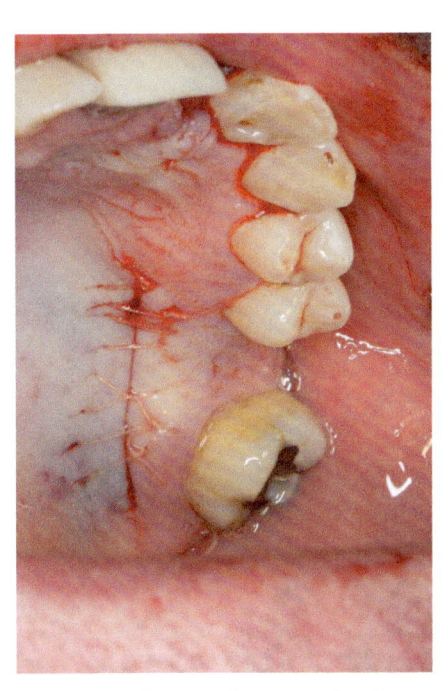

Figure 28.7 Flap was closed with single interrupted and cross-mattress suturing. Note the blanching of the tissue due to use of a local vasoconstrictor (epinephrine). Image by courtesy of Dr. George Kotsakis, Minneapolis, MN, USA.

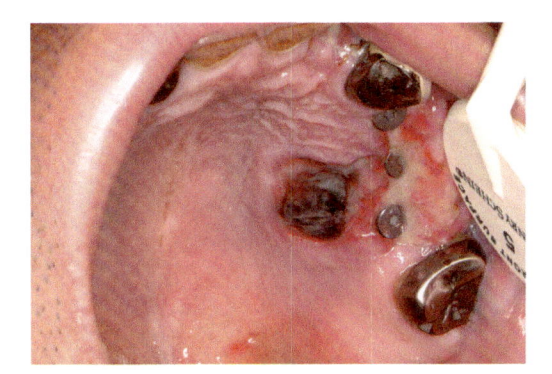

Figure 28.8 Case report demonstrating necrosis of the anterior palatal gingiva after the harvest of CTG a week prior. Image by courtesy of Dr. Len Tolstunov, San Francisco, CA, USA.

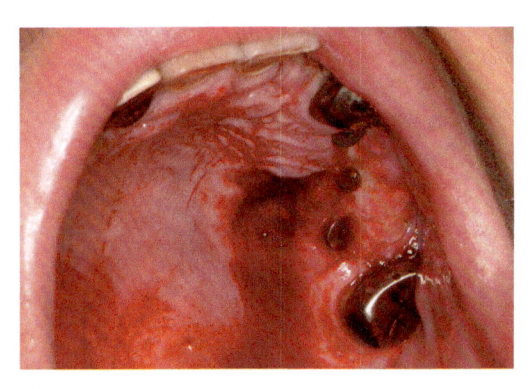

Figure 28.9 Bleeding that resulted from the debridement of the necrotic tissue. Bleeding was stopped with local measures. Image by courtesy of Dr. Len Tolstunov, San Francisco, CA, USA.

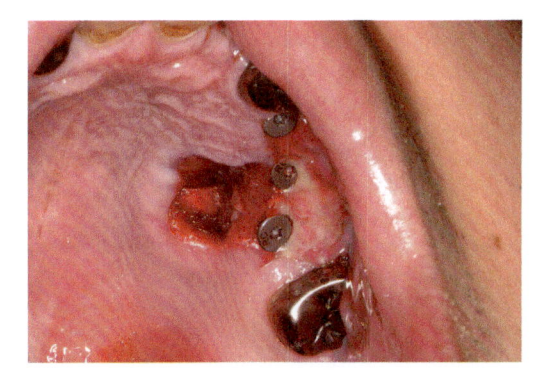

Figure 28.10 Condition of the debrided palatal donor site (day of debridement). Image by courtesy of Dr. Len Tolstunov, San Francisco, CA, USA.

vacuform stent was delivered to protect the site from trauma. Healing of the donor and recipient sites were uneventful.

Although this case was successfully managed intraoperatively, additional hemostatic agents such as absorbable gelatin or microfibrillar collagen can be considered at the bleeding site. Sutures may be used to hold the hemostatic agent in place in addition to ligating the vessels in the area. It is important that once hemostasis has been achieved, the patient should be observed for at least 30 minutes before being discharged and a post-operative appointment should be scheduled one week later to assess tissue healing.

In situations where patients are under a platelet inhibition treatment on a daily basis or have coagulation disorders, they are evidently more susceptible to bleeding during STG procedures. However, invasive treatments can be performed, as in the case of implantology procedures, without the interruption of medication, as long as meticulous pre-operative treatment planning has been performed, including contact with the physician and measurement of the international normalized ratio (INR) when indicated. When the INR is less than 3, adequate hemostatic measures are followed and efforts are made to use atraumatic surgery techniques, soft tissue and hard tissue grafting procedures, and implant surgery, which can be performed at the dental office with few problems.

Tissue necrosis at the donor site

Donor site necrosis is another potential complication of the palatal CTG. There are a few iatrogenic reasons why this can happen. Iatrogenic trauma of the greater palatine artery at the time of CTG harvest can cause ischemia of the anterior palatal gingival tissue and subsequent tissue necrosis. Another reason is perforation or extreme thinning of the gingival layer during the palatal CTG procedure. Excessively thin or even perforated palatal gingiva may not receive adequate vascularity and can become ischemic and then necrotic.

Figures 28.8 to 28.11 demonstrate a case report of a healthy 38-year-old man who developed necrosis of the donor palatal tissue. The necrosis was observed one week after the CTG harvest that was done to enhance buccal contours at the implant site in the anterior maxilla. Note the proximity of the donor and recipient sites that may comprise vascularity if a thin isle of tissue is only left to separate the two sites. At a one-week follow-up appointment, no pus or sign of infection were seen at the donor or recipient sites. The necrotic tissue was debrided, which led to some degree of bleeding that was

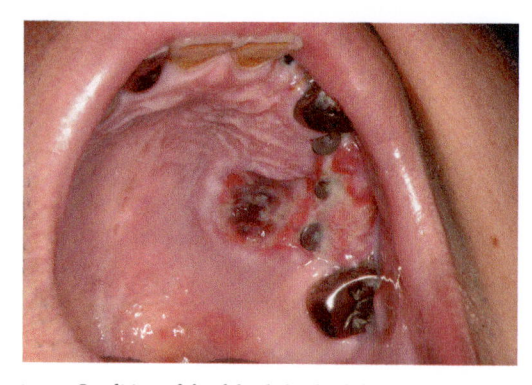

Figure 28.11 Condition of the debrided palatal donor site (the next day after debridement). Image by courtesy of Dr. Len Tolstunov, San Francisco, CA, USA.

stopped with local measures. This likely pointed to a hematoma accumulation under the closed wound (donor site) that could have been a cause of this donor site complication. Figure 28.11 shows the improving condition of the wound on the following day after debridement.

Prevention of tissue necrosis at the donor site is intrinsically related to a proper surgical technique of CTG harvest that includes atraumatic harvesting of the CTG avoiding perforation of the overlying epithelial layer, paying attention to the greater palatine artery patency during the surgery, and achieving an intraoperative hemostasis to prevent post-operative hematoma formation, which can lead to tissue ischemia and necrosis.

Conclusion

Complications associated with soft tissue grafting in implant dentistry are not frequent, but if they occur, they can lead to decreased patient satisfaction and success of the procedure. On the one hand, iatrogenic complications related to the surgical technique depend on the operator's experience and skills. On the other hand, complications related to success of these procedures are associated with the patient's overall health status. Appropriate selection of candidates for soft tissue grafting based on their current health status (e.g., diabetes mellitus under good control) should be a fundamental part of the pre-operative treatment planning. Additionally, modifiable behavioral factors that have a potential to compromise the success of the procedure, such as smoking or tobacco chewing, should also be addressed pre-operatively. If the surgical candidate is not willing to manage their exposure to these risk indicators, they should at least be carefully informed of the reduced success rate of these procedures. In some cases, even where the most ideal candidate undergoes soft tissue grafting, an arterial bleeding can occur due to anatomical variations. Thus, the implant surgeon should be well prepared and adept in the management of such complications.

References

1 Edel A: Clinical evaluation of free connective tissue grafts used to increase the width of keratinised gingiva. *Journal of Clinical Periodontology* 1974;**1**:185–196.
2 Edel A: The use of a free connective tissue graft to increase the width of attached gingiva. *Oral Surgery, Oral Medicine, and Oral Pathology* 1975;**39**:341–346.
3 Kotsakis GA, Salama M, Chrepa V, Hinrichs J, Gaillard P: A randomized, blinded, controlled clinical study of particulate anorganic bovine bone mineral and calcium phosphosilicate putty bone substitutes for alveolar ridge preservation. *Int J Oral Maxillofac Implants* 2014 Jan–Feb;**29**(1):141–151.
4 Pietrokovski J, Massler M: Alveolar ridge resorption following tooth extraction. *The Journal of Prosthetic Dentistry* 1967;**17**:21–27.
5 Morad G, Behnia H, Motamedian SR, et al: Thickness of labial alveolar bone overlying healthy maxillary and mandibular anterior teeth. *The Journal of Craniofacial Surgery* 2014;**25**:1985–1991.
6 Ioannou A, Kotsakis G, McHale M, Lareau DE, Hinrichs JE, Romanos GE: Soft tissue surgical procedures for optimizing anterior implant esthetics. *Int J Dentistry* 2015;**2015**:740–764.
7 Wiesner G, Esposito M, Worthington H, Schlee M: Connective tissue grafts for thickening peri-implant tissues at implant placement. One-year results from an explanatory split-mouth randomised controlled clinical trial. *European Journal of Oral Implantology* 2010;**3**:27–35
8 Kassab MM: Soft tissue grafting to improve implant esthetics. *Clinical, Cosmetic and Investigational Dentistry* 2010;**2**:101–107.
9 Covani U, Marconcini S, Galassini G, Cornelini R, Santini S, Barone A: Connective tissue graft used as a biologic barrier to cover an immediate implant. *Journal of Periodontology* 2007;**78**:1644–1649.
10 Sullivan HC, Atkins JH: Free autogenous gingival grafts. I. Principles of successful grafting. *Periodontics* 1968;**6**:121–129.
11 Kotsakis GA, Ioannou AL, Hinrichs JE, Romanos GE. A systematic eeview of observational studies evaluating implant placement in the maxillary jaws of medically compromised patients. *Clinical Implant Dentistry and Related Research* 2015 Jun;**17**(3):598–609.
12 Kotsakis GA, Javed F, Hinrichs JE, Karoussis IK, Romanos GE: Impact of cigarette smoking on clinical outcomes of periodontal flap surgical procedures: a systematic review and meta-analysis. *Journal of Periodontology* 2015;**86**:254–263.
13 Souza SL, Macedo GO, Tunes RS, et al: Subepithelial connective tissue graft for root coverage in smokers and non-smokers: a clinical and histologic controlled study in humans. *Journal of Periodontology* 2008;**79**:1014–1021.
14 Gurav AN: Advanced glycation end products: a link between periodontitis and diabetes mellitus? *Current Diabetes Reviews* 2013;**9**:355–361.
15 Xu J, Xiong M, Huang B, Chen H: Advanced glycation end products upregulate the endoplasmic reticulum stress in human periodontal ligament cells. *Journal of Periodontology* 2015;**86**:440–447.
16 Zizzi A, Tirabassi G, Aspriello SD, Piemontese M, Rubini C, Lucarini G: Gingival advanced glycation end-products in diabetes mellitus-associated chronic periodontitis: an immunohistochemical study. *Journal of Periodontal Research* 2013;**48**:293–301.
17 Allen EM, Matthews JB, O'Halloran DJ, Griffiths HR, Chapple IL: Oxidative and inflammatory status in Type 2 diabetes patients with periodontitis. *Journal of Clinical Periodontology* 2011;**38**:894–901.
18 Buczko P, Zalewska A, Szarmach I: Saliva and oxidative stress in oral cavity and in some systemic disorders. *Journal of Physiology and Pharmacology: An Official Journal of the Polish Physiological Society* 2015;**66**:3–9.
19 Galli C, Passeri G, Macaluso GM: FoxOs, Wnts and oxidative stress-induced bone loss: new players in the periodontitis arena? *Journal of Periodontal Research* 2011;**46**:397–406.
20 Koromantzos PA, Makrilakis K, Dereka X, et al: Effect of non-surgical periodontal therapy on C-reactive protein, oxidative stress, and matrix metalloproteinase (MMP)-9 and MMP-2 levels in patients with type 2 diabetes: a randomized controlled study. *Journal of Periodontology* 2012;**83**:3–10.
21 Monea A, Mezei T, Popsor S, Monea M: Oxidative stress: a link between diabetes mellitus and periodontal disease. *International Journal of Endocrinology* 2014;**2014**:917631
22 Tawil G, Younan R, Azar P, Sleilati G: Conventional and advanced implant treatment in the type II diabetic patient: surgical protocol and long-term clinical results. *The International Journal of Oral and Maxillofacial Implants* 2008;**23**:744–752.
23 Hinrichs JE, Kotsakis GA, Lareau D: Soft tissue augmentation surgery for dental implants, Chapter 27. In: Kademami D, Tiwana P (eds.), *Atlas of Oral and Maxillofacial Surgery*, 1st edn. Elsevier, 2015.
24 Reiser GM, Bruno JF, Mahan PE, Larkin LH: The subepithelial connective tissue graft palatal donor site: anatomic considerations for surgeons. *The International Journal of Periodontics and Restorative Dentistry* 1996;**16**:130–137.

SECTION VIII

Tissue Engineering of the Alveolar Complex

CHAPTER 29
Alveolar Bone Augmentation via In Situ Tissue Engineering

Robert E. Marx

Division of Oral and Maxillofacial Surgery, University of Miami Miller School of Medicine, Miami, Florida, USA

Introduction

In situ tissue engineering refers to the regeneration of missing tissue directly within a defect without the use of an autogenous graft. Related to ridge augmentation, it is capable of fulfilling the ideal criteria for dental implant placement, i.e.:

1 One hundred percent viable bone without residual non-viable particles.
2 Sufficient height for a 10-mm implant length.
3 Sufficient width for a 4.0-mm implant width without cortical dehiscence.
4 Sufficient mineral density to attain primary stability.

In situ tissue engineering, like all tissue engineering, must combine cells capable of tissue regeneration with a signal to promote proliferation and differentiation of these cells together with a matrix (scaffold), onto which the tissue can regenerate [1, 2]. This is frequently referred to as the tissue engineering triangle (Figure 29.1) [3]. In the case of bony ridge augmentation, the classic tissue engineering triangle is achieved by combining platelet rich plasma (PRP) (the cells) with recombinant human bone morphogenetic protein-2/absorbable collagen sponge (rhBMP-2/ACS) (the signal), and a crushed cancellous freeze-dried allogeneic bone (CCFDAB) (the matrix). Even with this, the host bone within the defect contributes substantially to the osteoprogenitor cells and stem cells in PRP and conversely the cell adhesion molecules in PRP (fibrin, fibronectin, and vitronectin) contributes to the matrix upon which the bone regenerates [4, 5].

Surgical approach to alveolar ridge augmentation (vertical and horizontal) in implant dentistry

General considerations

1 Because there is no need to harvest autogenous bone, in situ tissue engineered grafts can be accomplished under local anesthesia alone or complimented with intravenous sedation in a clinical/office setting.
2 Due to the particulate texture of in situ tissue engineered grafts space maintenance is required, which should also serve to stabilize and protect the graft from occlusal forces and/or pressure from provisional appliances during the healing period [6]. This may be achieved with the use of a reinforced membrane, titanium mesh, or resorbable mesh.
3 While the bone regeneration from in situ tissue engineering is predictable, the soft tissue healing is not. The surgery should realize that a bone deficiency is most always accompanied by a soft tissue deficiency that is often very subtle. The soft tissue is often contracted, scarred and is poorly vascular. The periosteum also cannot be relied upon to be osteogenic or angiogenic because it has been injured by tooth extraction, previous periodontal inflammation, and often previous flap reflections. Therefore, the surgeon must be prepared to design the incision in unaltered tissue and be prepared to extensively undermine the mucosa to gain a tension-free primary closure (Figures 29.2 and 29.3).
4 For ridge augmentation involving a focal defect of a three-tooth replacement area or less, 3 ml of PRP is adequate, which requires 20 ml of whole blood drawn through phlebotomy. For greater than a three-tooth replacement area, 7 ml or 10 ml of PRP should be used, using the guideline of 1 ml of PRP per tooth area. These quantities of PRP require 60 ml of whole blood drawn by phlebotomy.
5 The correct and most cost savings dose of rhBMP-2/ACS is 0.5 mg/tooth replacement area [7]. That is the smallest commercially available rhBMP-2/ACS dose, 1.05 mg, which may be used in a one- or two-tooth replacement area. The next higher dose of 2.1 mg is used for a three- to four-tooth replacement area and proportionally through the succeeding doses available of 4.2 mg and 8.4 mg.
6 Crushed cancellous mineralized allogeneic bone is the preferred primary matrix over demineralized allogeneic bone, cortical bone particles, or xenogeneic bone. This is due to the superior surface area of allogeneic cancellous bone and its ability to adhere to the cell adhesion molecules of fibrin, fibronectin, and vitronectin [7].

Specific approach for ridge augmentation in maxilla or mandible

The blood drawn for platelet-rich plasma is best accomplished immediately prior to the case or as part of the intravenous (IV) access, if IV sedation is used. A double-spin controlled centrifugation device (e.g., Harvest–Terumo, Denver, CO) is required as the only double-spin device that is proven to capture sufficient platelets for a four- to sevenfold increase over baseline to enhance stem cell proliferation [8].

Vertical Alveolar Ridge Augmentation in Implant Dentistry: A Surgical Manual, First Edition. Edited by Len Tolstunov.
© 2016 John Wiley & Sons, Inc. Published 2016 by John Wiley & Sons, Inc.

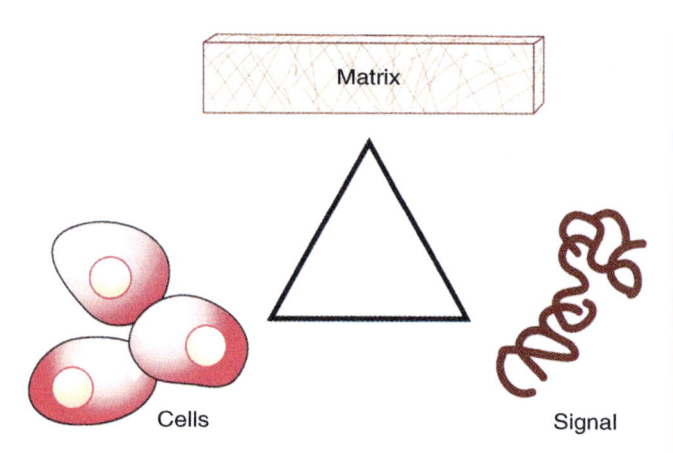

Figure 29.1 The classic tissue engineering triangle requires cells–signal matrix to regenerate tissue.

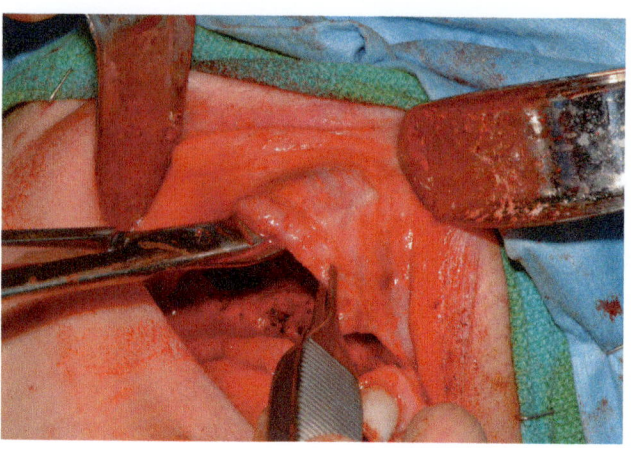

Figure 29.3 Significant undermining of the mucosa is required to gain a tension-free closure.

Although mid-crestal incisions are common and may be used, the author prefers a vestibular incision because the mid-crest is the most scarred and poorly vascular area and is the centerpoint of tension during the first few days of edema (Figure 29.2). A vestibular incision allows for closure and an unscarred area with better vascularity and one that is under less tension.

The mucosal reflection should reflect periosteum from the facial surface wound, the ridge crest, and include palatal periosteum. Since some scarred remnants of the periosteum often remain on the bony surface, it is prudent to remove it with a bur in the sense of roughing up the bony surface rather than decorticating it or placing bur holes in it. It is also prudent to reflect the flap thoroughly so as to facilitate the fitting of the space maintaining mesh or reinforced membrane (Figure 29.4).

Prior to fitting the mesh or membrane it is best to undermine the flap at this time for the eventual closure (Figure 29.3). This will allow a better access in which to try in and remove the mesh or membrane several times and will also allow for identification and control of bleeding points prior to the closure. The undermining is started by an incision in the periosteum followed by the introduction of sharp scissors. The scissor is used to bluntly make space beneath the mucosa followed by sharply cutting through septa created by the spreading maneuver. The plane of undermining should be superficial to the buccinator muscle just deep to the mucosa itself (Figure 29.3). In this manner, cheek movement during the postoperative period will not pull the tissue at the wound closure.

The next maneuver is to fit the mesh or reinforced membrane. However, while this is being accomplished one member of the surgical team should remove the PRP from the centrifugation device and place it into the crushed cancellous allogeneic bone so that the cell adhesion molecules can bind to the surfaces of the allogeneic trabecular bone network. Additionally, the PRP should be activated using 5 drops of a mixture obtained by placing 5 ml of 10% $CaCl_2$ into 5000 units of topical bovine thrombin. This activates the platelets to secrete their numerous growth factors into the environment of the graft material. It should be noted that the use of topical bovine thrombin is common today in a multitude of uses and represents a safe product. In the mid-1990s, some bovine thrombin products became contaminated with bovine factor Va, which produced antibodies that cross-reacted with human factor Va, resulting in excessive bleeding in a rare number of patients [8]. From 1998 forward, purification of bovine thrombin eliminated bovine factor Va, which eliminated this complication.

The author frequently uses resorbable mesh (e.g., Resorb-X, KLS Martin, Tuttlingen, Germany), which maintains rigidity for six months and slowly resorbs over six to nine months without excessive hydrolysis. This has the advantage of eliminating the

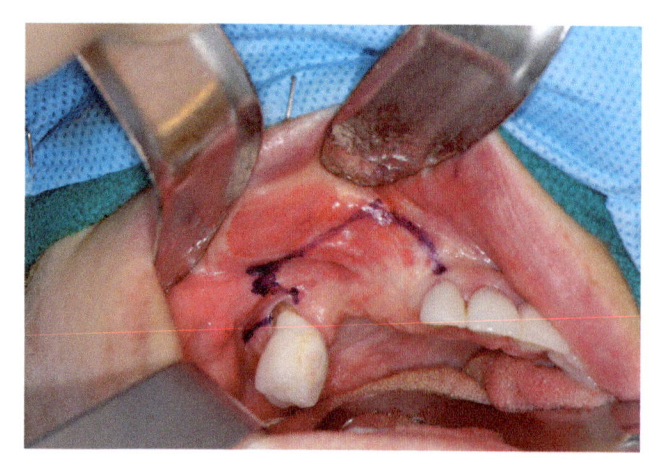

Figure 29.2 An incision design avoiding the crestal scar reduces the incidence of dehiscence.

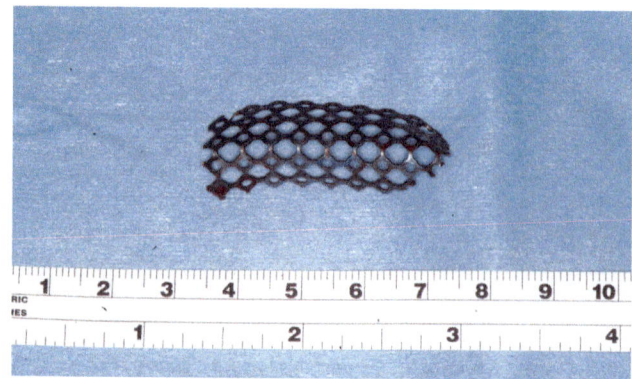

Figure 29.4 Titanium mesh crib contoured to the ideal ridge form will maintain the shape and space for the graft to regenerate new bone.

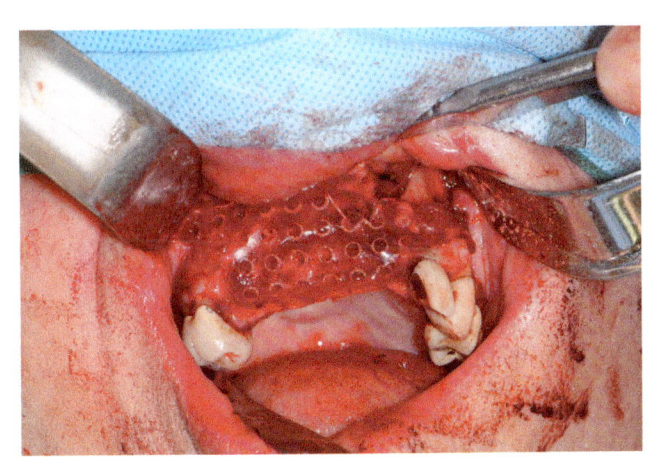

Figure 29.5 Resorbable cribs of PLA/PLGA ratios will maintain the shape and a space for the graft without negatively affecting bone regeneration and will obviate the need to remove the crib during implant placement.

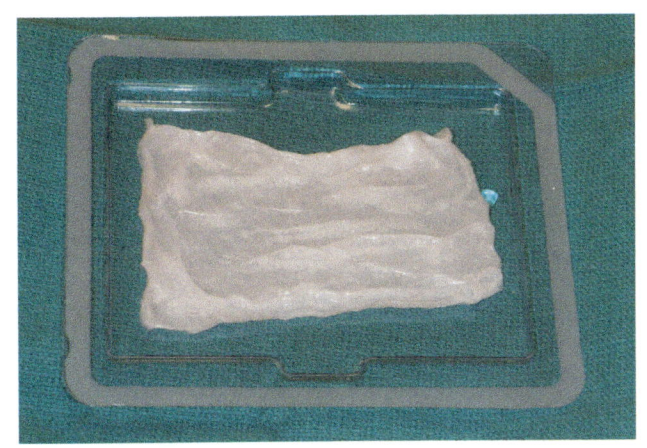

Figure 29.7 Absorbable (acellular) collagen sponge completely saturated with rhBMP-2; 93% saturation occurs in 15 minutes.

need to re-flap the tissue in order to remove a metal mesh and also eliminates the inherent recoil of metal meshes and reinforced membrane's that place a further tension on the closure (Figure 29.5).

Titanium mesh and reinforced membranes can be adapted in situ or on a pre-made model sterilized and modified for an ideal fit before being loaded with the graft. Resorbable cribs require in situ shaping using a hot water bath and flushing warm water over the mesh in situ for an ideal adaptation.

While the mesh or membrane is being fitted and after the PRP has been combined with the crushed cancellous allogeneic bone, the rhBMP-2/ACS is prepared. This requires combining the correct amount of sterile water into the vial of lyophilized rhBMP-2 powder until completely dissolved. It should be noted that only the prescribed amount of water as indicated on the package and only water should be used. Using other than water (e.g., saline, D5W, etc.) or a different amount changes the pH of the solution, reducing the rhBMP-2/ACS activity [9]. Additionally, rhBMP-2 is a protein with a specific tertiary structure. Therefore, shaking the vial rather than swirling it to gain dissolution may disrupt the active site of the protein and is discouraged. Once the rhBMP-2 is completely dissolved, it is placed evenly on the absorbable (acellular) collagen sponge (Figure 29.6) and allowed to bind to the sponge for 15 minutes, which binds 95% of the protein (Figure 29.7). After the 15-minute binding time, the rhBMP-2 loaded ACS is cut into squares of about 5 mm × 5 mm (Figure 29.8a) and mixed thoroughly into the activated PRP-CCFDAB composite (Figure 29.8b).

At this time, the mesh is loaded with the graft material, which now supports all three legs of the tissue engineering triangle

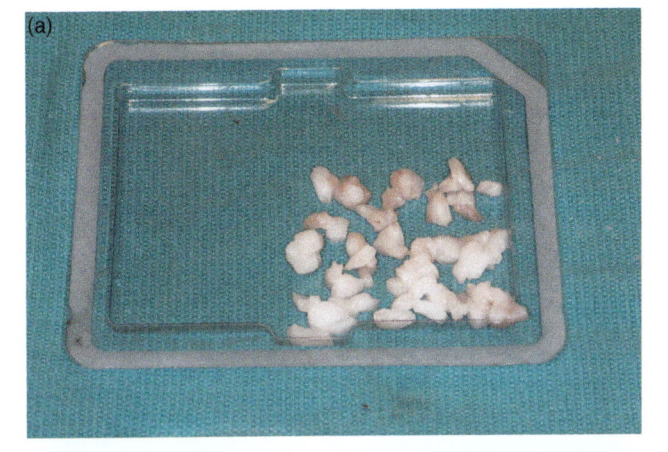

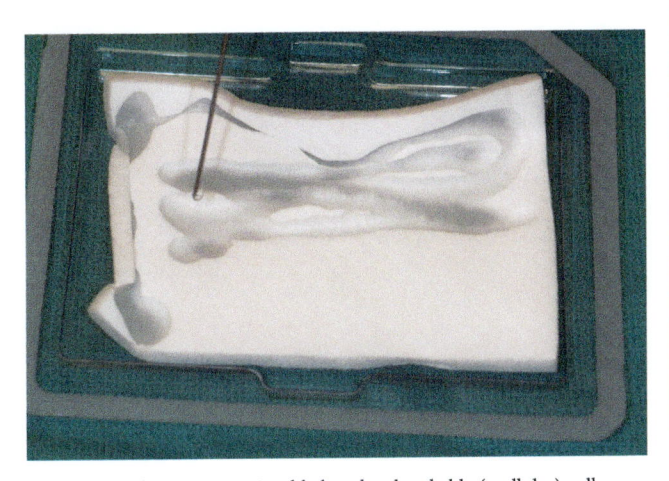

Figure 29.6 RhBMP-2 as it is added to the absorbable (acellular) collagen sponge (ACS).

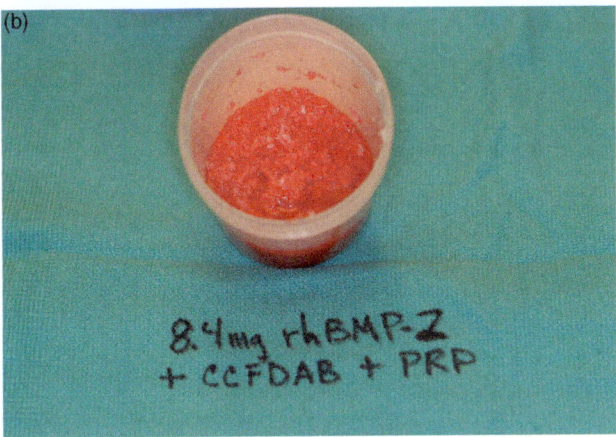

Figure 29.8 The rhBMP-2/ACS is (a) cut into small squares and (b) added to the crushed cancellous freeze-dried allogeneic bone (CCFDAB) and platelet-rich plasma (PRP).

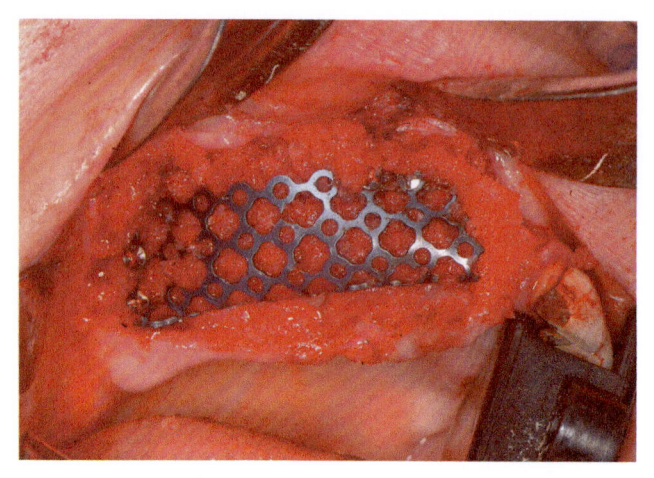

Figure 29.9 Composite graft of rhBMP-2/ACS–CCFDAB-PRP placed within the titanium crib.

(Figure 29.9). The mesh is then fixated with 1.5-mm titanium screws or with sonic weld screws, if a resorbable mesh is used. Additional bony defects or a sinus lift preparation may also be filled with the graft composite, if required.

The undermined flap is then advanced and closed over the graft using a double-layered closure consisting of a horizontal mattress closure and an overclosure of continuous running "baseball"-type sutures (Figure 29.10a). The regenerated bone is sufficiently mature for implant placements at 6 months (Figure 29.10b).

The author uses Unasyn 3 gm intravenously as an antibiotic of choice or Doxycycline 100 mg in the penicillin allergic patient during the surgery as well as 12 mg of Dexamethasone to reduce edema. For cases using local anesthetic only, similar antibiotic and Dexamethasone may be used orally one hour before the procedure.

The biology of the graft and its importance in the follow-up period

Because rhBMP-2/ACS attracts and proliferates osteoprogenitor cells and stem cells and it is essentially hypertonic, it will produce a greater amount of edema than most other grafts [10]. Therefore, provisional prostheses may not be possible for the first three weeks or, if it has been made, should be relieved and relined to avoid compressing the graft site.

The rhBMP-2 uncouples from the ACS over 21 days [11]. It chemo attracts osteoprogenitor cells and stem cells, it induces their proliferation and differentiation into functioning osteoblasts [12]. Because the rhBMP-2/ACS was mixed into the graft composite, this forms numerous centers of bone formation throughout the volume of the graft. rhBMP-2 also up-regulates vascular endothelial growth factor (VEGF) [10], which acts together with the VEGF from PRP, and together with participation of the platelet-derived growth factors (PDGFaa, PDGFbb, and PDGFab), transforming growth factors 1 and 2 (Tgfb-1, Tgfb-2), and stromal-derived activation factor 1-alpha (SDAF-1a) in PRP, the graft is rapidly revascularized.

The rapid revascularization and cellular proliferation induced by these growth factors allows the graft to get through the critical first two weeks of the graft life when a graft is most vulnerable to dehiscence, infection, and instability during this time. Therefore, the surgeon should caution the restorative team member about post-operative edema and to either defer provisional restoration or fabricate it off the graft site for the first three weeks. This becomes especially important when a wound dehiscence occurs, exposing the membranes or implanted mesh within the first 14 days. This early mesh or membrane exposure will most likely cause an infection with either partial or complete graft loss (Figure 29.11). If the dehiscence exposing a mesh or membrane occurs after 14 days, the graft revascularization is present and beyond a critical point. Epithelization then occurs under the exposure and does not negatively affect the graft outcome (Figures 29.12 and 29.13).

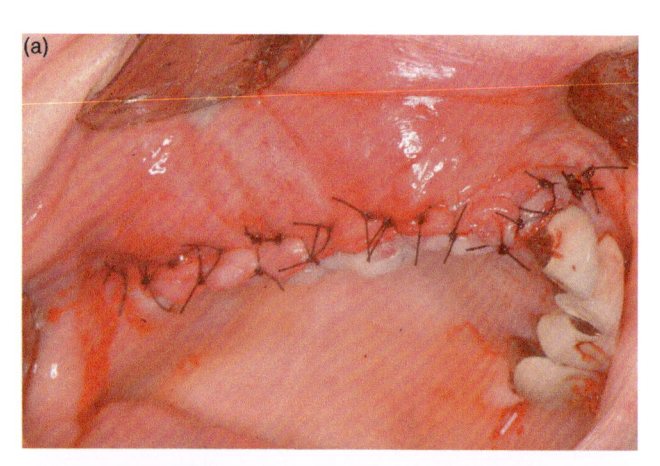

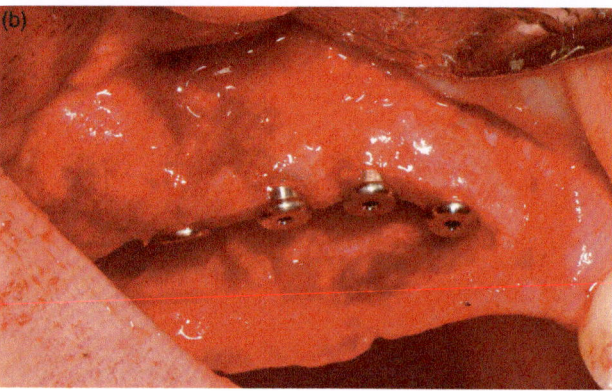

Figure 29.10 (a) Horizontal mattress closure is a preferred closure over cribs containing graft material. (b) Bone regenerated and implants placed from composite in situ engineered graft.

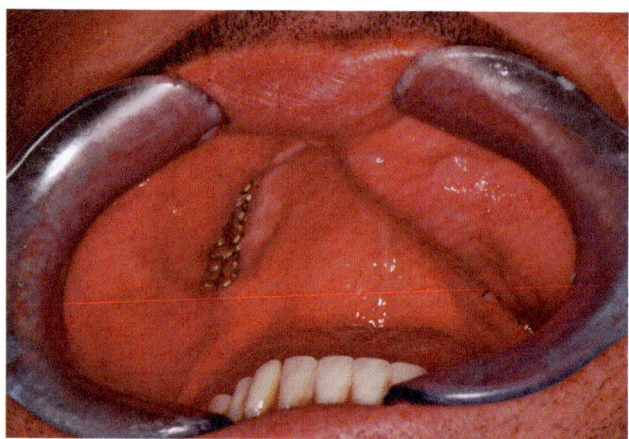

Figure 29.11 This mid-crestal dehiscence occurred on day 3 and resulted in loss of the graft due to infection.

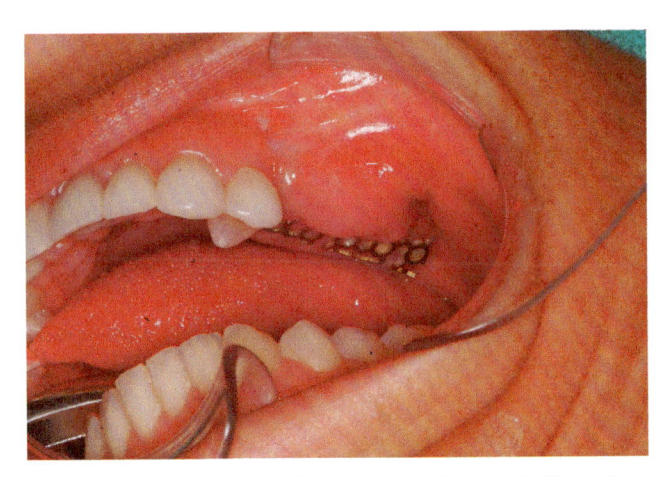

Figure 29.12 This mid-crestal dehiscence occurred on day 21. The graft had already revascularized under the mesh, resulting in complete bone regeneration.

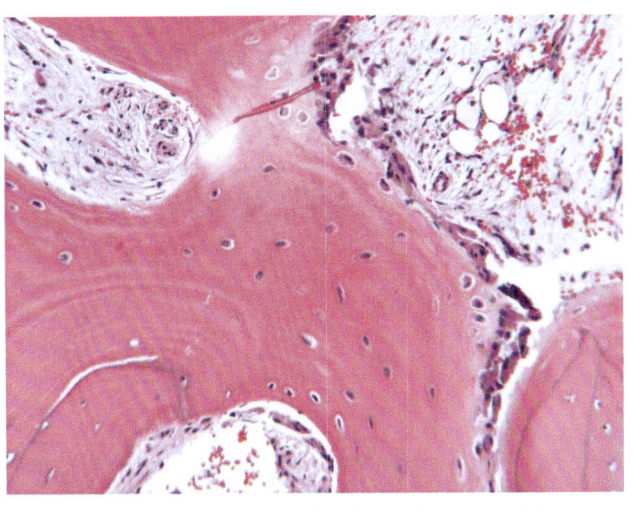

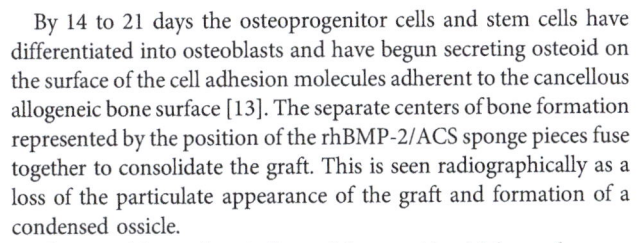

Figure 29.14 Viable osteoid forming (single arrow) on non-viable allogeneic bone (double arrows) by plump osteoblasts (triple arrows) induced by the rhBMP-2 seen in the first 2 months.

By 14 to 21 days the osteoprogenitor cells and stem cells have differentiated into osteoblasts and have begun secreting osteoid on the surface of the cell adhesion molecules adherent to the cancellous allogeneic bone surface [13]. The separate centers of bone formation represented by the position of the rhBMP-2/ACS sponge pieces fuse together to consolidate the graft. This is seen radiographically as a loss of the particulate appearance of the graft and formation of a condensed ossicle.

The initial bone that is formed is osteoid, which can be seen histologically as very cellular bone lacking in lamellar architecture and Haversian systems (osteon) (Figure 29.14). This bone resembles embryonic bone or the type of bone seen in a fracture callous (woven bone). This initial bone will undergo an obligatory osteoclast medicated resorption–remodeling cycle, which replaces this immature bone with a less cellular and more mineralized bone containing lamellar architecture and early Haversian systems (Figure 29.15). *At six months*, this graft represents type 2 or type 3 bone sufficient for implant primary stability (Figure 29.16).

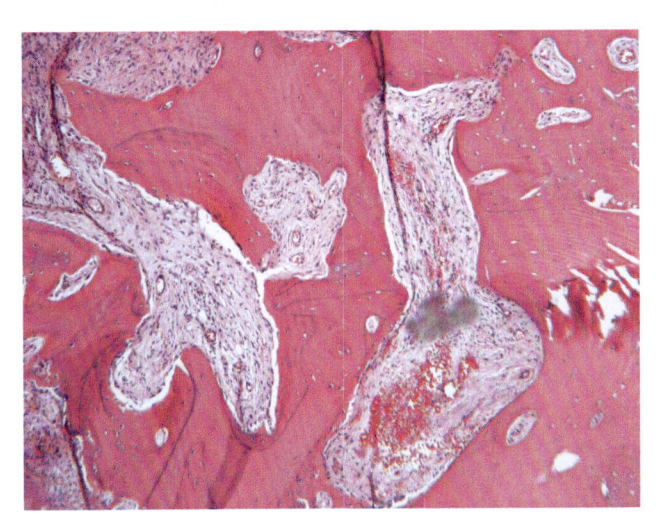

Figure 29.15 Between 2 and 6 months a mixture of mature and immature bone is seen along with some as yet unresorbed non-viable allogeneic bone particles.

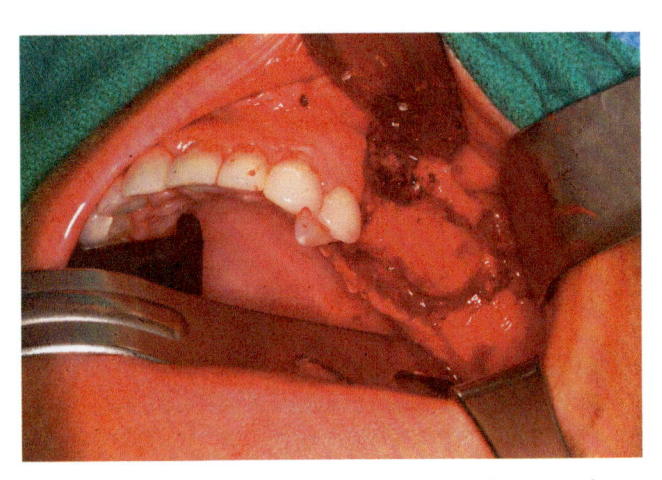

Figure 29.13 Complete bone regeneration despite the dehiscence and mesh exposure seen in Figure 29.12.

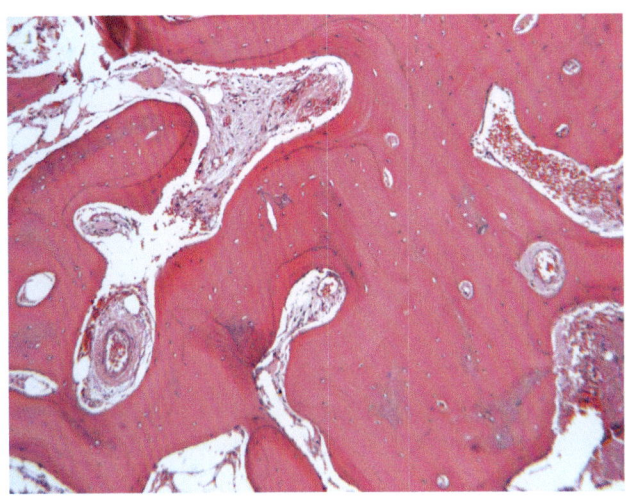

Figure 29.16 By 6 to 9 months the in situ tissue engineered graft is mature with no residual non-viable allogeneic bone particles.

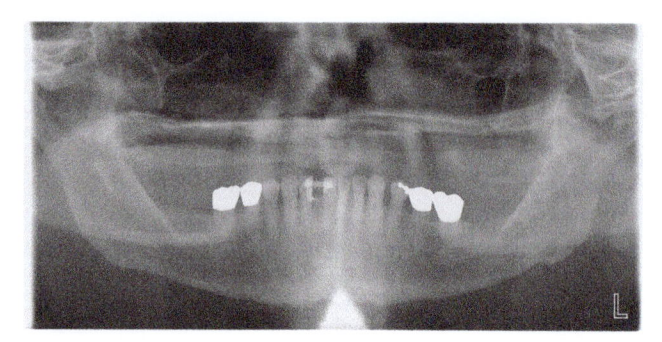

Figure 29.17 Severe maxillary vertical and horizontal bone loss from "combination syndrome".

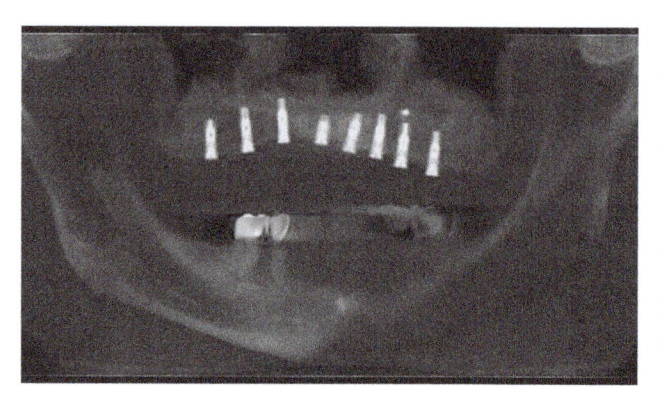

Figure 29.18 In situ tissue engineered bone graft just after implants were placed.

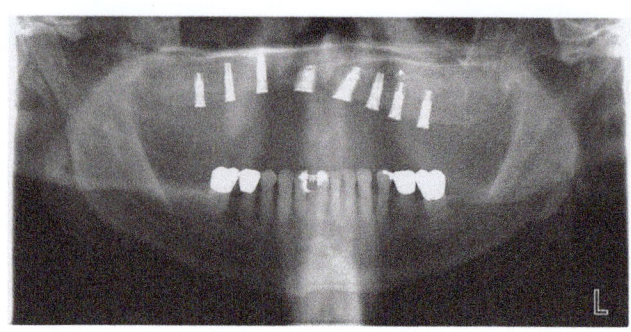

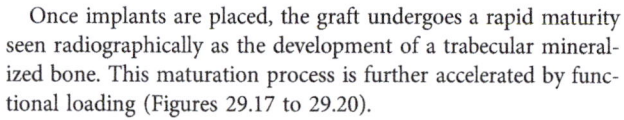

Figure 29.19 Stimulated bone maturation by the surgery of dental implants is evidenced by the emergence of a well-defined trabecular bone pattern.

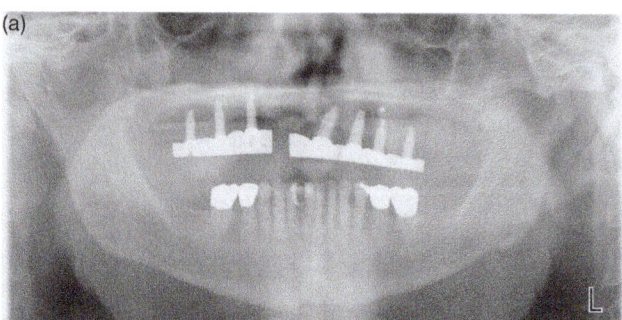

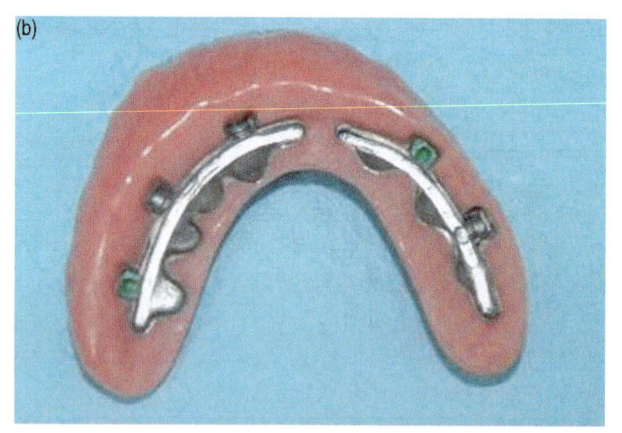

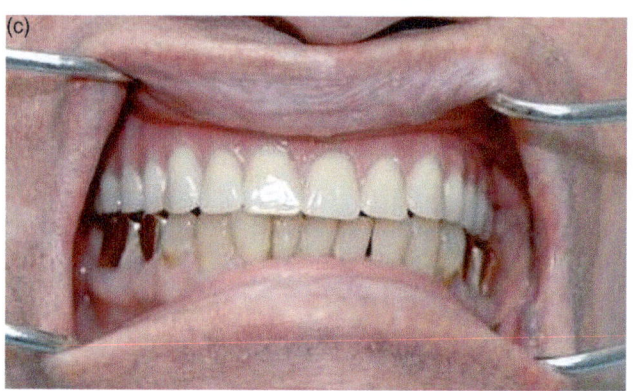

Once implants are placed, the graft undergoes a rapid maturity seen radiographically as the development of a trabecular mineralized bone. This maturation process is further accelerated by functional loading (Figures 29.17 to 29.20).

The value (advantages) of in situ engineered vertical and horizontal ridge augmentation is the avoidance of the time, second surgical site, pain, and morbidity of harvesting autogenous bone. The author accomplished a randomized open label study comparing the outcome of in situ tissue engineered grafts to similar autogenous grafts from the tibial plateau used specifically for ridge augmentation (Table 29.1). The results from this study clearly indicate equal outcomes related to bone regeneration, osseointegration of implants, bone maturity, and complications.

Table 29.1 Maxillary vertical ridge augmentation.

	Tissue engineered	Autograft	P value
N	40	40	0.99
Bone regeneration	37	37	0.99
Trabecular bone area	72%	64%	0.95
Osseointegrated implants	137/148 (92.6%)	140/156 (89.7%)	0.93
Donor sites	N/A	40/40	–
Average cost	$5700	$5200	0.09
Average time of procedure	48 minutes	78 minutes	$P = 0.05$

Figure 29.20 (a) Six-year follow-up of implants in an in situ tissue engineered graft supporting a milled maxillary appliance. (b) Milled bar complete denture fabricated for implants placed within in situ tissue engineered graft. (c) Clinical view of a stable maxillary appliance against natural dentition.

Moreover, there was no statistical difference in the cost of the procedure due to the time saving and/or second operator–second assistant savings inherent in in situ tissue engineered grafting.

A technique modification for defects requiring only horizontal ridge augmentation

Not infrequently a knife ridge presentation identifies the need for horizontal ridge augmentation without the need for a vertical ridge correction (Figure 29.21). This can be accomplished using another form of in situ tissue engineered bone grafting. In this situation a cortical-cancellous *allogeneic block* is used that is shaped and sized to fit into the defect with maximum bone contact and the desired amount of horizontal gain.

Once again, the recipient site is rough surfaced with a bur. The cancellous network side of the allogeneic cortical-cancellous block is saturated with activated PRP over which two layers of the rhBMP-2 loaded ACS is attached (Figure 29.22). The block graft is then placed with the PRP-rhBMP-2/ACS side on to the host bone surface and compressed using two 1.5-mm titanium screws in a lag screw fashion (Figure 29.23).

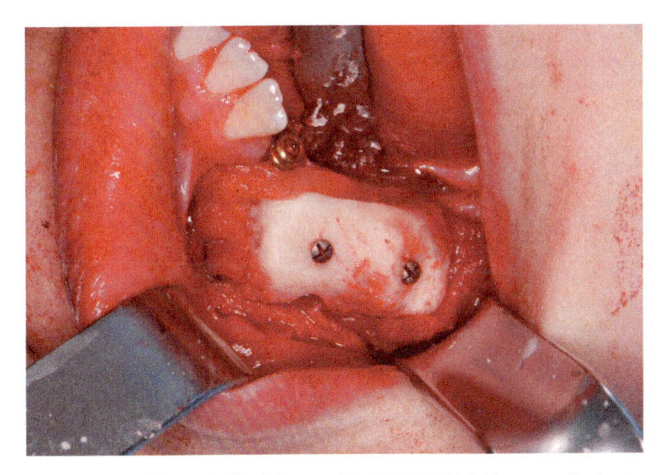

Figure 29.23 Allogeneic block bone with rhBMP-2/ACS between the host bone ridge and cancellous surface fixated with two screws using a lag screw technique.

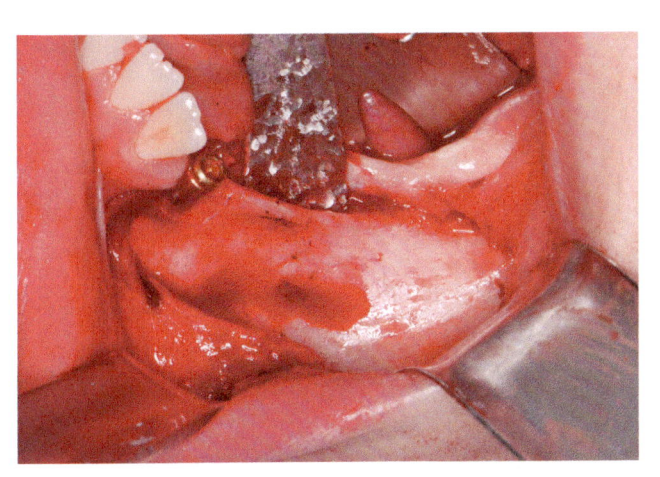

Figure 29.21 Thin "knife edge" edentulous mandibular ridge.

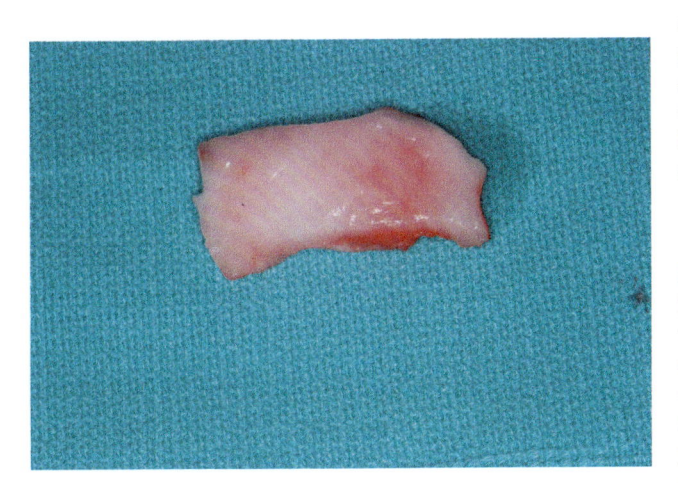

Figure 29.22 Allogeneic block bone with rhBMP-2/ACS draped over the cancellous surface prior to placement.

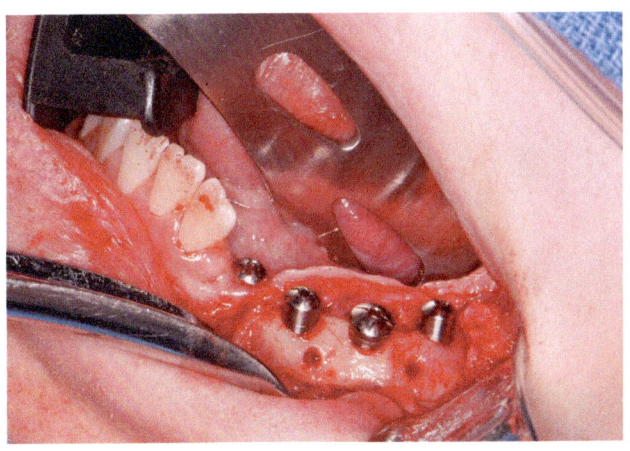

Figure 29.24 Re-entry into the graft site reveals a completely

This graft approach will ensure fusion of the allogeneic block to the host bone surface and reduce the volumetric contraction of the graft. Upon the re-entry, one will find the screw heads flush with the original bone surface and edges of the block graft rounded, indicative of bone remodeling (Figure 29.24). One will also observe the bleeding nature of the graft during implant site preparation, indicative of graft revascularization.

Conclusion

Directing bone regeneration in the very site were bone is needed using the patient's own cells combined with a proven safe and effective signal and matrix represents a straightforward approach achievable by almost all surgically trained dental providers today. Such in situ tissue engineering provides patients with the benefit of predictable bone regeneration and implant acceptable sites with a greatly reduced risk and morbidity that is inherent in open autogenous bone harvests.

References

1. Marx RE: Application of tissue engineering principles to clinical practice in tissue engineering. In: Lynch, SE, Marx RE, Nevins M, Lynch LAW (eds), *Tissue Engineering*. Quintessence Publishing, Chicago, IL, 2008, Ch. 4, pp. 47–63.
2. Spector M: Basic principles of scaffolds in tissue engineering. In: Lynch SE, Marx RE, Nevis M, Lynch LAW (eds), *Tissue Engineering*. Quintessence Publishing, Chicago, IL, 2008, Ch. 2, pp. 26–35.
3. Sander GK, Suuronen R: Combining adipose derived stem cells, resorbable scaffolds and growth factors. An overview of tissue engineering. *J Can Dent Assoc* 2008 Mar; 74(2):167–170.
4. Podor TJ, Campbell S, Chindemi P, Foulon DM, Farrell DH, Walton PD, Weitz JI, Peterson CB: Incorporation of vitronectin into fibrin clots. Evidence for a binding interaction between vitronectin and gamma A/gamma' fibrinogen. *J Biol Chem* 2002 Mar; **277**(9):7520–7528.
5. Marx RE, Carlson ER, Eichstadt RM, Schimmle SR, Strauss JE, Georgeff KR: Platelet rich plasma: growth factors enhancement for bone grafts. *Oral Surg, Oral Med, Oral Pathol, Oral Radiol, Endod* 1998;**85**:638–646.
6. Marx RE, Armentano L, Olivera A, Samaniego J: rhBMP-2/ACS grafts (vs) autogenous cancellous marrow grafts of large vertical defects of the maxilla; an unsponsored randomized open label clinical trial. *Oral Craniofac Tissue Eng* 2011;**1**(1):33–41.
7. Martin RB, Burr DB, Sharkey NA: Skeletal biology. In: Martin RG, Burr DB, Sharkey NA (eds), *Skeletal Tissue Mechanics*. Springer-Verlag, New York, 1998, pp. 29–78.
8. Marx RE: Platelet rich plasma: evidence to support its use. *J Oral Maxillofacial Surg* 2004;**62**:489–496.
9. Seekerman H: The influence of delivery vehicles and their properties on the repair of segmental defects and fractures with osteogenic factors. *J Bone Joint Surg Am* 2001;**83A** Suppl:S79–81.
10. Fu TS, Chang YH, Wong CB, Wang IC, Tsai TT, Lai PL, Chen LH, Chen WJ: Mesenchymal stem cells expressing baculovirus-engineered BMP-2 and VEGF enhance posterolateral spine fusion in a rabbit model. *Spine J* 2014 Nov 13;**Pii**: S1529–9430(14)01693-3.
11. McKay WF, Peckham SM, Marotta JS (eds): *The Science of rhBMP-2*. Quality Medical Publishing, Inc., St Louis, MO, 2006, pp. 70–73.
12. Theis RS, Bauduy M, Ashton BA: Recombinant human bone morphogenetic protein-2 induces osteoblastic differentiation in W-20-17 stromal cells. *Endocrinology* 1992;**130**:1318–1324.
13. Hollinger JO, Buck DC, Brudes S: Biology of bone healing. Its impact on clinical therapy. In: Lynch SB, Genco R, Marx RE (eds), *Tissue Engineering Applications in Maxillofacial Surgery and Periodontics*, vol. 107. Quintessence Publishing, Chicago, IL, 1999, pp. 50–54.

CHAPTER 30

Bone Marrow Aspirate: Rationale and Aspiration Technique

Dennis Smiler
Oral and Maxillofacial Surgeon, Encino, California, USA

Introduction

Successful bone grafts depend upon four main components: (1) a resorbable matrix scaffold that can be adequately stabilized, (2) nutrient support from adjacent tissues and blood, (3) soluble regulators such as cytokines and growth factors that modulate cell activity, and, most critically, (4) nucleated cells with active osteogenic and angiogenic competency.

An abundance of resorbable matrices are commercially available and can be stabilized with guided resorbable membranes, titanium mesh, bone tacks, and screws. Soluble regulators and nutrient support may be acquired from the recipient site or from circulating blood. Nucleated cells with osteogenic capacity may be circulating in peripheral blood [1, 2] or they may be obtained from the periosteum or from cancellous bone adjacent to the surgical site. However, if a sufficient quantity of osteoblasts or their precursor cells are not present, new bone will not form [3, 4].

Current opinion is that the use of autogenous bone for bone augmentation at implant-placement sites is one way of ensuring that enough osteoblasts will be present that the graft will succeed [5, 6]. However, a number of complications have been associated with this approach, including the need for a second surgical donor site, infection, hematoma, nerve damage, fracture, or weakening of the donor site. Complications associated with the harvest of iliac bone, more specifically, include gait disturbance, post-surgical pain, excessive blood loss, and paresthesia.

An alternative to using autogenous bone for grafting is to deliver to the bone graft matrix adult stem cells that will differentiate to osteoblasts [7, 8]. Such stem cells can be easily obtained using a simple aspiration technique. This chapter explains that technique, the use of which eliminates the need for a second surgical site. Post-operative morbidity is minimal and the adult stem cells populate the graft site with osteoblasts.

Aspiration sites

Bone marrow aspiration and injection can be performed as an outpatient procedure with the patient under oral sedation and local anesthesia, intravenous sedation, or general anesthesia. Hematopoietically active bone marrow, while distributed throughout the skeleton in children, is restricted to the axial bones of adults. A number of potential sites exist.

For maxillofacial outpatient procedures, the anterior iliac crest is optimum. This site offers ease of patient positioning, an adequate supply of bone marrow, and minimum post-operative morbidity. The posterior iliac crest site also offers safety for needle penetration and ease of obtaining the aspirate, but in the outpatient dental clinic it can be difficult to position the patient for the procedure while maintaining patient modesty. The posterior iliac crest nonetheless may be optimal for morbidly obese patients.

Alternative aspiration sites include the tibia and sternum, but both have disadvantages. The tibia typically is unsatisfactory in older patients because of variable cellularity and hardness of the cortical bone. The marrow also tends to contain more fat and aspirate volumes typically are smaller. The sternal site should be considered only if other sites prove unacceptable. Aspiration from the sternum must be performed by an experienced clinician to ensure that the aspiration needle passes only through the outer cortex into the marrow space and not through the inner cortex into the mediastinum or aorta.

The following section describes a technique for aspirating bone marrow cells from the anterior iliac crest.

Anterior iliac crest bone marrow aspiration

Since bone marrow aspiration is typically an outpatient procedure, appropriate supplies must be present. A compartmentalized tray or sterile towel wrapping can be carried to chairside. Table 30.1 presents a list of supplies that should be at hand.

The patient is directed to lie in a supine position and garments are positioned to expose one of the anterior iliac crest wings. Towels also can be placed under the patient's clothing to protect it during preparation of the aspiration site.

With non-sterile examination gloves, the clinician palpates the anterior, medial, and lateral crest walls in order to determine the optimal needle-puncture site (Figure 30.1). The center prominence of the crest should be the target; this is typically located the width of two fingers from the anterior spine (Figure 30.2). Stretching the skin over the anterior, medial, and lateral borders can facilitate assessment of the bone crest thickness and identification of the aspiration area. The anterior of the iliac crest and needle-puncture site can be outlined and marked with a marking pen.

The clinician dons sterile gloves and the aspiration site is prepared with three sterile swabs with 10% providone-iodine

---

Vertical Alveolar Ridge Augmentation in Implant Dentistry: A Surgical Manual, First Edition. Edited by Len Tolstunov.
© 2016 John Wiley & Sons, Inc. Published 2016 by John Wiley & Sons, Inc.

Table 30.1 Recommended supplies and equipment.

Betadine (Povidone-iodine, 10%) swab sticks
Isopropyl-soaked sterile swabs
Absorbent towels (2)
Gauze pads 3 × 4 inches (6)
Latex gloves, examination, non-sterile
Latex gloves, sterile
Lidocaine hydrochloride, injection, 1% 5 ml vial
Heparin (sodium heparin injection, 1000 USP units/ml, 2 ml vial
Needles, 20 gauge 1½ inch
Needles, 25 gauge 5/8 inch
Needles, 21 gauge 11/2 inch
Syringes, glass Luer lock 5 ml syringe for local anesthetic
Syringes, glass Luer lock 20 ml syringe for aspiration draw (2–4 ml)
Fenestrated drapes, sterile (30 inch × 30 inch with 1½ inch × 2 inch fenestration
Jamshidi bone biopsy needle, 8 inch length, 15 gauge with stylet
Specimen mixing container – glass or stainless steel, for matrix and aspirate
Bandage
Elastic tape

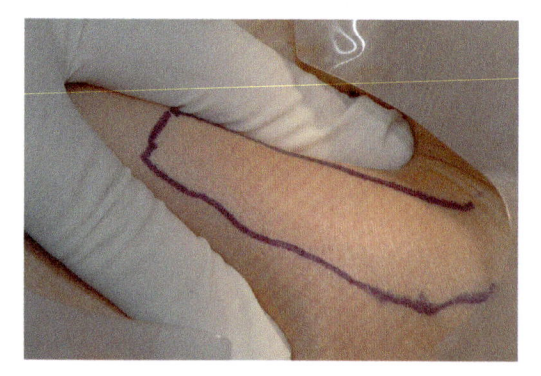

Figure 30.1 The skin is stretched between two fingers over the anterior iliac crest.

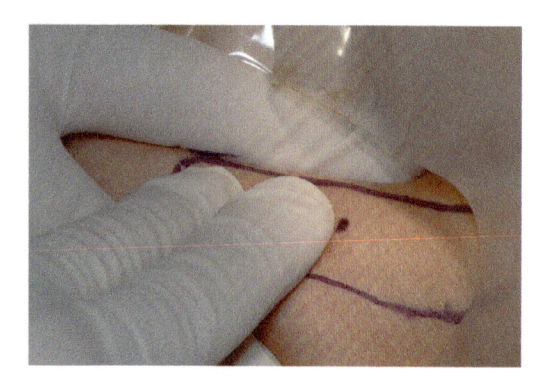

Figure 30.2 The center prominence of the iliac crest is located approximately the width of two fingers from the anterior spine.

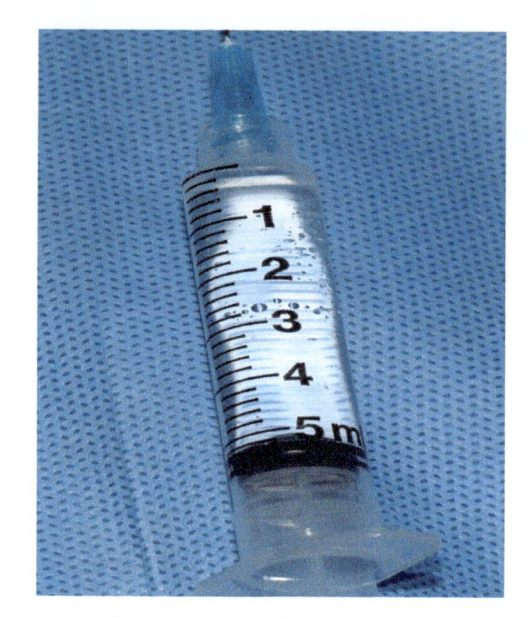

Figure 30.3 A 5 ml syringe is filled with 1% lidocaine.

solution or chlorhexidine gluconate. The skin is then wiped in a circular fashion with isopropyl-soaked sterile swabs and the site is isolated with sterile towels and drapes.

A 5 ml syringe is filled with lidocaine by aspiring from the ampule with the 20 gauge × 1 inch needle (Figure 30.3). A skin wheal is elevated with 1 ml lidocaine using the 25 gauge × 5/8 inch needle (Figure 30.4). A longer 21 gauge × 1 inch needle replaces the 25 gauge needle. After the skin is numb, the 21 gauge × 1 inch needle is inserted for deeper penetration and to confirm the crestal midpoint. The remaining 4 ml of lidocaine are deposited through the periosteum of the iliac crest and periosteum (Figure 30.5). The adequacy of the local anesthesia can be assessed by probing the periosteum with the 21 gauge × 1 inch needle.

With the patient remaining supine, the clinician holds the Jamshidi-type needle vertically and perpendicular to the iliac crest. Positioning the index finger near the needle's tip will control the depth of insertion and keep the needle in a centerline thrust through the cortical bone (Figure 30.6).

At the point where the local anesthesia was administered, the aspiration needle is inserted through the skin and into the anterior iliac wing. It should be rotated gently through the cortical bone, advancing approximately 1 cm into the marrow cavity. The stylet is

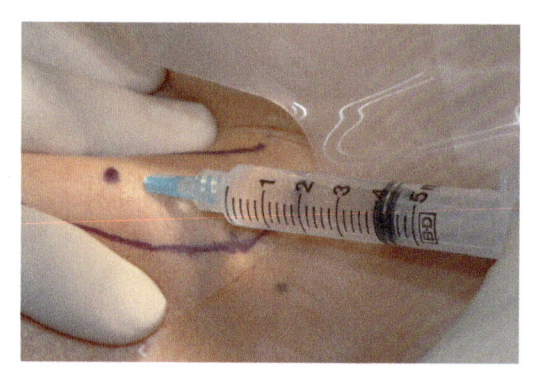

Figure 30.4 A skin wheal is elevated, using 1 ml of lidocaine in the 25 g × 5/8 inch needle.

Bone Marrow Aspirate: Rationale and Aspiration Technique

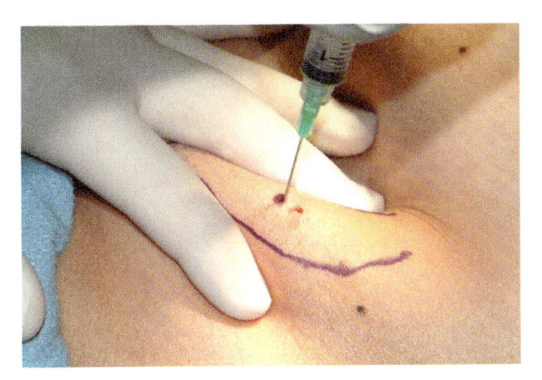

Figure 30.5 4 ml of lidocaine are deposited through the iliac crest and periosteum.

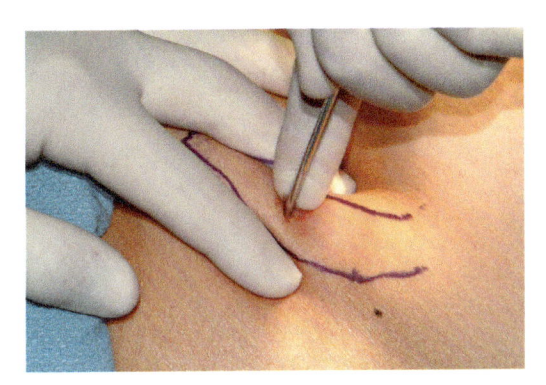

Figure 30.6 The index finger is positioned near the needle's tip to control insertion.

then removed from the needle (Figure 30.7) and the 20 ml syringe is attached. This provides a better vacuum pull than a 5 or 10 ml syringe.

Bone marrow is aspirated by retracting the syringe plunger (Figure 30.8). Typically, the first 2–4 ml of marrow contain the highest concentration of osteoprogenitor cells. If more marrow than that is required, the needle should be repositioned until a sufficient quantity of marrow has been obtained. This can be accomplished in one of two ways. The needle can be pulled out from the bone and reinserted through the same site and angled at a 30 to 45 degree angle for an additional blood draw or the needle can be completely

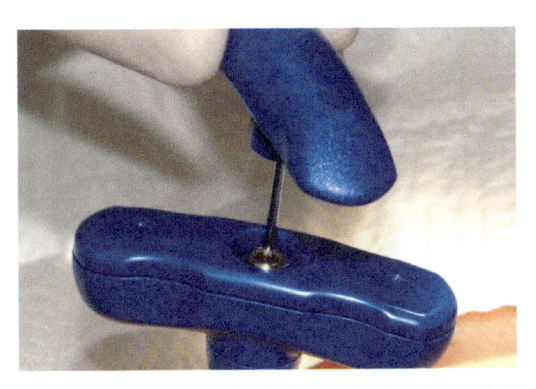

Figure 30.7 The stylet is removed and the 20 ml syringe is attached.

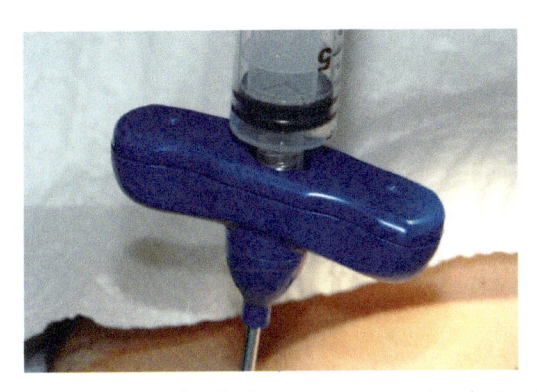

Figure 30.8 Between 2 and 4 ml of bone marrow are aspirated using the Jamshidi-type needle.

removed from the bone and skin and inserted through another site that is anterior and/or posterior to the first site. Changing the needle position helps to ensure that marrow is aspirated, rather than venous blood, which would dilute the concentration of stem cells.

The 20 ml syringe is removed from the Jamshidi-type needle and the aspiration needle is removed from the marrow space using an upward twisting motion (Figure 30.9). Typically this leaves only a small drop of blood (Figure 30.10). Pressure is placed over the aspiration site for five minutes and a bandage is placed on the site.

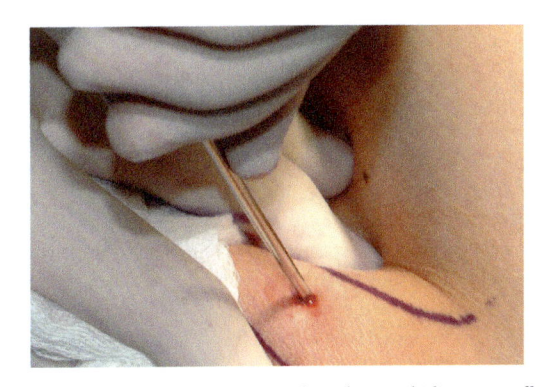

Figure 30.9 After the aspiration is complete, the Jamshidi-type needle is removed using an upward twisting motion.

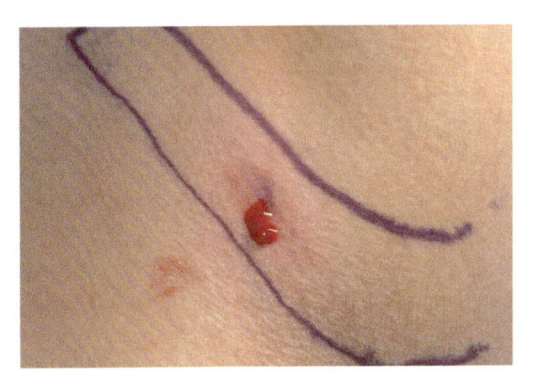

Figure 30.10 Typically, only a small spot of blood remains after the aspiration needle is removed. Pressure is applied for five minutes and the site is covered with a bandage.

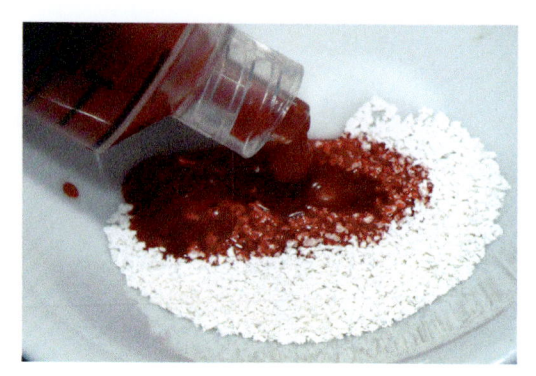

Figure 30.11 The bone marrow aspiration can be combined with a particulate graft (as seen here) or with an allograft bone block.

The aspirate is ejected into a specimen cup and mixed with the graft matrix (Figure 30.11).

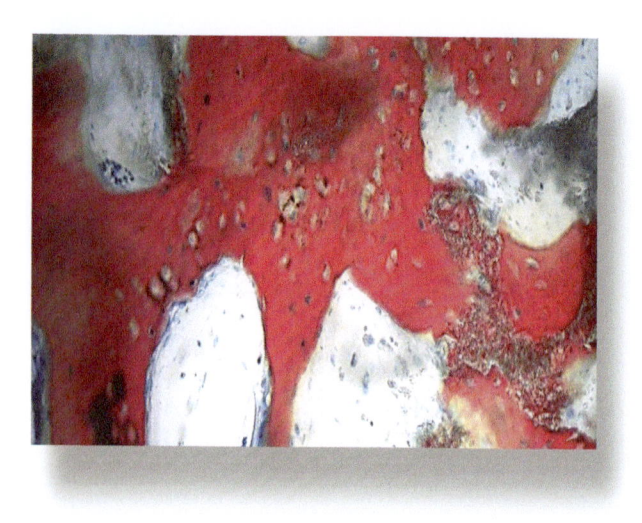

Figure 30.12 A bone core biopsy from a sinus lift augmentation site obtained after four months of healing.

Complications

The risks and complications of bone marrow aspiration of the anterior iliac crest are minimal; the technique has a very low incidence of morbidity. In reports of more than 900 bone marrow aspiration procedures, two patients experienced bruising. When the needle is pushed through the anesthetized skin into the bone, most patients feel pressure but not pain. After the stylet is replaced with the 20 ml syringe and the plunger is pulled to aspirate the bone marrow into the syringe, some patients report feeling deep pain or soreness, but this is immediately relieved when the draw ceases.

In several published reports of bone marrow aspiration procedures, no hematomas, infections, or chronic pain were documented [9–11]. The most frequently cited complication of iliac bone marrow aspiration harvesting is some tenderness at the site of perforation through the iliac crest, which usually resolves in one to two days. In the author's extensive experience using this procedure, no sensory disturbance within the dermatomal distribution of the lateral femoral cutaneous nerve occurred. Because the technique does not involve muscle dissection, blood loss is minimal to non-existent.

One problem that may occur is a failure to recover a significant quantity of marrow (a "dry tap"). This may occur for one of two reasons: improper positioning of the aspiration needle or age-related changes within the marrow cavity. When the Jamshidi-type needle perforates through the inner cortical plate and is not positioned within the cancellous compartment, the needle should be repositioned. Aspiration can then continue. With advancing age, patients' bone marrow cavity may be transformed from hematopoietic active "red" marrow to mostly yellow fatty marrow. It is estimated that this shift can result in a 60% change to fatty marrow by the age of 60 [12].

Application of the bone marrow aspirate

More than a dozen years ago, bone marrow delivered by injection or combined with other matrix material was demonstrated to significantly improve bone healing [13]. More recently, Smiler et al. [14] reported on the results of combining bone marrow aspirate with various commercially available bioengineered scaffold materials. A maximum of 4 ml of bone marrow was aspirated from the anterior iliac crest of five patients and used to saturate either xenograft or alloplast matrix scaffold material placed in seven graft sites in the five patients. (The sites included sinus lift augmentation, particulate onlay graft of the maxilla via a tunneling procedure, and particulate onlay graft of the maxilla stabilized with titanium mesh.) The xenograft scaffold was either PepGen Putty (DENTSPLY Friadent CeraMed, Lakewood, CO) or C-Graft resorbable algae material (Clinician's Preference, Golden, CO). The alloplast scaffold was beta-tricalcium phosphate (either Curasan AG, Kleinostheim, Germany, or Vitoss, Malvern, PA).

After 4–7 months of healing, core samples were biopsied for standard histologic (Figure 30.12) and histomorphometric analysis to determine the percentage of graft material converted into bone, percentage of vital graft matrix, percentage of unresorbed matrix, and percentage of remaining interstitial tissue (Figure 30.13). The authors concluded that bone marrow aspirate containing adult stem cells when mixed with bioengineered graft materials provide a scaffold to support the proliferation, differentiation, and maturation of the stem cells, as well as facilitating angiogenesis.

Bone marrow aspirate also has been demonstrated to produce a significant quantity of new bone growth when combined with slow-resorbing non-demineralized bone allograft particulate and resorbable hydroxylapatite matrix. Such materials require confinement and stabilization. Although this can be easily accomplished, it requires fairly invasive surgical removal of the mesh and screws. Soft-tissue dehiscences may result. An alternative is to use allograft bone blocks that can be impregnated with bone marrow aspirate and secured with easily removable screws (Figure 30.14). When allograft bone blocks impregnated with bone-marrow aspirate were placed in five patients and evaluated [15], all the grafts had integrated into the recipient bone after four to eight months, and implants placed in the sites all successfully osseointegrated. Histomorphometric analysis of a bone core obtained from one of the sites showed that 54% of the core consisted of bone and 46% of marrow; 89% of the bone was vital (Figure 30.15).

When bone marrow is aspirated with the intention of using it to infiltrate the trabecular region of a cortico/cancellous block of allograft material, it may be necessary to retard its clotting to

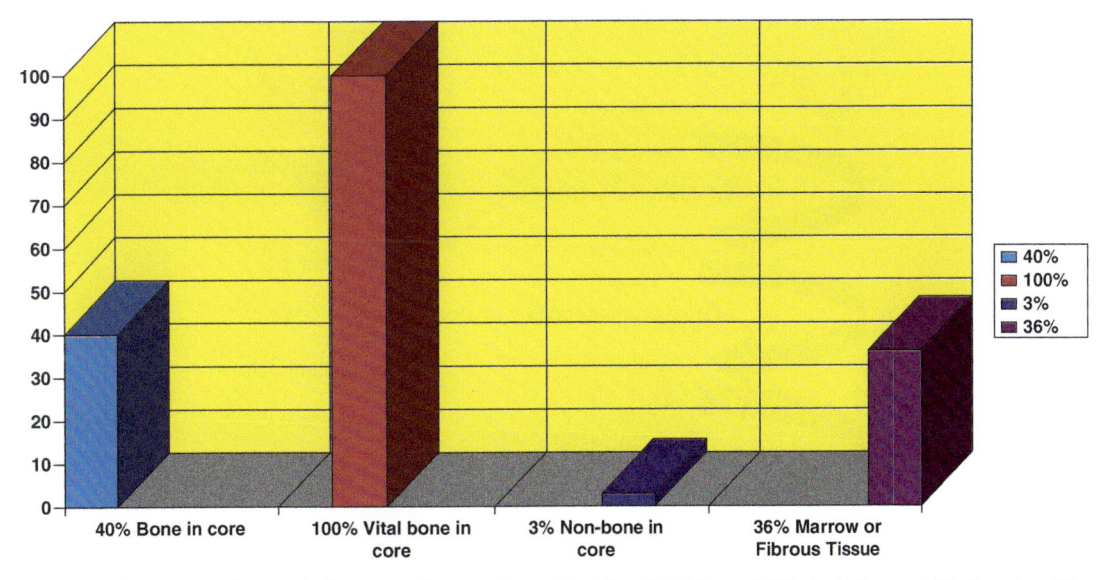

Figure 30.13 Histomorphometric analysis of the bone core shown in Figure 30.12 found 40% bone, 100% of which was viable. Less than 3% non-bone was found in the core.

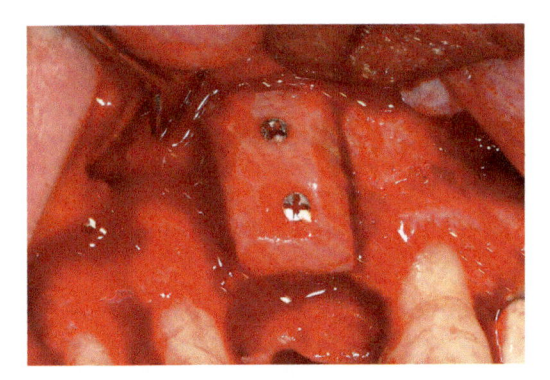

Figure 30.14 Corticocancellous bone block saturated with bone marrow aspirate and stabilized with bone screws.

facilitate dispersion. This can be accomplished by first drawing 2 ml of heparin solution into the 20 ml syringe before attaching it to the needle. The heparin washes the walls of the syringe and then is expelled before the syringe is attached to the Jamshidi-type needle.

Rationale for the application of bone marrow aspirate to graft sites

Adult bone marrow is a rich source of stem cells that have unique capabilities to self-renew, grow indefinitely, and differentiate or develop into multiple cell types and tissues [16]. They give rise to intermediate precursor or progenitor cell populations that differentiate and commit to various tissue lineages, including osteoblast precursors that can differentiate into the mature osteoblasts needed to promote osteogenesis [17, 18]. Compelling evidence exists that

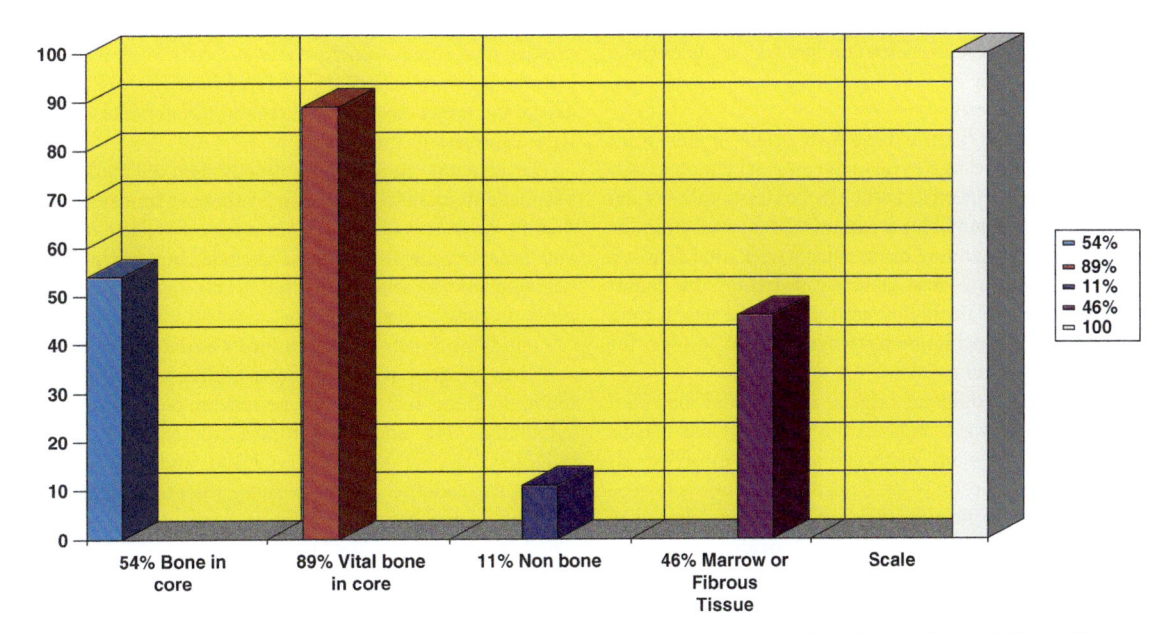

Figure 30.15 Histomorphometric analysis of block allograft saturated with bone marrow aspirate found 54% bone and 89% vital bone. The remaining 11% was non-resorbed cortical bone block.

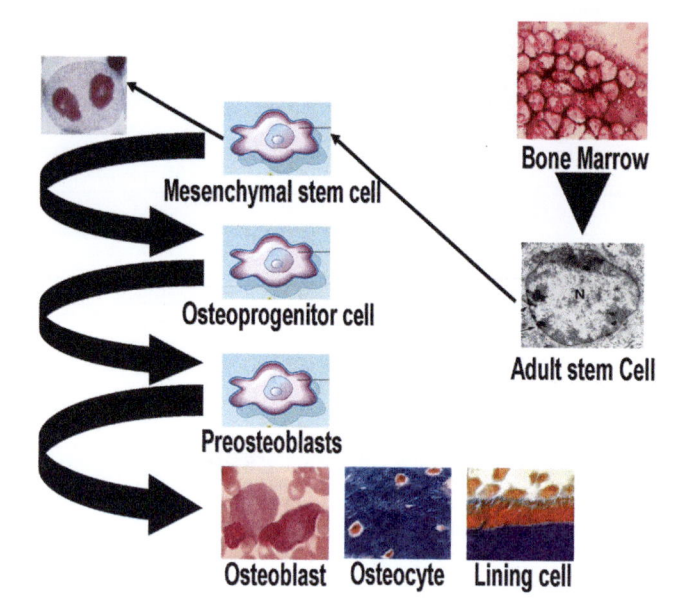

Figure 30.16 Bone marrow precursor cells can differentiate through the mesenchymal stem cell line to become osteoblasts.

bone formation occurs when marrow is implanted in osseous defects [19–23]. The marrow is the main source of pluripotent mesenchymal stem cells (MSCs) [24], which have been shown to be successful at inducing osteogenesis when delivered within a resorbable matrix [25] (Figure 30.16).

Although harvesting autogenous bone from the iliac crest and placing it in the maxilla or mandible is a common procedure for treating severely resorbed ridges, little attention has been given to the developmental origins of the extraoral donor bone or the intraoral recipient site(s). Many dental practitioners assume that bone is bone. In fact, iliac crest bone is a substantially different entity from alveolar bone, a distinction illuminated by the field of embryology.

Within the third week after fertilization, the human embryo develops three distinct germinal layers: the ectoderm, mesoderm, and endoderm. Each of these layers later undergoes a complex chain of development, branching off into the myriad components of the fully developed human body.

Iliac crest bone and its marrow have their origin in embryonic mesodermal cells. These cells give rise to the mesenchyme, a loosely organized embryonic connective tissue. In contrast, the alveolar bones (the maxilla and mandible) are ultimately derived from the ectoderm [26]. By the beginning of the fourth week after fertilization, the embryonic neural crest cells, derived from the neuroectoderm, migrate ventrolaterally on each side of the neural tube. They give rise to the branchial or pharyngeal arches to form the future head and neck region.

In addition to having different origins, alveolar and iliac crest bones form in different ways. Bone of the mandible and maxilla develop via intramembranous ossification. While most experts concur that the central portion of the large flat iliac bone is formed by intramembranous ossification, the outer portion (the ends) appear to form by means of endochondral ossification of the cartilaginous bone model [27–30]. It is from this outer portion that stem cells are harvested by needle aspiration.

The two different methods of bone formation also differ in their formation and mineralization processes [31–33]. Akintoye et al. have also demonstrated that bone marrow stem cells obtained from the iliac crest and the maxilla or mandible differ in regard to the type of bone they form. Stem cells from the iliac region form bone that is more closely packed, with histological observable hematopoietic marrow cells and an observable blood supply. Stem cells from the alveolar bone divide more actively and need induction. In contrast the iliac cells need growth factors to differentiate into bone cells [34].

Remarkably, when iliac crest marrow cells are placed into the mandible or maxilla, they form bone that is virtually indistinguishable from bone indigenous to that area [15]. The presence of a hypoxic environment at the surgical site, the change in vascular supply, the difference in functional load, and local growth factors influence the differentiation of stem cells to repair the defective sites [35–38]. This is possible in part because of the plasticity of the mesenchymal stem cells contained within the cancellous component of the iliac crest bone [39–41]. That plasticity allows the mesenchymal stem cells to differentiate into any tissue type regardless of their origin [42].

The advent of monoclonal antibody stem cell marker technology has made it possible to identify a variety of human stem cells and their progeny. Specific markers exist for cells related to bone healing and bone regeneration. These include, but are not limited to, hematopoetic, mesenchymal, endothelial, angiogenic, and vasculargenic precursor cells.

A study by Smiler et al. identified a variety of human stem cells and their progeny related to bone healing and bone regeneration found in bone marrow and peripheral blood [43]. Using flow cytometry [44] and six monoclonal antibody cell markers (CD14, CD34, CD36, CD105, CD106, and CD309, also known as vascular endothelial growth factor receptor (VEGFR) or KDR), stem cells were defined specific to bone marrow and peripheral blood. Results showed that bone marrow aspirate appears to contain a significantly greater percentage of hematopoietic, endothelial, and mesenchymal stem cells than peripheral blood (Figure 30.17).

The following case reports illustrate the use of bone marrow aspirate in three different situations.

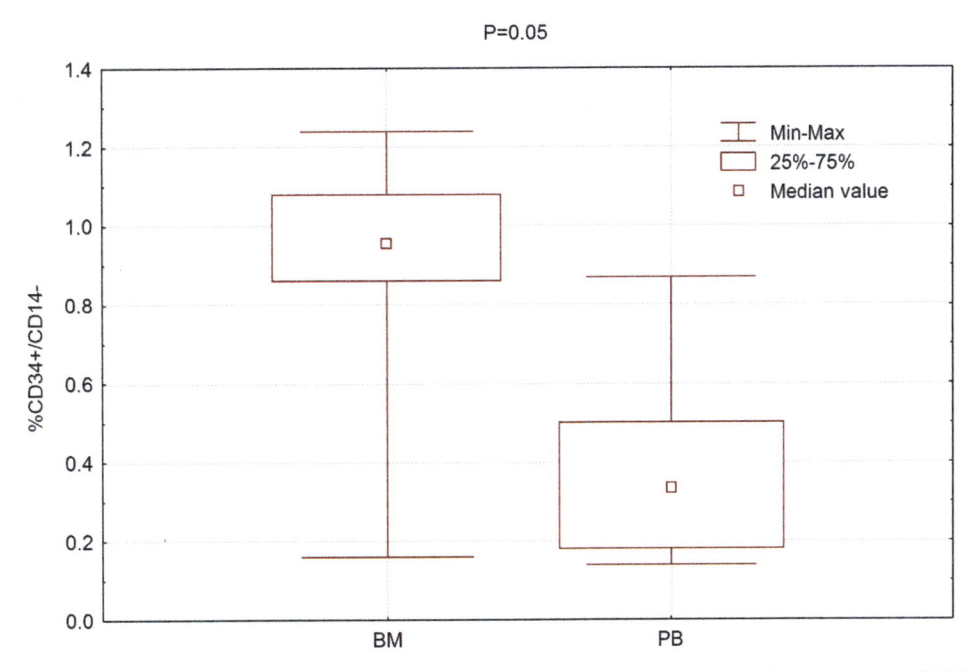

Figure 30.17 Percentage of CD34+/CD14− cells within all nucleated cells. Bone marrow aspirate contains a higher percentage of CD34+/CD14− cells, expressed by bone marrow stromal cells and osteoclast progenitors, than peripheral blood.

Case 1

SH, a 35-year-old female, presented with severe resorption of the anterior maxilla. The incisive papilla was at mid-crest, suggesting a minimum of 10 mm of horizontal bone loss. Measurement of the ridge suggested the bone width was no more than 3.0 mm (Figure 30.18).

Two allograft bone blocks (Musculoskeletal Transplant Foundation, University of Michigan Tissue Bank, MI) were stabilized with bone screws (ACE Bone Screws, ACE Surgical Supply Company, Inc., Brockton, MA) and contoured to fit the decorticated anterior maxilla recipient site (Figure 30.19). The prepared bone blocks were then removed, placed into a 20 ml syringe, and saturated with heparinized bone marrow aspirate (BMA) (Figure 30.20). The bone blocks were then decorticated, repositioned in the maxilla, and particulate graft matrix saturated with BMA was applied over and around the bone blocks (Figure 30.21).

After six months of healing, seven Nobel Replace Tapered Groovy implants (Nobel Biocare, Yorba Linda, California) were placed (Figure 30.22). All the implants osseointegrated and supported a fixed crown-and-bridge restoration.

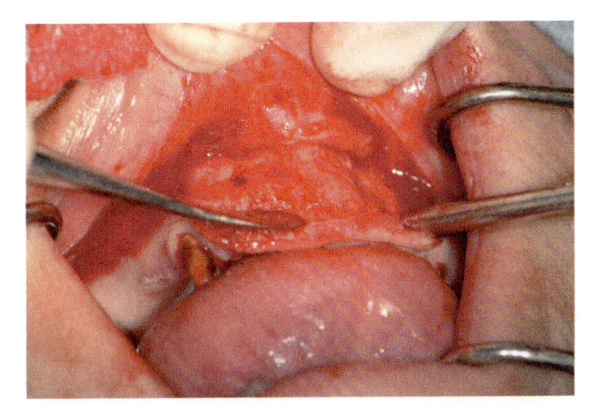

Figure 30.18 Case 1: the bone width in Case 1 measured a maximum of 3.0 mm.

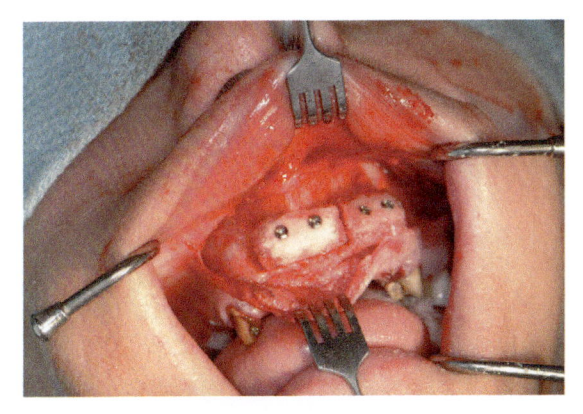

Figure 30.19 Bone blocks were contoured to fit the decorticated anterior maxilla recipient site.

(continued)

(Continued)

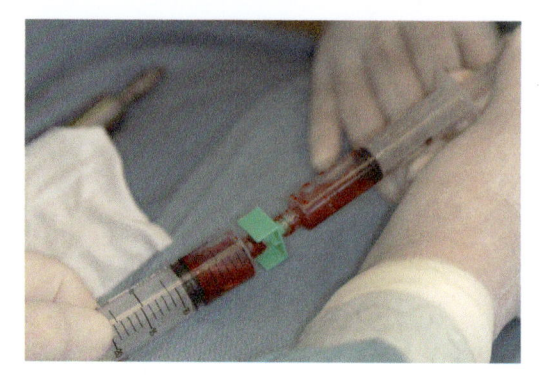

Figure 30.20 The prepared bone blocks were then removed, placed into a 20 ml syringe, and saturated with heparinized bone marrow aspirate.

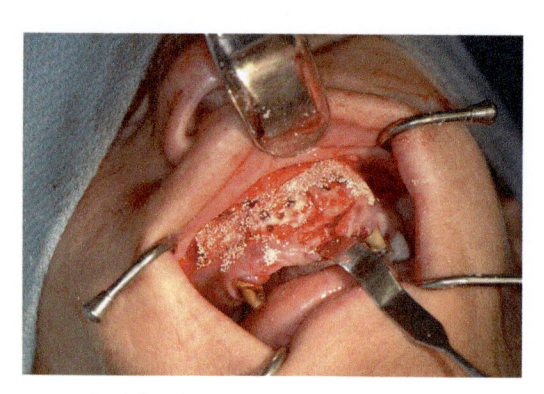

Figure 30.21 After being decorticated, the bone blocks were repositioned in the maxilla and particulate graft matrix saturated with BMA was applied to them.

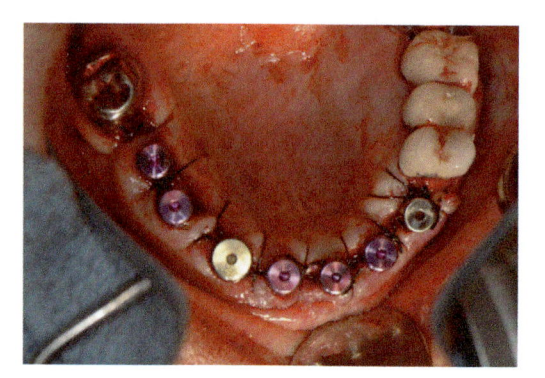

Figure 30.22 The implants are in place.

Case 2

MG, a 26-year-old female, presented with an osseous defect of the left lateral incisor site (Figure 30.23). Titanium mesh (ACE Titanium Mesh and Bone Screws, ACE Surgical Supply Company, Inc., Brockton, MA) was secured on the palatal and labial aspect of the defect. The crestal aspect of the mesh was then removed (Figure 30.24).

The crestal, palatal, and labial bones were decorticated with a 701 fissure bur. Particulate pure phase beta tricalcium phosphate graft matrix (SynthoGraft) saturated with bone marrow aspirate was loosely compacted between the labial and palatal titanium mesh (Figure 30.25). The mucoperiosteal flap was repositioned and sutured without tension and, after healing, a single Nobel Biocare Speedy implant was placed. It currently supports a successful provisional crown restoration.

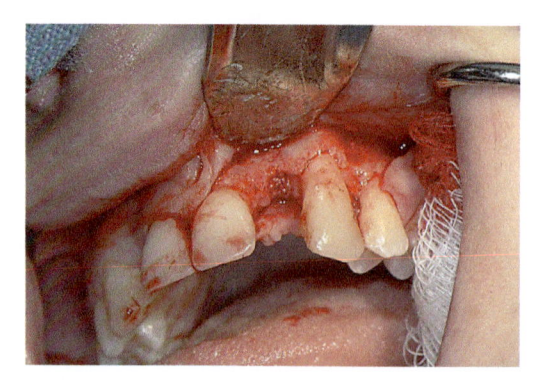

Figure 30.23 Case 2: osseous defect of the left lateral incisor site.

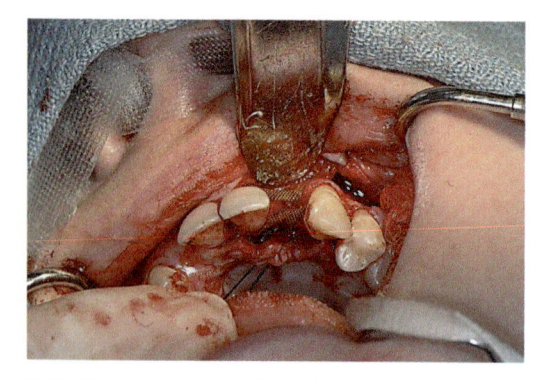

Figure 30.24 The crestal aspect of the mesh place on buccal and palatal sides was removed.

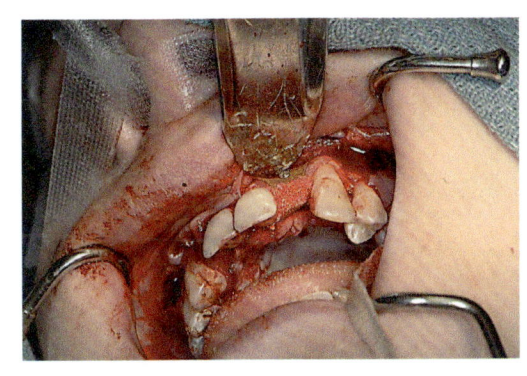

Figure 30.25 Particulate pure phase beta tri-calcium phosphate graft matrix saturated with bone marrow aspirate was loosely compacted between the labial and palatal titanium mesh.

Case 3

MB, a 41-year-old male, presented with a diminished alveolar bone around the right central incisor site (Figure 30.26). A piezosurgical bone incision was outlined and the labial bone was decorticated (Figure 30.27). The receptor site was then prepared, exposing the cancellous bone (Figure 30.28).

An allograft bone block secured with bone screws was contoured to fit the receptor site (Figure 30.29). The bone block was then saturated with bone marrow aspirate, secured with bone screws at the receptor site, and particulate graft matrix saturated with BMA was applied (Figure 30.30).

The mucoperiosteal flap was repositioned and sutured without tension on the incision (Figure 30.31).

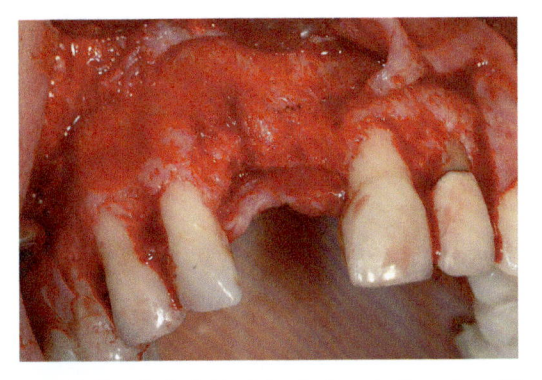

Figure 30.26 Case 3: diminished alveolar bone in the region of the right central incisor site.

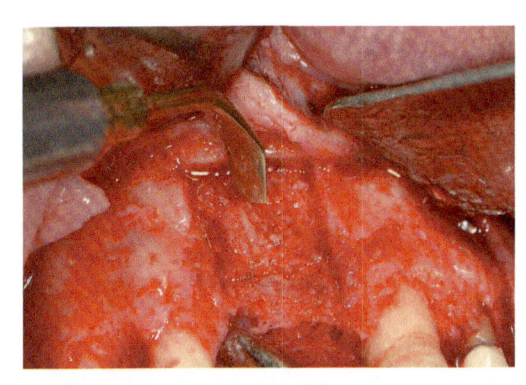

Figure 30.28 The receptor site was prepared exposing cancellous bone.

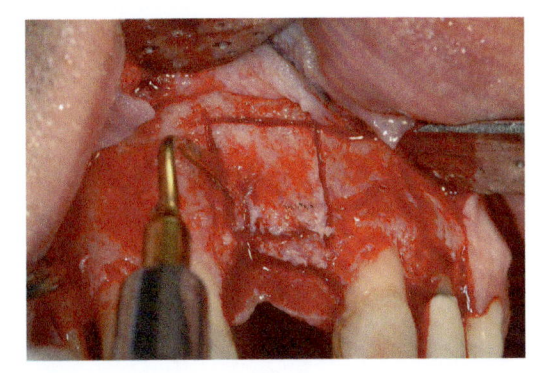

Figure 30.27 Piezosurgery instruments were used to outline and decorticate the labial bone.

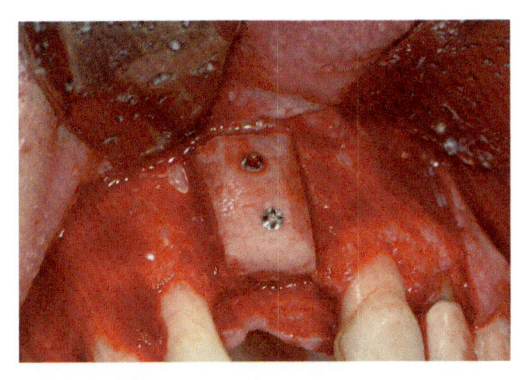

Figure 30.29 The allograft bone block secured with bone screws was contoured to fit the recipient site.

(continued)

(Continued)

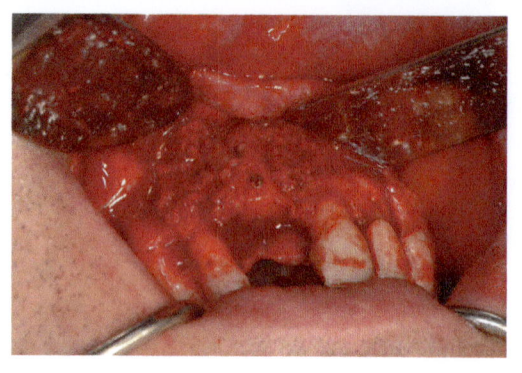

Figure 30.30 Bone block and particulate graft saturated with BMA.

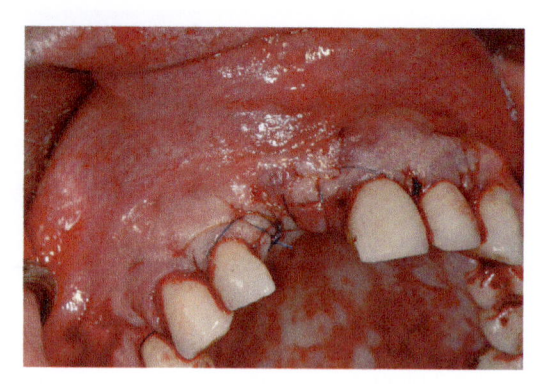

Figure 30.31 The mucoperiosteal flap was repositioned and sutured without tension.

Case 4

OS, a 29-year-old female, presented with missing teeth from the maxillary right first bicuspid to left first bicuspid. There was severe resorption of the anterior maxilla with the incisive papilla at mid-crest and crestal bone width of 2 mm (Figure 30.32).

An allograft rib with a cancellous/trabecular compartment of sufficient length to place within the edentulous anterior maxilla (Musculoskeletal Transplant Foundation, University of Michigan Tissue Bank, MI) was selected as the graft matrix (Figure 30.33). The allograft rib was placed in the anterior maxilla and the cortical bone scored with a thin fissure bur so that the graft could bend completely around the recipient graft site (Figure 30.34). The graft was contoured to fit the decorticated anterior maxilla recipient site, saturated with heparinized bone marrow aspirate and stabilized to the recipient site with bone screws (ACE Bone Screws, ACE Surgical Supply Company, Inc., Brockton, MA).

After six months of healing the bone screws were removed and a bone ridge was lightly contoured (Figure 30.35). Five 3.5 mm × 13 mm Nobel Replace Tapered Groovy implants (Nobel Biocare, Yorba Linda, California) were placed (Figure 30.36). After 5 months of healing all the implants osseointegrated and were used to support a cast primary bar (Figure 30.37). The teeth were processed to the secondary bar with retention using Hader clips (Figure 30.38). The final implant-supported restoration was stable, functional, and esthetic (Figure 30.39).

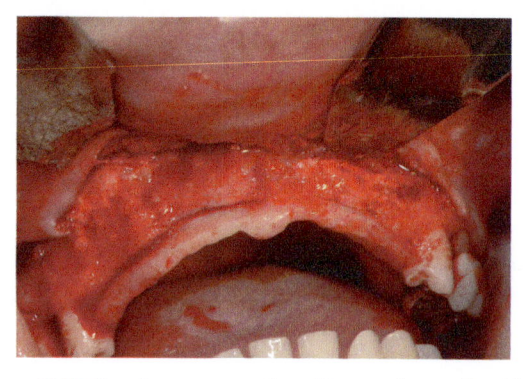

Figure 30.32 Case 4: severe resorption of the anterior maxilla with the incisive papilla at mid-crest and crestal bone width of 2 mm.

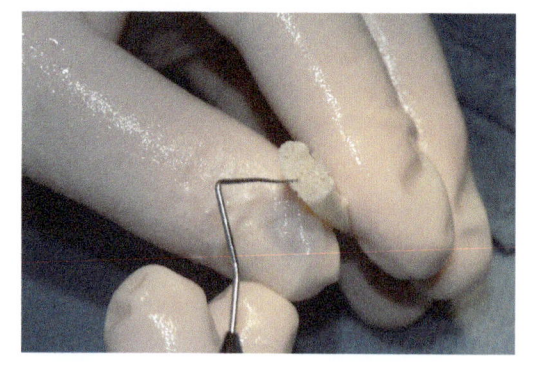

Figure 30.33 An allograft rib with a cancellous/trabecular compartment of sufficient length to place within the edentulous anterior maxilla was selected as the graft matrix.

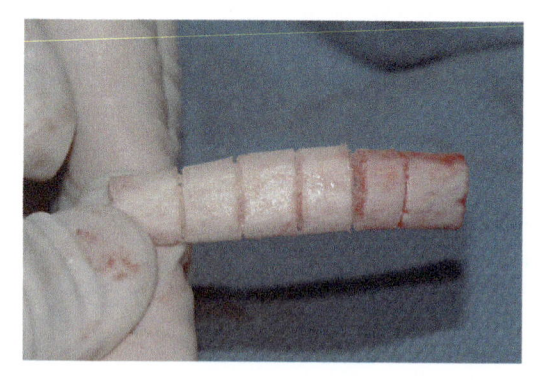

Figure 30.34 The allograft rib was placed in the anterior maxilla and the cortical bone scored with a thin fissure bur so that the graft could bend completely around the recipient graft site.

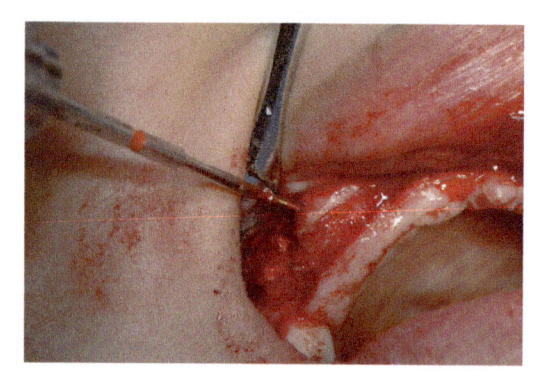

Figure 30.35 After six months of healing, the bone screws were removed.

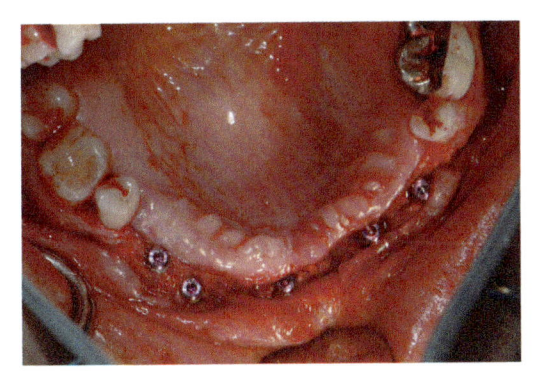

Figure 30.36 Five 3.5 mm × 13 mm Nobel Replace Tapered Groovy implants were placed.

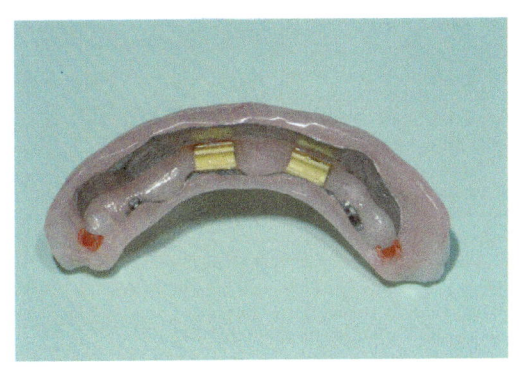

Figure 30.38 The teeth were processed to the secondary bar with retention using Hader clips.

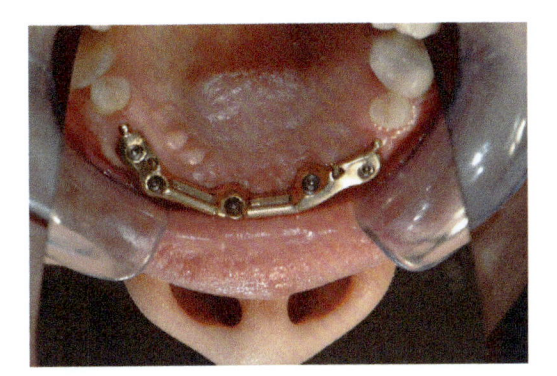

Figure 30.37 After 5 months of healing, all implants osseointegrated and were used to support a cast primary bar.

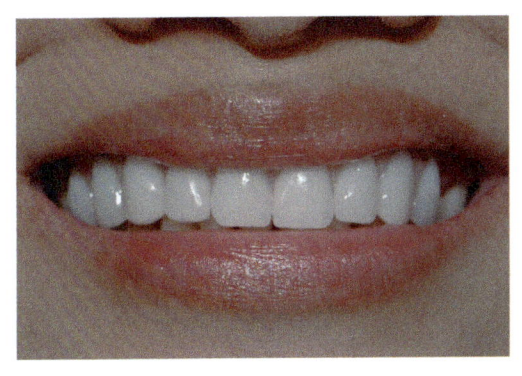

Figure 30.39 The final implant-supported restoration was stable, functional. and esthetic.

Conclusion

Bone tissue engineering in conjunction with bone graft surgery is an emerging approach in maxillofacial surgery. A suitable scaffold matrix in combination with soluble regulators (cytokines) and stem cells obtained from bone marrow aspirate may not only change the way bone graft surgery is done but also improve the success of graft procedures. Of all available sources of osteoblastic cells for bone grafting, the only one that does not require a second open surgical procedure is bone marrow harvested by aspiration. The iliac crest is an area rich in active marrow and it provides a source of cells with osteoinductive and osteogenic potential. Bone marrow aspirate can be easily obtained from the iliac crest with minimal morbidity.

The marrow aspiration technique described in this chapter has several advantages:

1. Aspirated autogenous bone marrow used in conjunction with a resorbable allograft or xenograft matrix has ideal properties for stimulating both osteoinduction and osteoconduction.
2. The aspiration technique is relatively simple and can be performed on an outpatient basis.
3. The need for an open surgical site to harvest autogenous bone is eliminated, along with any attendant complications.
4. The large quantity of stem cells available with bone marrow aspiration may prove this technique superior to grafting with autogenous bone.

References

1. Kawamura M, Urist MR: Induction of callus formation by implants of bone morphogenetic protein and associated bone matrix noncollagenous proteins. *Clin Orthop Relat Res* 1988;**236**:240–248.
2. Reddi AH, Hascall VC: Changes in proteoglycan types during Imatrix-induced cartilage and bone development. *J Biol Chem* 1978;**253**:2429.
3. Burwell RG: Studies in the transplantation of bone. The fresh composite homograft autograft of cancellous bone. *J Bone Joint Surg* 1964;**46B**:110–140.
4. Smiler DG, Soltan M: The bone-grafting decision tree: a systematic methodology for achieving new bone. *Implant Dent* 2006;**15**:122–128.
5. Burwell RG: Studies in the transplantation of bone. Treated composite homograft–autografts of cancellous bone: an analysis of inductive mechanisms in bone transplantation. *J Bone Joint Surg* 1966;**48B**:532–566.
6. Lindholm TS, Nilsson OS: Extraskeletal and intraskeletal new bone formation induced by demineralized bone matrix combined with marrow cells. *Clin Orthop Relat Res* 1982;**171**:251–255.
7. Smiler DG: Bone grafting: materials and modes of action. *Pract Periodontics Aesthet Dent* 1998;**8**:413–416.
8. Soltan M, Smiler D, Gallani F: A new platinum standard for bone grafting: autogenous stem cells. *Implant Dent* 2005;**14**:322–327.
9. Muschler GF, Boehm C, Easley K: Aspiration to obtain osteoblast progenitor cells from human bone marrow: the influence of aspiration volume. *J Bone Joint Surg Am* 1997;**79**:1699–1709. Erratum in: *J Bone Joint Surg Am* 1998;**80**: 302.
10. Majors AK, Boehm CA, Nitto H, et al: Characterization of human bone marrow stromal cells with respect to osteoblastic differentiation. *J Orthop Res* 1997;**15**:546–557.
11. Muschler GF, Nitto H, Matsukura Y, et al: Spine fusion using cell matrix composites enriched in bone marrow-derived cells. *Clin Orthop* 2003;**407**:102–118.
12. Bianco P, Riminucci M: The bone marrow stroma *in vivo*: ontology, structure, cellular composition and changes in disease. In: Beresford JN, Owen ME (eds.),

Marrow Stomal Cell Culture. Cambridge University Press, Cambridge, 1998, pp. 10–25.
13. Naughton G: From lab bench to market: critical issues in tissue engineering. *Ann NY Acad Sci* 2002;**961**:372–385.
14. Smiler D, Soltan M, Lee JW: A histomorphogenic analysis of bone grafts augmented with adult stem cells. *Implant Dent* 2007;**16**:42–53.
15. Soltan M, Smiler D, Prassad HS, et al: Bone block allograft impregnated with bone marrow aspirate. *Implant Dent* 2007;**16**:329–339.
16. Weissman H: Stem cells: units of development, units of regeneration, and units in evolution. *Cell* 2000;**100**:157–168.
17. Kassem M, Mosekilde I, Rungby J, et al: Formation of osteoclasts and osteoblast-like cells in long-term human bone marrow cultures. *APMIS* 1991;**99**:262–268.
18. Parfitt AM: The bone remodeling compartment: a circulatory function for bone lining cells. *J Bone Miner Res* 2001;**16**:1583–1585.
19. Bereford JN: Osteogenic stem cells and the stromal system of bone and marrow. *Clin Orthop* 1989;**240**:270–280.
20. Burwell RG: The function of bone marrow in the incorporation of a bone graft. *Clin Orthop* 1985;**200**:125–141.
21. Chase SW, Herndon CH: The fate of autogenous band homogenous bone grafts. *J Bone Joint Surg* 1955;**37**:809.
22. Connolly JF, Guse R, Lippiello L: Development of an osteogenic bone marrow preparation. *J Bone Joint Surg* 1989;**71A**:681–691.
23. Nade S: Clinical implications of cell function in osteogenesis. *Ann R Coll Surg Engl* 1979;**61**:189–194.
24. Zhang Yi, Li Chang, Jiang Xiao, et al: Comparison of mesenchymal stem cells from human placenta and bone marrow. *Chin Med J* 2004;**117**:882–887.
25. Helm GA, Dayoub H, Jane JA: Bone graft substitutes for the promotion of spinal arthrodesis. *Neurosurg Focus* 2001;**10**:E4.
26. Moore KL, Persaud TVN: *The Developing Human. Clinically Oriented Embryology*, 5th edn. WB Saunders, Philadelphia, PA, 1993, pp. 186–225.
27. Ponseti IV: Growth and development of the acetablum in the normal child. Anatomical, histological, and roentgenographic studies. *J Bone and Joint Surg* 1978;**60**:575–583.
28. Ogata S, Uhthoff HK: The early development and ossification of the human clavicle – an embryologic study. *Acta Orthop Scand* 1990;**61**:330–334.
29. Buckwalter JA, Glimcher MJ, Cooper RR, et al: Instructional course lecture. Bone biology. Part I: structure, blood supply, cells, matrix, and mineralization. *J Bone and Joint Surg* 1995;**77**:1256–1275.
30. Arey LB: *Developmental Anatomy: A Textbook and Laboratory Manual of Embryology*, 3rd edn. WB Saunders, Philadelphia, PA, 1934.
31. Dziedzic-Goclawska A, Emerich J, Grzesik W, Stachowicz W, et al: Differences in the kinetics of the mineralization process in endochondral and intramembranous osteogenesis in human fetal development. *J Bone Miner Res* 1988;**3**:533.
32. Bruder SP, Fink DJ, Caplan AI: Mesenchymal stem cells in bone development, bone repair, and skeletal regeneration therapy. *J Cell Biochem* 1994;**56**:283–294.
33. Fujii T, Ueno T, Kagawa T, et al: Comparison of bone formation in grafted periosteum harvested from tibia and calvaria. *Microsc Res Tech* 2006;**69**:580–584.
34. Akintoye S, Lam T, Shi S, et al: Skeletal site-specific characterization of orofacial and iliac crest human bone marrow stromal cells in same individuals. *Bone* 2006;**38**:758–768. Epub 2006 Jan 3.
35. Dennis JE, Caplan AI: *Bone Marrow Mesenchymal Stem Cells. Stem Cells Handbook*. Human Press Inc., Totowa, NJ, 2004, pp. 107–117.
36. Tepper OM, Capal JM, Galiano RD, et al: Adult vasculogenesis occurs through *in situ* recruitment, proliferation, and tubulization of circulating bone marrow-derived cells. *Blood* 2001;**105**:1068–1077.
37. Rafii S, Lyden D: Therapeutic stem and progenitor cell transplantation for organ vascularization and regeneration. *Nat Med* 2003;**9**:702–712.
38. Ceradini DJ, Gurtner GC: Homing to hypoxia: HIF-1 as a mediator of progenitor cell recruitment to injured tissue. *Trends Cardiovasc Med* 2005;**15**:57–63.
39. Barry FP, Murphy JM: Mesenchymal stem cells: clinical applications and biological characterization. *Int J Biochem Cell Biol* 2004;**36**:568–584.
40. Zipori D: Mesenchymal stem cells: harnessing cell plasticity to tissue and organ repair. *Blood Cells Mol Dis* 2004;**33**:211–215.
41. Verfaillie CM: Stem cell plasticity. *Graft* 2000;**3**:296–298.
42. Pittenger MF, Macay AM, Beck SC, et al: Multilineage potential of the adult human mesenchymal stem cells. *Science* 1999;**284**:143–147.
43. Smiler D, Soltan M, Albitar M: Toward the identification of mesenchymal stem cells in bone marrow and peripheral blood for bone regeneration. *Implant Dent* 2008;**17**:236–247.
44. Karin DF, McCoy JP Jr, Carey JL: *Flow Cytometry in Clinical Diagnosis*. ASCP Press, Chicago, IL, 2001.

CHAPTER 31
Alveolar Complex Regeneration

Nelson Monteiro and Pamela C. Yelick

Department of Orthodontics, Division of Craniofacial and Molecular Genetics, Tufts University School of Dental Medicine, Boston, Massachusetts, USA

Tooth development

To fully understand tooth development, one must consider the molecular signals that control cell growth, migration, and differentiation [1, 2]. Tooth development is the result of a complex and intricate cascade of gene expression patterns that direct cell migration to proper locations and toward proper differentiation pathways [1]. As for all organs, tooth formation is regulated by epithelial–mesenchymal interactions. Teeth are specialized in that the dental mesenchyme is derived from the neural crest, while the dental epithelium is derived from the ectoderm [3]. Figure 31.1 shows the principal stages of tooth morphogenesis.

Tooth development is characterized by discrete morphological stages. Initially, the dental lamina appears within the dental epithelium. Inside the dental lamina, within specific domains called placodes, localized proliferative activities lead to the formation of a series of epithelial outgrowths into the underlying ectomesenchyme at sites corresponding to the future positions of the teeth [1]. Next, tooth development proceeds in three stages: the bud, cap, and the bell stages [3]. In the bell stage, species-specific cusp patterns emerge (single cusped tooth or multicusped teeth), followed by final growth and matrix secretion. The inner enamel epithelium differentiates into ameloblasts that produce enamel, while the adjacent mesenchymal cells differentiate into odontoblasts that secrete dentin [2, 3].

The tooth is attached to the jaw by specialized supporting tissues that consist of the periodontal ligament (PDL), the cementum, and the alveolar bone, all of which are derived from the dental mesenchyme and are protected by the gingiva (see Figure 31.2) [1]. Enamel is the most highly mineralized tissue in the body, consisting of more than 96% hydroxyapatite and a complex crystalline lattice organization [1, 3]. Ameloblasts, which cover the entire surface of the enamel as it forms, almost entirely undergo apoptosis prior to the time that the tooth emerges into the oral cavity. A few dental epithelial cell remnants remain in the PDL as the epithelial Rests of Malassez (ERM). Dentin is a resilient (approximately 70% mineralized) and elastic tissue that forms the bulk of the tooth, supports the enamel, and compensates for its brittleness. Dentin is a sensitive tissue that is capable of repair, because odontoblasts and dental mesenchymal cells present in the pulp can be stimulated to deposit more dentin in response to mechanical injury [1]. Dental pulp, the soft connective tissue enclosed by dentin (the central pulp chamber), serves a variety of functions, including: (i) to support nerves that provide sensitivity to dentin; (ii) to nourish the avascular dentin; and (iii) to produce the dentin that surrounds it. When human adult teeth are damaged or lost, they cannot be regenerated or regrown. Thus, to solve the problem of limited tooth renewal in mammals, the development of technologies to allow for the regeneration and repair of lost or damaged teeth has become one of the major goals of dental tissue engineering and regenerative medicine in recent years.

Tooth-bone (alveolar complex) regeneration approaches

Particularly, tooth-bone (alveolar complex) engineering is difficult because both teeth and bone must be restored [4]. One of the approaches used to repair jaw defects is autologous bone graft techniques followed by the placement of dental implants. Although these techniques may result in a significantly improved quality of life, there are some drawbacks, including associated donor-site morbidity, limitations on the quantity of bone stock available, poor bone quality (density), and difficulties in dental implant placement because of severe alveolar ridge atrophy present in many edentulous situations or the need for several complex surgical procedures to achieve the optimal prosthetically driven result [4, 5].

Both severe tooth decay and extensive periodontal disease necessitate tooth extraction. Alveolar bone is also susceptible to inflammation induced by an often high rate of progressive periodontitis or extensive bone resorption due to tooth loss (edentulism), which alters alveolar bone morphology and destroys surrounding tooth-supporting tissues. Moreover, the alveolar ridge often continues to resorb following tooth removal even if a dental implant is placed into the extraction socket, due to continuous bone remodeling in response to mechanical loading changes that occur with alterations in the applied force and strain distribution to the osseous tissue during mastication that is often observed in cases of implant overdentures [5]. Thus, tooth-bone bioengineering strategies are needed to repair jaw defects. Tooth formation (engineering) is a good place to start. The ability to regenerate tooth as a quick replacement for the natural failing tooth (due to advanced caries or periodontal disease) would help to prevent subsequent bone loss.

Highly complex molecular signaling pathways drive natural tooth formation. In order to engineer a tooth, it is necessary to reproduce *in vitro* or *in vivo* the necessary processes of tooth-bone formation.

Vertical Alveolar Ridge Augmentation in Implant Dentistry: A Surgical Manual, First Edition. Edited by Len Tolstunov.
© 2016 John Wiley & Sons, Inc. Published 2016 by John Wiley & Sons, Inc.

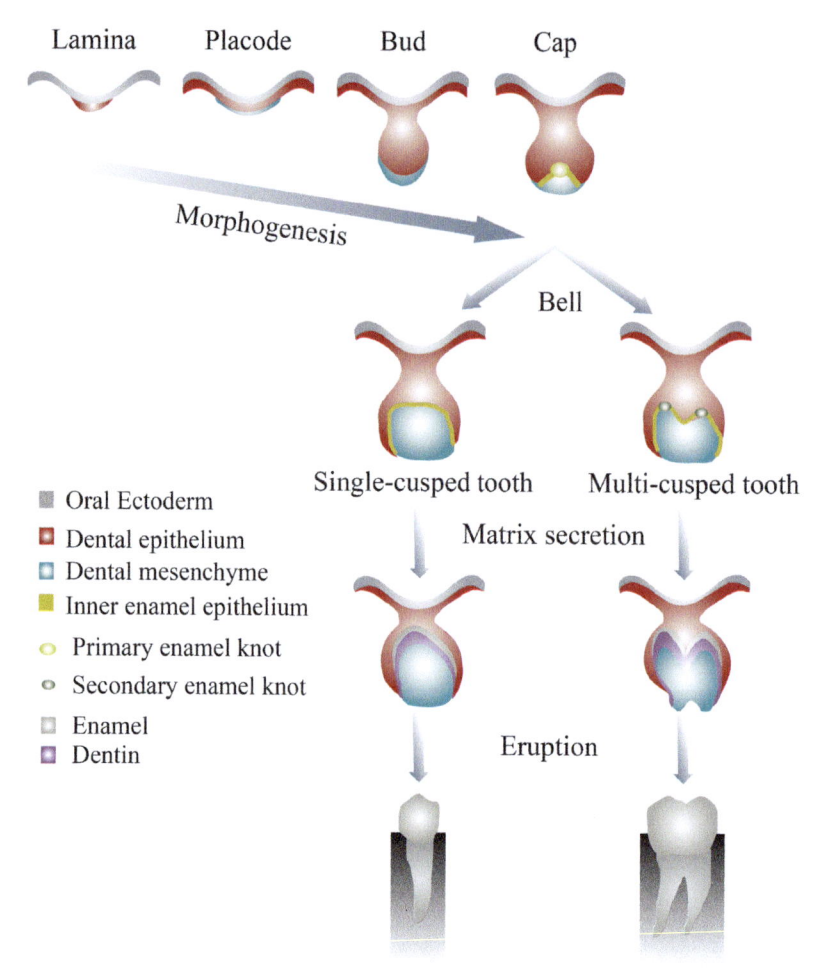

Figure 31.1 Principal stages of tooth formation. Adapted from Jernvall and Thesleff [3].

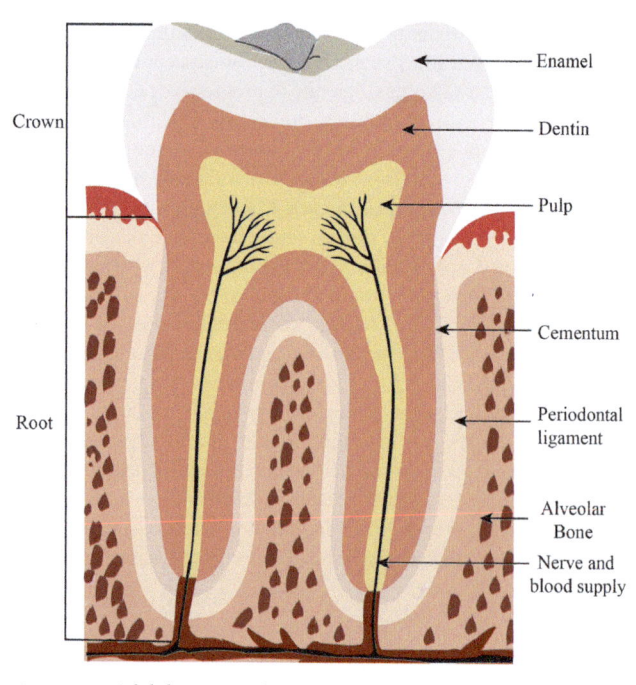

Figure 31.2 Adult human tooth morphology.

The spatiotemporal expression and interactions of a variety of signaling molecules, such as growth factors and cytokines, regulate the macromorphological (crown size and tooth length) and micromorphological (the number and position of cusps and roots) aspects of a tooth. Therefore, proper control of these interactions is required to generate a biotooth with the desired identities of incisor, canine, premolar, or molar teeth [2]. To date, several approaches to engineer or regenerate an entire biological tooth have been proposed. These include stimulation of the formation of a third dentition, use of tooth tissue engineering scaffolds, dental cell tissue recombinations, chimeric tooth tissue engineering, and gene-manipulated tooth regeneration [2, 6].

Presently, the two major approaches used for tooth regeneration are dental cell tissue recombination and tissue engineering scaffold approaches. Dental cell tissue recombination approaches rely on replicating the signaling processes involved in embryonic tooth development, where the cultured cell tissue construct is directly implanted in the defect site (Figure 31.3) [7]. Several studies have shown that functional teeth can be formed from embryonic tooth germ cells (embryonic stem cells, orESCs) cultured *in vitro* and also implanted *in vivo* [8–10]. Although these studies demonstrate the potential of using ESCs for tooth regeneration, several major issues need to be considered, including possible tumorigenesis when transplanted, ethical issues regarding the use of human embryos, and allogeneic immune rejection [7, 11].

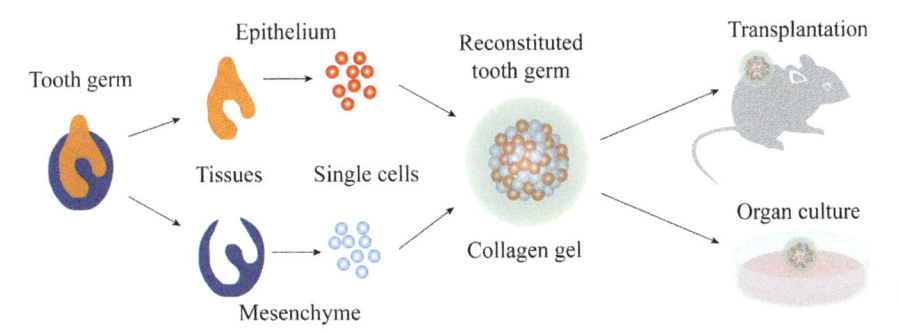

Figure 31.3 Cell tissue recombination approach. Adapted from Nakao et al. [9].

Tissue engineering approach

The goal of tissue engineering (TE) and regenerative medicine (RM) is the development of biological substitutes for the repair, restoration, or regeneration of tissue and organ function, and to reestablish the regenerative niche at sites of damage [12, 13]. Tissue engineering involves three basic components – cells, scaffolds, and bioactive agents [12]. Figure 31.4 depicts the tooth tissue engineering approach. In this section, we will describe the use of dental stem cells, a variety of different scaffolds materials and techniques employed for dental tissue engineering, and current efforts being used to develop highly multifunctionalized systems for teeth-bone regeneration.

Adult dental stem cells: factor 1

One of the main components of TE are cells. Adult stem cells have been identified in many tissues and organs and have been shown to undergo self-renewal, to differentiate for the maintenance of normal tissue, and to repair injured tissues. Adult dental stem cells (DSCs) are a relatively new stem cell population that have been isolated from various dental tissues [14]. Post-natal dental pulp stem cells (DPSCs) produced only sporadic, but densely calcified, nodules and did not exhibit the capacity to form adipocytes, as compared to bone marrow stromal cells (BMSCs), which routinely calcified throughout the adherent cell layer with dusters of lipid-laden adipocytes [15]. Moreover, DPSCs transplanted into immunocompromised mice generated a dentin-like structure lined with human odontoblast-like cells that surrounded a pulp-like interstitial tissue. Stem cells from human exfoliated deciduous teeth (SHED) were identified as a population of highly proliferative, clonogenic cells capable of differentiating into a variety of cell types including neural cells, adipocytes, and odontoblasts [16]. SHED were found to

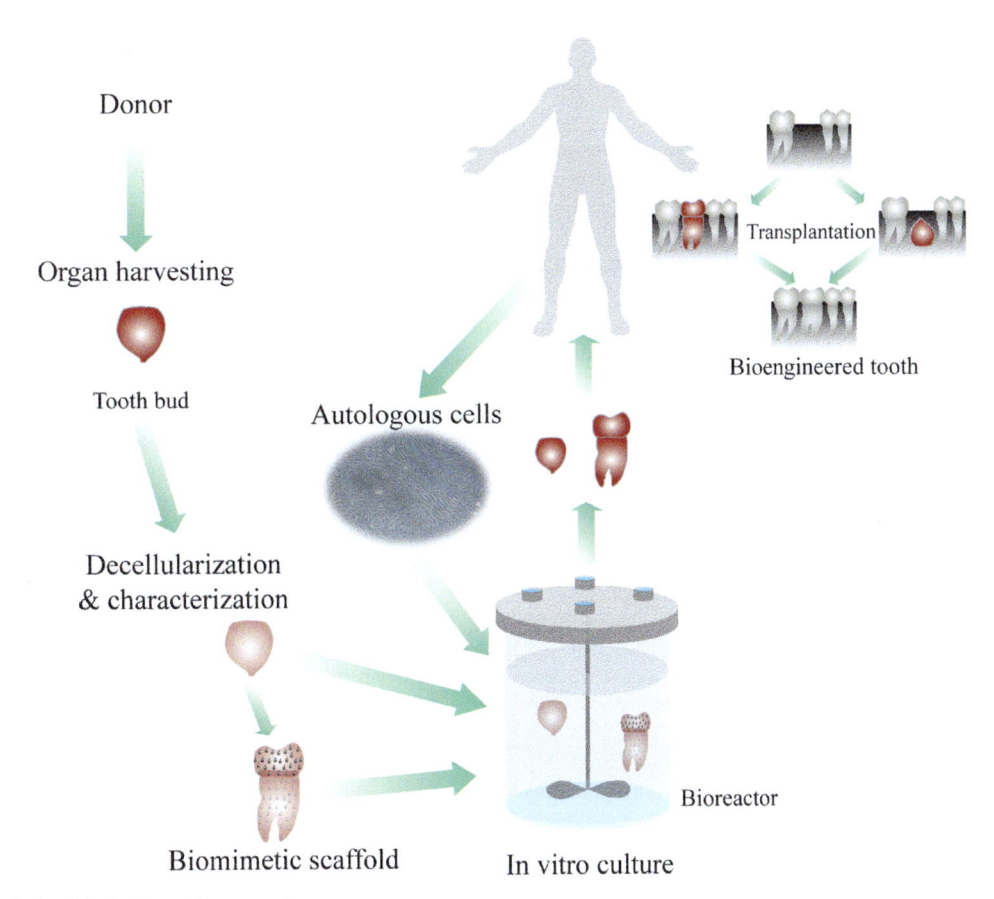

Figure 31.4 Tooth decellularized scaffold approach.

be able to induce bone formation, generate dentin, and to survive in the mouse brain after *in vivo* transplantation. SHED are a quite promising type of stem cell, in that they are not only derived from a very accessible tissue resource (autologous baby teeth) but are also potentially capable of providing enough cells for potential clinical applications [16]. Periodontal ligament stem cells (PDLSCs) can differentiate into adipocytes, cementoblast-like cells, and collagen-forming cells, and have the capacity to generate a cementum/PDL-like structure and contribute to periodontal tissue repair [17]. DE cells present in PDL tissue as ERMs exhibit the capacity to form enamel-producing ameloblasts. Dental follicle progenitor stem cells (DFPCs) expressed higher amounts of insulin-like growth factor-2 (IGF-2) transcripts than human BMSCs and after *in vivo* transplantation in immunocompromised mice, DFPCs expressed osteocalcin and bone sialoprotein, but without any sign of cementum or bone formation [18]. Stem cells from the apical papilla (SCAP) proliferate two- to threefold greater than those obtained from the pulp organ, and are as potent in osteo/dentinogenic differentiation as BMSCs but are weaker in adipogenic potential [19]. Based on these promising characteristics, tooth tissue engineering efforts are focused on creating tooth-bone and supporting structures using adult dental stem cell populations combined with non-dental stem cells (i.e., BMSCs and umbilical cord MSCs).

Scaffolds: factor 2

In a typical TE methodology, progenitor cells are encapsulated within or seeded on to a scaffold prior to transplantation in order to repopulate a defect and restore function. Thus, a scaffold provides a physical support for the development of new tissues in a manner that mimics the function of the natural extracellular matrix (ECM). Tissue engineering strategies based on the combination of scaffolds, cells, and bioactive agents have grown remarkably in recent years, leading to significant advances in the field of tooth regeneration [20, 21]. It is of extreme importance to consider the physical aspects and composition of the biomaterial scaffold for successful tissue regeneration [21]. The scaffolds must be designed to ensure mechanical integrity and functionality, and the scaffold surface needs to have appropriate properties for proper cell adhesion, proliferation, and differentiation. Therefore, the selection of biomaterials is a critical factor to consider when determining the suitability of a scaffold to mimic the ECM.

Several natural and synthetic biomaterials have been examined for their utility for bioengineered tooth regeneration [2,20,21]. Scaffolds can be made of different forms such as fibers, foams and gels. The main requirements of biomaterials used as TE scaffolding are that they must be inherently biocompatible and biodegradable. The major advantage of using natural material-based synthetic scaffolds is the ability to tune their degradation rates, which can be readily achieved by varying the concentration of the polymer and/or cross-linking agents. The most commonly used natural biomaterials in TE scaffolding for tooth regeneration include collagen, alginate, fibrin, chitosan, gelatin, silk, peptides, and hyaluronic acid [20, 21]. Synthetic scaffolds also have been examined, mainly due to their ability to be manufactured in many desired shapes and sizes, their processing flexibility, and the ability to predefine scaffold architecture and structural parameters [21]. The most commonly used synthetic polymers for TE scaffolding include polylactic acid (PLA), polyglycolic acid (PGA), poly-L-lactic acid (PLLA), poly-lactic-co-glycolic acid (PLGA), and polycaprolactone (PCL) [20, 21]. Inorganic materials such as calcium phosphate (CaP) ceramics, bioactive glass, and ceramic/polymer composites have also been especially developed for tooth and bone TE applications [5, 22]. Commercial synthetic CaP bone substitutes include hydroxyapatite (HA) ceramics, β-tricalcium phosphate (β-TCP) cements, and biphasic calcium phosphates (BCPs) [5]. Although they lack mechanical bone characteristics, osteoinductive, or osteogenic abilities, ceramics gradually acquire mechanical strength similar to cancellous bone after their incorporation [5, 23].

For alveolar bone regeneration, biodegradable granule forms of ceramics, such as β-TCP, are preferred because they are easy to shape and they adapt into the three-dimensional structure of the bone defect, which is important for esthetic reasons [23]. The advantages of combining ceramics with polymers are biocompatibility, biodegradability, and the ability to readily bind growth factors critical for osteoinduction. It has been shown that PCL scaffolds coated with CaP or HA increase osteoblast adhesion, spreading, proliferation, and promote alveolar bone formation in periodontal defects [5].

The manufacturing methods for fabricating a polymeric 3D scaffold for TE applications have been widely reviewed in the literature. The conventional methods include solvent casting, particulate leaching, high-pressure processing, fiber bonding, melt molding, phase separation, gas foaming, electrospinning, and rapid prototyping [20, 21]. Hydrogels are a particular class of scaffolds exhibiting significant potential for applications in tooth regeneration, as smart and stimuli responsive systems. They can be used as injectable materials, which offer several advantages, namely: easy incorporation of therapeutic agents, such as cells, under mild conditions; minimally invasive local delivery; and high contourability, which is essential for filling in irregular defects [20, 21].

Our group has been working to define methods to establish proper dental epithelial (DE) and dental mesenchymal (DM) cell interactions using a variety of scaffold materials [24–28]. Our published results showed that dental cells obtained from dissociated porcine or rat tooth buds were capable of generating multiple, small, organized tooth crowns [24–26]. The tooth scaffolds used in these studies lacked the ECM molecule gradients that are present in naturally formed teeth, and which provide essential cues for proper tooth development, periodontal tissues, and surrounding alveolar bone [28]. In these studies, hybrid tooth-bone tissues were bioengineered using pig third molar tooth bud cells seeded on to PGA and PLGA scaffolds [25]. Bone implants also were generated from osteoblasts induced from bone marrow progenitor cells obtained from the same pig, which were seeded on to PLGA fused wafer scaffolds. The tooth and bone implants were grown in the omenta of adult rat hosts for 8 weeks. Histological and immunohistochemical analyses revealed the presence of tooth tissues, including primary and reparative dentin and enamel in the tooth portion of hybrid tooth-bone implants and osteocalcin and bone sialoprotein-positive bone in the bone portion of hybrid tooth-bone constructs. Moreover, collagen type III-positive connective tissue resembling periodontal ligament and tooth root structures were present at the interface of bioengineered tooth and bone tissues. These results demonstrate that the hybrid tooth-bone TE constructs could be used for the eventual clinical treatment of tooth loss accompanied by alveolar bone resorption [25]. In another study, *tooth-bone constructs* were prepared from third molar tooth tissue and iliac crest bone marrow-derived osteoblasts isolated from, and implanted back into, the same pig as an autologous reconstruction [4]. The results showed that small tooth structures were identified and consisted of organized dentin, enamel, pulp, and periodontal ligament tissues, surrounded by new bone [4].

However, we are still unable to bioengineer teeth of predetermined size and shape. It is likely that detailed functional characterization of ECM molecule gradients present in natural tooth scaffolds will provide insight on how to achieve this goal [29]. Along these lines, we have described methods to effectively decellularize and demineralize porcine molar tooth buds, while at the same time preserving natural ECM protein gradients [29]. These results showed that collagen I, fibronectin, collagen IV, and laminin gradients were detected in natural tooth tissues and retained in decellularized samples. Also, decellularized tooth scaffolds reseeded with dental progenitor cells exhibited distinctly improved collagen content and organization as compared to decelluarized scaffolds. These results demonstrate the potential for natural decellularized molar tooth ECM to instruct dental cell matrix synthesis. This could be the foundation for future use of biomimetic scaffolds for dental tissue engineering applications.

Bioactive agents for tooth-bone regeneration: factor 3
Odontogenesis is initiated by factors resident in the first arch dental epithelium, which influence the underlying ectomesenchyme [1]. The molecular signals that control the position and the number of teeth along the oral surface are still not entirely clear, and fully deciphering the network of regulatory events directing this process will be quite challenging. Several bioactive agents, including growth and transcription factors from several signaling families, have been identified as critical regulators throughout all stages of tooth development. At least 12 transcription factors are expressed in odontogenic mesenchyme [1] and more than 200 genes have been identified that are expressed in the oral epithelium, dental epithelium, and dental mesenchyme during the initiation of tooth development [6]. Therefore, controlled release of selected bioactive agents from biodegradable scaffolds may be useful to enhance the efficacy of tooth TE approaches [2]. Indeed, TE scaffolds can be used as bioactive agent reservoirs combined with the delivery cells. Bioactive scaffolds can provide a multitude of advantages such as safe delivery profiles, protection of bioactive agents from biodegradation, and the ability to deliver the bioactive agents locally where the cells are attached [30]. This type of multifunctionalized system may be used to create a highly regulated network of signals able to orchestrate dental cell proliferation, migration, and differentiation, directing the development of a fully functional tooth.

Presently, growth factors (GFs) are the most commonly used bioactive agents. GFs are critical to the development, maturation, maintenance, and repair of craniofacial and dental tissues, because they establish the communication between cells/tissues [1]. GFs are secreted proteins known for their roles in cell migration, differentiation, proliferation, gene expression, and organization of functional tissues [31]. Important for the use of stem cells in TE strategies is understanding which of the many GFs resident in the dental stem cell niche provide the essential cues that control their fate. For instance, dentin retains its regenerative capacity to a certain degree throughout adulthood, which is thought to be attributed to the production of certain GFs by dental stem cells, thus maintaining their proliferation and differentiation potential [1]. In response to injury, dental mesenchymal progenitor cells present in the tooth pulp can be stimulated to differentiate into odontoblasts that deposit dentin. Therefore, GFs can be incorporated into TE scaffolds to attract and direct stem cell differentiation. Many GFs such as bone morphogenetic proteins (BMPs), transforming growth factor (TGF)-beta1, fibroblast growth factor (FGF-2), and vascular endothelial growth factor (VEGF) have been found to be expressed during tooth formation and repair [1, 2]. Cai et al. studied which differentiation approach (e.g., maintenance of stemness, osteogenic or chondrogenic induction) is most suitable for periodontal regeneration in vivo using rat BMSC seeded on o PLGA/PCL electrospun scaffolds. The results showed that the chondrogenic differentiation approach promotes regeneration of alveolar bone and ligament tissues. The retention of multilineage differentiation potential supported only ligament regeneration, while the osteogenic differentiation approach boosted alveolar bone regeneration [32]. Comparison of DPSCs cultured on PLLA nanofiber scaffolds in medium containing dexamethasone, or BMP7 plus dexamethasone, both resulted in DPSCs differentiation into odontoblast-like cells [33]. However, DPSCs cultured in the BMP7 plus dexamethasone medium exhibited greater capacity to form extracellular matrix and hard tissue formation after 8 weeks of ectopic implantation in nude mice. Therefore, PLLA nanofiber scaffolds combined with odontogenic inductive factors may provide an excellent environment for DPSCs to regenerate dental pulp and dentin [33].

Gene therapy has also been proposed as a means to control stem cell differentiation and tissue formation. The principle of gene therapy is the insertion of a gene containing a sequence that encodes for a specific protein into the host cell genome to replace a hereditary genetic defect or to provide a new function in a cell, such as overexpressing GFs or killing cancer cells [34]. Therefore, the gene therapy treatment must enter the nucleus of the host cell in order to be transcribed into messenger RNA (mRNA) and ultimately translated into protein in the cytoplasm. This strategy relies on activating or repressing endogenous dental cell gene expression. In support of this approach, efficient gene transfection of neural crest cell (NCC)-derived dental mesenchymal cells has been reported [35]. It was reported that porous chitosan/coral composites were combined with plasmid encoding the PDGFB gene, seeded with human PDLCs, and subcutaneously implanted into mice [36]. The results showed that the PDLCs proliferated better on the gene-loaded scaffolds than on the pure scaffolds, in the presence of increased expression of PDGFB in vivo [36]. In another study, chitosan/collagen scaffolds were loaded with adenoviral vector encoding human TGFβ1 and seeded with human PDLCs [37]. In vitro analyses showed that an adenoviral vector TGFβ1-loaded scaffold exhibited the highest PDLC proliferation rate. Successful regeneration of alveolar bone and surrounding periodontal tissues using gene therapy vectors such as adenoviral BMP-7 (Ad-BMP-7) was achieved in vivo [38]. Bone regeneration and bridging was observed with the use of ex vivo BMP-7 gene transfer using a gelatin-based scaffold seeded with syngeneic dermal fibroblasts (SDFs) and implanted in a rat wound model consisting of a large mandibular alveolar bone defect. Transduction of SDFs using green fluorescent protein (Ad-GFP) or noggin (Ad-noggin) did not result in ectopic bone formation. Mature cartilage and newly formed bone was observed using Ad-BMP-7 gene transfer after 21 days [38]. Mesoporous bioglass (MBG)/silk fibrin scaffold combined with BMP7 and/or PDGF-B adenovirus synergistically promoted periodontal regeneration by allowing up to two times greater regeneration of the periodontal ligament, alveolar bone, and cementum when compared to each adenovirus used alone [39]. Transcription factors, which drive gene expression and native protein production, can offer advantages over strategies that require the delivery of DNA encoding sets of proteins [40]. The successful delivery of transcription factors could ensure that the expression of all natural splice variants occurs in a coordinated time and sequence, and may regulate a cascade of multiple genes, all of which may be advantageous for tooth regeneration. Thus, transcription factor gene delivery approaches may exhibit utility for tooth regeneration.

A relatively new way to induce stem cell differentiation is through the delivery of interference RNA (RNAi) [41]. RNAi is a specific gene silencing mechanism mediated by the delivery of chemically synthesized small interfering RNA (siRNA), small hairpin RNA (shRNAs), or micro RNA (miRNAs). Briefly, plasmid DNAs can be delivered to continuously transcribe shRNAs, which are then spliced by endogenous dicer proteins to release the corresponding siRNA. Tissue engineering scaffold systems can be used to deliver genes in a controlled and spatially localized manner [41]. This strategy has been widely used for tendon, ligament, skin, nerve, muscle, bone, cartilage, and periodontal regeneration [30].

Summary

Maxillofacial injuries, diseases, and conditions such as advanced and progressive periodontitis, edentulism-related ridge atrophy and sinus pneumatization, facial and dentoalveolar trauma, benign and malignant jaw lesions and defects related to their excision/resection and reconstruction, certain systematic diseases (like diabetes), and medication-related alveolar bone complications (like bisphosphonate-linked osteonecrosis of the jaws) can result in both tooth loss and alveolar bone resorption. The resulting craniofacial defects are often three-dimensional and involve loss of many tissue types (tooth, bone, and soft tissues), making functional repair of craniofacial deformities an especially intricate task. Even in healthy and dentate individuals, gradual bone resorption occurs and even endosseous implant restorations may not always stop this process. Optimal restoration of craniofacial bones and teeth requires multiple surgical procedures, and in certain cases bone and soft tissue defects have to be repaired first to provide sufficient support for subsequent tooth implant placement. The need for multiple surgeries results in prolonged duration and recovery time for the patient, resulting in extended periods of pain and suffering. Moreover, multiple surgical procedures introduce additional risks associated with the repeated tissue manipulation, administration of anesthesia, and perioperative medications.

Therefore, strategies to bioengineer functional tooth and alveolar bone that would efficiently develop in a coordinated manner with the surrounding and associated soft tissues would be a welcome solution. For example, the demonstrated successful use of autologous stem cells derived from an individual's tooth and bone, combined with suitable scaffold materials, could theoretically eventually be used to bioengineer functional teeth containing supporting roots, periodontium, and alveolar bone, in a single implantation surgery in the jaw. The interactions of scaffolds and bioactive agent-loaded delivery systems (i.e., nanoparticles and microparticles) is an interesting option for future directions. The demonstrated efficacy of biomaterial scaffolds, combined with drug and growth factor delivery systems for connective tissue regeneration, is a promising indication that similar approaches can eventually be used in alveolar complex regeneration.

Acknowledgments

This work was supported by NIH/NIDCR R01DE016132 (PCY).

References

1. Nanci A, Cate ART: *Ten Cate's Oral Histology: Development, Structure, and Function.* Mosby, 2003.
2. Lai WF, Lee JM, Jung HS: Molecular and engineering approaches to regenerate and repair teeth in mammals. *Cellular and Molecular Life Sciences* 2014;**71**(9):1691–1701.
3. Jernvall J, Thesleff I: Tooth shape formation and tooth renewal: evolving with the same signals. *Development* 2012;**139**(19):3487–3497.
4. Abukawa H, Zhang W, Young CS, Asrican R, Vacanti JP, Kaban LB, et al: Reconstructing mandibular defects using autologous tissue-engineered tooth and bone constructs. *Journal of Oral and Maxillofacial Surgery* 2009;**67**(2):335–347.
5. Pilipchuk SP, Plonka AB, Monje A, Taut AD, Lanis A, Kang B, et al: Tissue engineering for bone regeneration and osseointegration in the oral cavity. *Dental Materials* 2015;**31**(4):317–338.
6. Takahashi K, Kiso H, Saito K, Togo Y, Tsukamoto H, Huang B, Besho K: Feasibility of gene therapy for tooth regeneration by stimulation of a third dentition. In: Martin F. (ed.), *Gene Therapy: Tools and Potential Applications.* InTech, Rijeka, Croatia, 2013, pp. 727–744.
7. Otsu K, Kumakami-Sakano M, Fujiwara N, Kikuchi K, Keller L, Lesot H, et al: Stem cell sources for tooth regeneration: current status and future prospects. *Frontiers in Physiology* 2014;**5**:36.
8. Oshima M, Ogawa M, Yasukawa M, Tsuji T: Generation of a bioengineered tooth by using a three-dimensional cell manipulation method (organ germ method). *Methods in Molecular Biology (Clifton, NJ)* 2012;**887**:149–165.
9. Nakao K, Morita R, Saji Y, Ishida K, Tomita Y, Ogawa M, et al: The development of a bioengineered organ germ method. *Nature Methods* 2007;**4**(3):227–230.
10. Hirayama M, Oshima M, Tsuji T: Development and prospects of organ replacement regenerative therapy. *Cornea* 2013;**32**:S13–S21.
11. Zhang W, Ahluwalia IP, Yelick PC: Three dimensional dental epithelial-mesenchymal constructs of predetermined size and shape for tooth regeneration. *Biomaterials* 2010;**31**(31):7995–8003.
12. Liao S, Chan CK, Ramakrishna S: Stem cells and biomimetic materials strategies for tissue engineering. *Materials Science and Engineering C – Biomimetic and Supramolecular Systems* 2008;**28**(8):1189–1202.
13. Langer R, Vacanti JP: Tissue engineering. *Science* 1993;**260**(5110):920–926.
14. Yang MB, Zhang HM, Gangolli R: Advances of mesenchymal stem cells derived from bone marrow and dental tissue in craniofacial tissue engineering. *Current Stem Cell Research and Therapy* 2014;**9**(3):150–161.
15. Gronthos S, Mankani M, Brahim J, Robey PG, Shi S: Postnatal human dental pulp stem cells (DPSCs) *in vitro* and *in vivo*. *Proceedings of the National Academy of Sciences of the United States of America* 2000;**97**(25):13625–13630.
16. Miura M, Gronthos S, Zhao MR, Lu B, Fisher LW, Robey PG, et al: SHED: Stem cells from human exfoliated deciduous teeth. *Proceedings of the National Academy of Sciences of the United States of America* 2003;**100**(10):5807–5812.
17. Seo BM, Miura M, Gronthos S, Bartold PM, Batouli S, Brahim J, et al: Investigation of multipotent postnatal stem cells from human periodontal ligament. *Lancet* 2004;**364**(9429):149–155.
18. Morsczeck C, Gotz W, Schierholz J, Zellhofer F, Kuhn U, Mohl C, et al: Isolation of precursor cells (PCs) from human dental follicle of wisdom teeth. *Matrix Biology* 2005;**24**(2):155–165.
19. Sonoyama W, Liu Y, Yamaza T, Tuan RS, Wang S, Shi S, et al: Characterization of the apical papilla and its residing stem cells from human immature permanent teeth: a pilot study. *Journal of Endodontics* 2008;**34**(2):166–171.
20. Yuan ZL, Nie HM, Wang S, Lee CH, Li A, Fu SY, et al: Biomaterial selection for tooth regeneration. *Tissue Engineering Part B – Reviews* 2011;**17**(5):373–388.
21. Zhang L, Morsi Y, Wang Y, Li Y, Ramakrishna S: Review scaffold design and stem cells for tooth regeneration. *Japanese Dental Science Review* 2013;**49**(1):14–26.
22. Sowmya S, Bumgardener JD, Chennazhi KP, Nair SV, Jayakumar R: Role of nanostructured biopolymers and bioceramics in enamel, dentin and periodontal tissue regeneration. *Progress in Polymer Science* 2013;**38**(10–11):1748–1772.
23. Matsuno T, Omata K, Hashimoto Y, Tabata Y, Satoh T: Alveolar bone tissue engineering using composite scaffolds for drug delivery. *Japanese Dental Science Review* 2010;**46**(2):188–192.
24. Young CS, Terada S, Vacanti JP, Honda M, Bartlett JD, Yelick PC: Tissue engineering of complex tooth structures on biodegradable polymer scaffolds. *Journal of Dental Research* 2002;**81**(10):695–700.
25. Young CS, Abukawa H, Asrican R, Ravens M, Troulis MJ, Kaban LB, et al: Tissue-engineered hybrid tooth and bone. *Tissue Engineering* 2005;**11**(9–10):1599–1610.
26. Duailibi MT, Duailibi SE, Young CS, Bartlett JD, Vacanti JP, Yelick PC: Bioengineered teeth from cultured rat tooth bud cells. *Journal of Dental Research* 2004;**83**(7):523–528.
27. Zhang W, Abukawa H, Troulis MJ, Kaban LB, Vacanti JP, Yelick PC: Tissue engineered hybrid tooth-bone constructs. *Methods* 2009;**47**(2):122–128.

28 Zhang W, Ahluwalia IP, Literman R, Kaplan DL, Yelick PC: Human dental pulp progenitor cell behavior on aqueous and hexafluoroisopropanol based silk scaffolds. *Journal of Biomedical Materials Research Part A* 2011;**97**(4):414–422.

29 Traphagen SB, Fourligas N, Xylas JF, Sengupta S, Kaplan DL, Georgakoudi I, et al: Characterization of natural, decellularized and reseeded porcine tooth bud matrices. *Biomaterials* 2012;**33**(21):5287–5296.

30 Monteiro N, Martins A, Reis RL, Neves NM: Liposomes in tissue engineering and regenerative medicine. *Journal of the Royal Society Interface* 2014;**11**(101).

31 Chen FM, An Y, Zhang R, Zhang M: New insights into and novel applications of release technology for periodontal reconstructive therapies. *Journal of Controlled Release* 2011;**149**(2):92–110.

32 Cai X, Yang F, Yan X, Yang W, Yu N, Oortgiesen DAW, et al: Influence of bone marrow-derived mesenchymal stem cells pre-implantation differentiation approach on periodontal regeneration in vivo. *Journal of Clinical Periodontology* 2015;**42**(4):380–389.

33 Wang J, Liu X, Jin X, Ma H, Hu J, Ni L, et al: The odontogenic differentiation of human dental pulp stem cells on nanofibrous poly(L-lactic acid) scaffolds *in vitro* and *in vivo*. *Acta Biomaterialia* 2010;**6**(10):3856–3863.

34 Winn SR, Chen JC, Gong X, Bartholomew SV, Shreenivas S, Ozaki W: Non-viral-mediated gene therapy approaches for bone repair. *Orthodontics and Craniofacial Research* 2005;**8**(3):183–190.

35 Takahashi K, Nuckolls GH, Tanaka O, Semba I, Takahashi I, Dashner R, et al: Adenovirus-mediated ectopic expression of Msx2 in even-numbered rhombomeres induces apoptotic elimination of cranial neural crest cells *in ovo*. *Development* 1998;**125**(9):1627–1635.

36 Zhang Y, Wang Y, Shi B, Cheng X: A platelet-derived growth factor releasing chitosan/coral composite scaffold for periodontal tissue engineering. *Biomaterials* 2007;**28**(8):1515–1522.

37 Zhang Y, Cheng X, Wang J, Wang Y, Shi B, Huang C, et al: Novel chitosan/collagen scaffold containing transforming growth factor-β1 DNA for periodontal tissue engineering. *Biochemical and Biophysical Research Communications* 2006;**344**(1):362–369.

38 Jin QM, Anusaksathien O, Webb SA, Rutherford RB, Giannobile WV: Gene therapy of bone morphogenetic protein for periodontal tissue engineering. *Journal of Periodontology* 2003;**74**(2):202–213.

39 Zhang YF, Miron RJ, Li S, Shi B, Sculean A, Cheng XR: Novel MesoPorous BioGlass/silk scaffold containing adPDGF-B and adBMP7 for the repair of periodontal defects in beagle dogs. *Journal of Clinical Periodontology* 2015;**42**(3):262–271.

40 Monteiro N, Ribeiro D, Martins A, Faria S, Fonseca NA, Moreira JN, et al: Instructive nanofibrous scaffold comprising runt-related transcription factor 2 gene delivery for bone tissue engineering. *ACS Nano* 2014;**8**:8082–8094.

41 Yau WWY, Rujitanaroj P-O, Lam L, Chew SY: Directing stem cell fate by controlled RNA interference. *Biomaterials* 2012;**33**(9):2608–2628.

Index

A
ABBG. *see* autogenous block bone graft (ABBG)
absorbable collagen sponge (ACS), 262, 317
acellular dermal connective tissue grafts (ADCTs), 292
acellular dermal matrix (ADM), 291, 295
active osteogenic, 323
ADCTs. *see* acellular dermal connective tissue grafts (ADCTs)
ADM. *see* acellular dermal matrix (ADM)
ADO. *see* alveolar distraction osteogenesis (ADO)
adult dental stem cells (DSCs), 337
age-related changes
  in maxilla and mandible, 71
aging, 71
  changes associated with, 71
  craniofacial, 72
AIC. *see* anterior iliac crest (AIC)
algisorb™, 113, 114, 117
algorithm for risk factor, 73
allogeneic block, 321
  bone, 321
allogeneic bone, 270
allografts, 75, 82, 295
alloplasts, 82, 270
alveolar bone, 30, 33, 34
  distraction, 222
  resorption, 338
alveolar complex, 335
alveolar defect, 62
alveolar distraction osteogenesis (ADO), 5, 222, 229, 233
  advantage, 224, 233
  alveolar width
    for implant placement, 242
  anterior maxillary post-traumatic defect, 226
  biological rationale of, 222, 223
  block graft, 242
  case report, 241, 242
  complications
    management of, 238
    rates, 225–227
    time line of, 239
  contraindications, 223
  cutting jig, 240
  deficient bone width, 242
  devices
    extraosseous distractors, 224
    intraosseous devices, 225
  disadvantages, 224
  distraction rod, 239
  distractor arm plate, 240
  implant placement, 225
  indications, 223
  intraoperative complications
    bone osteotomies, 240
    failed osteotomy, 239
    hardware failure, 239, 240
    poor incision design, 239
    poor soft tissue management, 240
  orthodontic wire, 239
  phases of
    consolidation (phase 4), 224
    distraction (phase 3), 223, 224
    latency (phase 2), 223
    surgery (phase 1), 223
  post-consolidation complications
    inadequate bone formation, in distraction chamber, 241
    inadequate height, 241
  post-operative complications, 240
    device dehiscence, 240
    device failure, 240
    incorrect vector, 239, 240
    infection, 240
    pain, 240
  pre-operative complications
    failure to control, 238
    failure to diagnose, 238
    failure to execute, 238
    wrong distractor, 239
  protocol for, 231
  radiograph, 242
  screws and distractor failure, 239
  surgical principles and treatment planning, 223
  surgical rationale of, 222
  vector control, 225
  wound dehiscence
    at beginning of distraction, 241
    distraction rate, 241
alveolar distraction process, 232
alveolar distraction surgery, for implant site development
  choosing a distractor, 203, 204
  clinical examination, 203
    evaluation of hard tissue, 203
    evaluation of soft tissue, 203

alveolar distraction surgery, for implant site development (*Continued*)
   prosthetic requirements for final prosthesis, 203
   radiographs, 203
  contraindications, 202
  diagnosis and treatment planning, 203
  distraction osteogenesis (*see* distraction osteogenesis (DO))
  Garcia-Garcia classification of post-distraction defects, 219
  indications, 202
  osteotomy design, 204, 205
  planning implant placement into distracted alveolar bone, 219
   type II distracted bone, 219
   type III distracted bone, 219, 220
   type I shaped bone, 219
   type IV distracted bone, 220
  planning surgery, 203
  preparing distractor for surgery, 204
  regional anatomic considerations, 203
   anterior mandible, 203
   anterior maxilla, 203
   posterior mandible, 203
   posterior maxilla, 203
  screw size, 205
  steps of distraction osteogenesis surgery, 204, 205
  stereolithic models, 203
  vector in alveolar distraction, 203
alveolar mucosa, 3
alveolar ridge, 33, 34
alveolar ridge augmentation, 31, 83, 84
  classification of, 4
alveolar ridge reconstruction techniques, 3
alveolar ridge/socket preservation, 83
  with moderate buccal bone destruction, 83
  with no or minimal buccal bone destruction, 83
  with severe buccal bone destruction, 83
anatomy of mandible, 7
  anatomic variation of mandibular canal, 9
  coronal cross-section of cone beam computed tomography, 8
  critical vascular structures, 11, 12
  facial nerve, 11
  foramina and canals, 7
  glossopharyngeal nerve, 11
  lingual nerve, 11
  lingual nerve and lingual crest of mandible, 11
  major sensory nerves located within, 9
  mental nerve with the overlying depressor anguli oris muscle, 10
  neurovascular structures, 8–11
  orthopantomogram of implant, 8
  sublingual artery, 11
anatomy of maxilla, 12
  foramina and canals, 12
  maxillary sinus, 12
  palatine foramen, 12
  Schneiderian membrane, 12
angiogenesis, 326
angiogenic competency, 323
angular bone defect, 31
Ankylos®, 126
anterior iliac crest (AIC), 251, 323
  bone marrow aspiration, 323

anterior inferior iliac spine (AIIS), 251
anterior mandible, 19
  implants positioned in, 19
anterior maxilla
  after extraction illustrates thin interseptal and buccal bone, 73
  buccal view after extractions, 86
  facial and lingual grafting with autogenous bone to reconstruct, 75
  flap advanced and closed primarily, 76
  flaps elevated and bone exposed, 76
  grafting crestally with symbios non-resorbable OsteoGraf LD-300 and, 76
  for a male patient, 73
  reconstructed to compensate for facial resorption, 76
  residual defect subsequent to implant removal in, 74
anterior maxilla, vertical alveolar distraction of, 234
anterior–posterior component, 229
anterior–posterior (AP) maxillary bone projection, 232
anterior/posterior (AP) spread, 18, 19
anterior superior iliac spine (ASIS), 251
ASIS. *see* anterior superior iliac spine (ASIS)
aspiration sites, 323
associated vertical alveolar bone loss, 33
atrophic edentulous mandible, 102
atrophic jaws, 14
atrophic posterior maxilla, 161
atrophy, 15, 71
augmentation, 3, 270
  alveolar ridge, 7
  performed on sinus side, 16
augment deficient, 286
augmented bone, 125
autogenous block bone graft (ABBG), 121, 222, 229
autogenous block grafts, in implant dentistry
  "A III" defect, 257
  anatomic repositioning, 260
   distraction osteogenesis (DO), 260
   inferior alveolar nerve lateralization, 260, 261
  anterior iliac crest bone grafting
   for vertical ridge augmentation, 266–269
  anterior iliac crest schematic, 254, 255
  anterior maxilla, defects, 260
  anterior maxillary defect, with missing central incisor, 249
  BiCAT, 259
  bone grafting materials
   allogeneic bone, 256, 257
   alloplastic bone, 257
   autogenous bone, 256
   xenogeneic bone, 257
  bone grafting techniques, 257–260
  bone harvest site, from anterior mandible, 250
  bone marrow, derived MSCs, 265
  bone regeneration, cell therapy for, 264
  case reports, 266–270
  CAT, posterior mandible, 258
  CAT, vertical/horizontal, 258
  CTA, bilateral, 258
  CTA, simultaneous implant placement, 259
  defect analysis, 247
  distraction osteogenesis (DO)
   advantages and disadvantages of, 261

donor sites, for block bone, 248
  extraoral harvest, 250
    anterior iliac crest (AIC), 251, 252
    calvarium, 252–254
    posterior iliac crest (PIC), 250, 251
  graft preparation/fixation
    bone grafting principles, 255, 256
  HA/TCP for, 265
  history of bone grafting, 247
  inferior alveolar nerve lateralization (IANL)
    advantages and disadvantages of, 261
  intraoral harvest, 248
    chin, 248–250
    ramus, 248
  Le Fort I osteotomy and block bone, 270
  mesenchymal stem cells, 263
  MSCs, morphologic characteristics of, 263
  nerve skeletonization, 262
  onlay block graft (OBG)
    advantages and disadvantages of, 260
  position of facial nerve, 256
  posterior iliac crest harvesting, 252, 253
  recipient site classification, 247
  regenerative techniques, in bone grafting, 261
    mesenchymal stem cells, 263–270
    RhBMP-2, 261–263
  stellate adherent MSCs, under light microscopy, 263
  tibial bone grafting for vertical ridge augmentation, 269, 270
  wall defect, 248
autogenous bone, 20, 323
  grafting, 222, 270
autogenous epithelized palatal grafts, 291
autogenous onlay grafts, 19
autografts, 82
autologous concentrated growth factors, 167

B
baseball type sutures, 318
benign paroxysmal positional vertigo (BPPV), 149
beta tricalcium phosphate, 99
bidirectional crest distractor, 230
bilateral CAT (biCAT), 257
bioactive agent reservoirs, 339
bioactive agents, 339
  for tooth-bone regeneration, 339
biocompatibility, 81
biodegradable scaffolds, 339
bioengineer teeth, 339
biologic width
  around implants, 23
  and soft tissue esthetics, 22–24
bleeding, 309
block allograft, 327
  histomorphometric analysis of, 327
block bone grafting, 5, 26, 93, 257, 321
  cortical autogenous tenting (CAT) technique, 257
  three-dimensional reconstruction technique, 257
bone atrophy, 3
bone augmentation, 3, 291, 323
bone biopsy, 129
bone classification, 110

bone deficiency, 229
bone elongation, 231
bone graft(ing), 4, 14, 135, 323
  history of, 247
  materials, 82
  selection, 82
  studies, 247
bone loss, due to trauma, 231
bone marrow aspiration, 323
  application of, 326
  complications, 326
    aspiration needle, improper positioning, 326
    needle repositioning, 326
  rationale for, 327
bone marrow stromal cells (BMSCs), 337, 338
bone maturity, 320
bone morphogenetic proteins (BMPs), 232, 261, 339
bone preservation, 3
bone quality, 52
  classification, 53
bone regeneration, 110, 320
  cell therapy for, 264
bone remodeling, 321
bone replacement materials, 14
bone resorption, 33, 121
bone shape, classification, 53
bone sialoprotein-positive bone, 338
bone splitting, 93
bone trimming, 15
bovine-derived porous mineral, 86
bovine factor Va, 316
BPPV. *see* benign paroxysmal positional vertigo (BPPV)
bridge
  design, 21
  prostheses, 15
  splint, 20
buccal bone surface defect, 227
buccolingual ridge width atrophy, 34

C
CAD/CAM titanium metal frames, 15
CAF. *see* coronally advanced flap (CAF)
calcium sulfate, 82
Caldwell-Luc approach, 135, 178, 198
Cantilever length formula, for implant-supported
    prostheses, 20
cantilever lengths, 19
case reports, 328
  advanced periodontal disease with soft tissue loss, need for
      temporary fixed restoration, 53–55
  alveolar distraction osteogenesis procedure, 241, 242
  anterior maxilla, resorption of, 328
  atrophic edentulous mandible at right premolar–molar side
      region, 105–108
  autogenous block grafts, in implant dentistry, 266–270
  complications, 183
  diminished alveolar bone, 331
  distraction osteogenesis (DO)
    ankylosed teeth, 216–218
    anterior mandible, 205–210
    posterior maxilla, 211–216

case reports (*Continued*)
    fractured upper right central incisor root resulting in acute abscess and bone loss, need for autogenous bone graft, 55, 56
    implant fenestration, 87–89
    lateral approach to sinus floor elevation for delayed implant placement, 181–183
    lateral incisor site, osseous defect, 330
    management of atrophic
      anterior maxilla, 98, 99
      posterior maxilla, 99–101
    management of severely atrophic edentulous mandible, 102–105
    mandible, 234, 235
    maxillary, 234, 235
    maxillary/mandibular post-traumatic alveolar bone defects, 234, 235
    peri-implantitis treatment with bone regeneration, 89–91
    piezoelectric sandwich technique with interpositional bone graft for vertical augmentation of severely atrophic
      anterior mandibular alveolar ridge, 127–131
      posterior mandibular alveolar ridge, 122–127
    socket preservation, 85, 86
    tonsillar squamous cell carcinoma, 278, 279
CAT. *see* category scales (CAT)
category scales (CAT), 17
cavitation effect, 121
CBCT. *see* cone beam computed tomography (CBCT)
CCFDAB. *see* crushed cancellous freeze-dried allogeneic bone (CCFDAB)
cell delivery methods, 264
cellular proliferation, 318
ceramic restoration, 130
CGF. *see* concentrated growth factors (CGF)
chlorhexidine gluconate, 324
chromic gut sutures, 86
clindamycin, 145, 309
clinical
    risks, 76
    training, 7
coagulation disorders, 311
collagen, 82
    plug, 86
complications, 308
    post-operative, 309
computed tomography (CT), 39, 238, 277
    maxillary left lateral incisor area prior to implant placement, 87
    maxillary right central incisor area prior to implant placement, 87
    for vertical/horizontal bone defect in mandibular left canine and premolar area, 122
computer-aided design/computer-aided machining (CAD/CAM) abutment, 33
computer-assisted design (CAD) software, 277
concentrated growth factors (CGF), 163, 176
    case report, 164–167
    centrifuge to prepare CGF and sticky bone, 172
    minimally invasive ridge augmentation
      using CGF membrane and growth factor-enriched putty, 171
    preparation of fibrin-rich block with, 163, 164

cone beam computed tomography (CBCT), 38, 39, 138, 238
    coronal section showing nasal cavity and maxillary sinuses, 43
    cross-sectional image to evaluate implant placed in mandibular right premolar region, 51
    crosssections through mandibular edentulous area, 42
    cross-section through edentulous region, 46
    effective doses and dentomaxillofacial radiographic examinations, 51
    guidelines and position statements on, 49–51
    image, 33
      of alveolar bone of edentulous right maxillary second premolar, 145
    mandibular canal and opening of mental foramen, 45
    midsagittal section showing nasopalatine canal and, 43
    ocations of mandibular canal and exit of mandibular canal, 46
    pneumatization of maxillary sinus following tooth loss, 136
    pneumatized maxillary sinus and decreased vertical height of residual alveolus, 138
    principles of, 39
    radiation risks from examinations, 48, 49
    sagittal and coronal images demonstrating patency of ostium/osteomeatal complex (OMC), 136
    sagittal and coronal sections
      through premolar and molar teeth, 43
    sagittal sections through anterior mandible, 46
    section large area of osteosclerosis in edentulous ridge., 47
    sections for implant planning in the maxillary right molar region, 44
    sinus pathology seen on, 138
    technical parameters, 39
      field of view (FOV), 40
      image detector, 39
      number of basis projections, 39, 40
      voxel size, 40
      X-ray exposure parameters, 40
congenital tooth agenesis, 36
connective tissue (CT), 304
connective tissue graft (CTG), 304
contemporary periodontology, 292
conventional denture, 20
conventional maxillary prostheses, 17
conventional radiography, 38
coronally advanced flap (CAF), 291, 295
cortical autogenous tenting, 5
corticocancellous bone, 19
corticosteroids, 95
craniofacial changes, 72
craniofacial variations, 73
crestal bone remodeling, 24
crestal incision, 33
crestal sinus floor elevation, 144
    applied surgical anatomy, 144, 145
    complications, 148, 149
    contraindications, 144
    graft sources, 145
    history, 144
    indications, 144
    indirect/transalveolar, with implant placement, 145–147
      CBCT scan demonstrating implant position, 147
    location of osteomeatal complex (OMC), 145
    subantral maxillary alveolar bone

compressed apically and laterally with progressively larger osteotomes, 145
trans-socket sinus floor elevation
  with bone grafting after extraction, 147, 148
  completion of a socket bone grafting, 150
  interseptal bone and socket after, 149
  management of a pinpoint perforation during, 149
  postoperative CBCT after implant placement, 150
  post-operative imaging confirming, 150
  radiographic image of a "snow capped peak," 150
crown design, 21
crown fracture, 34
crushed cancellous freeze-dried allogeneic bone (CCFDAB), 315
CT. see computed tomography (CT); connective tissue (CT)
CTG. see connective tissue graft (CTG)
cutaneous–vermillion junction, 7
cutting guides, 240

D

decalcified freeze-dried bone allografts (DFDBAs), 82
decortication, 94, 106
defects, types of, 61
definitive implant-supported primary bar, 20
definitive mandibular resin to titanium CAD/CAM hybrid denture prosthesis, 24
definitive maxillary ceramometal screw-retained fixed prosthesis, 24
definitive maxillary overpartial denture prosthesis, 25
definitive "wrap around" CAD/CAM hybrid denture prosthesis design, 26
delayed orthodontic space opening, 34
dental follicle progenitor stem cells (DFPCs), 338
dental implants, 3, 14, 81, 135, 278
  placed in anterior mandible, 19
  surgery, 7
dental mesenchymal progenitor cells, 339
dental prosthesis, 14
dental pulp stem cells (DPSCs), 337, 339
  cultured on PLLA nanofiber scaffolds, 339
dentin, 335
dentistry, 3
deproteinated bovine bone mineral, 33
deproteinized bovine bone matrix (DBBM), 93
design and construction, of prosthesis, 21
DFDBAs. see decalcified freeze-dried bone allografts (DFDBAs)
diagnostic imaging objectives, 40–48
  anatomical structures and variations and pathological conditions, 41
    anatomic variants, 45
    mandibular canal, 44
    maxillary sinus, 41
    nasal cavity, 41
    nasopalatine canal and incisive foramen, 41
  architecture and quality of trabecular and cortical bone, 41
  morphology of edentulous site and, 41
  post-surgical implant complications, 47
  pre-surgical/post-surgical evaluation of bone augmentation, 46
  specific diagnostic objectives of radiographic imaging, 40
diagnostic wax-up., 139
digital imaging, 17
distraction, 231

poor vector control/direction of, 227
distraction osteogenesis (DO), 65, 93, 110, 113, 201, 260
  advantages, 67, 261
  anterior mandible, 67
  basic principles of, 201
    distraction period, 201
    injury (osteotomy) to the bone via, 201
    latency period, 201
    period of consolidation, 201
  case reports
    ankylosed teeth, 216–218
    anterior mandible, 205–210
    posterior maxilla, 211–216
  disadvantages, 67, 261
  plan for, 203
  steps of surgery, 204, 205
divergent implants, 58
DO. see distraction osteogenesis (DO)
donor site necrosis, 311
DPSCs. see dental pulp stem cells (DPSCs)
d-PTFE. see Titanium reinforced dense-polytetrafluoroethylene (d-PTFE)

E

edema, 316
edentulous mandible, 20
  treatment options, 18
    conventional denture, 18
    fixed hybrid denture, 18
    implant-retained overdenture, 18
    implant-supported overdenture, 18
edentulous maxilla, 20
  treatment options for, 19
edentulous patient, 16
embryologically bone development, 254
endochondral bone formation, 254
endosseous bone loading (EBL), 3
endosseous dental implant, 14
endosseous implants, 7, 14, 19, 20
endosteal, 5
epithelial–mesenchymal interactions, 335
esthetic challenges, 14
esthetic demands, 72
evaluation, of patient, 61
expanded polytetrafluoroethylene (e-PTFE), 81
  suture, 305
extensive alveolar defect, 231
extracellular matrix (ECM), 337, 338

F

fabrication of removable prostheses, 14
facial vein, 135
fenestration/dehiscence formation, 32
FGGs. see free gingival grafts (FGGs)
fibroblast growth factor (FGF-2), 339
fibula free flap, 275, 276, 280
  anterior incision, 276
  distal and proximal osteotomies, 276
  fibula osteocutaneous free flap, 279
    inset of, 279
  flap debulking and placing of dental implants, 278

fibula free flap (*Continued*)
   free double skin paddle fibula flap, 278
   pre-operative markings of, 276
fibula osteocutaneous flap, 275, 281
fixed bridges, 3
fixed crown, 15, 20
fixed–detachable hybrid prosthesis, 15
fixed hybrid denture, 20
fixed, one-piece full-arch prosthesis, 19
fixed partial denture, 88
fixed restorations, 16, 21
   options, for edentulous maxilla, 21
fixed toothborne prostheses, 3
flapless crestal sinus floor augmentation procedure, 152
   advantages, 157
     in patients with antral septum, 157
     in patients with severely atrophic maxillae, 157
   CBCT scans
     immediately after surgery, 157, 159
     of severely atrophic ridge, 158
   grafting material, 157–159
   specimen of Bio-Oss collagen sponge, 159
   surgical instruments, 152
     bone plugger, 152
     digital surgical guide, 153
     dome-shaped crestal approach bur, 152
     hydraulic membrane lifter, 152
     osteotomy drill, 152
     sinus curette, 152
     stopper, 152
   technique, 153
     pre-operative protocol, 153, 154
     surgical protocol, 154
       drill osteotomy, 154
       expanding the opening hole of the sinus floor, 156
       grafting procedure, 156
       immediate restoration/installing a healing abutment, 156
       implant placement, 156
       membrane elevation, 154
       membrane integrity test, 155
       penetrating bony sinus floor, 154
       radiographic evaluation, 157
flapless surgery, 55
"flat-thick" gingival architecture., 54
four-dimensional (4D) tissue augmentation, 4
free connective tissue graft, 304
free distant bone flap transfer, 5
free fibula osteocutaneous flap harvest technique, 276, 277
free gingival grafts (FGGs), 291, 305
freeze-dried bone, 257
freeze-dried bone allografts (FDBAs), 82

G

GBR. *see* guided bone regeneration (GBR)
gene silencing mechanism, 340
gene therapy, 339
GFs. *see* growth factors (GFs)
gingival architecture, 52, 74
gingival soft tissue, 23
goblet cells, 137
graft destabilization, 308

grafted bone, 19
graft harvesting, 292
graft infection, 309
grafting, 144
   material, 14
     selection of, 75
   sources, categories, 179
graft necrosis, 309
graft revascularization, 5, 321
growth factors (GFs), 339
growth of alveolar process, 12
guided bone regeneration (GBR), 3, 31, 62, 66, 93, 121, 222
   advantages, 62
   anterior maxilla, 66
   disadvantages, 62
   posterior mandible, 66

H

hard–soft palate junction, 7
hard tissue management, 56
Haversian systems, 319
healing abutments, and sutured flap, 88
hemangioendothelioma
   case report, 279, 280
histomorphometric analysis, 326
horizontal augmentation, 14, 33
horizontal bone deficiency, 201
horizontal crest distractor, 230
horizontal defects
   within alveolar housing, 84
   that require augmentation, 84
horizontal osseous grafts, 25
horizontal widening of alveolar crest (horizontal PSP), 115
   clinical examples, 116
     horizontal two-step PSP in posterior mandible, 116
   one-step method, 116–118
   osteotomies, 119
   two-step method, 115, 116, 118
horseshoe design, 21
HPISE. *see* hydrodynamic piezoelectric sinus augmentation (HPISE)
HV-type defect, 96
hybrid denture, 21
   prostheses, 17, 19, 21
hybrid dentures, 19
hybrid mandibular denture prosthesis, 19
hybrid tooth-bone TE constructs, 338
hybrid tooth-bone tissues, 338
hydraulic sinus condensing (HSC) technique, 167
hydrodynamic piezoelectric sinus augmentation (HPISE), 167
   bone graft optional after elevation of sinus mucosa, 169
   case report, 169–171
   first step, 168
   second step, 168
   simultaneous implant placement, 169
   surgical procedure of, 168
hydrogels, 338
hygiene, 15
hyperglycemia, 309
hypertrophy, 71
hypoxia-inducible factor 1α (HIF-1α), 232

I

iliac crest free flap, 281
Ilizarov effects, 229
implant abutment junction, 25
implant dentistry, 3, 315
    dental implants depend on factors, 3
implant-driven bone augmentation procedures, 3
implant macrostructure considerations, 74
implant placement, 144
    using osteotome technique, 144
implant-placement sites, 323
implant-retained
    mandibular overdenture, 18
    maxillary overdenture, 20
    maxillary prostheses, 21
implants into residual bone with/without hard tissue
        augmentation, 58, 59
implant site development
    protocol, 289
implants osseointegration, 320
implants positioned at angles, up to, 19
implant-supported
    ceramometal prosthesis, 17
    fixed prostheses, 19
    mandibular overdenture, 18
    maxillary overdentures, 21
    overdentures, 19, 20, 21
        primary bar, 15
    prostheses, 19, 21, 125
implant tenting, 5
implant therapy, keys to success in, 53
implant thread geometry, 74
implant treatment
    challenges, 52
    planning, 72
improved crown–implant ratio, 229
indications
    for particulate grafts after implant placement, 84
    for particulate grafts in conjunction with implant
        placement, 84
induce stem cell differentiation, 340
inferior alveolar nerve lateralization (IANL), 260, 261
    advantages and disadvantages of, 261
inferior border grafts, 19
INFUSE® bone graft, 262
INLAY grafts, 5
innate immunity, 7
INR. see international normalized ratio (INR)
intaglio
    of definitive implant-supported mandibular overdenture
        prosthesis, 20
    of definitive maxillary implant
        -retained overdenture prosthesis, 21
        -supported overdenture prosthesis, 22
    of definitive maxillary prosthesis, 16
    of maxillary overpartial denture prosthesis, 25
interdental papilla, 52, 53
interference RNA (RNAi), 340
intermolar distance, 71
international normalized ratio (INR), 311
international team for implantology (ITI), 288

interpositional alveolar bone graft, 121
interpositional bone graft, 19, 65, 186
interproximal bone on adjacent central
        incisor, 27
interproximal papilla, 33
interproximal soft tissue, 25
intraosseous alveolar distractor, 226
intraosseous distraction
    with distraction device, 231
    with implants, 231

J

Jamshidi-type needle, 324
jawbone augmentation techniques, classiication, 111

K

Kaplan–Meier analysis, 97
keratinization, 32, 33
keratinized gingiva (KG), 293, 302
keratinized tissue (KT), 286, 287
KG. see keratinized gingiva (KG)
KT. see keratinized tissue (KT)

L

labial inclination, 304
lactide/glycolide copolymers, 82
lateral ramus cortical bone (LRCB), 257
lateral sinus augmentation, 162
    using autologous concentrated growth factors
        alone, 162
lateral sinus floor elevation and grafting, 178
    applied surgical anatomy, 178, 179
    CBCT images, 180
    contraindications, 178
    for delayed implant placement, 179, 180
        case report:, 181–183
    indications, 178
    intraoperative photograph of a sinus perforation, 183
    pre-operative and post-operative radiographs, 184
    surgical technique, 179
LEAD distractor system, 225
Le Fort I osteotomy, 65
ligament, 340
lithotripsy, 121
localized defects, 247
lymphatic drainage, 135

M

macrophages, 137
malocclusion, mandibular reconstruction, 276
management
    atrophic anterior maxilla, case report, 98, 99
    complications associated with particulate grafts, 84, 85
        encapsulation of particulate grafts and need for
            retreatment, 85
        infection, 85
        membrane exposure, 85
    maxillary and mandibular
        post-traumatic alveolar bone defects, 229–236
    severely atrophic edentulous mandible, case report,
        102–105

mandibular
    algorithm of alveolar bone augmentation, 64
    angle, 71
    atrophy, 19
    body, vertical alveolar distraction of, 235
    fracture, 233
    immediate load prostheses, 24
    implants, 17
    and maxillary cross-sectional shapes, 52
    premolars, 34
    reconstruction, double-barrel approach, 275
    ridge, knife edge edentulous, 321
mastication, 7
maxillary
    algorithm of alveolar bone augmentation, 63
    anterior alveolar ridge, 226
    arches, 15, 17, 20, 21
    bones, 135
    case report, 234, 235
    complete dentures, 17
    dentition, 16
    fixed and removable prostheses, 17
    immediate load prostheses, 24
    implant prostheses, 17
    implants with large AP spread, 21
    lateral incisors, 34
    left central incisor, 33
    ostium, 135
    overdentures prosthesis, 17
    prosthesis implant retained, 280
    screw retained implant-supported ceramometal splints, 24
    sinus, 135
        grafting, 178
        lift with particulate graft, 65
    teeth, 135, 136
    tuberosity, 291
    vertical ridge augmentation, 320
maxillary/mandibular post-traumatic alveolar bone defects
    alveolar distraction osteogenesis (ADO), 229
        complications and disadvantages of, 233
        description of method, 231
    bidirectional crest distractor, 230
    bone resorption, 232
    case report, 234, 235
    consolidation period, 231, 232
    different distraction devices, 230, 231
    distraction osteogenesis, 229, 232
        advantages of, 232, 233
    distraction, vector controlling, 232
    guided bone regeneration (GBR), 229
    latency period, 231, 232
    osteogenic molecules/stem cells, use of, 232
    rate of bone elongation, 231, 232
    survival of implants, 232
    unidirectional/bidirectional/horizontal, 229
    unidirectional extraosseous distraction osteogenesis, 230
maxillectomy, surgical defect, 279
maxillomandibular complex, 7
mCAT. *see* multiple cortical autogenous tenting (mCAT)
MDCT. *see* multidetector computed tomography (MDCT)
medication-related osteonecrosis of the jaws (MRONJ), 178

membrane materials, 81
mental foramen, 18
    osteotomy, 261
mentalis muscle, 128
mesenchymal stem cells (MSCs), 232, 263, 328
    on HA/TCP, 265
    morphologic characteristics, 263, 265
mesh pores, 93
mesialization, 36
metal housings, 15
micrometric cut, 121
micro RNA (miRNAs), 340
microvascular anastomosis, 5
microvascular free flaps
    discussion, 280, 281
mild-to-moderate alveolar bone, 229
Miller class 3 recession defect, 33
mineralization processes, 328
minimal alveolar reduction, 19
minimally invasive ridge augmentation
    case report, 173–175
    preparation of sticky bone, 172
    using CGF membrane and growth factor-enriched putty conditioned bone, 171, 172
missing or failing teeth, 3
moderate-to-severe alveolar bone deficiency, 229
molecular signals, 339
morbidity, 7
MSCs. *see* mesenchymal stem cells (MSCs)
mucogingival junction, 249
mucoperiosteal dissection, 123
mucoperiosteal reflection, 231
mucous membrane, 136
multidetector computed tomography (MDCT), 39
multiple cortical autogenous tenting (mCAT), 257
multiple implant supported crowns, 26–28

N
natural bone modeling and remodeling, 81
natural dentition, 3
natural ECM protein gradients, 339
natural teeth, 23
nerve relocation, 261
nerve skeletonization, 261
neural crest cell (NCC)-derived dental mesenchymal cells, 339
neurosensory dysethesia (NSD), 260
next generation titanium mesh. *see* Ultraflex mesh plate®
non-resorbable hydroxylapatite (HA) particles, 178
nonresorbable membranes, 81
non-splinted stud attachments, 18
non-vascular block bone, 247

O
occlusal interference, 233
occlusal tooth reduction, 33
odontoblasts, 339
odontogenesis, 339
OISS. *see* orthodontic implant site switching (OISS)
OMC. *see* osteomeatal complex (OMC)
one-piece three BioHorizons implants, 130
onlay block grafting, 68

advantages, 68
anterior and posterior distant (extraoral) maxillary block grafts, 68
anterior maxillary
   localized block graft, 68
   ramus graft, 68
disadvantages, 69
mandibular continuity defect, 68
posterior mandible: block graft, 68
onlay (veneer) extraoral (hip, rib, calvarium), 3
ONLY grafts, 5
oral cavity, 7
oral hygiene, 285
orthodontic extrusion, 31–34
   for implant site development, 33
   of maxillary left central incisor, 33
   treatment protocols, 31
orthodontic extrusive remodelling, 31
orthodontic implant site development, 30, 31
orthodontic implant site switching (OISS), 34–36
orthodontic retention, 36
orthodontic therapy, 30, 34
orthodontic tooth movement, 36
osseointegrated dental implants, 277
osseointegration, 3, 14, 125, 137
osseous tissue, 14, 25
   around an endosseous implant, 25
   preservation, 15
ossification, 4, 5, 67, 233, 328
   maxilla, 135
osteoblasts, 255, 318
osteocalcin, 338
osteomeatal complex (OMC), 135, 138, 178
osteoperiosteal flap ridge-split procedure, 62
   advantages, 62
   disadvantages, 65
osteoprogenitor cells, 315, 319
osteoradionecrosis
   pre-operative CT scan, 278
osteotomies, 62, 144, 275, 277
   bone and appropriate execution of, 225
   design, 238
   instruments, 121
otolaryngology, 178
overdenture prostheses, 21

P

Palacci–Ericsson classification of alveolar ridge, 52
palatal base materia, 21
palatal placement, 34
palatine artery, 311
palatine nerves, 135
papillae regeneration technique, 57
partially edentulous patient, 22
   general treatment options, 22
particulate bone and marrow (PCBM), 93
particulate bone grafts, 5, 88, 90
   indications for, 83
particulate grafts combined with GBR
   in ridge preservation, 83
pathologic diseases, 30

patient preparation, 61
patient selection, 61
pedicle flap, 293
pedicle grafts, 57
penicillin allergy, 309
periodontal ligament, 136
periodontal ligament stem cells (PDLSCs), 338
periodontal plastic surgery, 291, 309
   procedures, 288
periodontal regeneration *in vivo* using rat BMSC, 339
periosteal, 5
   tenting, 5
periosteum, 95, 113, 293
permanent teeth, 34, 136
phlebotomy, 315
physiologic dentistry, era of, 3
physiologic treatment, 3
piezoelectric approach, 121
piezoelectric bone surgery, 121, 131
piezoelectric inserts, for sinus augmentation, 161
   round carbide tip, 161
   round diamond-coated tip, 161
   saw insert, 161
piezoelectric instruments, 181
piezoelectric internal sinus elevation (PISE), 167
piezoelectric sandwich osteotomy, 131
piezoelectric sandwich technique
   with interpositional bone graft for vertical augmentation of severely atrophic
      anterior mandibular alveolar ridge, 127–131
      posterior mandibular alveolar ridge, 122–127
piezoelectric surgery, 121
   device, 121, 131, 161, 162
piezoelectric surgical instruments, 121
   advantages of, 121
pink esthetic score (PES), 285
pink prosthetic material, 21
plaque accumulation, 285
platelet-derived growth factor (PDGF), 176
platelet rich plasma (PRP), 315
plating, 277
PLGA scaffolds, 338
PLLA nanofiber scaffolds, 339
pneumatization, 135, 136
   maxillary sinus, 136
polyethyleneglycol, 82
polyglactice-910, 82
polyglycolic acid, 82
polylactic acid, 82
polymeric 3D scaffold for TE applications, 338
polyurethane, 82
poor esthetics, resulting from vertical tissue loss, 27
porcine collagen matrix, 291
posterior atrophy, 18
posterior iliac crest (PIC), 250
   harvesting with muscular attachments and cluneal nerves marked, 252
posterior iliac crest bone graft (PICBG), 250
posterior mandible, 74
   tendency for movement of bone is from medial to lateral, 75

posterior maxilla, 74, 135, 186
    craniofacial changes over time influence on, 75
posterior maxillary sandwich osteotomy, 186
    CBCT image, 191
    clinical application, 186
    combined with sinus floor grafting, 186
    intraoperative photograph
        depicting a segment of bone, 190
        placement of three endosseous implants, 191
        removal of hardware, 191
        secondary buccal grafting with xenograft, 191
        showing curved lateral osteotomy, 189
        of wound closure, 190
    palatal osteotomy, 187
    post-operative periapical radiographs of placed dental
            implants, 192
    pre-operative
        lateral view, 189
        panoramic image, 189
    technique, 186
    vertically deficient maxilla approached via vestibular
            incision, 187
posterior segmental osteotomy, biological rationale, 186
post-natal dental pulp stem cells (DPSCs), 337
postoperative morbidity, 323
post-treatment smile, 25
precision in implant placement, 56–58
pre-implant era, 3
primary bar, secured implants with a large AP spread, 22
primary bar secured to four interforaminally positioned
        implants, 18
progenitor cells, 337, 338
prophylactic antibiotics, 309
prosthetic appliances, 81
prosthetic designs, 15, 18
prosthetic material, 21
prosthetic teeth, 14
PRP. see platelet rich plasma (PRP)
psychometric measurements, 17
pterygoid plexus, 135
punch technique, 303

Q
quality of life, 81

R
radial forearm fasciocutaneous free flap, 281
radiological evaluation of jaws, 38
radiological information, 38
ramus block graft
    surgical technique for, 248
reconstructive ridge preservation/augmentation procedures, 81
reconstructive surgeries, 30
reduced surgical noise, 121
regenerative material selection, 81
regenerative medicine (RM), 337
removable dentures, 3
removable toothborne prostheses, 3
reserve implant-based dental rehabilitation, 277
resorbable membranes, 81, 82, 85, 88
    adapted over the grafted area, 90
    advantages, 82
    disadvantages, 82
restorative (reconstructive) dentistry, 3
restorative designs, 21
restorative dimension, 15
revascularization, 318
rhBMP-2, mesenchymal stem cells, 270
ridge augmentation, 315
    horizontal, 321
        technique modification, 321
    surgical approach, 315
        general considerations, 315
        graft importance, 318
        in mandible, 315
        in maxilla, 315
    vertical, 315
ridge defects
    classification, 53
    in edentulous regions, 52
ridge preservation procedures, 285
ridge-split/bone graft, 3
ridge splitting, 229
roll flap, 303
    occlusal view, 304
root canal treatment, 33
rotary bur, 161

S
salivary lubricants, 7
sandwich bone augmentation, 121
sandwich osteotomy, 121, 131, 186
sandwich technique, 121
    anterior maxilla, 67
scaffolds, 338, 339
    synthetic, 338
"scalloped-thin" gingival architecture, 54
scapular free flap, 281
Schneiderian membrane, 99, 100, 137, 146, 179, 180
screw tenting, 5
SCTG. see subepithelial connective tissue graft (SCTG)
SDAF-1a. see stromal-derived activation factor 1-alpha
        (SDAF-1a)
Simplant® simulation data from a CT scan, 103
single implant supported crown, 24–26
sinus augmentation, 15
sinus elevation and grafting, 14
    through a lateral window approach, 178
sinus elevation plus implant placement, 59
sinus lift, 135
    biological basis of, 137
    contraindications, 137, 138
    crestal approach, 140, 141
        osteotome for crestal sinus lift, 140
    diagnosis and treatment planning, 138, 139
    history of, 135
    indications, 137
    lateral window technique, 139
    post-operative care, 142
        panoramic radiograph, 142
        post-operative CBCT scan, 142
    simultaneous vs. delayed implant placement, 141, 142

advantages and disadvantages, sinus grafting techniques, 141
  at time of tooth removal, 142
sinus lift procedures, complications associated with, 194
  bleeding during lift procedure, 196, 197
  evaluation by CBCT scans, 196
  flap dehiscence and graft exposure, 197
  functional endoscopic sinus surgery (FESS), 196
  hematoma, 197
  implant loss, 197
  infection, 194
  injury to adjacent teeth, 197
  mucocele formation, 197
  neurosensory changes, 197
  oroantral fistula, 197
  perforation, 194
  post-operative antibiotics, 196
  post-operative sinusitis, 194
  use of pre-operative chlorhexidine, 196
skin elasticity, 71
skin incision, posterior, 277
skin paddle, 281
  design, 276
small hairpin RNA (shRNAs), 340
smoking, 137
soft-tissue, 27, 33, 71
  biotype, 72
  changes, 71
  considerations, success factors, 289
  dehiscences, 31, 326
  loss, 33
  management, 56
  periodontal plastic surgery, 285
  vs. hard tissue augmentation, 4
soft tissue augmentation, 299
  bone resorption, 299
  with implant placement, 299
  implant placements, 301
  keratinized gingiva, 301
  mineralized allograft, 300
  native gingiva, color discrepancy from, 300
  palatal donor sites, 300
  revascularization, 300
  at second implant stage, 301
  surgical bed, 299
  tenting screws, 300
  titanium reinforced dense-polytetrafluoroethylene (d-PTFE), 300
soft tissue grafting, 288, 290, 291, 304, 308
  complications, 308
    excessive bleeding, 309
    graft destabilization, 308
    graft infection and necrosis, 309
    post-operative, 309
    tissue necrosis, 311
  connective soft tissue graft, 287
  considerations, 289
  contraindications, 287, 288
  diagnosis/treatment planning, 288–290
  esthetic complications, 304
  evolution of, 292
  gingival biotype, 287
  for implant site development, 285
  implant site development, during tooth extraction, 288
  indications, 285, 286
    biotype and color discrepancies, 287
    bone and soft tissue deficiency, 285, 286
    keratinized tissue (KT), 286, 287
    rescue procedures, 287
    tooth extraction – implant site development, 287
  maxillary left central incisor, 286
  protocol for implant site development, 289
  rescue procedure, 304
  stable peri-implant bone levels, 286
  types, 291
    free gingival graft, 291
    subepithelial connective tissue graft, 291
  vertical and horizontal bone loss, 286
speech, 7
sphenopalatine vein, 135
stable peri-implant bone, 225
static vs. dynamic bone augmentation, 4
stem cells, 315
  from the apical papilla (SCAP), 338
  from human exfoliated deciduous teeth (SHED), 337
  maturation of, 326
stromal-derived activation factor 1-alpha (SDAF-1a), 318
subepithelial connective tissue graft (SCTG), 291
subperiosteal implants, 14
subperiosteal tunnel, 33
subtractive surgical procedures, 15
subtractive tissue procedures, 18
superior–posterior border, 7
supraeruption, 33
surgical additive tissue procedures, 18
surgical stent, 139
SurgyBone®, 123
sutured flap, 91
symmetrical implant placement, 72
symphyseal bone harvest anesthesia, 249
symptomatic dentistry, era of, 3
syngeneic dermal fibroblasts (SDFs), 339
  transduction, 339
synthesized small interfering RNA (siRNA), 340
synthetic polymers for TE scaffolding, 338

T
TADs. see temporary anchorage devices (TADs)
taste sensations, 7
temporary anchorage devices (TADs), 30, 31, 232
  orthodontic elastics connect, 232
temporary restoration, 57
tendon, 340
tension–stress effect, 229
tenting technique, 19
  for particulate graft, 5
three-dimensional (3D) tissue augmentation, 4
Ti-mesh tenting, 5
TIME technique, 93
tissue engineering (TE), 337
  adult stem cells, 337
  scaffold systems, 340
tissue necrosis, 311

tissue preservation technique, 303
titanium, 14
titanium (Ti) mesh, 93, 94
  device, 93
titanium-reinforced barrier membrane, 93
titanium reinforced dense-polytetrafluoroethylene (d-PTFE), 300
titanium-reinforced non-resorbable membranes, 81
tooth-bone, 335
  cell tissue recombination approach, 337
  constructs, 338
  regeneration approaches, 335, 336
  tissue engineering approach, 337
tooth decellularized scaffold approach, 337
tooth development, 335
tooth extraction, 285
  implant site development, 288
tooth preservation, 34
tooth regeneration, 338
trabecular mineralized bone, 320
transcription factors, 339, 340
transforming growth factor (TGF)-beta1, 176, 339
trauma, 25, 26
"tunneling" procedure, 62
Tutoplast pericardium®, 124
two-dimensional (2D) tissue augmentation, 4

U
Ultraflex mesh plate®, 105
  conventional mesh *vs.*, 105
ultrasonic energy, 121
unidirectional distraction device, 229
unidirectional extraosseous distraction osteogenesis, 230
upper lip length, 71

V
vascular endothelial growth factor (VEGF), 176, 232, 339
vasoconstriction, 310
venous drainage, 135
vertical alveolar ridge augmentation, 93
  autogenous bone chips harvested from, 94
  bone quality/quantity of augmented area, by titanium mesh and particulate bone graft, 96
  complications, 96, 97
  crestal incision, 94
  decortication, 94
  defect size and augmentation procedure, 97
  disadvantage of procedure, 108, 109
  indications and timing of implant placement, 97
  management of the mesh exposure, 108
  mesh removal, 95
  periosteum released along facial vestibule to, 95
  pre-operative intraoral view, 94
  surgical procedure, 93
  titanium mesh fixed with, 94
  titanium mesh was trimmed and adjusted to the desired shape, 94
  with titanium-reinforced devices, 93
vertical alveolar ridge defects, 223
vertical augmentation of maxillary and/or mandibular alveolus, 7
vertical bone volumes, 21
vertical crown height, 33
vertical grafting, 19, 27
vertical pedicled sandwich plasty (vertical PSP), 110
  clinical example
    in anterior (interforaminal) mandibular region, 114, 115
    in posterior mandible, 112–114
  for mandible, 111
  for maxilla, 111
  panoramic radiographs/cephalometric radiograph, 116
  sequence of vertical pedicled sandwich plasty in posterior mandibular situation, 112
vertical prosthetic space, 15
vertical restorative space, 15, 21
vertical space, 15
  requirements, 15
vessel traverses, 310
vestibular incision subperiosteal tunnel access (VISTA) technique, 32, 33
vicryl sutures, 251
virtually designed CAD/CAM abutment, 32
VISTA technique. *see* vestibular incision subperiosteal tunnel access (VISTA) technique
visual analog scales (VAS), 17

W
whether grafting, 27

X
xenogeneic bone, 257, 270
xenografts, 75, 82
  scaffold, 326

Y
Yucatan minipig model, 222